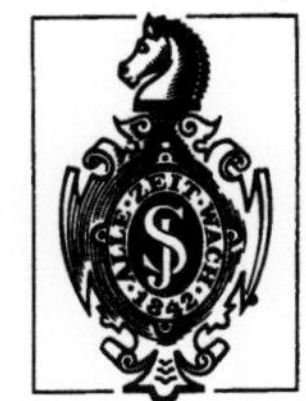

E.R. Heitzman

The Mediastinum

Radiologic Correlations with Anatomy and Pathology

Completely Revised Second Edition

With 302 Figures
in 733 Separate Illustrations

Springer-Verlag
Berlin Heidelberg New York
London Paris Tokyo

Professor Dr. E. Robert Heitzman
State University of New York
Health Science Center
University Hospital
Department of Radiology
750 East Adams Street
Syracuse, New York 13210
USA

ISBN-13:978-3-642-73303-1   e-ISBN-13:978-3-642-73301-7
DOI: 10.1007/978-3-642-73301-7

Library of Congress Cataloging-in-Publication Data. Heitzman, E. Robert, 1927 –. The mediastinum: radiologic correlations with anatomy and pathology / E.R. Heitzman. – Completely rev. 2nd ed. p. cm. Bibliography: p. Includes index. ISBN-13:978-3-642-73303-1 1.Mediastinum–Diseases–Diagnosis. 2. Mediastinum–Imaging. 3. Mediastinum–Anatomy. I. Title. RC754.H44 1988. 616.2'70757–dc19. 88-15630 CIP

2121/3130-543210

*To my wife Betty
and my children
Beth, Anne, Rob, and Carol*

Preface to the Second Edition

Over 10 years have passed since the first edition of *The Mediastinum* was published in 1977. I have been very gratified by the response to the first edition and determined to do a second edition as soon as possible. However, good intentions are sometimes difficult to achieve and a decade has passed.

This period has been one of enormous growth in the discipline of diagnostic imaging. In the study of the mediastinum, computed tomography, and more recently magnetic resonance, have revolutionized our diagnostic capabilities. This second edition of the mediastinum is intended to emphasize the importance of these modalities to the evaluation of mediastinal disease. In addition, an attempt will be made to integrate into the text the many new and important observations relating to all aspects of mediastinal imaging which have appeared in the literature since 1977.

The overall emphasis, however, will remain the same: that accurate radiologic diagnosis is based upon a thorough understanding of correlated radiographic anatomy and pathology. No matter what the imaging modality, this principle remains fundamental to each and every radiographic interpretation.

I would like to express once again my deep appreciation to Dr. Stephen A. Kieffer, Chairman of the Department of Radiology at the State University of New York Health Science Center at Syracuse for his continued support and encouragement.

Mrs. Margo Flood somehow found the time to provide secretarial support. To her and to others in the department who assisted her in this effort I extend my sincere appreciation.

The new photographic work for the second edition was performed by John G. Hodgson. It is typical of his artistry and I also thank him sincerely.

Once again, I would also like to express my deep and loving appreciation to my wife for her unwavering support and constant tolerance during this and other similar projects over the years.

E. Robert Heitzman

Preface to the First Edition

This book on the mediastinum has been developed as a companion to an earlier volume, *The Lung: Radiologic-Pathologic Correlations.* It proposes the same basic philosophy emphasized in *The Lung*–that radiologic interpretation must be based on a thorough understanding of the anatomy of the region under study and an appreciation of the ways in which the anatomy is altered by disease. This concept seems particularly appropriate to radiologic analysis of the mediastinum, an area of intricate anatomy commonly harboring a wide variety of pathologic lesions. Despite its complexities, the mediastinum can and should be viewed as a dynamic region whose component parts can be recognized by careful analysis of the radiograph rather than as an inert mass of unit density structures that cannot be separated radiologically.

The material presented in the book has been organized along regional anatomic lines. In general, basic anatomic considerations are discussed first, followed by radiologic correlations with these anatomic points. Subsequently, pathologic conditions occurring in the region are discussed, and the dependence of their diagnosis on anatomy is emphasized. No attempt has been made to develop an all-inclusive compendium of diseases of the mediastinum. It is felt, however, that most common conditions have been covered; some rarer entities also are included.

As is the case with most books, the illustrations have been selected to amplify the discussions in the text. Additionally, an attempt has been made here to arrange the illustrations and the content of their captions in such a manner that they would be meaningful if studied independently of the text.

This radiologic study, correlating mediastinal anatomy and pathology, could not have been undertaken without the availability of a large quantity of gross anatomic material specifically prepared with such correlations in mind. Many cadavers have been radiographed and sections prepared in various planes to elucidate the complexities of mediastinal anatomy as seen on radiographs. Specific effort has been made to produce teaching material that would illustrate anatomic points with the greatest possible clarity. Over the years these specimens have been used in several scientific exhibits, papers, and lectures; these presentations form the nucleus about which this volume has been developed.

The anatomic correlations presented in this book reflect the great cooperation of the staff of the Department of Anatomy of SUNY Health Science Center under the Chairmanship of Dr. Donald Goodman. The ready willingness of these individuals to provide their expertise, time, and materials has been remarkable. Dr. Henry S. DiStefano, Professor of Anatomy, was particularly helpful. Very special thanks must go also to Ludwig J. Rimmler, Jr., technical specialist in the Department of Anatomy. The techniques used to produce the gross anatomic material were developed by Mr. Rimmler and result in specimens of unmatched quality. Over the years, Mr. Rimmler has given unstintingly of his time and effort to many collaborative efforts between the Departments of Radiology and Anatomy.

The contributions of the attending and resident staffs of the Department of Radiology of the SUNY Health Science Center to the development of this book have been immeasurable. I am especially indebted to Dr. Stephen A. Kieffer, Chairman of the Department, for his advice and encouragement. Drs. Edward J. Lane and Anthony V. Proto were constant sources of information and stimulation. Many other department members also assisted in the development of materials and ideas that appear in the book. They are William N. Cohen, W. Martin Dinn, Richard L. Goldwin, David B. Hammack, Bedros Markarian, Joseph Martino, Joseph Moro, Thomas W. Phillips, John C. Sanborn, and Joseph V. Scrivani.

Mrs. Diane Pajak provided outstanding secretarial support, retyping multiple drafts of the manuscript and organizing the bibliography.

Rob Heitzman assisted in the compilation of the bibliography and in review of the galley proofs.

Mr. Richard Fellion performed most of the photographic work. I am deeply indebted to him for his interest and cooperation and, of course, for the illustrations, which reflect the high quality of his work. Some of the photographs were done by John G. Hodgson and by Charles G. Reiner, R.B.P. Drawings were produced by Allen G. Ayres. I extend to each of these professionals sincere appreciation for their fine efforts.

And finally, I would like to thank my wife and children once again for their help, encouragement, and forbearance during the preparation of the manuscript.

E. ROBERT HEITZMAN

Contents

1 Introduction

1.1 General Comments

Chapter 1 of the first edition of this volume opened with the following statement:

"All too often, the mediastinum is considered to be a radiologic "blind spot" – an area composed of a multiplicity of structures that are hidden from X-ray view because they are all of the same radiographic density. In some quarters this attitude has led to a rather superficial approach to the mediastinum, which in turn has stultified radiologic investigation of this vital area. For example, it is popular to divide the mediastinum anatomically into four compartments-superior, anterior, middle, and posterior. If a lesion can be localized to one these regions, many observers consider the job done, and even problem cases often do not seem to stimulate an interest in any greater degree of anatomic analysis of the problem."

In the decade which has passed since that negative comment was made, interest in the radiographic investigation of the mediastinum has heightened significantly. Undoubtedly the catalyst in this renewal has been computed tomography. Not only does it demonstrate excellent anatomic detail in the axial plane but the improved contrast resolution it provides over that resulting from radiographs made with conventional film/screen combinations permits discrimination between anatomic structures and pathologic processes which was never before achievable. The advent of magnetic resonance imaging has been a further stimulus to the study of the normal and abnormal mediastinum.

As these new diagnostic modalities have established their place in our diagnostic armamentarium, they have required us to be knowledgeable about anatomy, especially cross-sectional anatomy, as never before. The second edition of this book is a renewed attempt to provide in-depth roentgen-anatomic correlations in the mediastinum which, it is hoped, will lead to more accurate radiologic evaluation. The content of the first edition will be updated to include many new and cogent observations made in the last 10 years. A major effort will be made to emphasize radiologic correlations with anatomy and pathology derived from computed tomography, since relatively little material of this type was included in the first edition which was written when computed tomography was in its infancy.

As in the first edition, pathologic conditions in the mediastinum will be discussed, not always in great depth, but as "vignettes" in which the major emphasis is placed on the role of correlative roentgen anatomy in the establishment of the correct diagnosis.

A great deal has been written about mediastinal lines – so much that each new publication discussing a mediastinal line is greeted with apathy and a feeling that another abstract and not very practical fact must be committed to memory. The various lines of the mediastinum are discussed in considerable detail in this volume not because knowing their names is so important but because they are a reflection of mediastinal anatomy. An understanding of the significance of these lines is vital to accurate radiologic analysis of the mediastinum.

This exposition of anatomy and its correlation with radiographs will rely on relationships as they are demonstrated in cadaver sections – transverse, coronal, and, in some instances, sagittal. Many years ago, Lachman [4, 5] pointed out that anatomy as it is seen in the cadaver does not always reflect accurately the situation in life; he emphasized the importance of radiology to the study of anatomy in the living subject. Therefore, although some radiographs of cadaver slices are included in this book, most of the anatomic correlations will be made with in vivo radiographs including plain films and conventional and computed tomograms. Sagittal body sections showing left-sided thoracic structures will be displayed as though are being viewed from the left; sagittal sections showing right-sided structures will be displayed as though they are being viewed from the right. A similar orientation will be used for all lateral radiographs. Computed tomograms and magnetic resonance images will be displayed as being viewed from below [2].

In the chapter on the supra-azygos area, a number of azygograms are shown. They have been used only to clarify certain anatomic points, and their inclusion should not be construed as an endorsement of this now outmoded technique.

Finally, it should be stated that few, if any, of the observations included in the following chapters are mine. The enormous contributions made to the radiologic study of the mediastinum by a host of workers have provided the basis for the discussions that follow.

It is hoped that the studies of the mediastinum recorded here will stimulate even greater interest in the radiologic investigation of this region so that interpretation of roentgen studies of the mediastinum will become even more analytic and deductive in future years.

1.2 An Anatomic Classification of the Mediastinum

Over the years, anatomists have devised various schemes for subdividing the mediastinum. A brief historical review of these classifications can be found in the book by Leszczynski [6]. Clearly, the most popular breakdown of the mediastinum today continues to be a simple separation into superior, anterior, middle, and posterior compartments [7, 10]. In fact, this scheme has become standard despite its many drawbacks. In this classification the superior compartment is defined as that part of the mediastinum lying above a line drawn from the lower aspect of the manubrium of the sternum posteriorly through the lower edge of the body of the fourth thoracic vertebra. The anterior mediastinum lies below the superior, between the sternum and pericardium. The posterior mediastinum is generally said to lie behind a coronal plane through the posterior aspect of the pericardium [9]. The middle mediastinum lies between the anterior and posterior compartments. Some observers feel that the posterior mediastinum should be considered to extend backward only to the anterior margins of the vertebral bodies, and that the extrapleural space behind the posterior mediastinum should be termed the "paraspinal area". One of the inadequacies of the subdivision just described is the lack of unanimity of opinion concerning the boundaries of the posterior mediastinum and the paraspinal regions. There are, however, many other deficiencies of this classification as Berne et al. [1] and Felson [3] have pointed out. These limitations can be summarized as follows:

1. It is based on mediastinal anatomy in only a limited way. In fact, the only mediastinal structure used as a reference point in this classification is the pericardium. Therefore, it has little radiologic relevance because it is insufficiently based on anatomy.
2. It tends to constrict thinking and minimizes more detailed anatomic analysis, an approach to radiologic interpretation that is mandatory if correct diagnosis is to be achieved.
3. It has virtually no application to the gross pathologic diagnosis of mediastinal lesions. It is true that this classification can be used to recall that thymic and thyroid masses are found in the anterior mediastinum and that most neurogenic tumors are situated posteriorly. This approach is too simplistic, for surely such basic facts can be remembered without resort to any mediastinal subdivision. Ideally, a mediastinal classification should provide a basis for dividing pathologic processes into more specific groupings based on their anatomic point of origin.

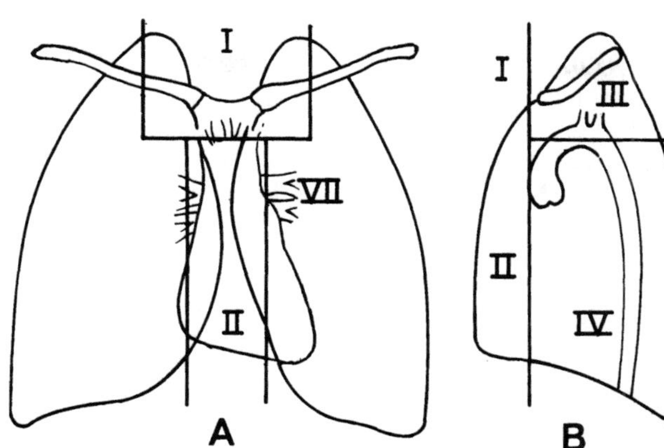

Fig. 1.1 Anatomic classification of mediastinum in frontal (*A*), left lateral (*B*), and right lateral (*C*) perspectives. Roman numerals correspond to sections of mediastinum outlined in Table 1.1

As the first edition of this volume was being prepared, it became apparent at once that some subdivision of the mediastinum had to be offered, if only to provide chapter headings and to divide the material into workable units. As a result, a new classification is offered here. It is hoped that this scheme will not be used as the standard classification has been – to develop gamut lists of various pathologic conditions found in each area – but rather as a rational approach to an understanding of anatomic relationships and their radiologic significance. This proposal is shown in Table 1.1 and Fig. 1.1.

This scheme is based on an earlier subdivision, which according to Leszczynski [6], was offered by Tillier, who likewise used the aortic and the azygos arches as anatomic boundaries for mediastinal compartments [8]. This approach seems a reasonable one, providing a division of the right and left sides of the mediastinum into areas of somewhat similar size separated by a major vascular channel. Furthermore, the arches actually serve as functional anatomic boundaries in certain disease states; for example, the azygos arch often limits the caudal extension of posterior intrathoracic goiters (Figs. 4.20 and 4.21) and localized mediastinal abscesses (Fig. 4.26). A classification based on the aortic and azygos arches is very practical since these structures are usually easy to identify on radiographs and since the X-ray appearance of each side of the mediastinum is predicated largely upon the way in which the left and right mediastinal pleurae are subtended from the arches. Differential diagnosis is aided by the classification since it offers a means by which pathologic processes involving the mediastinum can be categorized on the basis of their anatomic site of origin.

Recently the American Thoracic Society offered a new classification of mediastinal lymph nodes [9] (see Chapter 3) and it also used the

Table 1.1. An anatomic classification of the mediastinum

I. Thoracic inlet	A region with a narrow cephalocaudad dimension marking the cervicothoracic junction and lying immediately above and below a transverse plane through the first rib
II. Anterior mediastinum	A region extending from the thoracic inlet to the diaphragm, in front of the ascending aorta and the superior vena cava

Behind the anterior medastinum are situated:

III. Supra-aortic area	A region above the aortic arch
IV. Infra-aortic area	A region below the aortic arch
V. Supra-azygos area	A region above the azygos arch
VI. Infra-azygos area	A region below the azygos arch
VII. The hila	Regions containing major bronchi and blood vessels in a connective tissue compartment that is continuous with the infra-aortic and infra-azygos areas

aortic and azygos arches as reference points. The arches are used as dividing lines between several of the nodal stations newly developed by them.

It is hoped this classification will have one other major advantage: that of providing a way of considering the mediastinum that facilitates the learning of structural relationships because they "hang together" as anatomic units.

One might question whether it is appropriate to include the hilum in a mediastinal classification. In standard terminology the hilum is not usually considered to be a part of the mediastinum, but it is included here because of the anatomic continuity of the two regions and their frequent concomitant involvement by disease.

It is recognized that this breakdown, like others, is arbitrary to a degree. For example, the paraspinal regions are discussed with the supra- and infra-aortic areas and with the supra- and infra-azygos areas, although they lie behind both the aorta and the azygos vein. However, the classification is less arbitrary than most, is soundly based on anatomic principles and, above all, is practical.

References

1. Berne AS, Gerle RD, Mitchell GE (1969) The mediastinum – normal roentgen anatomy and radiologic techniques. Semin Roentgenol 4:3–21
2. Eyler WR, Figley MM (1976) Computed tomography display. Radiology 119:487–488
3. Felson B (1973) Chest roentgenology. Saunders, Philadelphia
4. Lachman E (1942) Comparison of the posterior boundaries of the lungs and pleura as demonstrated on the cadaver and on the roentgenogram of the living. Anat Rec 83:521–542
5. Lachman E (1946) The dynamic concept of thoracic topography: a critical review of present day teaching of visceral anatomy. Am J Roentgenol 56:419–440
6. Leszczynski SZ (1972) Purulent and fibrous mediastinitis: radiological diagnosis. Polish Medical Publishers, Warsaw
7. Lyons HA, Calvy GL, Sammons BP (1959) The diagnosis and classification of mediastinal masses. I. A study of 782 cases. Ann Intern Med 51:897–932
8. Tillier JG (1947) Anatomie radiologique du mediastin postérieure. Algerie Med 5:205
9. Tisi GM, Friedman PJ, Peter RM, Pearson G, Carr D, Lee RE, Selawry O (1983) Clinical staging of primary lung cancer. Am Rev Respir Dis 127:659–664
10. Warwick R, Williams PL (1973) Gray's anatomy, edn 35. Saunders, Philadelphia

2 Preparation of Body Sections for the Study of Mediastinal Anatomy

The anatomy of the mediastinum is exceedingly complex, and therefore clinical and radiologic problems encountered daily require a knowledge of structural relationships that may not always be firmly in mind. Many excellent texts of anatomy and correlated radiographic anatomy are available to provide such information [1–8]. Obviously, the advent of computed tomography and magnetic resonance imaging has been a major stimulus for the development of many of these works and has resulted in a renewal of interest in such classical texts as authored by Eycleshymer and Schoemaker [4] and by Pernkopf [7].

Clearly, however, the best study material is a series of cadaver sections sliced in different planes. Such material is not available commercially, but the development of one's own collection of body sections is not difficult. Since it is felt that some readers may wish to prepare their own specimens, a brief description of the technique used at the Health Science Center, Syracuse, New York to produce body sections for anatomic study is included here.

Following a prearranged agreement with the department of anatomy, the radiology department receives a body donated for medical research immediately after it arrives at the morgue or the anatomy laboratory. Bodies should preferably be fresh, not emaciated, and should be without known significant disease that might alter the anatomy of the portion of the body to be prepared.

Radiographs of the thorax should be made prior to embalming so that radiologic correlations of the unaltered postmortem anatomy with the body sections can be performed. The best X-ray examinations result when the lungs are in an expanded state; this can be accomplished by inflating the lungs through an endo-

tracheal tube or a tracheotomy tube. Cuffed tubes facilitate the maintenance of the lungs in an expanded state for the relatively long period of time necesssary to perform all of the radiologic studies. Plain radiographs, tomograms, computed tomograms, and esophagrams may be done. Esophagrams require the use of a tube; usually a neck incision provides easier access to the esophagus than does the mouth or the nose.

Following completion of the radiologic studies, the body is returned to the laboratory for preparation. The technique used at the Upstate Medical Center has been developed by L. Rimmler and has undergone considerable refinement over the years as the result of accumulated experience. The method produces uniform study material of the highest quality.

Two methods may be used to fix the tissue: the body may be arterially embalmed and packed in dry ice, or it may be packed in dry ice without embalming. The latter method requires that the sections be fixed in formalin after sectioning. The body should be frozen in the dry ice for a period of no less than 48 h. Sections are made with a commercial band saw at arbitrarily selected levels. If sections are to be made for comparison with computed tomograms, transverse slices can be made at 10-mm intervals, using skin markers as reference points to assure that the scan and the body section represent comparable levels. Coronal slices provide excellent correlation with conventional frontal tomograms, and sagittal slices are instructive as well. Slices as thin as 6.25 mm can be produced without difficulty. After slicing, surface debris prevents visualization of anatomic detail; the sections must be cleaned carefully using lukewarm water and a fine brush. The sections are stored ultimately in formalin.

Formalin-stored sections are certainly not practical for the correlative study of radiographs in the X-ray reading room. Preferably, the individual slices are X-rayed and photographed in color using transparency film. Paper prints can also be produced. Sections should be photographed promptly after preparation to avoid the deterioration of tissue color that occurs with the passage of time. Such tissue color is of great benefit in the differentiation of one structure from another when the slices are studied.

Selected body sections may be embedded in plastic for permanence and convenience of use. Although embedding is time consuming and rather expensive, the preparation of at least a few slices demonstrating key anatomic points is valuable and greatly facilitates the learning of mediastinal anatomy. Embedded slices have an advantage over photographs in that they show three-dimensional anatomic relationships more clearly.

The embedding technique, also developed by Rimmler, utilizes a material called Castolite (The Castolite Co., Woodstock, IL, USA), a thermosetting type of plastic. This substance, of syrup-like consistency in the liquid form, hardens when cured into a transparent state that is heat and solvent resistant.

The body section is first placed on a glass plate that has been coated with wax to facilitate the subsequent separation of the slice from the plate. This section is steeped in a solution made up of half formalin and half glycerin for 3–4 h and then in glycerin alone for the same length of time. Following this, the section is immersed in liquid Castolite for 24 h; the material is then poured off, and fresh liquid Castolite is used to cover the section for another 24 h. Previously used Castolite should be saved and can be utilized again for the first immersion of other slices. When the reused Castolite darkens appreciably, it should be discarded. Following the two baths in liquid Castolite, the surfaces of the slice are cleaned, and the section is placed in a stainless steel frame. The slice again rests on a waxed glass plate, and a weight is placed on top of the slice. The final phase of the embedding process begins by the addition of a hardener to the liquid Castolite. Following a waiting

period during which all of the air bubbles should have risen to the surface, the Castolite is poured into the stainless steel frame to a depth of 12.5–18.75 mm and allowed to set for 24 h. Subsequent layers are poured at 24-h intervals until the section is almost covered. The weight is then removed and a top layer of plastic is poured so that the superior surface of the slice is totally immersed. Since the Castolite surface cures slowly, preparation of the final product can be speeded up if the tacky exterior surface layer is cut off using a band saw. The surface of the slice that was resting on the glass plate is then subjected to a coarse and a fine sanding and cleaned with acetone. The section is turned over, and the bottom surface (now facing upward) is then steeped in liquid Castolite; the material is poured into a well that is constructed around the bottom of the section using masking tape. After 24 h the final layer of Castolite with added hardener is poured. The Castolite edges of the embedded section are then trimmed and given rough, medium, and fine sandings. Finally, the surfaces are buffed using a silicone polish and a cloth wheel.

The body sections prepared in this manner are extremely durable. The plastic retains its clear transparency for years, and the surfaces are quite resistant to chipping and cracking.

References

1. Bo WJ, Meschan I, Krueger WA (1980) Basic atlas of cross sectional anatomy. Saunders, Philadelphia
2. Cahill DR, Orland MJ (1984) Atlas of human cross sectional anatomy. Lea and Febiger, Philadelphia
3. Carter BL, Morehead J, Wolpers SL, Hammerschlag SB, Griffiths HJ, Kahn PC (1977) Cross-sectional anatomy: computed tomography and ultrasound correlation. Appleton-Century-Crofts, New York
4. Eycleshymer AC, Schoemaker DM (1970) A cross-section anatomy. Appleton-Century-Crofts, New York
5. Kieffer SA, Heitzman ER (eds) (1979) An atlas of cross-sectional anatomy. Computed tomography, ultrasound, radiology, gross anatomy. Harper and Row, New York
6. Ledley RS, Huang HK, Mazziotta JC (1977) Cross sectional anatomy – an atlas for computed tomography. Williams and Wilkins, Baltimore
7. Pernkopf E (1963) Atlas of topographic and applied human anatomy, vol 2. Saunders, Philadelphia
8. Peterson RR (1980) A cross-sectional approach to anatomy. Year Book Medical Publishers, Chicago

3 General Radiologic Considerations

3.1 Radiologic Examination of the Mediastinum

An in-depth discussion of radiologic techniques for the evaluation of the mediastinum is beyond the scope of this book, which has as its main objective the development of radiologic correlations with mediastinal anatomy and pathology. A brief discussion is included for the sake of completeness. For a more thorough review of this topic the reader is referred to the works of Berne et al. [9], Felson [29], and Fraser and Pare [31].

3.1.1 The Plain Film Examination

Posteroanterior and lateral radiographs constitute the basic radiographic examination of the chest. One of the major limitations of this conventional X-ray study, when films are made at 125 kV or less, is suboptimal demonstration of the mediastinum. With lower kilovoltage technique many lung-mediastinal interfaces are not visualized and anatomic detail as well as pathologic findings can be lost behind the diaphragm, the heart, and the great vessels. As a result, there has been a trend in recent years toward higher kilovoltage films, in the 125–150 kV range, that show the mediastinum more satisfactorily while still demonstrating the lung parenchyma adequately. If X-ray units with such kilovoltage capability are not available, overpenetrated radiographs using lower kilovoltages are valuable as a supplement to standard films. Some radiologists have added such a film to their standard chest examination. Certainly, whenever plain radiographs raise any suspicion of a mediastinal

abnormality, overpenetrated films of the thorax should be made.

The most valuable film projections for evaluation of the mediastinum are the frontal and lateral; occasionally films made in slight obliquity or with lordotic projection will be helpful in clarifying confusing shadows. For example, lordotic films can be useful to prove that questionable shadows at the thoracic inlet or in the supra-aortic or supra-azygos areas are vascular in nature by demonstrating the shadows to arch laterally over the lung apices in the characteristic course of the great vessels (see Fig. 4.21).

3.1.2 The Esophagram

Berne et al. have aptly stated that "the air-containing lungs serve to define the rind of the mediastinum, the barium-filled esophagus delineates its 'core'" [9]. Esophagrams are not invasive, are simple to perform, and often provide a great deal of information at relatively low cost. It is unfortunate that the esophagram is so frequently bypassed today in favor of examinations such as computed tomography and magnetic resonance imaging. Ideally, the esophagus should be demonstrated in frontal, lateral, and oblique projections throughout its entire intrathoracic course. It should be moderately distended to bring it into contact with contiguous mediastinal structures. Impressions upon the esophagus as well as loss of its normal outpouchings should be looked for with care [14, 39] (Fig. 3.1). The radiographic appearance of the normal and abnormal esophagus is discussed on a regional basis in the ensuing chapters.

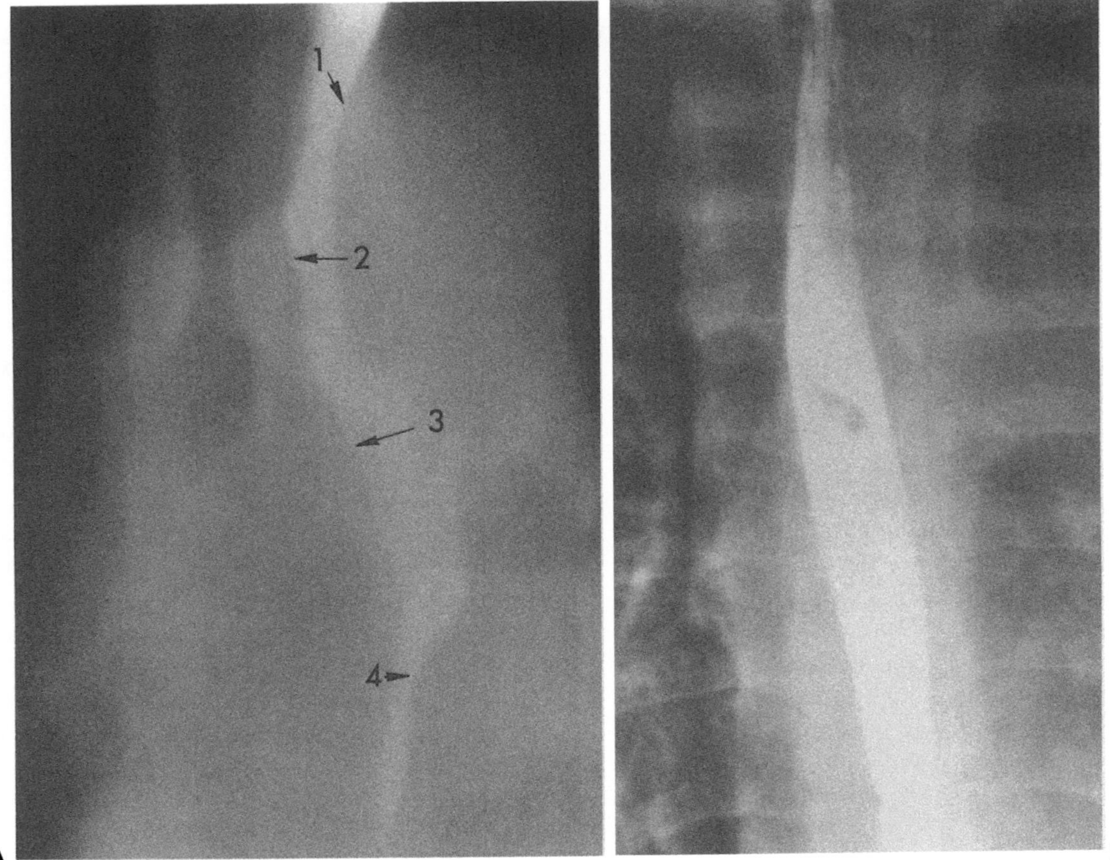

A   B

Fig. 3.1A, B. Loss of normal mediastinal impressions on esophagus and lung caused by diffuse mediastinal disease. **A** AP tomogram. **B** AP radiograph. AP tomogram demonstrates many of the impressions that normal structures make on esophagus: aortic arch (*1*), posterior portion of the azygos arch (*2*), right lower lobe in the azygoesophageal recess (*3*), and confluence of left pulmonary veins (*4*). Neither these impressions nor any others are seen in **B** a case in which the mediastinum is diffusely infiltrated by lymphoma. Note also that impressions made by normal anatomic structures on lung in **A** are totally obliterated in **B**

3.1.3 Fluoroscopy

The mediastinum is a dynamic area that changes its position and configuration with changes in body position, intrathoracic pressure, and phase of respiration. Such changes seen under fluoroscopic vision are often very significant to the establishment of a correct diagnosis. A great many of these observations could be listed, but the following are among the most important:

1. Abnormal mediastinal contours that change their shape with change in body position or intrathoracic pressure are not due to solid tumors. Among such lesions are vascular masses, pericardial cysts, and occasionally lipomas. Pedunculated pleural tumors lying against the mediastinum may show similar findings due to their movement in the pleural space [8].
2. Masses that move significantly with the lung during respiration are not mediastinal in location.

In addition, turning the patient under fluoroscopic control will often clarify the nature of a questionable mediastinal contour by placing the shadow exactly tangential to the X-ray beam, thus permitting it to be viewed optimally. The demonstration of epicardial fat is helpful in the diagnosis of pericardial effusion [13, 63] (see Fig. 5.23) and the assessment of heart size in large left pleural effusions [36]. In some cases, epicardial fat may be seen better at fluoroscopy, cinefluorography [60] or TV taping than on plain films. When radiographs of the barium-filled esophagus are not ideal, fluoroscopy is valuable to obtain spot films of the esophagus in the optimal obliquity and degree of distention. Cinefluorography or videotaping of barium swallows offers a similar advantage. Most observers who have attempted to distinguish intrinsic from transmitted pulsations in the mediastinum concede that this distinction can be made only rarely; a similar opinion is held here. It is unfortunate that, like the esophagram, fluoroscopic examination for the elucidation of mediastinal disease is rather infrequently employed.

3.1.4 Conventional Tomography

Just a few years ago, conventional tomography was an integral part of the radiographic workup of almost all thoracic problems. Today, it is used rarely, having been supplanted by computed tomography for a wide variety of applications [20, 101, 103, 112, 114, 116, 136, 137] especially in the mediastinum [4, 19, 24, 35, 61, 68, 77] and to some extent by magnetic resonance imaging [53, 130]. Conventional tomography still has some advantages and it is the opinion of this author that it remains preferable to computed tomography for the study of the trachea and central airways in many instances.

Fig. 3.2 A, B. Angled tomography of normal right hilum. **A** Right posterior oblique tomogram made at an angle of 55°. **B** Drawing of this projection. Angled tomography in posterior oblique projection with plane of patient's back forming angle of 55° with the table top clearly lays out bronchial bifurcations and often permits a distinction to be made between shadows of hilar vessels and those of enlarged hilar lymph nodes. *V* indicates lower lobe pulmonary vein. Technique is in limited use. (**B** reproduced from [25]). *MB* main bronchus; *UL* upper lobe bronchus; *PA* pulmonary artery; *LL* lower lobe bronchus; *ML* middle lobe bronchus; *V* inferior pulmonary vein; *1–10* B1 bronchus–B10 bronchus (Boyden system)

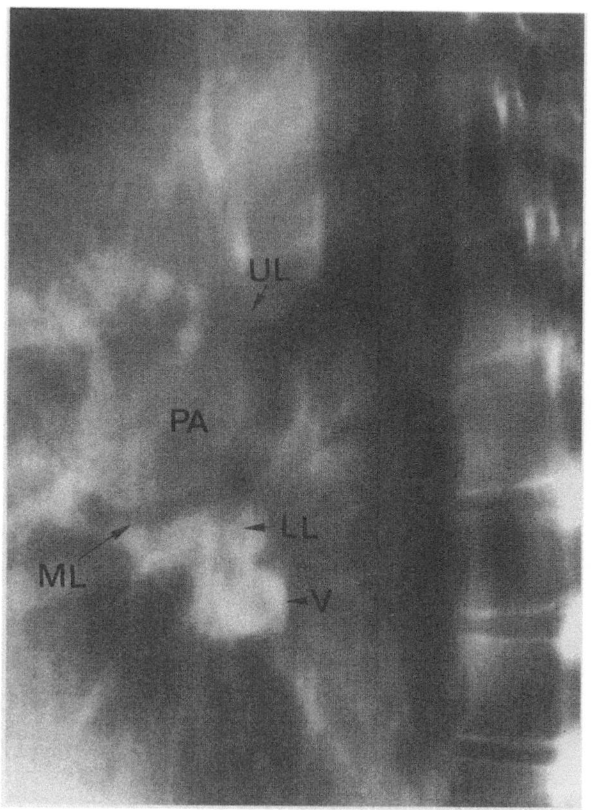

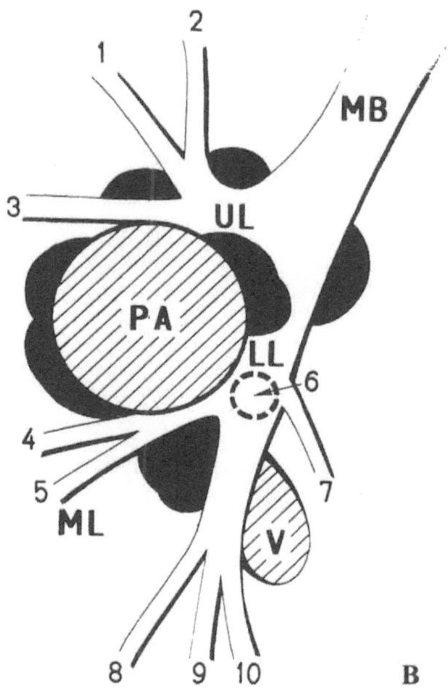

The standard tomographic examination is made in an AP projection. To obtain the optimum demonstration of mediastinal detail, a contoured filter with vertically oriented trough has been used. We have felt that in general a linear tube sweep has produced the best examinations, although occasionally (and seemingly unpredictably) pluridirectional motion has proven superior. Tomograms at 1-cm levels are made, and frequently the frontal examination is supplemented by lateral cuts. Angling the coronal plane of section by tilting the film tray or placing the patient obliquely across the table has proven of little benefit and is rarely done.

Tomography at an angle of 55° has been advocated for the study of the hila [25]. The patient is placed on the table so that the angle formed by his back with the table top is 55°. The right posterior oblique films clearly demonstrate right hilar detail (Fig. 3.2); the left posterior oblique films show the left. A principal advantage of the oblique projection is that it "lays out" the major bronchi in profile, simplifying the evaluation of endobronchial disease. Perhaps more importantly, this projection demonstrates hilar nodes in the bronchial angles more clearly and facilitates their distinction from shadows caused by vessels. These advantages not withstanding, today angled tomography to study the hilum has been largely replaced by computed tomography [40, 87, 88, 127, 128, 129] (see chapter 10). Likewise, xerotomography occasionally employed in the past for the study of mediastinal pathology [16, 51, 133, 134] (Fig. 3.3), is rarely employed at present.

3.1.5 Computed Tomography

In the last decade, computed tomography has become the major complement to PA and lateral chest radiographs for the study of mediastinal anatomy and pathology. Two factors have been responsible for the rapid emergence of computed tomography for this purpose. These are the transverse display of the image which it provides and the enhanced contrast resolution (about twice that of conventional film-screen combinations) inherent in the examination.

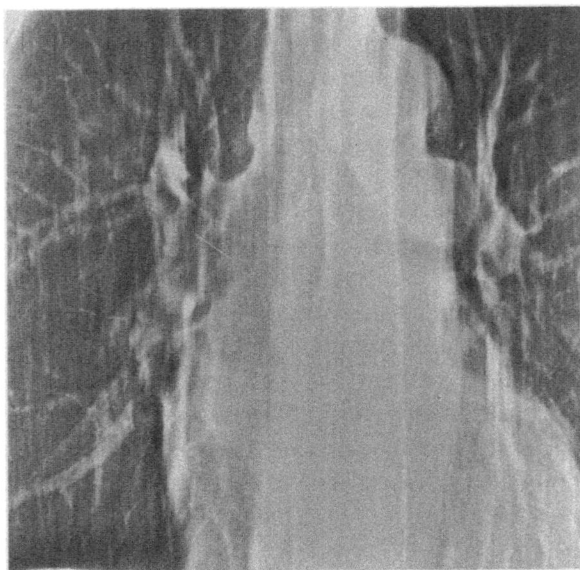

Fig. 3.3. Xerotomography (AP xerotomogram). Xerotomography of thorax offers advantages of considerable edge enhancement and wide exposure latitude. Note excellent demonstration of mediastinal detail and lung detail on same tomogram resulting from these two factors. Technique is in limited use. (Courtesy of G. Tricomi, Rome, Italy)

As an adjunct to frontal examinations, transverse studies are often superior to lateral projections for evaluation of the mediastinum because they afford another profile view of mediastinal detail. Such detail may not be seen well on lateral films because in this projection most mediastinal structures are viewed en face by the incident X-ray beam. The impressions of these structures upon lung are usually seen in better profile in the frontal and transverse projections.

The transverse display of the image and the increased contrast resolution afforded by computed tomography combine to permit demonstration of anatomic structures that were not visible or only rarely visible with older noninvasive techniques. In fact, computed tomography usually demonstrates mediastinal detail with exceptional clarity.

Ideally, computed tomography should be performed with a state-of-the-art fourth generation scanner. Images should be made from apex to diaphragm to include the entirety of the mediastinum and each lung. Contiguous sections are usually made and most are often 1 cm in thickness. Thinner sections may be required on occasion as for study of detailed bronchial or vascular anatomy. Contrast enhancement is desirable but is not always necessary. Images should invariably be photographed with settings to show both mediastinal and pulmonary parenchymal detail.

General indications for computed tomographic examination of the body have been discussed by several authors [55, 115, 118]. In the first edition of this book a table of specific indications for the use of computed tomography in the study of the mediastinum was offered. At present it seems sufficient to say that any mediastinal problem is amenable to, and constitutes an indication for, performance of the study. Individual indications will be discussed and illustrated throughout this volume.

3.1.6 Magnetic Resonance Imaging

Shortly after the introduction of magnetic resonance imaging, the role of this modality became firmly established in neuroradiology. Its usefulness in other areas of the body has been the subject of intensive study and only now is its superiority for evaluating some clinical problems outside the central nervous system coming to be recognized. In the mediastinum and hilum (see chapter 10) the utility of magnetic resonance remains essentially undetermined as data is being accumulated [53, 130].

Most studies are now performed using spin echo technique to obtain T1 and T2 weighted images. The capability of magnetic resonance imaging to provide sagittal and coronal images of a quality equal to axial images would seem to provide considerable additional diagnostic potential but, in early experience, this adjunct has not been found to be as valuable in the thorax as might have been anticipated [92, 130]. In the chest, respiratory and cardiac motion have been vexing problems although cardiac gaiting and the introduction of newer techniques for faster data acquisition have done much to improve image quality.

Contrast resolution of magnetic resonance imaging is superior to that of computed tomo-

graphy. For this reason small nodes or masses may stand out against mediastinal soft tissues better than they do on computed tomography. On the other hand, spatial resolution is not as good on magnetic resonance examinations and computed tomography is to be preferred for evaluation of bronchi and vessels. Contrast material is currently not used for magnetic resonance studies; the study therefore offers an alternative to computed tomography for those patients in whom contrast enhancement might be risky because of iodine sensitivity. On the negative side, the study poses difficulty for claustrophobic patients and is, in general, more expensive than computed tomography.

As the technology of magnetic resonance develops and overcomes some of the previously mentioned problems and with the development and authorization for use of paramagnetic contrast agents, it is likely that magnetic resonance will assume a major role in imaging the thorax.

3.1.7 Special Procedures

Over the years, a number of special radiographic examinations of the mediastinum have been developed using air and iodinated agents as contrast materials. Pneumomediastinography has virtually disappeared from use with the advent of mediastinoscopy and limited anterior thoracotomy. The indications for angiography in the mediastinum are now virtually restricted to the demonstration of aneurysms and other forms of congenital and acquired vascular malformations. The use of pulmonary angiography or azygography for the evaluation of the extent of mediastinal tumor has all but disappeared in most areas. Lymphography for the evaluation of mediastinal disease has a limited range of applications. This topic as it relates to the thoracic duct is discussed further in chapter 7.

3.2 Factors Affecting the Demonstration of Mediastinal Anatomy and Pathology

3.2.1 The Lung-Mediastinum Interface

The mediastinum lies in the midplane of the thorax between the lungs, from which it is separated only by the visceral and parietal pleurae. It is clear that air in the lungs provides the contrast that outlines the mediastinal contents. Those structures immediately beneath the mediastinal pleura groove or otherwise indent the air-filled lungs to a variable degree [9, 30]. The classic illustrations in standard books of anatomy showing the impressions made by mediastinal structures on the medial surfaces of the lungs are graphic demonstrations of this point [1, 18] (Fig. 3.4). The deeper the indentation the structure makes on the lung, the better is its visualization. An ectatic aorta and a dilated esophagus are better seen because they are enlarged and intrude more deeply into lung. Conversely, greater mediastinal detail is usually apparent when the lungs are of large volume, as in patients with emphysema, since the hyperexpanded lungs intrude more deeply into mediastinal recesses. From the technical point of view, the best mediastinal examinations are obtained in full inspiration when the lungs are tightly packed against the mediastinum.

The diffuse infiltration of the mediastinum that occurs in mediastinitis and occasionally with neoplasm prevents lung from contacting normal mediastinal structures and thereby causes the mediastinum to have a straight, formless contour (Fig. 3.1). This type of mediastinal appearance on radiographs should raise the suspicion of widespread, infiltrative mediastinal abnormality.

3.2.2 Mediastinal Fat

Another anatomic characteristic of the mediastinum that facilitates its radiographic evaluation is the presence of fat, often found normally in rather large quantity. Major locations of fat deposition are in the anterior mediastinum extending downward into each cardiophrenic angle, over the epicardium, especially along the coronary arteries, and in the atrioventricular grooves, along the base of the heart extending into the area of the aortic-pulmonic window and paraspinally behind the aorta (Fig. 3.5). Genereux [37] has also studied the distribution of mediastinal fat and commented that fat distribution depends upon the habitus and nutritional state of the patient. While confirming the above-stated distribution, he noted that fat accumulations were in general located in the superior, anterior, and lower posterior mediastinum. He pointed out, further, that there is symmetry in the quantity of fat lateral to the vertebral bodies above the aortic arch but asymmetry is the rule below the arch; with left-sided position of the descending aorta, there is always more fat on the left than there is on the right. The radiologic appearances caused by these normal accumulations of fat and by abnormal collections of fat as well are considered in the chapters that follow.

The contact of lung and mediastinal pleura usually creates a simple interface. When left lung contacts right lung across the pleurae, a true line is produced – a linear shadow of increased density outlined between two more radiolucent areas. At times, a line is also produced when lung contacts mediastinal pleura that immediately overlies mediastinal fat (Fig. 3.6). This is the anatomic situation that so often causes the aortic-pulmonary line to appear as a true line. Local conversion of such a line to an interface suggests that the mediastinal fat has been changed to water density, and therefore mediastinal pathology should be suspected.

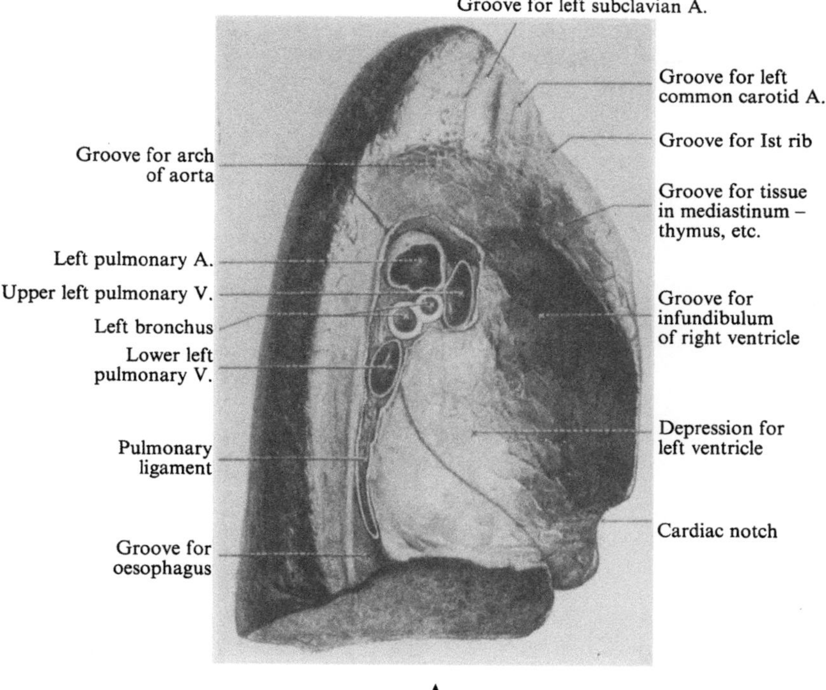

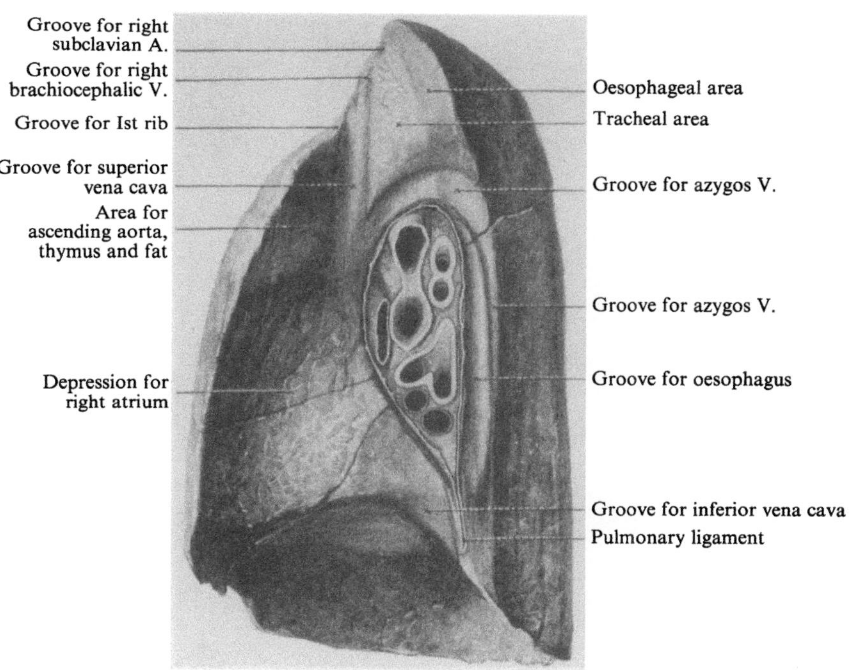

Fig. 3.4 A, B. Impressions made by mediastinal structures on left and right lungs. Photographs of medial surfaces of the left (**A**) and right (**B**) lungs hardened in situ. These pictures demonstrating the impressions made by mediastinal structures on the medial surfaces of each lung serve to emphasize why these mediastinal structures are visible on chest radiographs. The aerated lungs, in intimate contact with many of these mediastinal structures, provide contrast causing structures to be visible radiographically. The more deeply these structures indent lung and the more tightly lung is packed against mediastinum, the better is the demonstration of mediastinal detail (see Fig. 3.1). (From [18]).

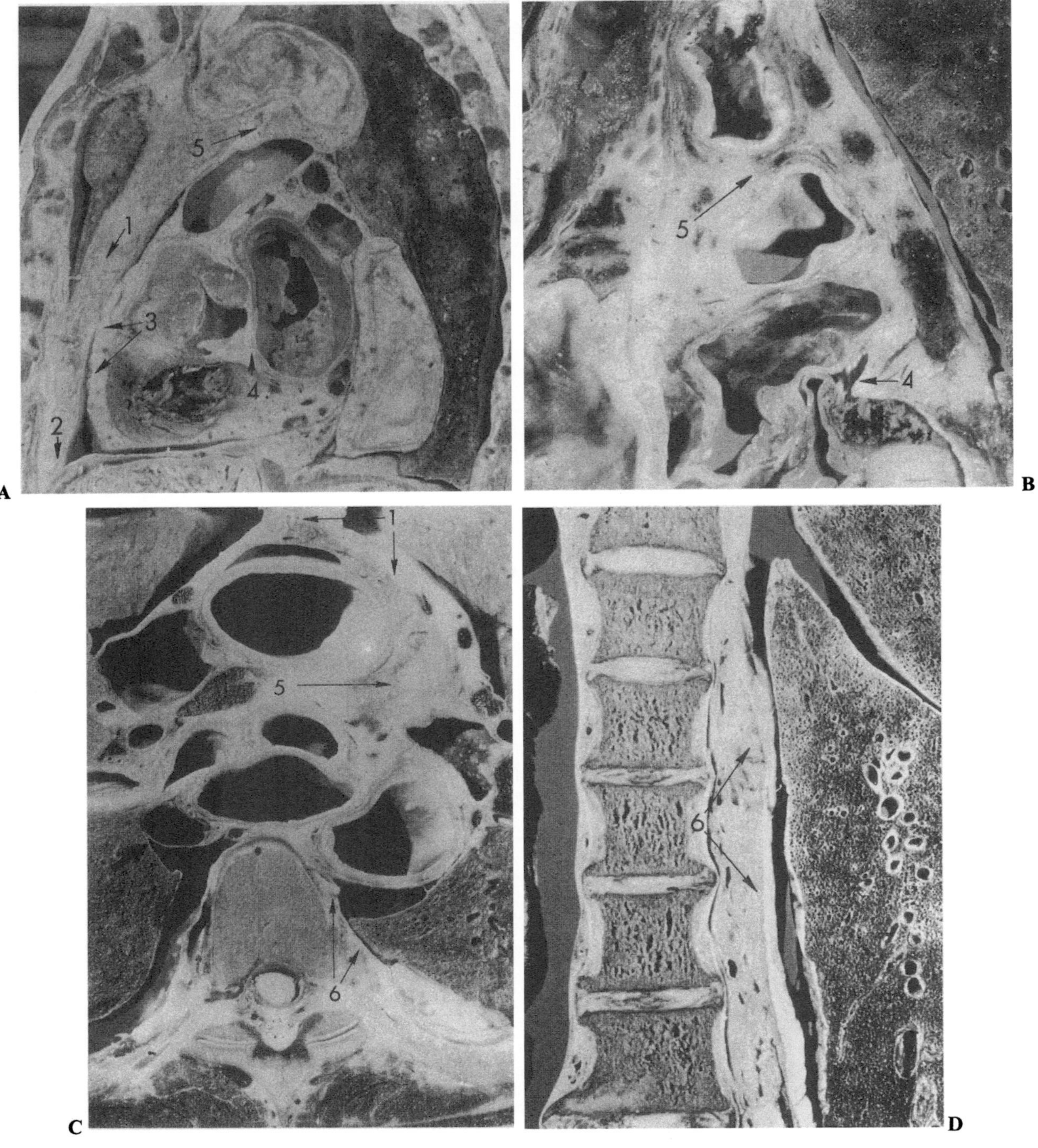

Fig. 3.5A–D. Anatomic location of mediastinal fat. **A** Sagittal body section. **B** and **D** Coronal body sections. **C** Transverse body section. Major locations of fat deposition in mediastinum are retrosternally in the anterior mediastinum (*1*), extending downward into each cardiophrenic angle (*2*), over the epicardium (*3*), especially along the coronary arteries and in the atrioventricular grooves (*4*), along the base of the heart extending into the area of the aortic pulmonic window (*5*), and paraspinally behind the aorta (*6*)

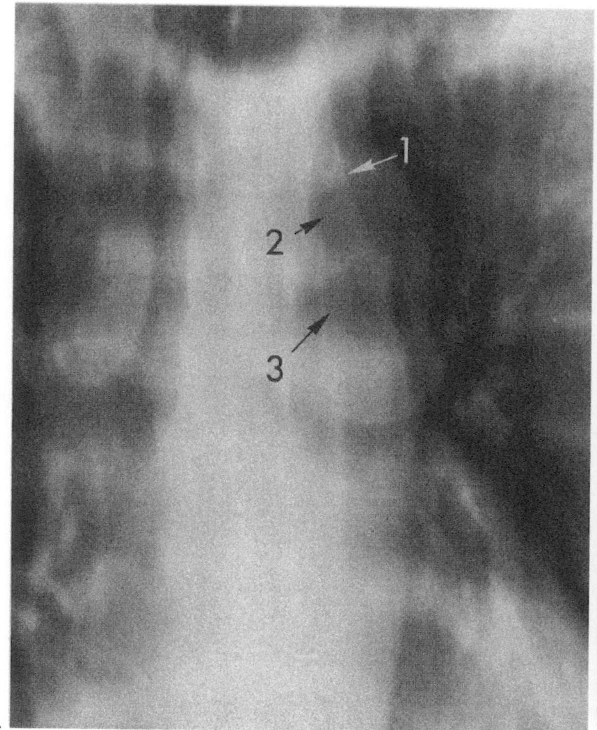
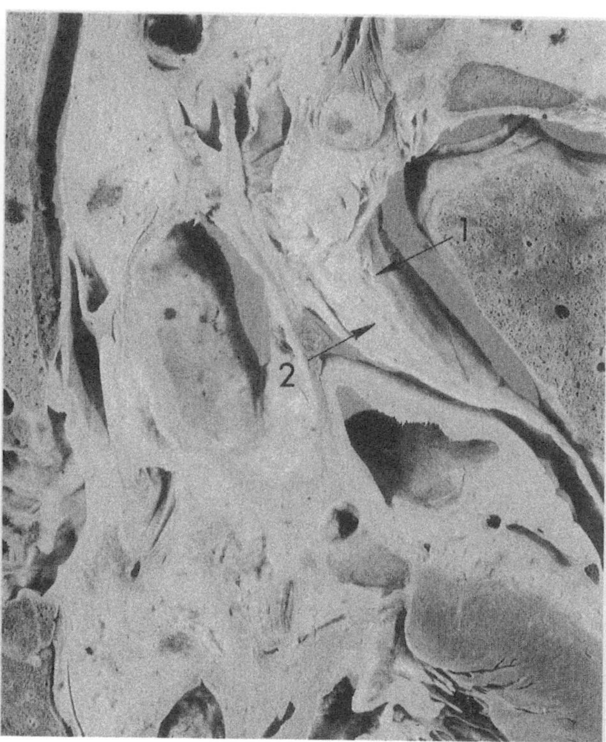

Fig. 3.6A, B. Radiologic demonstration of mediastinal fat. **A** AP tomogram. **B** Coronal body section. Mediastinal fat cannot usually be appreciated as being more radiolucent than other soft tissues of the mediastinum, possibly due to high contrast provided by adjacent aerated lung. Occasionally, however, mediastinal fat can be identified as it causes apposed visceral and parietal pleurae to appear as a line (*1*) between fat (*2*) and aerated lung. At times it can be difficult to distinguish this appearance from that caused by the Mach effect without photodensitometry. Note also that there appears to be some fat in the aortic-pulmonic window (*3*) (see also Fig. 7.3)

3.2.3 Mach Effect

The "Mach effect" is a normal visual phenomenon elucidated in the previous century by Ernst Mach [73]. Although many aspects of the Mach effect remain to be explained, it is recognized as a form of visual edge enhancement produced by the normal physiologic processes of the eye [107]. For a complete review of this subject the interested reader is referred to the book *Mach Bands* by Ratliff [106]. The radiologic implications of the Mach effect have been discussed in depth by Lane et al. [64].

For practical radiologic purposes the Mach effect can be considered to accentuate the margins of structures or lesions. As a result, it often makes contours on radiographs easier to see, just as it does other images in everyday visual experience. If a structure or lesion is bordered by a white halo, this halo is called a "positive Mach band"; a black halo is a "negative Mach band" (Fig. 3.7). Positive Mach bands are produced when a convex surface of lesser luminance meets a concave surface of greater luminance; negative Mach bands are caused when these physical conditions are reversed. The cardiac silhouette, for example, frequently appears to be edged in black – a negative Mach band; the convex left ventricular border of greater luminance is received by the concave left lung of lesser luminance (Fig. 3.8). Utilization of this concept can be helpful in telling the paraspinal line from the edge of the descending aorta when such a distinction causes a problem. The paraspinal line will seem to be edged by white – a positive Mach band – whereas the aorta will seem edged in black – a negative Mach band (see Figs. 3.7 and 6.26). The paraspinal line is

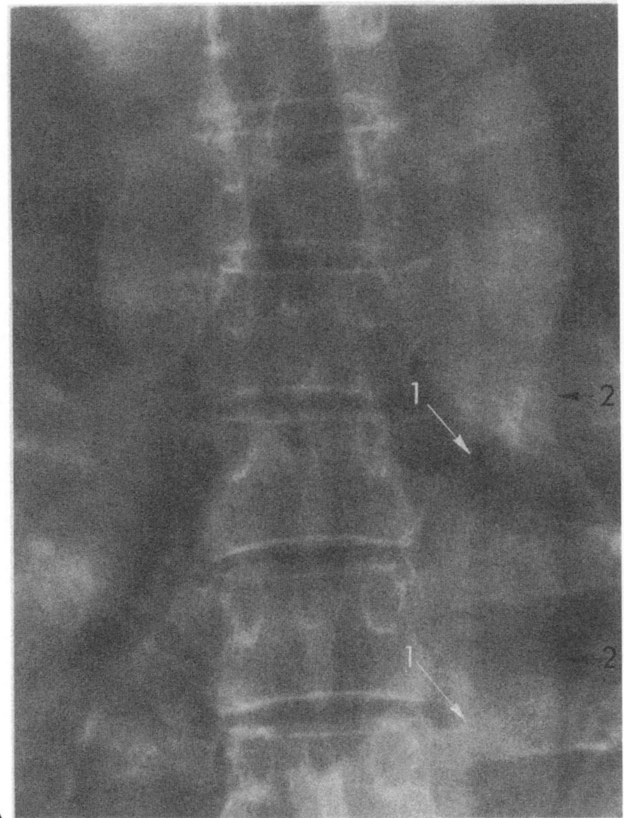

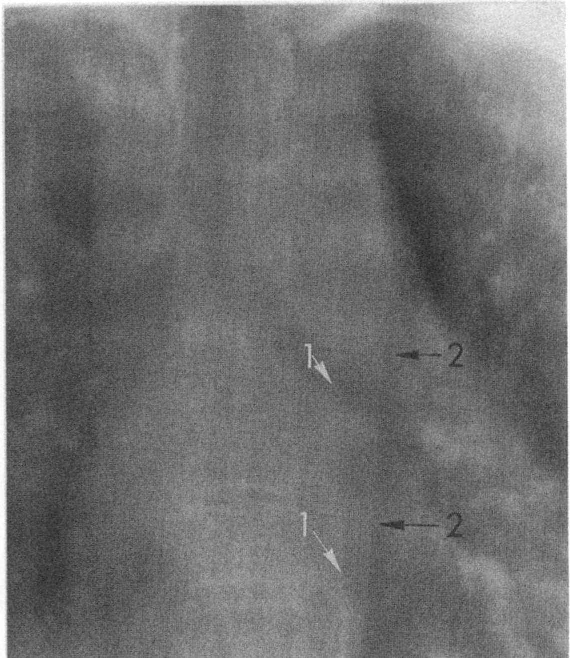

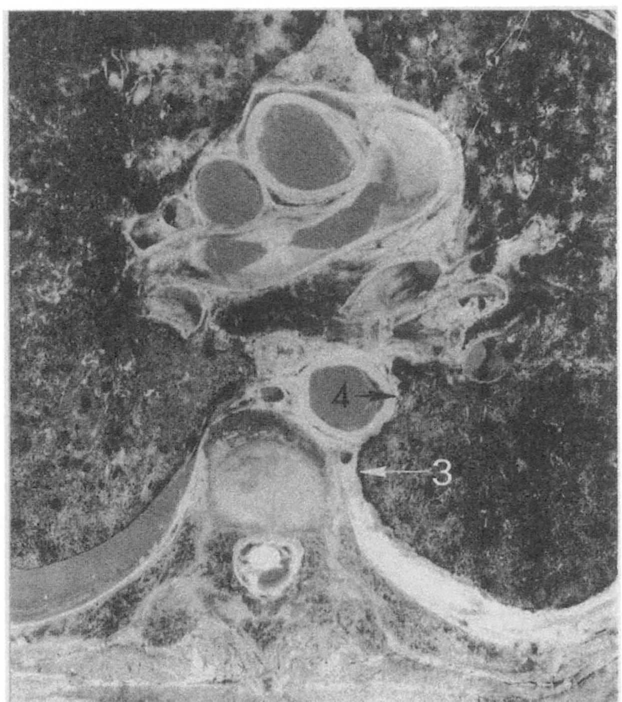

Fig. 3.7A–C. Mach effect. **A** Overpenetrated AP radiograph. **B** AP tomogram. **C** Transverse body section. Note that paraspinal line seems to be edged by white, a positive Mach band (*1*), whereas the descending aorta appears to be edged by black, a negative Mach band (*2*). The positive Mach band edging paraspinal line is produced by contact of convex lung of lesser luminance with concave surface of mediastinum of greater luminance (*3*). The negative Mach band about aorta is produced by contact of concave lung of lesser luminance with convex aorta of greater luminance (*4*). Use of Mach effect can be used in this manner to determine physical characteristics of the lung-mediastinal interface

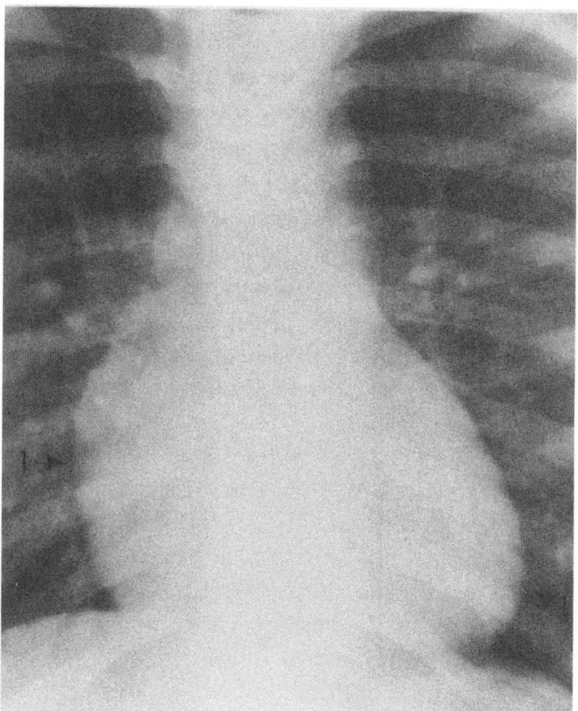

Fig. 3.8. Mach effect (PA radiograph). Black border around cardiac shadow (*1*) on this PA radiograph is due to Mach effect. Mach effect can be considered a form of visual edge enhancement produced by the normal physiologic processes of the eye. Mach effect is an important factor in causing interfaces of lung and mediastinum to be better seen. (Courtesy A. Proto, Richmond, VA)

not infrequently seen as a white line rather than an interface, even though photodensitometry shows that no true line is present. The spurious line is a positive Mach band.

How does one tell whether the paraspinal line is a Mach band or a real line representing the pleurae between mediastinal fat and lung? Without photodensitometry, one cannot tell with absolute certainty, although if the line disappears when one masks the film on either side of it, it is very likely to be a Mach band. Genereux [37] contends that what is seen as the paraspinal line is never the apposition of the visceral and parietal pleura causing a visible line but is always the result of the Mach effect. Arguments for and against this contention are elaborated in chapter 7. The appearance of the paraspinal line as a line rather than an interface can still be useful in radiologic interpretation wheth-

er it is real or not. If, along its course, the paraspinal line can no longer be seen as a line but rather becomes an interface, paraspinal disease medial to this point should be inferred. If the line was a real one, it can be assumed that paraspinal fat is infiltrated, rendering it of soft tissue density. If the line was spurious, the same conclusion must be drawn since the Mach effect should not occur at one point along the paraspinal line and not at another unless the physical conditions affecting its visualization were different at the two points. Mach bands commonly aid in the visualization of radiographic images; less frequently they can be misinterpreted as evidence of pathology. Swischuk has pointed out that the Mach effect can at times allow a medial pneumothorax to be more visible, whereas at other times it may cause a simulated pneumothorax [121]. The distinction is made by covering the cardiac silhouette with dark paper; if the black paramediastinal area disappears, no pneumothorax is present and the visual phenomenon can be ascribed to the Mach effect. Friedman [32] has suggested that the Mach effect may assist in the diagnosis of minimal pneumomediastinum. Mach bands rarely simulate disease in the mediastinum. For further discussion of these pitfalls in other areas the reader is referred to the work of Lane et al. [64].

3.3 Radiologic Characteristics of Mediastinal Masses

One of the most difficult problems in pulmonary radiology can be the determination of whether a centrally situated chest mass lies in the mediastinum, the pleural space, or the lung parenchyma. Although in some cases the lesion may defy accurate localization, correct assessment of the position of the lesion is usually possible with careful attention to radiologic criteria.

There are three radiologic findings pointing to a mediastinal location of a mass lesion. The first is a smooth, sharply defined interface with contiguous lung. As a mediastinal mass grows, it pushes the parietal and visceral pleurae ahead of it into lung. The pleurae become a connective

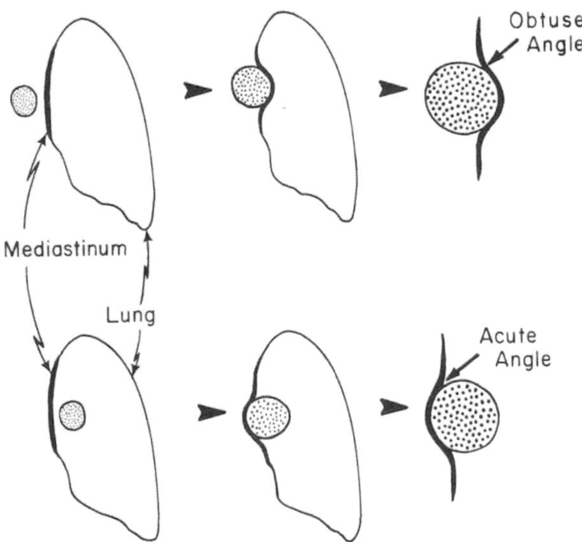

Fig. 3.9. Comparison of angles made with mediastinal pleura by mediastinal masses and pulmonary masses. Assuming a concentric growth of the mediastinal mass, it lifts mediastinal pleura away from mediastinal structures; therefore angles formed by reflection of pleura over mass are obtuse when viewed in profile (*top row*). Lung masses form acute angles with pleura when they have grown sufficiently to contact mediastinum (*bottom row*). This finding can be useful in distinguishing mediastinal from pulmonary lesions but is far from infallible

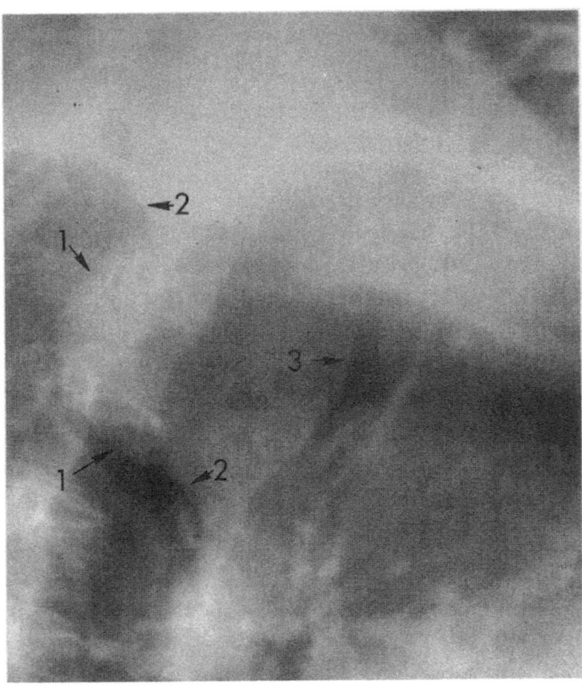

tissue coat of double thickness covering the lesion and cause the mass to be smooth and sharply outlined (Figs. 3.10 and 3.11). This is not to say that parenchymal lung lesions cannot be smooth and well defined – they often are. Perhaps the corollary of this principle is a better way of thinking about it: a poorly defined mass is infrequently mediastinal in location. This sign has good reliability, although occasionally a primary mediastinal process such as Hodgkin's disease will cross the pleurae to invade the lung [54], resulting in a poorly marginated lesion of mediastinal origin.

The second important finding is the formation of obtuse angles between the margin of the lesion and contiguous lung. If concentric growth of a mediastinal mass is assumed, the mass should gently lift the mediastinal pleura away from mediastinal structures, and the angles produced by the reflection of the pleura over the mass should therefore be obtuse when viewed in profile (Figs. 3.9 and 3.10). Again assuming concentric growth, lung masses should form acute angles with the pleurae when they have grown sufficiently to contact the mediastinum (Fig. 3.9). This principle is analogous to the criteria used for distinguishing mucosal lesions from submucosal lesions in gastrointestinal radiology. The application of this radiologic finding should be approached with caution since at times mediastinal lesions will produce acute angles with the mediastinal pleura (Fig. 3.11). Its reliability as a single radiologic criterion is therefore somewhat limited; in conjunction with a smooth, sharply defined surface it is quite high. The combination of a sharp convex outline and tapering margins is called the "extrapleural sign" by Felson [27–29] (Fig. 3.10).

Fig. 3.10. Extrapleural sign (right anterior oblique radiograph). This mass lesion in the supra-azygos area presents two features that characterize the extrapleural sign: lesion is very sharply marginated (*1*), and angles formed by mass with mediastinum are obtuse (*2*). In combination these two findings are called the "extrapleural sign" by Felson [27–29]. This sign is strongly indicative of extrapleural location of mass. Note also localized impression on trachea (*3*). This intimate effect of mass on mediastinal structure further supports mediastinal location of mass. The lesion is a posterior goiter

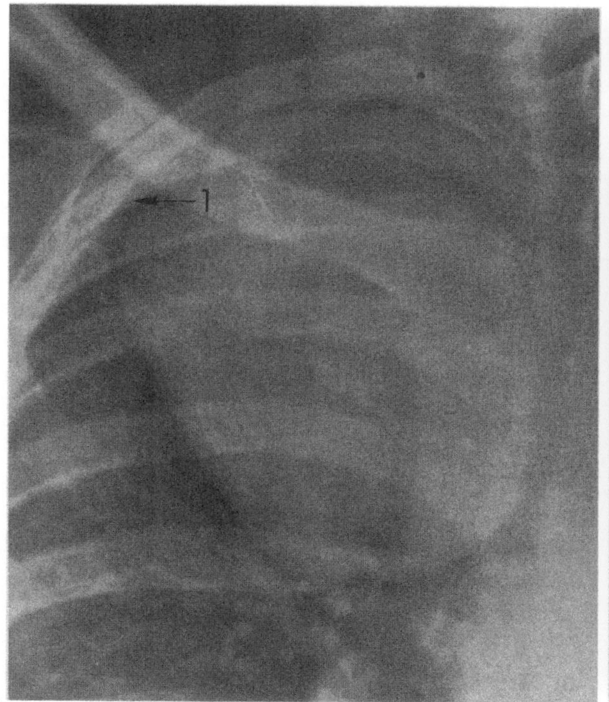
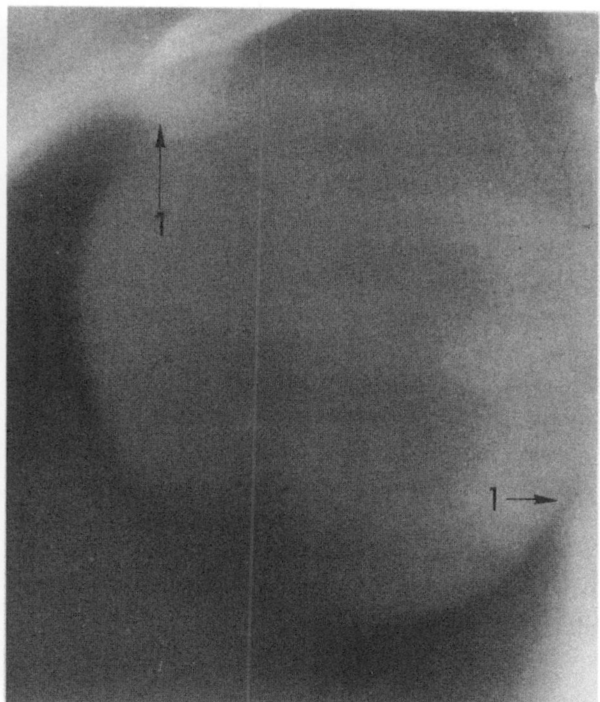

A   B

Fig. 3.11A, B. An extrapleural mass forming acute angles with adjacent lung. **A** PA radiograph. **B** AP tomogram. This large apical mass was proven to be a neurofibroma. There is no associated bone involvement. Lesion presents very sharp margin against lung, but angles formed by lesion with lung are acute rather than obtuse (*1*). Not infrequently, extrapleural lesions will invaginate lung so deeply that such acute angles will be produced. In attempting to distinguish whether a mass is mediastinal, pleural, or pulmonary, only limited reliance should be placed on angle formed by mass with pleura as a sole finding

The third finding of importance in differential diagnosis is intimate effect on mediastinal contents. Lesions that closely contact or locally displace mediastinal structures such as the esophagus or trachea are very likely mediastinal in location. The more localized the effect, the more likely the mass is to be mediastinal. It is for this reason that careful inspection of the trachea and the barium-filled esophagus is so important to correct film analysis.

The three factors just described should be considered the primary ones indicating a mass lesion to be mediastinal in location. Other findings, however, may be supportive. Sometimes,

the simple expedient of identifying the epicenter of the mass as being within the mediastinum or the lung can be the most valuable clue to the site of origin of the process. Central lesions that show the characteristic calcifications of a teratoma or that are composed of fat are almost certainly in the mediastinum. Lesions that move with the lung during respiration are not mediastinal and almost certainly reside in lung.

Frequently, it is not possible to distinguish a mediastinal lesion from a pleural one. Among localized pleural masses, mesothelioma is common. If a central chest mass changes its position in relation to the mediastinum and the lung during respiration or with change in body position, it is likely to be a pedunculated pleural mesothelioma [8]. Most of these tumors are on the stalk and move about freely in the pleural space. Aside from this point, radiologic investigation will distinguish a mediastinal mass from a pleural one only rarely. Most often surgery will be required to make the distinction. Exceptionally, diagnostic pneumothorax may be worthwhile.

Finally, evaluation can be complicated by the tendency of some pathologic processes to cross the pleurae; Hodgkin's disease shows a definite propensity to extend from the mediastinum into the lung along the bronchovascular sheaths and even directly through the pleurae [54].

It should be concluded that it is frequently difficult to determine from radiographs whether a central thoracic mass lesion is mediastinal, pleural, or pulmonary in location. The general signs just described are helpful, but a thorough knowledge of radiographic anatomy and of the often subtle changes caused by disease in various areas of the mediastinum is the most reliable way of localizing the process to the mediastinum. Findings such as distortion of the azygoesophageal recess, the preaortic line or the paraspinal line cannot only prove the process to be mediastinal but can pinpoint its position with precision. Discussions of this correlated anatomic-radiologic approach form the basis of subsequent chapters.

3.4 Lymph Nodes of the Mediastinum

Evaluation of mediastinal lymph node enlargement is one of the most important and challenging tasks in pulmonary medicine. Radiologic examination is at the forefront of this effort. Although mediastinoscopy has developed into a very effective tool for the study of mediastinal disease and especially mediastinal adenopathy, it is an invasive technique that results in a small but definite incidence of morbidity [46]. More significantly, this procedure has definite limitations, since only a portion of the mediastinal lymph nodes can be visualized [59, 100]. The relative roles of mediastinoscopy and radiologic examination are discussed more completely in Chapter 4. Suffice it to say that the radiologic examination remains the keystone in the diagnostic evaluation of the lymph nodes of the mediastinum. Findings that permit a diagnosis of mediastinal lymph node enlargement are covered on a regional basis in subsequent chapters. The anatomic organization of the nodes of the mediastinum and the general significance of their involvement by tumor will be included in this chapter.

3.4.1 Anatomy of the Lymph Nodes of the Mediastinum

Lymph nodes can be distinguished from other lymphoid aggregates in the thorax by the presence of trabeculation and clear-cut encapsulation [86]. A true node is found in the lung parenchyma only rarely; on occasion it may be seen on radiographs as a pulmonary nodule [47, 102]. Nodes are common in the hilar regions and in the mediastinum. Beck and Beattie [6], who cleared a group of mediastinums at postmortem examination, found that the average number of mediastinal nodes was 64; most of them, about 50, were paratracheal in position, and about a dozen were paraesophageal. Nodes may adopt round, oval, or pyramidal shapes [21]; normal nodes rarely exceed 2 cm in any dimension and most of them are less than 15 mm in diameter [38]. In the mediastinum, nodes usually appear in clusters, several of them being surrounded by a single connective tissue envelope.

Many investigators have studied the organization of the lymph nodes in the mediastinum, and almost all of them have offered classifications that subdivide the nodes into various groups. These classifications are in general rather similar: only two of the older ones will be considered here. A comprehensive historical review of the subject can be found in the book *Functional Anatomy and Histology of the Lung* by Nagaishi [86] and in other works [21, 76, 90, 91, 109, 120]. Table 3.1 presents a comparison of the most frequently quoted older classification authored by Rouviere in 1932 [109], with a more recent subdivision proposed by Nagaishi [86] some 40 years later. The similarities between the two schemes are immediately apparent; the differences between them are largely semantic except for their handling of the nodes of the anterior mediastinum. These nodes, sometimes called "prevascular nodes" because of their position anterior to the aortic arch and left common carotid artery on the left and the superior vena cava on the right, are included in Rouviere's classification but are not given that designation in Nagaishi's system. Nagaishi doubtlessly includes them among the groups he called the "pretracheal and the aortic arch

Table 3.1. A comparison of the bronchopulmonary lymph node classifications of Rouviere [109] and Nagaishi [86]

Rouviere (1932)	Nagaishi (1972)

Intrapulmonary nodes
  Lobar
  Interlobar
	Bronchopulmonary nodes

Peritracheobronchial nodes of the pulmonary root	Bronchopulmonary nodes Pulmonary ligament nodes Aortic arch nodes Botallo's ligament nodes
Nodes of the tracheal bifurcation Retrotracheal nodes Paratracheal nodes	Tracheal bifurcation nodes Tracheobronchial nodes Paratracheal nodes Pretracheal nodes Aortic arch nodes
Nodes of the anterior mediastinum Nodes of the posterior mediastinum	Innominate vein angle nodes

Table 3.2. Classification of bronchopulmonary lymph nodes as proposed in the first edition of this book

1	Nodes of the thoracic inlet and anterior mediastinum
1.1	Innominate vein angle nodes
1.2	Internal mammary nodes
1.3	Cardiophrenic angle nodes
2	Tracheobronchial nodes
2.1	Aortic-pulmonic window nodes
2.1.1	Ductus nodes
2.2	Paratracheal nodes
2.3	Subcarinal nodes
3	Periesophageal nodes
4	Hilar nodes
4.1	Inferior pulmonary ligament nodes

nodes." In their study, Beck and Beattie [6] state: "Only a few lymph nodes were observed in the anterior part of the mediastinum."

Neither the classification of Rouviere nor that of Nagaishi is totally applicable to radiologic diagnosis, and the terminology used is certainly not common parlance.

In the first edition of this book a compromise between existing classifications was offered (Table 3.2). This outline was suggested as being simple and employing terminology that was in common usage. At the time this classification

Table 3.3. Proposed definitions of regional nodal stations for prethoracotomy staging. (From [122])

X	Supraclavicular nodes
2R	Right upper paratracheal (suprainnominate) nodes: nodes to the right of the midline of the trachea between the intersection of the caudal margin of the innominate artery with the trachea, and the apex of the lung (includes highest R mediastinal node). Radiologists may use the same caudal margin as in 2 L.)
2L	Left upper paratracheal (supra-aortic) nodes: nodes of the left of the midline of the trachea between the top of the aortic arch and the apex of the lung (includes highest L mediastinal node)
4R	Right lower paratracheal nodes: nodes of the right of the midline of the trachea between the cephalic border of the azygos vein and the intersection of the caudal margin of the brachiocephalic artery with the right side of the trachea (includes some pretracheal and paracaval nodes). (Radiologists may use the same cephalic margin as in 4L.)
4L	Left lower paratracheal nodes: nodes of the left of the midline of the trachea between the top of the aortic arch and the level of the carina, medial to the ligamentum arteriosum (includes some pretracheal nodes)
5	Aortopulmonary nodes: subaortic and para-aortic nodes, lateral to the ligamentum arteriosum or the aorta or left pulmonary artery, proximal to the first branch of the left pulmonary artery
6	Anterior mediastinal nodes: nodes anterior to the ascending aorta or the innominate artery (includes some pretracheal and preaortic nodes)
7	Subcarinal nodes: nodes arising caudal to the carina of the trachea but not associated with the lower lobe bronchi or arteries within the lung
8	Paraesophageal nodes: nodes dorsal to the posterior wall of the trachea and to the right or left of the midline of the esophagus (includes retrotracheal, but not subcarinal nodes)
9	Right or left pulmonary ligament nodes: nodes within the right or left pulmonary ligament
10R	Right tracheobronchial nodes: nodes to the right of the midline of the trachea from the level of the cephalic border of the azygos vein to the origin of the right upper lobe bronchus
10L	Left peribronchial nodes: nodes to the left of the midline of the trachea between the carina and the left upper lobe bronchus, medial to the ligamentum arteriosum
11	Intrapulmonary nodes: nodes removed in the right or left lung specimen plus those distal to the main stem bronchi or secondary carina (includes interlobar, lobar, and segmental nodes)[a]

[a] Post-thoracotomy staging: nodes could be divided into stations 11, 12, 13 according to the AJC classification.

was proposed there was no agreement as to which nodes constituted the hilar group. Some authors felt that only those nodes located in the major bronchial bifurcations should be called "hilar," whereas others included nodes somewhat more peripheral in lung in this category. Still other observers preferred to designate some of the nodes in the lower tracheobronchial chain as being hilar in location.

In addition to the problems raised by this controversy, another concern over classification has been raised. Relatively extended survival in some patients classified by the TNM system as having Stage III disease because of mediastinal lymph node involvement has been reported by several observers [89, 100]. This fact has led to the recent development of a modification in the TNM system [82] (see section 3.4.3.1). Additionally, however, Tisi [122] has commented:

"In drawing attention to improved survivorship ... each of these series raises the question as to whether the N characteristics require further refinement ... they simultaneously draw attention to a glaring deficiency in the classification of regional lymph node involvement in lung cancer, i.e. commonly accepted, specific anatomic definitions of each nodal station are lacking."

As an outgrowth of these concerns the American Thoracic Society (ATS) charged a committee to: "develop a map of regional pulmonary lymph nodes that would be acceptable to all physicians who care for the patient with lung cancer" [122]. This new classification is summarized in Table 3.3 and Figs. 3.12 and 3.13 taken from the article by Tisi [122]. Note that the boundaries of the lower paratracheal areas are now clearly defined and that the designation "hilar" has been dropped from the ATS classification. Glazer et al. [42] have recently reported a computed tomographic study of the size and number of normal lymph nodes in the various stations of the ATS classification and H.S. Glazer [44] has discussed the computed tomographic appearance of calcified mediastinal

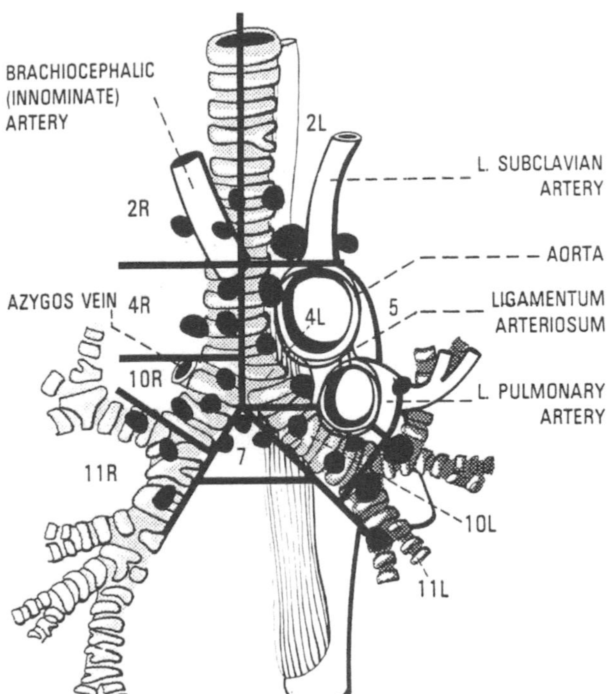

Fig. 3.12. American Thoracic Society's classification of regional pulmonary lymph nodes (see text and Table 3.3). (From [122])

nodes relative to the classification. Application of this classification will have increasing radiologic relevance. Classification is important; some years ago Strauss [119] commented that sophisticated staging of bronchogenic carcinoma would hopefully lead to improved survival as it did in patients with Hodgkin's disease, perhaps it yet will.

Fig. 3.13A, B. American Thoracic Society's classification of regional pulmonary lymph nodes. **A** Six representative transverse sections through areas of regional pulmonary lymph nodes as obtained by computed tomographic scanning. **B** Designation of the nodal stations at each of the six computed tomographic scans. (From [122])

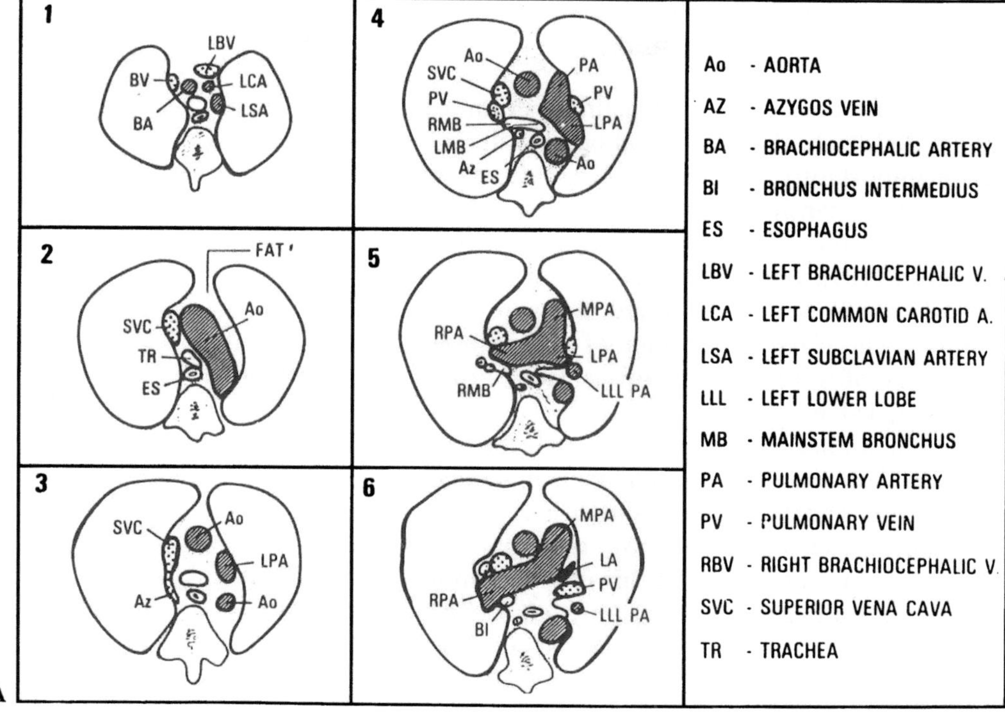
1
LBV
BV
LCA
BA
LSA
2
FAT
SVC
Ao
TR
ES
3
SVC
Ao
LPA
Az
Ao
4
Ao
SVC
PA
PV
PV
RMB
LPA
LMB
Az ES
Ao
5
MPA
RPA
LPA
RMB
LLL PA
6
MPA
LA
PV
RPA
LLL PA
BI
Ao   - AORTA
AZ   - AZYGOS VEIN
BA   - BRACHIOCEPHALIC ARTERY
BI   - BRONCHUS INTERMEDIUS
ES   - ESOPHAGUS
LBV - LEFT BRACHIOCEPHALIC V.
LCA - LEFT COMMON CAROTID A.
LSA - LEFT SUBCLAVIAN ARTERY
LLL - LEFT LOWER LOBE
MB   - MAINSTEM BRONCHUS
PA   - PULMONARY ARTERY
PV   - PULMONARY VEIN
RBV - RIGHT BRACHIOCEPHALIC V.
SVC - SUPERIOR VENA CAVA
TR   - TRACHEA
A

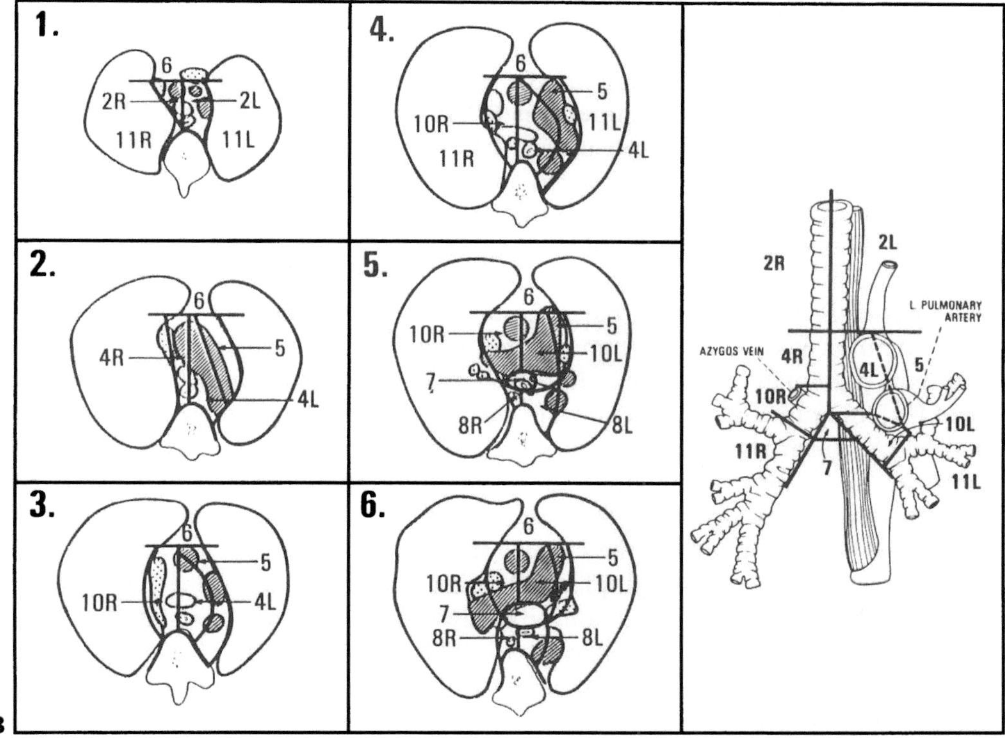
1.
6
2R
2L
11R
11L
2.
6
4R
5
4L
3.
6
5
10R
4L
4.
6
10R
5
11R
11L
4L
5.
6
10R
5
10L
7
8R
8L
6.
6
10R
5
10L
7
8R
8L
2R
2L
L. PULMONARY ARTERY
AZYGOS VEIN
4R
4L
5
10R
10L
11R
7
11L
B

3.4.2 Patterns of Metastatic Spread to Mediastinal Lymph Nodes

The lymph nodes of the mediastinum drain the upper abdomen, the breast and chest wall, and more importantly, the lungs. The patterns of metastatic extension to the mediastinum from the various lung lobes were clearly described by Rouviere [109], whose observations were subsequently confirmed by Nohl [90, 91] and other authors. This classic description of the anatomic pathways of spread of tumor is summarized briefly in Table 3.4.

Recent studies have pointed out that the concept of the spread of tumor to mediastinal nodes outlined in Table 3.4 is too simplistic [46, 84]. It does, of course, explain how right paratracheal nodes result from a left lower lobe tumor. However, drainage occurs not only left to right but right to left as well; communication can occur through the subcarinal nodes and also between the paratracheal nodes [31, 46]. In the series reported by Goldberg [46], mediastinoscopy showed that left-sided tumors spread to the contralateral side of the mediastinum in 55% of cases, whereas right lung tumors spread to the left side of the mediastinum in 62% — about the same figure. All too often, there is contralateral spread through left-sided and subcarinal nodes even when the tumor is right-sided in origin. The traditional concept does explain on an anatomic basis the reason why contralateral metastasis without ipsilateral metastasis is more common with left lung tumors than it is with right pulmonary neoplasms. In Goldberg's series [31], only one of 57 patients with mediastinal spread from right-sided tumors had contralateral nodes only, compared to seven of 29 patients whose tumor originated on the left. Murray [84] has summarized the current status of our understanding of the lymphatic drainage of the lungs as follows: "It is no longer believed that the right lymphatic duct drains 80% of the total pulmonary lymph and the remaining 20%, mainly from the left upper lobe, drains through the left lymphatic duct; it is now agreed that pulmonary lymph drainage patterns are complex and variable ..."

Table 3.4. Pathways of lymphatic drainage from the lobes of the lung (after McCort and Robbins [76], Nohl [90, 91] and Rouviere [109]). This classic description is now recognized as being too simplistic (see text)

Right upper lobe	
Anteromedial aspect	→ Right paratracheal nodes
Posterolateral aspect	→ Right paratracheal nodes ↑ → Subcarinal nodes
Right middle lobe	→ Right paratracheal nodes ↑ → Subcarinal nodes
Right lower lobe	
Superior aspect	→ Right paratracheal nodes
Inferior aspect	→ Right paratracheal nodes ↑ → Subcarinal nodes ↑ → Periesophageal nodes
Left upper lobe	
Superior aspect	→ Left paratracheal nodes
Inferior aspect	→ Left paratracheal nodes → Subcarinal nodes → Right paratracheal nodes
Left lower lobe	
Superior aspect	→ Left paratracheal nodes → Subcarinal nodes → Right paratracheal nodes
Inferior aspect	→ Subcarinal nodes → Right paratracheal nodes ↑ → Periesophageal nodes

3.4.3 Significance of Mediastinal Lymph Node Metastasis in Carcinoma of the Lung

The presence of lymph node spread in carcinoma of the lung has long been known to affect prognosis in a very significant way. Whereas apparent complete resections in patients without mediastinal nodal metastases produce 5-year survivals of between 30% and 45%, depending upon the cell type of the tumor, fewer than 10% of patients live 5 years if mediastinal nodes are involved [81]. It is interesting that the presence of positive segmental or interlobar nodes without nodal involvement elsewhere does not appear to affect prognosis adversely [7, 91]. In Mountain's experience [82], 33% of all patients with lung cancer have mediastinal lymph node involvement when first seen. Other investigators have confirmed this figure [23, 34, 77, 95]. It is obviously very important to find such metastatic involvement during the diagnostic work-up, not only to evaluate prognosis, but also to decide upon the best form of management for the patient.

Evaluation of lymph node metastases to the mediastinum is clearly important in the selection of patients for surgery. Some surgeons feel that the demonstration of mediastinal lymph node metastases in a case of carcinoma of the lung contraindicates surgery. All concur that contralateral lymph node involvement rules out surgery. Radical pneumonectomy with lymph node dissection is sometimes advocated when only low ipsilateral and/or subcarinal nodes are present, especially if the tumor is of the squamous cell type. Few surgeons would operate upon a patient with high ipsilateral nodal involvement [81]. Anaplastic small cell (oat cell) carcinoma is not, in general, treated by surgery in most clinics.

3.4.3.1 Staging of Bronchogenic Carcinoma

In 1959, the American Committee for Cancer Staging and End Results Reporting was formed. Shortly thereafter, this committee adopted the Tumor-Nodal Involvement-Metastasis (TNM) system of cancer staging advocated by the committee on clinical stage classification of the International Union Against Cancer [122–124]. This action popularized the TNM system and led to an upturn of interest in the evaluation of mediastinal lymph node metastases in lung cancer. Under the TNM system the extent of the local tumor and its spread is recorded; T characterizes the gross features of the primary tumor, N the extent of regional lymph node metastases, and M the presence or absence of distant metastases. Recently, a modification of the TNM system has been developed [82]. For a complete review of TNM staging, interested readers are referred to the papers of Carr and Mountain [12], Mountain [82, 83], and others [3, 123, 124].

Evaluation of mediastinal lymph nodes is required in the TNM staging of lung cancer. The N part of the classification, the extent of regional lymph node metastases, is very relevant to the present discussion. The new TNM system stages the presence or absence of extension to regional lymph nodes in the following manner [82]:

Nodal Involvement (N)

N_0 No demonstrable metastases to regional lymph nodes

N_1 Metastasis to lymph nodes in the peribronchial or the ipsilateral hilar region, or both, including direct extension

N_2 Metastasis to ipsilateral mediastinal lymph nodes and subcarinal lymph nodes

N_3 Metastasis to contralateral mediastinal lymph nodes, ipsilateral or contralateral scalene or supraclavicular nodes

N_1 involvement places the case in Stage II or in Stage III a depending upon other parameters. N_2 involvement places the case in Stage III a, whereas N_3 involvement requires placement of the case in Stage III b [82].

The objectives of TNM staging of lung cancer as summarized by Mountain [81] are as follows:

1. To aid in treatment planning
2. To make an assessment of prognosis
3. To add validity to end-result evaluation that serves for continuing self-assessment
4. To facilitate exchange of information between centers of study

Observations growing out of the initial TNM staging system demonstrated its clinical importance. Of 1568 cases (excluding undifferentiated small cell carcinoma) studied in this way to relate prognosis to the extent of regional lymph node metastases, those categorized as N_0 had a 25%–30% 5-year survival, N_1 cases a 10% – 15% 5-year survival, and N_2 cases a 2%–4% 5-year survival [83]. Some N_2 patients had long-term survival [89, 100] leading in part to the development of the new modifications in the system.

Obviously, factors not considered in staging of lung cancer by the TNM system also influence patient management. Among these are cell type and the general condition of the patient.

3.4.4 Radiologic Assessment of Metastases to Mediastinal Lymph Nodes

Discussion of the diagnosis of mediastinal lymph node enlargement by conventional radiography and by conventional and computed tomography is an integral part of each chapter in this book. Nevertheless, it is important to discuss here some general precepts in the computed tomographic diagnosis of mediastinal lymphadenopathy in bronchogenic carcinoma.

Computed tomography has now emerged as the principal adjunct to plain film radiography in the diagnosis of mediastinal adenopathy in patients with lung cancer or suspect lung cancer [52, 68, 78]. It is possible that, in the future, magnetic resonance imaging may prove to equal or exceed computed tomography in its capacity to demonstrate adenopathy. At present the sensitivity and specificity of the two modalities is relatively comparable [131].

Early in our experience with computed tomography, it was hoped that density criteria based on the Hounsfield number might prove to be helpful to distinguish malignant nodes from benign nodes. Unfortunately, this hope has not been realized and the only criterion now used for making this distinction is node size.

3.4.4.1 Factors Affecting Lymph Node Size

At least three, and perhaps four, factors should be considered in evaluating the size of mediastinal lymph nodes.

Location of the Node

Nodes vary in size depending upon their location in the mediastinum. The largest nodes are in the paratracheal regions near the carina. Nodes higher in the mediastinum, in the subcarinal areas and in the paraesophageal areas, are on an average, smaller [38].

Axis in Which the Node is Imaged

Nodes in the paratracheal area are arranged such that their long axis is in a cephalocaudad plane. Since images displayed at computed tomography are axial, they do not demonstrate the long axis of the node. Node size determined from normal computed tomographic examinations is therefore somewhat less than node size determined from anatomic studies which have generally recorded the long axis of the node.

The Association of Lung Collapse and/or Infection

An important factor to consider in the evaluation of mediastinal adenopathy in patients with bronchogenic cancer is whether there is collapse and/or infection accompanying the tumor. Chronic infection behind an obstructed bronchus frequently results in enlargement of mediastinal lymph nodes on a reactive basis [70]. Under these circumstances, mediastinal nodes may well be larger than the established upper limit of normal and yet not harbor tumor.

Nodal Calcification

It has been stated that if mediastinal lymph nodes are shown to be calcified and therefore likely to have been involved in a past granulomatous process, they may very well be larger in size than noncalcified nodes found in normal individuals [70]. Glazer [42], however, failed to show any relationship between node calcification and node size or number.

3.4.4.2 Size Criteria for Mediastinal Adenopathy

What size criteria are to be used for the determination of mediastinal lymph node involvement? Genereux [38] found that among 225 lymph nodes imaged by computed tomography, 99% measured less than 16 mm in greatest diameter. In the precarinal and subcarinal area 90% of the nodes were in the 6–10 mm range. Glazer [42] stated: "Our data suggests that at present the size threshold for an abnormal node should be set at one cm in the short axis." Quint [104] has suggested from autopsy studies that computed tomograms size right-sided nodes more accurately than they do left-sided ones.

At the present time, it would appear that nodes smaller than 1 cm in diameter should be considered normal, realizing, of course, that such nodes may harbor microscopic foci of tumor. Nodes between 1 cm and 1.5 cm should be considered suspicious, and nodes greater than 1.5 cm should be considered abnormal, realizing, of course, that some nodes in this category may ultimately prove to be reactive, particularly if the lung harbors pneumonia in addition to tumor.

3.4.4.3 Efficacy of Computer Tomographic Assessment of Involvement of Mediastinal Nodes by Tumor

The practical value of the assessment of mediastinal adenopathy by computed tomography has been and continues to be the subject of lively debate. Libshitz [69] reviewed eight studies reported in the literature and found that, as expected, sensitivity was high but specificity was low when 1 cm was used as the upper limit of normal size for a normal node; sensitivity was low and specificity was high when nodes were not considered abnormal unless they were over 2 cm in size. Baron et al. [4] studied a group of patients retrospectively using 2 cm as the upper limit of size for a normal node. They, too, found high specificity and justified the use of this larger size criterion on the basis that all patients judged to be abnormal would indeed be abnormal and that no patient with histologically normal nodes would be denied surgery, either mediastinoscopy or thoracotomy, if size criteria were relied upon heavily by the surgeon. This philosophy, however, resulted in a very large percentage of patients (approximately $^1/_3$) being considered indeterminate for mediastinal lymph node involvement in this series. The ideal benchmark would be criteria which result in both high sensitivity and high specificity. Obviously, this cannot be achieved, and a compromise must be found which permits reasonably satisfactory sensitivity and specificity figures.

Radiologists might consider the following proposal: nodes less than 1 cm in diameter should be reported as having low probability of tumor involvement; nodes between 1 cm and 1.5 cm, intermediate probability of tumor involvement; and nodes greater than 1.5 cm, high probability of tumor involvement.

Despite the practical utility of the determination of mediastinal node size by computed tomography and its rather good predictability of tumor involvement, Libshitz [70] feels that these size criteria should be used cautiously, offering the following comment: "On the basis of present information, nodal size alone should not be used to deny the possible benefits of surgical exploration." Osborne et al. [95] in an earlier report came to the same conclusion. A somewhat more positive view of the value of computed tomography in the assessment of mediastinal lymphadenopathy is held by Faling et al. [23]. An interesting debate between Osborne and Korobkin and Faling et al. was published in *Radiology* in 1982 [24, 94].

Determination of mediastinal involvement in bronchogenic carcinoma by any radiographic modality including computed tomography is an important responsibility. The opportunity for surgical cure may be lost if false-positive diagnosis of mediastinal involvement is rendered. Glazer [43] has emphasized some of the pitfalls in the diagnosis of lymph node enlargement at computed tomography. Radiologic interpretations should be made conservatively and should be as precise as possible in terms of the anatomic structures or areas involved. Criteria used for establishing the extent of disease should have high specificity and should be meticulously and consistently applied. Furthermore, as Friedman [34] has stated: "There must be locally accepted and implemented criteria for operation. Staging by non-invasive sizing of lymph nodes is an expensive exercise unless clinical management is responsive to diagnostic findings."

3.4.4.4 Implications for Mediastinoscopy

The role of computed tomography in determining whether or not mediastinoscopy should be performed is another controversial topic. Glazer et al. [41] state that, in their experience, negative computed tomography is "highly accurate in excluding mediastinal metastases and makes screening mediastinoscopy unnecessary." Positive computed tomography is less reliable and should not be considered evidence of inoperability. Rather, positive computed tomography should locate enlarged nodes for biopsy before attempted curative resection. In a recent presentation, Friedman [34] concurred with these observations.

3.4.4.5 Implications for Limited Anterior Thoracotomy

There are no data available concerning the value of computed tomography to determine whether or not a limited anterior thoracotomy should be performed. It is presumed that at least in some cases, the demonstration of enlarged lateral aortic nodes or nodes in the aortic pulmonic window will suggest that biopsy be performed by limited anterior thoracotomy.

3.5 Connective Tissue Planes of the Mediastinum

Although some discussion of the fascial planes of the mediastinum is included in almost every chapter of this book, a review of the general organization of these connective tissue planes seems indicated in this chapter on general radiologic considerations since it is so relevant to the spread of blood, infected material, and air throughout the mediastinum. Surprisingly little has been written about this important facet of anatomy [117]; the few authors who have touched on the subject refer to the original work of Marchand [75]. The following descriptions are based heavily on his observations.

The anatomy of the mediastinal connective tissue itself is not complex. The mediastinal fascia does, however, extend in continuity across the thoracic inlet where it merges with the cervical fascia. A practical understanding of the mediastinal fascia requires a knowledge of this cervicothoracic continuum [93], and the anatomic

considerations involved here are complicated. Archer [2] states that the descriptions of the cervical fascia are "utterly confusing". There is discrepancy in the descriptions of the anatomy of the spaces delineated by the fascial planes, and there is particular controversy over which spaces communicate with one another. Many years ago, Grodinsky and Holyoke [48] provided a comprehensive study of the subject and more recently Levitt [66, 67] has offered two contemporary reviews. Levitt has described the fascial spaces of the neck as being encompassed by leaves of the middle and deep cervical fascia and has divided them into three major groups (Table 3.5).

The middle cervical fascia surrounds the trachea, pharynx, and esophagus to form the visceral space. This space is divided into two compartments by a dense band of tissue extending laterally from the esophagus to the carotid vessels which it encompasses as the carotid sheath or the visceral vascular space.

The anterior aspect of the visceral space is sometimes referred to as the "pretracheal space" and the anterior aspect of the middle cervical fascia is also called the "pretracheal fascia." The anterior visceral space extends cephalad only as far as the hyoid bone but inferiorly is in free communication with the mediastinum.

Table 3.5. Clinically potential neck spaces. (From [66])

I. Spaces involving the entire length of the neck
   A. Retropharyngeal space (posterior visceral space, retrovisceral space, retroesophageal space)
   B. "Danger" space
   C. Prevertebral space
   D. Visceral vascular space

II. Spaces above the hyoid bone
   A. Submandibular space
     1. Sublingual
     2. Submaxillary
       a) Submental (central)
       b) Submaxillary (lateral)
   B. Pharyngomaxillary (lateral pharyngeal) space
   C. Masticator space
   D. Parotid space
   E. Peritonsillar space

III. Spaces below the hyoid bone (anterior only)
   A. Anterior visceral (pretracheal) space

The posterior aspect of the visceral space is sometimes referred to as the "retropharyngeal space" or "retroesophageal space." It extends cephalad to the base of the skull and caudad into the mediastinum where, according to Levitt [66, 67], the middle and deep cervical fascia fuse at the level of T-1 or T-2. Behind the posterior visceral space lies the so-called danger space said to lie between the alar and prevertebral layers of the deep cervical fascia. This space also extends to the skull base and inferiorly is in free communication with the mediastinum. Behind the prevertebral fascia lies the prevertebral space. The suprahyoid spaces are not directly related to the mediastinum and will not be discussed here.

Thus, the neck and the mediastinum communicate freely. The visceral compartments of the neck and the danger space are in continuity with the perivisceral space within the mediastinum. As Marchand [75] has pointed out and Oliphant et al. [93] have reemphasized, the key to an understanding of the fascial planes of the mediastinum is the concept that the trachea and the esophagus are enveloped in a loose connective tissue sheath termed the "mediastinal perivisceral fascia" (Fig. 3.14). Behind the perivisceral fascia lies the prevertebral fascia.

3.5.1 The Perivisceral Fascia

The perivisceral fascia of the mediastinum was given this designation by Marchand [75] because it encompasses the trachea and the esophagus (see Fig. 3.14). Around these structures it produces a potential space termed the "visceral compartment" [1, 93]. The perivisceral fascia of the mediastinum extends cephalad into the neck where it is commonly given the name "middle cervical fascia." Anteriorly in the neck it surrounds the larynx and trachea, whereas posteriorly it is continuous with the fascia that covers the pharynx and the esophagus. The spaces it encloses, the visceral spaces, and the space behind the middle cervical fascia, the danger space, communicate with the perivisceral space of the mediastinum. This continuum provides the avenue along which retropharyngeal

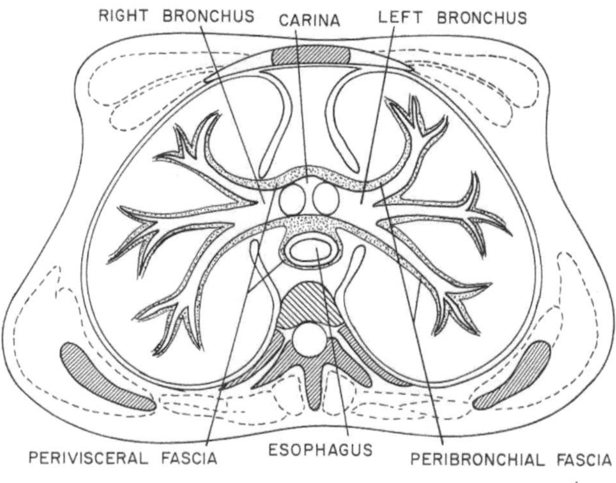

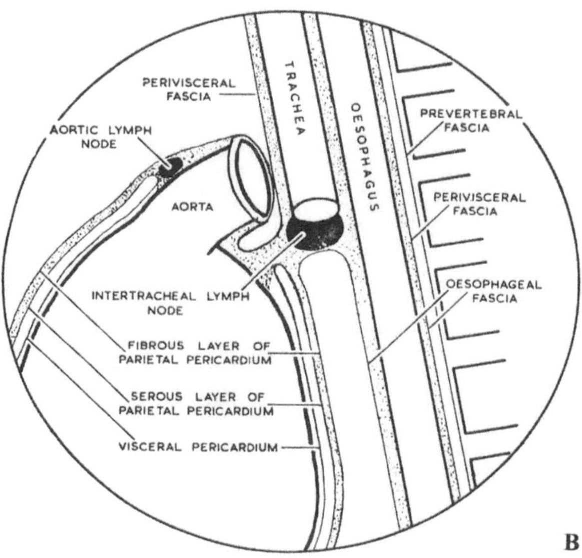

Fig. 3.14A, B. Connective tissue planes of mediastinum. **A** Transverse body section. **B** Sagittal body section. These two classic drawings show essentials of connective tissue planes of the mediastinum. Visceral compartment of the mediastinum (*stippled*) is enclosed by the perivisceral fascia that encompasses the esophagus and trachea. At its cephalad extent it is continuous with fascial spaces of neck, while inferiorly it fuses with fibrous pericardium anteriorly. Behind heart it encompasses esophagus all the way to diaphragm and is continuous with aortic adventitia. Note that laterally perivisceral fascia extends over major bronchovascular trunks. Behind tough prevertebral fascia lies the prevertebral space. (Modified from [75])

abscesses extend into the mediastinum (see Fig. 4.26). Retropharyngeal abscess also may involve the prevertebral space secondary to involvement of lymph nodes lying in front of the second cervical vertebra [57]. At mediastinoscopy, the instrument is inserted into the cervical visceral compartment, which it traverses as it passes into the mediastinum [46] (see Fig. 4.27). Tumor masses such as intrathoracic goiters cross the thoracic inlet through the anterior visceral space, as do infectious processes.

A very common occurrence is the extension of air from mediastinum to neck or vice versa through these spaces (Fig. 3.17). A curious, and unexplained, fact is the infrequency of extension of pneumomediastinum into the neck in infants [97, 98, 110]; no anatomic explanation has been offered. Quottromani et al. [105] have described the fascia encompassing the thymus and feel it to be an extension of the perivisceral fascia (Fig. 3.15). It may be responsible for the loculation of anterior pneumomediastinum. Since the perivisceral fascia invests the esophagus, fluid content dissects along this sheath following spontaneous esophageal rupture and may enter the neck through the visceral compartment. The mediastinal visceral compartment is crossed at random by connective tissue septa, some of which are continuous with the adventitia of the aorta (Fig. 3.16). The aortic adventitia can be surprisingly tough and often contains hematomas that develop following traumatic aortic rupture (see Figs. 7.38 and 7.39). Sometimes, however, blood dissects throughout the perivis-

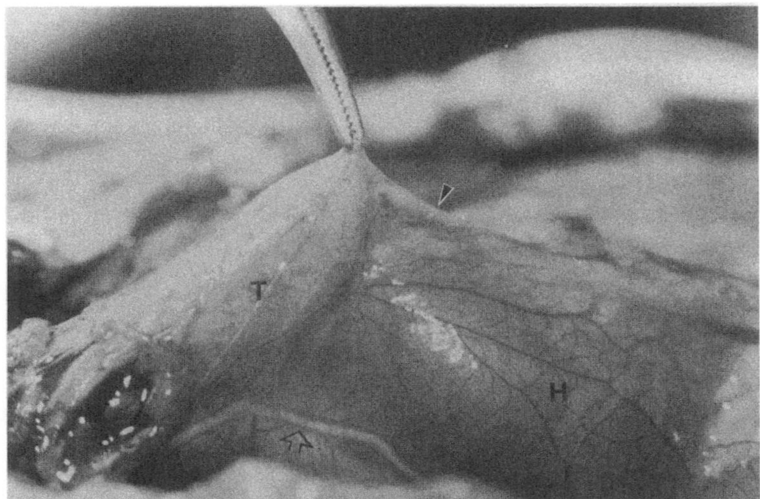

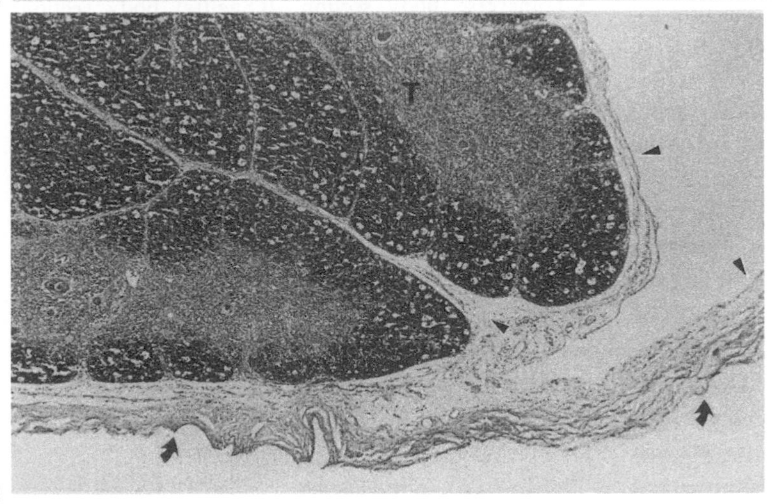

Fig. 3.15A, B. A Lateral views of anterior mediastinum. Fibrous connective tissue extends over thymus and heart tenting outward from forceps at inferior pole of thymus (*arrowhead*); it extends laterally to the parietal pleural reflection (*arrow*). *T*, thymus; *H*, heart. B Lateral micrograph. Connective tissue (*arrowheads*) envelops thymus (*T*) extending into thymic lobules and inferiorly over fibrous pericardium (*curved arrows*). (From [105])

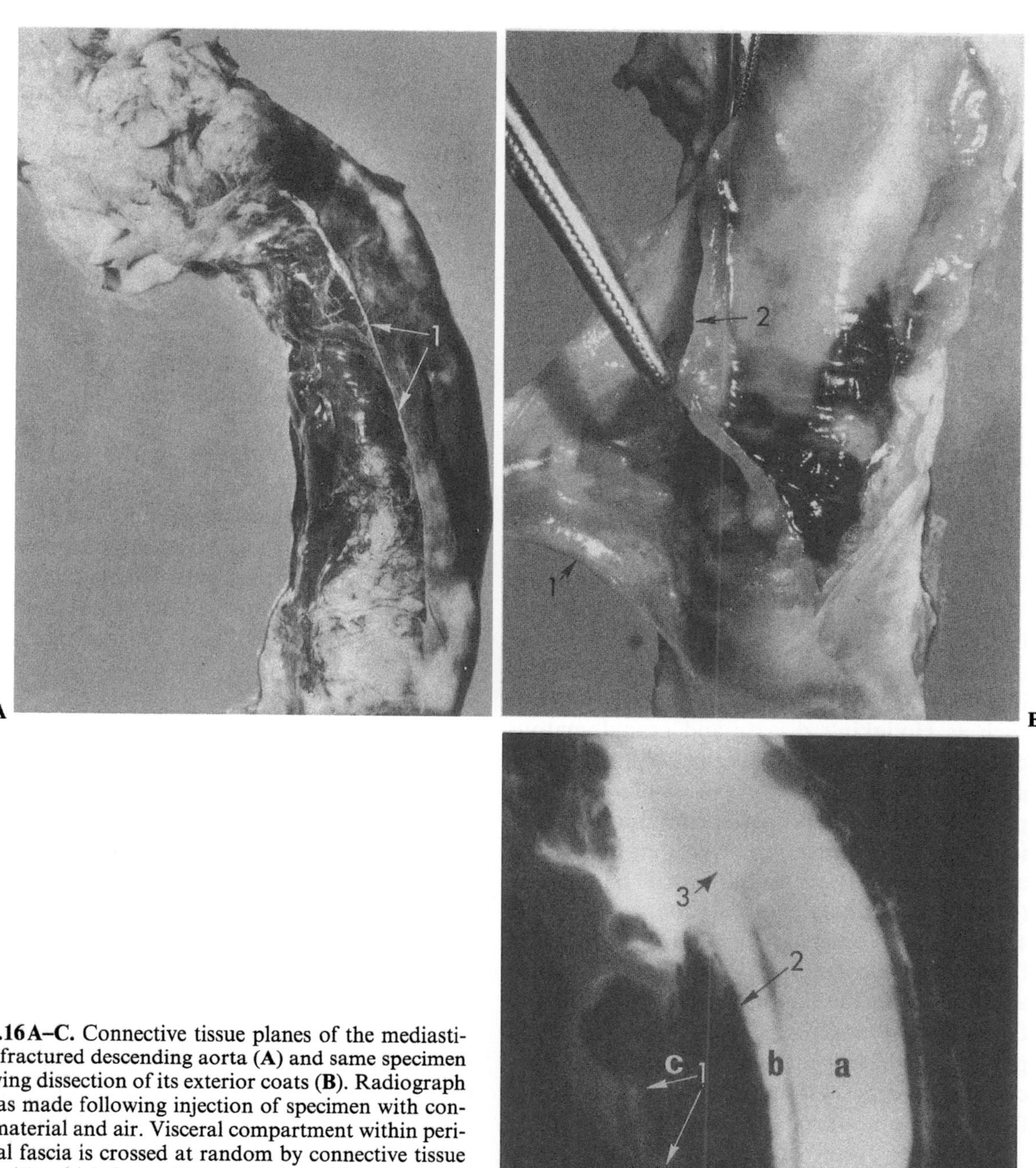

Fig. 3.16 A–C. Connective tissue planes of the mediastinum: fractured descending aorta (**A**) and same specimen following dissection of its exterior coats (**B**). Radiograph (**C**) was made following injection of specimen with contrast material and air. Visceral compartment within perivisceral fascia is crossed at random by connective tissue planes (*1*), which fuse with aortic adventitia (*2*). Aortic adventitia is frequently strong and may contain and control bleeding following traumatic rupture of aortic intima and media. Radiograph (**C**) shows fracture (*3*). Contrast can be seen in lumen (*a*) and between media and adventitia (*b*). Air outside adventitia is contained by connective tissue septa (*1*). Connective tissue planes through perivisceral compartment are, however, frequently filamentous or incomplete and often permit free dissection of material such as esophageal content, blood, or pus throughout mediastinum. (**B** and **C** from [111])

ceral space following aortic tears (see Fig. 7.40). Laterally, the perivisceral fascia of the mediastinum is prolonged over the major bronchi and blood vessels (Fig. 3.14). A potential connective tissue space exists around these structures peripherally to the third or fourth bronchial divisions. Distal to this point the connective tissue sheath is so closely applied to the bronchi and vessels that it cannot be separated even by sharp dissection. Despite this apparent fusion, it is now generally accepted that interstitial emphysema, resulting from alveolar wall rupture, tracks back along bronchovascular sheaths sometimes within lymphatics [135] to the mediastinum to produce pneumomediastinum [74] (Fig. 3.17). It may well be that air also dissects along the connective tissue sheaths around the veins. Bronchogenic carcinoma extends centrally along these bronchovascular bundles [56]. It is along this space around the arteries and bronchi that fluid resulting from purulent mediastinitis or mediastinal hemorrhage extends into lung [75, 99]. Similarly, neoplastic processes such as Hodgkin's disease and granulomatous diseases such as sarcoidosis extend into the lung along this pathway [54]. At its caudal limit, the perivisceral fascia becomes continuous anteriorly with the fibrous pericardium (Fig. 3.14) and posteriorly with the aortic adventitia (Fig. 3.16), forming multiple connective tissue septa that are loosely applied to the prevertebral fascia over the anterior longitudinal ligament all the way to the diaphragm. The perivisceral fascia can be easily separated from the tough prevertebral fascia covering the paraspinal musculature; the mediastinal structures are removed from the thorax through this plane at autopsy.

The lower extent of the perivisceral space is in continuity with the retroperitoneal space through the aortic hiatus and the lumbocostal arches (see chapter 7). Gas may also enter the abdomen by an anterior route between the sternocostal origins of the diaphragm [62].

3.5.2 The Prevertebral Fascia

The prevertebral fascia serves to separate the visceral compartment from the paravertebral tissues (Fig. 3.14). It extends from the base of the skull to the sacrum. The prevertebral space, lying behind the prevertebral fascia, can provide a pathway for processes such as osteomyelitis of the cervical spine to dissect into the thorax. Apparently, however, such extension is uncommon because the prevertebral space so often is obliterated at the T-1 level by the fusion of the prevertebral fascia with the anterior longitudinal ligament [93].

The prevertebral fascia of the neck is prolonged laterally where it becomes continuous with the suprapleural membrane and with the sheath of the subclavian vessels. Exceptionally, prevertebral infectious processes in the cervical area will extend along these vascular sheaths to present in the axilla or even at the elbow [93].

3.6 Air in the Mediastinum

3.6.1 Pneumomediastinum

Air in the mediastinum is a highly significant finding. Its cause must be ascertained immediately since prompt treatment can be life saving in some situations [74].

Air may enter the mediastinum via the deep fascial planes of the neck or rarely by dissection from the retroperitoneal space or by transit through a patent foramen from the peritoneal cavity. Pneumomediastinum also results from perforation of the trachea or bronchi [5] or esophagus (see chapter 7) and as a sequela of interstitial emphysema. The latter condition, sometimes referred to as "spontaneous pneumomediastinum," is the result of alveolar wall rupture secondary to high intra-alveolar pressure caused by artificial ventilation, cough, straining, etc. (Fig. 3.17). The gas dissects centrally along bronchovascular trunks to reach to mediastinum [74, 96], sometimes within lymphatics [135]. The reverse situation apparently never occurs; gas in the mediastinum does not

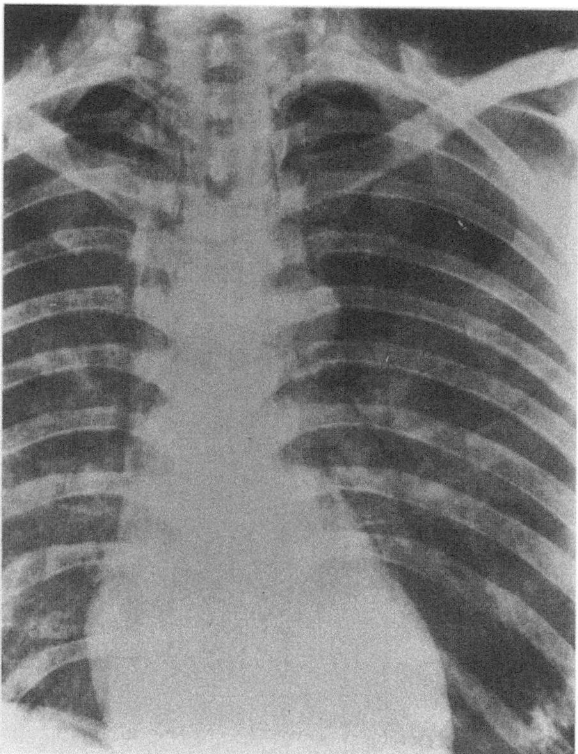

Fig. 3.17. Pneumomediastinum, PA radiograph. In this patient, barotrauma has caused pneumomediastinum. Gas is tracking along the left pulmonary artery and over the pulmonary outflow tract. Gas has dissected through the perivisceral fascial space into the neck

extend into the lung. Pneumothorax is a common complication of pneumomediastinum [71], but pneumothorax never causes pneumomediastinum.

The radiologic diagnosis of pneumomediastinum is usually not difficult if frontal and lateral radiographs are available for study. It has been stated that without a lateral film, the diagnosis will be missed in about half of the cases [71] (see Fig. 4.25). The signs of pneumomediastinum are a lifting of the mediastinal pleura off the heart and other mediastinal structures, linear streaks of gas in the mediastinum often extending into the neck (Fig. 3.17), retrosternal gas collections sometimes termed "pneumoprecardium," and extrapleural dissection along the diaphragm [71] (Figs. 3.18 and 3.19). Friedman et al. [32] feel that minimal pneumomediastinum may, in some cases, be visible because of the

Mach effect. On occasion, interstitial emphysema is present to support the diagnosis. In infants and children mediastinal air may elevate the thymic lobes to produce the "spinnaker sail" sign [29, 50, 79]. Quottromani et al. [105] have described the fascial relationships about the thymus which, they feel, are responsible for the spinnaker sail sign. They further suggest that the perithymic fascia is an extension forward of the perivisceral fascia (Fig. 3.15). Levin has described the "continuous diaphragm" sign of pneumomediastinum [65]. Normally the central portion of the diaphragm is not visible because it is in contact with the heart, which is of the same radiographic density. In some cases of pneumomediastinum, the entire diaphragm, including its central part, is visible – the continuous diaphragm sign (Fig. 3.18). Sometimes demonstration of the sternal origins of the diaphragm permits the diagnosis on a lateral film [62]. Naclerio [85], in reporting two cases of esophageal rupture, described a sharply angulated radiolucent shadow usually seen where the left diaphragm meets the paraspinal tissues. This shadow represents a combination of paraspinal air and extrapleural diaphragmatic air, which he called the "V sign" of pneumomediastinum (Fig. 3.19).

Although pneumomediastinum is usually easily diagnosed, it can be missed if only a frontal radiograph is available (see Fig. 4.25). Cimmino [17] has pointed out that pneumothorax should loculate anteriorly on supine radiographs; sizeable pneumothoraces can be missed on such radiographs. If the patient's position cannot be changed, across-table lateral film will establish or exclude the diagnosis [80]. Moskowitz and Griscom [80] have emphasized that pneumothorax will lie not only anteriorly but also medially on supine films, especially in infants. The pleural air may be mistaken for pneumomediastinum. The distinction between paramediastinal pneumothorax and pneumomediastinum is not easy to establish or clinical grounds. Many authors have pointed out that it is not possible clinically to distinguish left-sided pneumomediastinum from a left paramediastinal pneumothorax on the basis of Hamman's sign (a localized auscultatory "crunch") [49], since gas

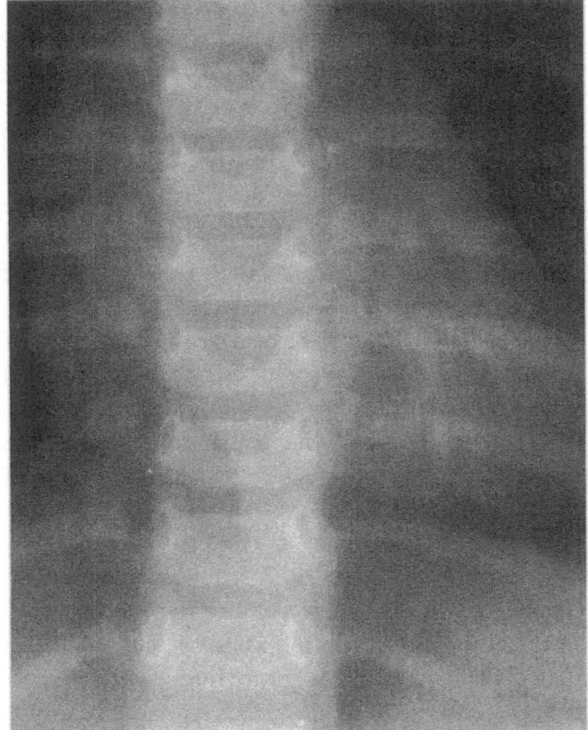

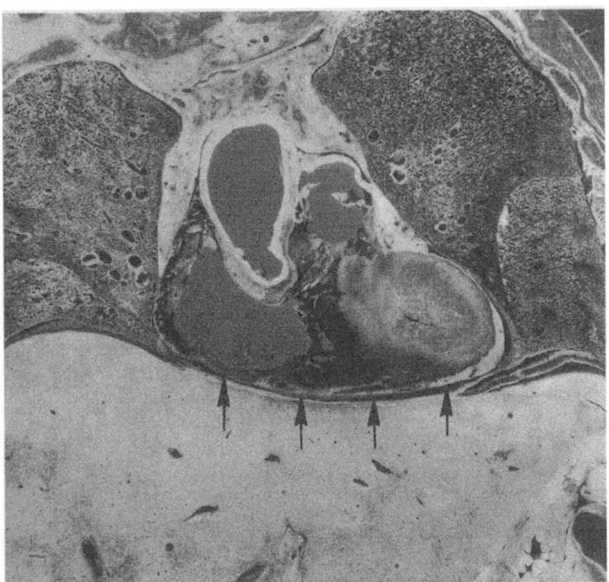

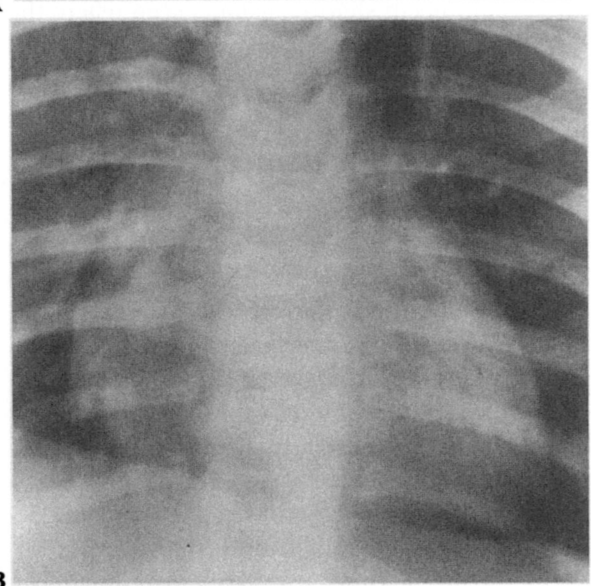

Fig. 3.18A–C. Pneumomediastinum. Continuous diaphragm sign. **A** and **B** PA radiographs. **C** Coronal body section. Note that in **B** diaphragm can be seen as continuous infracardiac line that was not present on film made 1 day earlier (**A**). Mediastinal air collected below pericardium (*arrows*) has served to outline superior surface of diaphragm. Radiographic appearance has been termed "continuous diaphragm" sign by Levin [65]

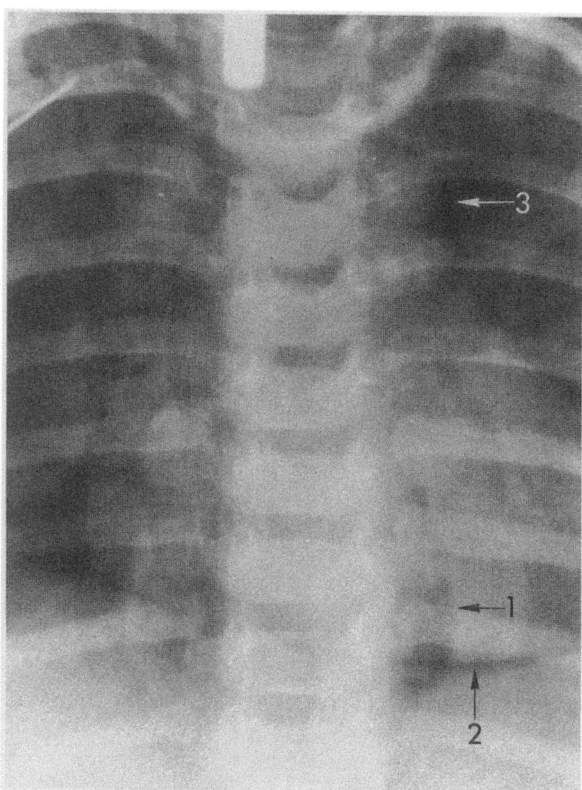

Fig. 3.19. Pneumomediastinum. "V" sign of Naclerio [85] (AP radiograph). Linear streak of mediastinal air is seen in paraspinal position on left side immediately above diaphragm (*1*). This is crossed by extrapleural air under parietal pleura (*2*) of diaphragm producing so-called V sign described by Naclerio as characteristic of pneumomediastinum. Note also there is gas about aortic knob (*3*)

in the pleural space is as capable of producing this finding as is gas in the mediastinum [17, 29, 96, 113]. At times it may be difficult to distinguish subpulmonary pneumothorax from extrapleural gas collections along the diaphragm [71]. The fact that subpulmonary pneumothorax is very commonly associated with lower lobe disease simplifies the differential diagnosis [71]. In the final analysis, it may not be possible, on a supine film, to distinguish pneumomediastinum from pneumopericardium or paramediastinal pneumothorax if the gas shadow in question is minimal [17]. Decubitus films will usually resolve the dilemma. Air in the pericardium and pleural space will move away from the dependent side, gas in the mediastinum does not usually move.

Air in the mediastinum may also loculate in rather large collections. In these circumstances, as with large generalized mediastinal air collections, the gas may be under tension and venous return may be impeded. Neonates and young infants with this condition may be in grave distress. With large collections the diagnosis of pneumomediastinum is usually not a problem. Collections are usually anterior, where they may be loculated by extensions of the perivisceral fascia as described by Quottromani et al. [105], or posterior where they often are found beneath the azygos arch and are referred to as "infra-azygos pneumomediastinum" by Bowen and Quottromani [10] (Fig. 3.20). They emphasize that anterior pneumomediastinum often remains loculated whereas infra-azygos pneumomediastinum frequently decompresses itself by cephalad or caudad dissection.

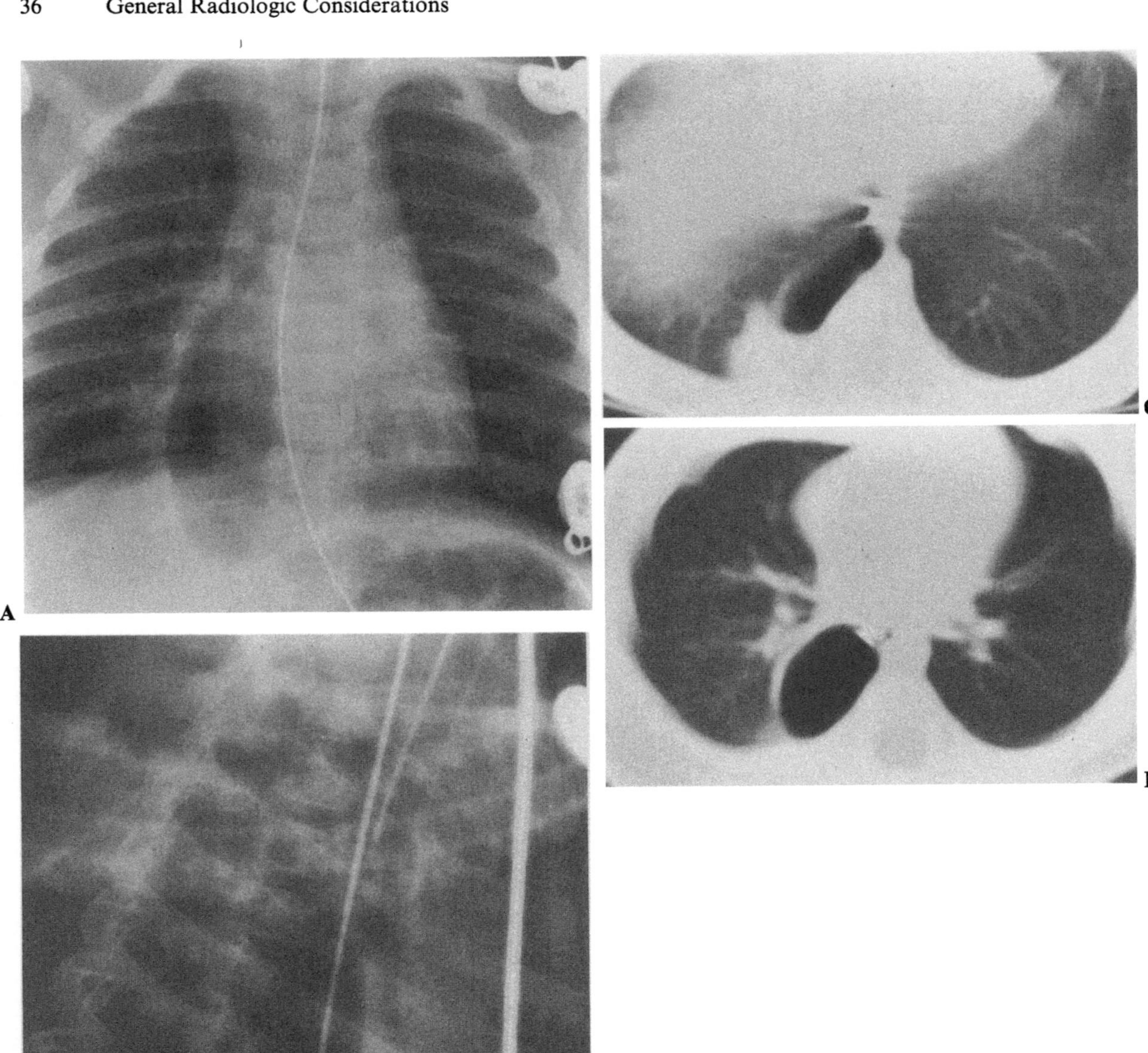

Fig. 3.20 A–D. Infra-azygos pneumomediastinum. **A** AP radiograph. **B** Lateral radiograph. **C** and **D** Computed tomograms. A 3-month-old child dropped from second floor window of burning building to grass below. Loculated pneumomediastinum sometimes occurs posteriorly, collecting under the azygos arch where it has been called "infra-azygos pneumomediastinum" by Bowen and Quottromani [10]. Unlike pneumomediastinum loculated anteriorly, infra-azygos pneumomediastinum tends to decompress cephalad or caudad. Review of the computed tomograms shows the air collection to be behind the position of the inferior pulmonary ligament

3.6.2 Paramediastinal Pneumatocoel

An excellent example of the difficulty in distinguishing a localized collection of mediastinal air from a localized collection of air in the pleural space is the entity referred to as "paramediastinal air cyst" or "pneumatocoel" [22, 26, 45, 58] (Fig. 3.21).

Such inferomedial air collections occur most commonly in children or young adults and are the result of blunt trauma or barotrauma [45].

When they are due to blunt trauma, they present the following features outlined by Godwin et al. [45] (Fig. 3.21):

1. Present on initial radiographs
2. Almost always left sided
3. Demonstrate an air-fluid level
4. Have no associated pneumomediastinum
5. Clear spontaneously in days or weeks

When they are due to barotrauma, the following features are encountered [45]:

1. Usually left sided; sometimes right sided or bilateral
2. Demonstrate no air-fluid level
3. Usually have associated pneumomediastinum or pneumothorax

Early articles on this subject raised the likelihood that the air resided within the leaves of the inferior pulmonary ligament [22, 26, 58, 108, 125]. More recently, Friedman [33] pointed out that in his cases, and those in the literature in which lateral films were available, the air collection was too far posterior to be in the ligament (Fig. 3.20). Based on this observation and the appearance of the pneumatocoels on computed tomograms, he feels that in the adult and per-

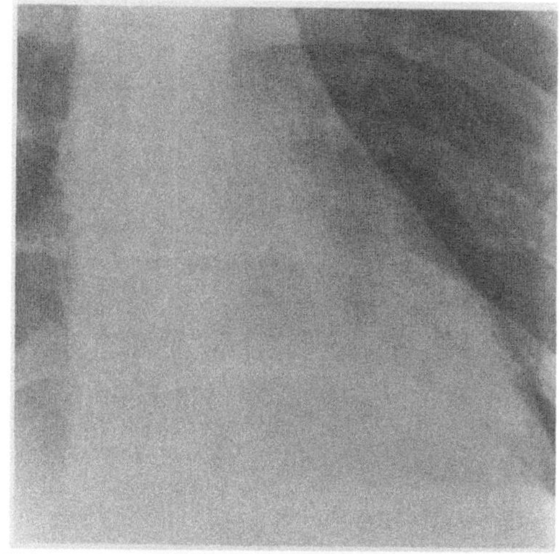
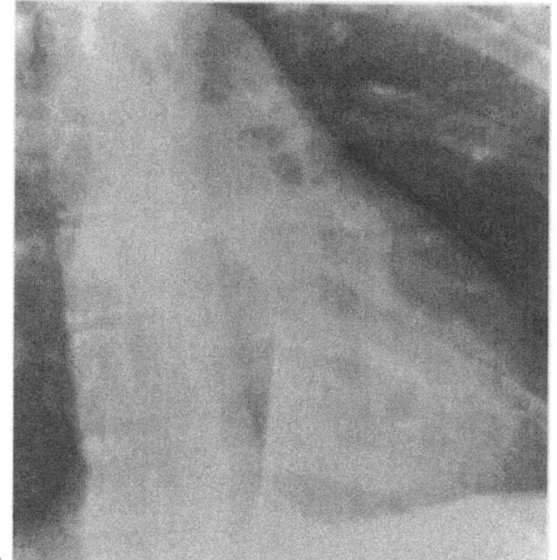
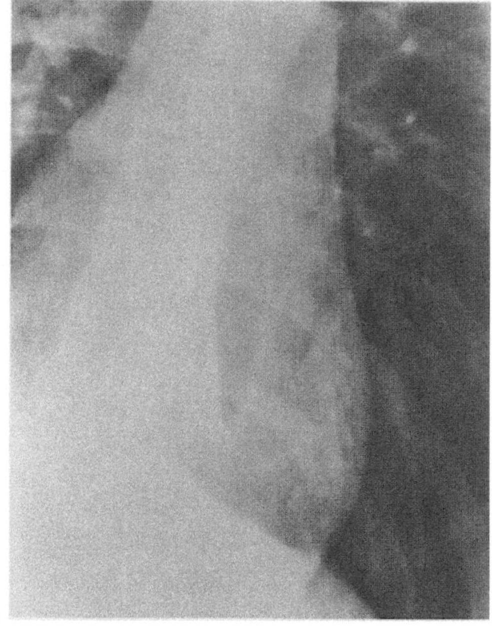

Fig. 3.21 A–C. Paramediastinal pneumatocoel. **A** PA radiograph. **B** Decubitus film made with left side down. **C** Decubitus film made with right side down. An 18-year-old man who dove into water from a 12-m cliff. Immediate onset of hemoptysis. Note left-sided air-fluid collection. Collection is infrequently, if ever, within the inferior pulmonary ligament but may be due to loculated pneumomediastinum or loculated pneumothorax. Fluid level and absence of other findings of pneumomediastinum supports diagnosis of loculated pneumothorax [45] (see text)

haps in children they represent posteromedially loculated pneumothoraces. Godwin et al. [45] state that paramediastinal penumatocoel sometimes represents loculated pneumothorax and, on occasion, loculated pneumomediastinum and they also present supporting computed tomograms.

Godwin et al. [45] feel that loculated pneumothorax will show an air-fluid level (Fig. 3.21) with a longer dimension from front to back than from side to side. Loculated pneumomediastinum does not show an air-fluid level and is round or oval in shape.

Why these pneumatocoels are loculated and lie posteromedially is not clear. In the cause of paramediastinal pneumothorax adhesions are commonly indicted [33, 45]. Whether gas collections in the inferior pulmonary ligament ever occur remains uncertain.

3.6.3 Pneumopericardium

Pneumopericardium is a rare condition almost always associated with trauma, surgical procedures, or infection. Exceptionally large quantities of air may be demonstrated in the pericardium following blunt trauma without an evident mechanism for its entry. Theories to explain this phenomenon are several but consensus opinion seems to be that a pericardial tear in juxtaposition to a laceration of a bronchus or lung is required to cause the pneumopericardium [132]. Introduction of air into the pericardium after pericardiocentesis has been used to evaluate the pericardial and cardiac surfaces [15]. When pneumopericardium occurs secondary to surgical procedures (Fig. 3.22) or infection, the clinical setting usually makes the diagnosis obvious and in each case air-fluid levels are usually visible on films made at right angles to the plane of gravity; such levels can be shown to be confined to the anatomic boundaries of the pericardial sac. Of practical importance to radiologic interpretation is the relationship of the pericardial sac to the aorta, the pulmonary artery, and their branches. The main pulmonary artery is entirely intrapericardial. The right pulmonary artery exits the pericardial sac just after giving

off the truncus anterior branch to the right upper lobe, whereas the left pulmonary artery has a shorter course within the pericardium and exits from the sac before dividing. The pericardium also invests the ascending aorta, reaching almost to the level of the innominate artery where it merges with the aortic adventitia (Fig. 3.23).

The pericardium can bee divided into an outer fibrous layer and an inner serous one. The serous layer of the pericardium does not extend as far cephalad along the aorta and the pulmonary artery as does the fibrous layer; thus pneumopericardium confined by the serous pericardium does not extend as high as the pericardial reflection is depicted in many textbooks of anatomy [126] (Fig. 3.23). The upper edge of the gas shadow is characteristically dome shaped (Fig. 3.23). The pericardial sac also encompasses the central portion of the superior vena cava, extending cephalad to a point just below the entry of the azygos vein, and extends over the inferior vena cava and the pulmonary veins for a short distance. Gas that outlines the aortic knob or more than 1–2 cm of the superior vena cava is not within the pericardium. Sometimes, as following stab wounds, the differential diagnosis of pneumopericardium versus pneumomediastinum may be considered. Ancillary signs of pneumomediastinum and extension of gas beyond the confines of the pericardial sac are obvious important differential points, but if these findings are not demonstrated, it may be necessary to obtain films in other projections. Gas in the pericardium should move freely away from the dependent portion of the sac, whereas mediastinal air should show little movement. With infection the pericardial air often outlines a thickened pericardium (Fig. 3.23).

Pneumopericardium apparently does not result from interstitial emphysema in adults. In the experimental work of Macklin and Macklin, interstitial air in the lung never entered the pericardium [74]. Loftis et al. [72], however, reported six cases of pneumopericardium in infants under 5 months of age, all receiving assisted ventilation; no similar example occurred in older children. By way of explanation, Cimmino [17] suggested that in the young infant

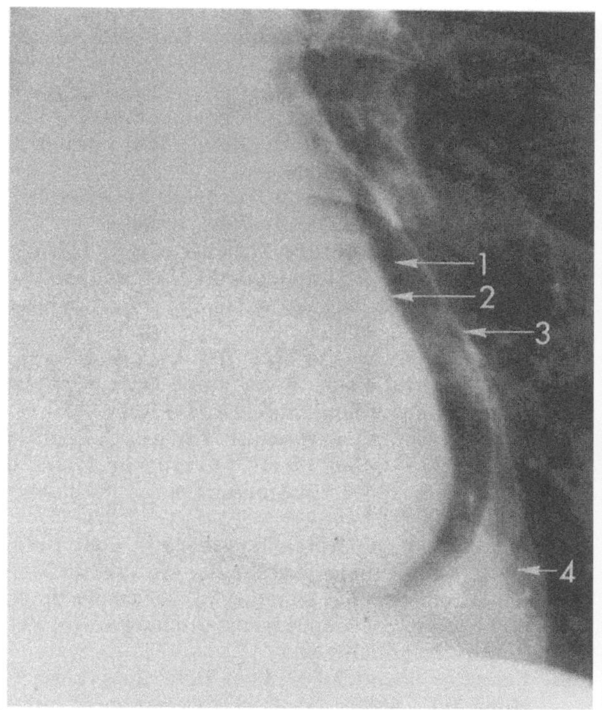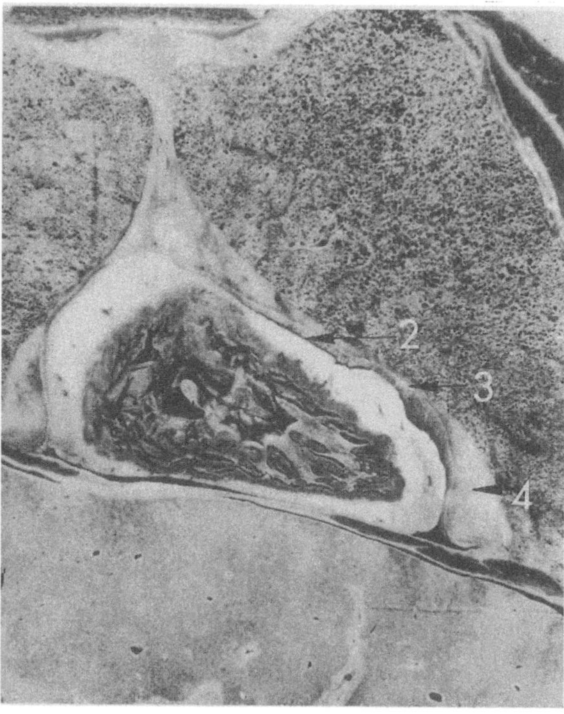

A   **B**

Fig. 3.22 A, B. Pneumopericardium. A PA radiograph.
B Coronal body section. Gas in pericardial sac (*1*) is
seen outlining left ventricle (*2*) in this postoperative patient. Normal pericardium, 1–2 mm thick, is easily identified (*3*). Note lateral displacement of left pericardial
fat pad (*4*)

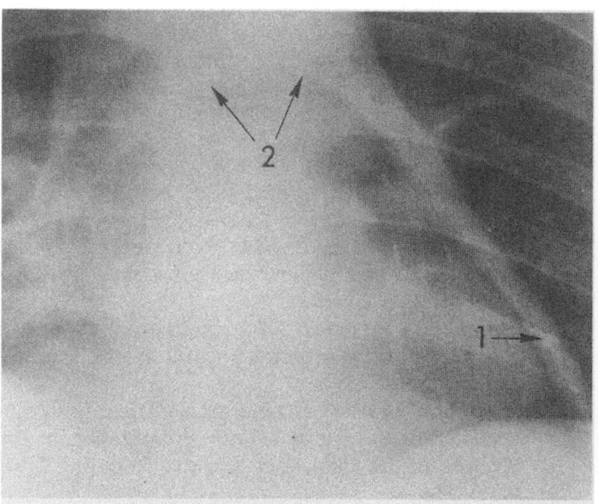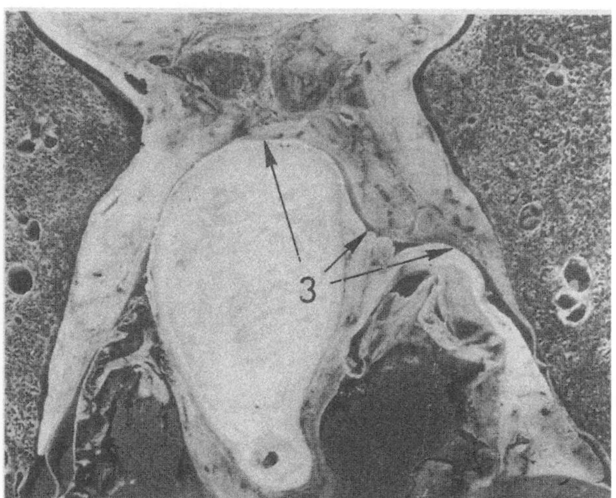

A   **B**

Fig. 3.23 A, B. Pneumopericardium. A Erect PA radiographs. B Coronal body section. In this patient with
pericarditis, air entered pericardium following drainage
of pericardial sac. Pericardium is thickened (*1*). Note
dome-shaped configuration of upper portion of pericardial sac (*2*). Serous pericardium, which limits air, does
not extend as high onto great vessels as does fibrous
pericardium (*3*) (see text)

the serosal layer of the pericardium is more susceptible to dissection. In a recent study by Burt and Lester [11], 36 of 50 neonates with pneumopericardium had some procedural event, most often abnormal endotracheal tube placement, as a probable cause for the intrapericardial air. Of these infants, 92% showed evidence for extraventilatory air. In some of the children, pneumopericardium appeared to be "spontaneous."

References

1. Anson BJ (1966) Morris' human anatomy, edn 12. McGraw-Hill, New York
2. Archer WH (1975) Oral, face and neck infections. In: Archer WH (ed) Oral and maxillofacial surgery, edn 5. Saunders, Philadelphia, pp 438–517
3. Armstrong JD, Bragg DG (1975) Radiology in lung cancer: problems and prospects. CA 25:242–263
4. Baron RL, Levitt RG, Sagel SS, White MJ, Roper CL, Marbarger JP (1982) Computed tomography in the preoperative evaluation of bronchogenic carcinoma. Radiology 145:727–732
5. Bates M, Beard HJ (1956) Six cases of traumatic rupture of the bronchus. Thorax 11:312–323
6. Beck E, Beattie EJ Jr (1958) The lymph nodes in the mediastinum. J Int Coll Surgeons 29:247–251
7. Bergh NP, Schersten T (1965) Bronchogenic carcinoma. A follow-up study of a surgically treated series with special reference to the prognostic significance of lymph node metastasis. Acta Chir Scan [Suppl] vol 347
8. Berne AS, Heitzman ER (1962) The roentgenologic signs of pedunculated pleural tumors. Am J Roentgenol 87:892–895
9. Berne AS, Gerle RD, Mitchell GE (1969) The mediastinum-normal roentgen anatomy and radiologic techniques. Semin Roentgenol 4:3–21
10. Bowen A, Quottromani FL (1980) Infraazygous pneumomediastinum in the newborn. AJR 135:1017–1021
11. Burt TB, Lester PD (1982) Neonatal pneumopericardium. Radiology 142:81–84
12. Carr DT, Mountain CF (1974) The staging of lung cancer. Semin Oncol 1:229–234
13. Carsky EW, Azimi F, Mauceri R (1980) Epicardial fat sign in the diagnosis of pericardial effusion. JAMA 244:2762–2764
14. Chasen MH, Rugh KS, Shelton DK (1984) Mediastinal impressions on the dilated esophagus. Radiol Clin North Am 22:591–605
15. Chen JTT, Peter RH, Orgain EJ, Lester RG (1972) The pitfalls in interpreting artificial pneumopericardium. Am J Roentgenol 116:91–96
16. Chuang VP, Doust BM, Ting YM (1974) Xerotomography of the mediastinum and tracheobronchial tree. Radiology 111:475–477
17. Cimmino CV (1967) Some radio-diagnostic notes on pneumomediastinum, pneumothorax, and pneumo-pericardium. Virginia Med Monthly 94:205–212
18. Cunningham DJ (1972) Textbook of Anatomy, edn 11. Oxford University Press, London
19. Ekholm S, Albrechtsson U, Kugelberg J, Tylen U (1980) Computed tomography in preoperative staging of bronchogenic carcinoma. J Comput Assist Tomogr 4:763–765
20. Emami B, Melo A, Carter BL, Munzenrider JE, Piro A (1978) Value of computed tomography in radiotherapy of lung cancer. AJR 131:63–67
21. Engel S (1962) Lung structure. Thomas, Springfield
22. Fagan CJ, Swischuk LE (1976) Traumatic lung and paramediastinal pneumatoceles. Radiology 120:11–18
23. Faling LJ, Pugatch RD, Jung-Legg Y, Daly BDT, Hong WK, Robbins AH, Snider GL (1981) Computed tomographic scanning of the mediastinum in the staging of bronchogenic carcinoma. Am Rev Respir Dis 124:690–695
24. Faling LJ, Pugatch RD, Daly BDT, Jung-Legg Y, Hong WK, Snider GL (1982) Detection of intrathoracic lymph node metastases from lung cancer. Radiology 144:187
25. Favez G, Willa C, Heinzer F (1975) Posterior oblique tomography at an angle of 55 degrees in chest roentgenology. Am J Roentgenol 120:907–915
26. Felman AH, Rodgers BM, Talbert JL (1976) Traumatic para-mediastinal air cyst. Pediatr Radiol 4:120–121
27. Felson B (1958) Some special signs in chest roentgenology. In: Ravin CV (ed) Roentgenology of the chest. Thomas, Springfield
28. Felson B (1969) The mediastinum. Semin Roentgenol 4:41–58
29. Felson B (1973) Chest roentgenology. Saunders, Philadelphia
30. Figley MM (1969) Mediastinal minutiae. Semin Roentgenol 4:41–58
31. Fraser RG, Pare JAP (1970) Diagnosis of diseases of the chest. An integrated study based on the abnormal roentgenogram. Saunders, Philadelphia
32. Friedman AC, Lautin EM, Rothenberg L (1981) Mach bands and pneumomediastinum. J Can Assoc Radiol 32:232–235
33. Friedman PJ (1985) Adult pulmonary ligament pneumatocoel: a loculated pneumothorax. Radiology 155:575–576
34. Friedman PJ (1984) The radiological determination of resectability of lung cancer. Presentation at the Meeting of the Fleischner Society, Santa Fe, NM, June 1984
35. Friedman PJ, Feigin DS, Liston SE, et al. (1984) Sensitivity of radiography, computed tomography and gallium scanning to metastasis of lung carcinoma. Cancer 54:1300–1306

36. Frolich DJ, Clements JL Jr, Weens HS (1975) Epicardial fat line in left pleural effusion. Am J Roentgenol 124:394–396
37. Genereux GP (1983) The posterior pleural reflections. AJR 141:141–149
38. Genereux GP, Howie JL (1984) Normal mediastinal lymph node size and number: CT and anatomic study. AJR 142:1095–1100
39. Gladnikoff H (1948) A radiographic study of the mediastinum in health and pulmonary carcinoma. Acta Radiol [Suppl] (Stockh) 73:1–87
40. Glazer GM, Francis IR, Shirazi KK, Bookstein FL, Gross BH, Orringer BH (1983) Evaluation of the pulmonary hilum: comparison of conventional radiography, 55° posterior oblique tomography, and dynamic computed tomography. J Comput Assist Tomogr 7:983–989
41. Glazer GM, Orringer MB, Gross BH, Quint LE (1984) The mediastinum in non-small cell lung cancer: CT-surgical correlation. AJR 142:1101–1105
42. Glazer GM, Gross BH, Quint LE, Francis IR, Bookstein FL, Orringer MB (1985) Normal mediastinal lymph nodes: number and size according to American Thoracic Society mapping. AJR 144:261–265
43. Glazer HS, Aronberg DJ, Sagel SS (1985) Pitfalls in the recognition of mediastinal lymphadenopathy. AJR 144:267–274
44. Glazer HS, Aronberg DJ, Sagel SS, Friedman PJ (1986) CT demonstration of calcified mediastinal lymph nodes: a guide to the new ATS classification. AJR 147:17–25
45. Godwin JD, Merten DF, Baker ME (1985) Paramediastinal pneumatocoel: alternative explanations to gas in the pulmonary ligament. AJR 145:525–530
46. Goldberg EM, Shapiro CM, Glicksman HS (1974) Mediastinoscopy for assessing mediastinal spread in clinical staging of lung carcinoma. Semin Oncol 1:205–215
47. Greenfield H, Jelaso DV (1965) Peripheral intrapulmonary lymph node metastasis. Br J Radiol 38:955–956
48. Grodinsky M, Holyoke A (1938) The fasciae of the head and neck. Am J Anat 63:367–408
49. Hamman L (1939) Spontaneous mediastinal emphysema. Bull John Hopkins Hosp 64:1–21
50. Han SY, Rudolph AJ, Teng CT (1963) Pneumodiastinum in infancy. J Pediatr 62:754–762
51. Harle TS, Hevezi JM, Rogers LF, Martin JE, Jing B (1975) Xerotomography of the tracheobronchial tree. Am J Roentgenol 124:353–357
52. Harper PG, Houang M, Spiro SG, Geddes D, Hodson M, Southami RL (1981) Computerized axial tomography in the pretreatment assessment of small cell carcinoma of the bronchus. Cancer 47:1775–1780
53. Heelan RT, Martini N, Westcott JW, Bains MS, Watson RC, Caravelli JF, Berkmen YM, Henschke CI, McCormack PM, McCaughan BC, Zaman MB (1985) Carcinomatous involvement of the hilum and mediastinum: computed tomographic and magnetic resonance evaluation. Radiology 156:111–115
54. Heitzman ER (1984) The lung: radiologic-pathologic correlations 2nd ed. Mosby, St. Louis
55. Heitzman ER (1981) Computed tomography of the thorax. Current perspectives. AJR 136:3–12
56. Heitzman ER, Markarian B, Raasch BN, Carsky EW, Lane EJ, Berlow ME (1982) Pathways of tumor spread through the lung: radiologic correlations with anatomy and pathology. Radiology 144:3–14
57. Hora JF (1963) Deep neck infections. Arch Otolaryngol 77:129–136
58. Hyde I (1971) Traumatic para-mediastinal air cysts. Br J Radiol 44:380–383
59. Jolly PC, Hill LD, Lawless PA, West TL (1973) Parasternal mediastinotomy and mediastinoscopy adjuncts in the diagnosis of chest disease. J Thorac Cardiovasc Surg 66:549–556
60. Jorgens J, Kundel R, Lieber A (1968) Cinefluorographic approach to diagnosis of pericardial effusion. Radiology 91:1–5
61. Khan A, Gersten KC, Garvey J, Khan FA, Steinberg H (1985) Oblique hilar tomography, computed tomography, and mediastinoscopy for the prethoracotomy staging of bronchogenic carcinoma. Radiology 156:295–298
62. Kleinman PK, Brill PW, Whalen JP (1978) Anterior pathway for transdiaphragmatic extension of pneumomediastinum. AJR 131:271–275
63. Lane EJ, Carsky EW (1968) Epicardial fat: lateral plain film diagnosis in normals and pericardial effusion. Radiology 91:1–5
64. Lane EJ, Proto AV, Phillips TW (1976) Mach bands and density perception. Radiology 121:9–18
65. Levin B (1973) The continuous diaphragm sign – a newly recognized sign of pneumomediastinum. Clin Radiol 24:337–338
66. Levitt GW (1970) Cervical fascia and deep neck infections. Laryngoscope 80:409–435
67. Levitt GW (1976) Cervical fascia and deep neck infections. Otolaryngol Clin North Am 9:703–716
68. Lewis JW Jr, Madrazo BL, Gross SC, et al. (1982) The value of radiologic and computed tomography in the staging of lung carcinoma. Ann Thorac Surg 34:553–558
69. Libshitz HI (1983) CT of mediastinal lymph nodes in lung cancer: is there a "state of the art"? AJR 141:1081–1085
70. Libshitz HI, McKenna RJ Jr (1984) Mediastinal lymph node size in lung cancer. AJR 143:715–718
71. Lillard RL, Allen RP (1965) The extrapleural air sign in pneumomediastinum. Radiology 85:1093–1098
72. Loftis JW, Susen AF, Marcy JH, Sherman FE (1962) Pneumopericardium in infancy. Am J Dis Child 103:61–65
73. Mach E (cited in) Ratliff F (1965) Mach bands: quantitative studies on neural networks in the retina. II. Mach's papers on the interdependence of retinal points. Holden-Day, San Francisco

74. Macklin NT, Macklin CC (1944) Malignant interstitial emphysema of lungs and mediastinum as important occult complications in many respiratory diseases and other conditions. Medicine 23:281–358

75. Marchand P (1951) The anatomy and applied anatomy of the mediastinal fascia. Thorax 6:359–368

76. McCort JJ, Robbins LL (1951) Lymph node metastases in carcinoma of lung. Radiology 57:339–360

77. Mintzer RA, Malave SR, Neiman LH, Michaelis LL, Vanecko RM, Sanders JH (1979) Computed versus conventional tomography in evaluation of primary and secondary pulmonary neoplasms. Radiology 132:653–659

78. Modini C, Passariello R, Iascone C, et al. (1982) TNM staging in lung cancer: role of computed tomography. J Thorac Cardiovasc Surg 84:569–574

79. Moseley JE (1960) Loculated pneumomediastinum in the newborn. A thymic spinnaker sail sign. Radiology 75:788–790

80. Moskowitz PS, Griscom NT (1976) The medial pneumothorax. Radiology 120:143–147

81. Mountain CF (1974) Surgical therapy in lung cancer: biologic, physiologic and technical determinants. Semin Oncol 1:253–258

82. Mountain CF (1986) A new international staging system for lung cancer. Chest 89:225S–233S

83. Mountain CF, Carr DT, Anderson WAD (1974) Clinical staging of lung cancer. Am J Roentgenol 120:130–138

84. Murray JF (1976) The normal lung; the basis for diagnosis and treatment of disease. Saunders, Philadelphia

85. Naclerio EA (1957) The "V" sign in the diagnosis of spontaneous rupture of the esophagus (an early clue). Am J Surg 93:291–298

86. Nagaishi C (1972) Functional anatomy and histology of the lung. University Park Press, Baltimore

87. Naidich DP, Khouri NF, Scott WW Jr, Want K, Siegelman S (1981) Computed tomography of the pulmonary hila. I. Normal anatomy. J Comput Assist Tomogr 5:468–475

88. Naidich DP, Khouri ND, Stitik FD, McCauley D, Siegelman S (1981) Computed tomography of the pulmonary hila. II. Abnormal anatomy. J Comput Assist Tomogr 5:485–490

89. Naruke T, Suemasu K, Ishikawa S (1978) Lymph node mapping and curability at various levels of metastasis in resected lung cancer. J Thorac Cardiovasc Surg 76:832

90. Nohl HC (1956) An investigation into the lymphatic and vascular spread of carcinoma of the bronchus. Thorax 11:172–185

91. Nohl HC (1962) The spread of carcinoma of the bronchus. Year Book Medical Publishers, Chicago

92. O'Donovan PB, Ross JS, Sivak ED, O'Donnell JK, Meaney TF (1984) Magnetic resonance imaging of the thorax: advantages of coronal and sagittal planes. AJR 143:1183–1188

93. Oliphant M, Wiot JF, Whalen JP (1976) The cervicothoracic continuum. Radiology 120:257–262

94. Osborne DR, Korobkin M (1982) Detection of intrathoracic lymph node metastases from lung carcinoma. Radiology 144:187–188

95. Osborne DR, Korobkin M, Ravin CE, et al. (1982) Comparison of plain radiography, conventional tomography, and computed tomography in detecting intrathoracic lymph node metastases from lung carcinoma. Radiology 142:157–161

96. Ovenfors CO (1964) Pulmonary interstitial emphysema – experimental roentgen diagnostic study. Acta Radiol [Suppl] (Stockh) vol 224

97. Ozonoff MB (1965) Pneumomediastinum associated with pneumonia and asthma in children. AJR 95:112–117

98. Ozonoff MB, Rudhe U (1966) Some theoretical aspects of pneumomediastinum in infants and children. Ann Radiol 9:295–303

99. Panicek DM, Ewing DK, Markarian B, Heitzman ER (1987) Interstitial pulmonary hemorrhage from mediastinal hematoma secondary to aortic rupture. Radiology 162:165–166

100. Pearson FG, Nelems JM, Henderson RD, Delarue NC (1972) The role of mediastinoscopy in the selection of treatment for bronchial carcinoma with involvement of superior mediastinal lymph nodes. J Thorac Cardiovasc Surg 64:382–390

101. Prasad SC, Pilepich MV, Perez CA (1981) Contribution of CT to quantitative radiation therapy planning. AJR 136:123–128

102. Pripstein S, Culliner MM, Brody PA (1976) Roentgenographic demonstration of peripheral intrapulmonary lymphadenopathy. Radiology 121:280

103. Proto AV, Thomas SR (1985) Pulmonary nodules studied by computed tomography. Radiology 156:149–153

104. Quint LE, Glazer GM, Orringer MB, Francis IR, Bookstein FL (1986) Mediastinal lymph node detection and sizing at CT and autopsy. AJR 147:469–472

105. Quottromani FL, Foley LC, Bowen A, Weisman L, Hernandez J (1981) Fascial relationship of the thymus: radiologic-pathologic correlation in neonatal pneumomediastinum. AJR 137:1209–1211

106. Ratliff F (1965) Mach bands: quantitative studies on the neural networks of the retina. Holden-Day, San Francisco

107. Ratliff F (1972) Contour and contrast. Sci Am 226:90–101

108. Ravin CE, Smith GW, Lester PD, McLoud TC, Putman CE (1976) Posttraumatic pneumatocele in the inferior pulmonary ligament. Radiology 121:39–41

109. Rouviere H (1932) Anatomie des lymphatiques de l'homme. Masson, Paris

110. Rudhe V, Ozonoff MB (1966) Pneumomediastinum and pneumothorax in the newborn. Acta Radiol [Diagn] (Stockh) 4:193–205

111. Sanborn JC, Heitzman ER, Markarian B (1970) Traumatic rupture of the thoracic aorta. Roentgenpathological correlations. Radiology 95:293–298

112. Sandler MA, Pearlberg JL, Madrazo BL, Gitschlag KF, Gross SC (1982) Computed tomographic eval-

uation of the adrenal gland in the preoperative assessment of bronchogenic carcinoma. Radiology 145:733–736

113. Scadding JG, Wood P (1939) Systolic clicks due to left sided pneumothorax. Lancet 2:1208–1211

114. Schaner E, Chang AE, Doppman JL, Conkle DM, Flye MW, Rosenberg SA (1978) Comparison of computed and conventional whole lung tomography in detecting pulmonary nodules: a prospective radiologic-pathologic study. Am J Roentgenol 131:51–54

115. Sheedy PF II, Stephens DH, Hattery RR, Muhm JR, Hartman G (1976) Computed tomography of the body: initial clinical trial with the EMI prototype. Am J Roentgenol 127:23–51

116. Siegelman SS, Zerhouni EA, Leo FP, Khouri NF, Stitik FP (1980) CT of the solitary pulmonary nodule. AJR 131:1–130

117. Sone S, Higashihara T, Morimoto S, Yokota K, Ikezoe J, Oomine H, Arisawa J, Monden Y, Nakahara K (1982) Potential spaces of the mediastinum. CT pneumomediastinography. AJR 138:1051–1057

118. Stanley RJ, Sagel SS, Levitt RG (1976) Computed tomography of the body: early trends in application and accuracy of the method. Am J Roentgenol 127:53–67

119. Strauss MJ (1974) Lung cancer. Semin Oncol 1:285–287

120. Sukiennikow W (1903) Topographische Anatomie der bronchialen und trachealen Lymphdrüsen. Berl Klin Wochenschr 40:316, 347, 369

121. Swischuk L (1976) Two lesser known but useful signs of neonatal pneumothorax. Radiology 127:623–627

122. Tisi GM, Friedman PJ, Peters RM, Pearson G, Carr D, Lee RE, Selawry O (1983) Clinical staging of primary lung cancer. Am Rev Respir Dis 127:659–664

123. TNM classification of malignant tumors (1972) Joint publication of the International Union Against Cancer and American Joint Committee on Cancer Staging and End Results Reporting, Geneva

124. TNM classification of malignant tumors (1974) International Union Against Cancer, Geneva

125. Volberg FM, Everett CJ, Brill PW (1979) Radiologic features of inferior pulmonary ligament air collections in neonates with respiratory distress. Radiology 130:357–360

126. Warwick R, Williams PR (1973) Gray's anatomy, edn 35. Saunders, Philadelphia

127. Webb WR, Glazer G, Gamsu G (1981) Computed tomography of the normal pulmonary hilum. J Comput Assist Tomogr 5:476–484

128. Webb WR, Gamsu G, Glazer G (1981) Computed tomography of the abnormal pulmonary hilum. J Comput Assist Tomogr 5:485–490

129. Webb WR, Gamsu G, Speckman JM (1983) Computed tomography of the pulmonary hilum in patients with bronchogenic carcinoma. J Comput Assist Tomogr 7:219–225

130. Webb WR, Gamsu G, Stark DD, Moore EH (1984) Magnetic resonance imaging of the chest. Normal and abnormal. Radiology 153:729–735

131. Webb WR, Jensen BG, Sollitto R, deGeer G, McCowin M, Gamsu G, Moore E (1985) Bronchogenic carcinoma: staging with MR compared with staging with CT and surgery. Radiology 156:117–124

132. Westaby S (1977) Pneumopericardium and tension pneumopericardium after closed chest injury. Thorax 32:91–97

133. Wolfe JN (1969) Xeroradiography of bones, joints and soft tissues. Radiology 93:583–587

134. Wolfe NJ (1973) Xeroradiography: image content and comparison with film roentgenograms. Am J Roentgenol 117:690–695

135. Wood BP, Anderson VM, Mauk JE, Merritt TA (1982) Pulmonary lymphatic air: locating "pulmonary interstitial emphysema" of the premature infant. AJR 138:809–814

136. Zerhouni EA (1984) CT of the pulmonary nodule: initial results of a cooperative study. Paper presented at the Annual Assembly of the Radiological Society of North America, Washington DC, November 1984

137. Zerhouni EA, Boukadoum M, Siddiky MA, et al. (1983) A standard phantom for quantitative analysis of pulmonary nodules by CT. Radiology 149:767–775

4 The Thoracic Inlet

4.1 General Anatomic Considerations

The thoracic inlet is the junctional region between the structures of the root of the neck and the contents of the thoracic cavity. The transverse plane through the thoracic inlet parallels the first rib and is tilted so that it is higher posteriorly than it is anteriorly (Fig. 4.28a). The anatomic structures in this plane will be considered from front to back.

The thymus is found at the extreme anterior aspect of the thoracic inlet in front of the innominate veins. It is a fairly large structure in infants and children and often persists as a relatively sizeable structure into adult life [5, 9, 18, 22, 25, 30, 38, 47]. It is composed of two distinct lobes that extend through the plane of the thoracic inlet from the lower pole of the thyroid gland above to the level of the fourth costal cartilage below. Since its greatest bulk, especially when enlarged, lies below the junction of the manubrium and the body of the sternum, the correlated radiographic anatomy of the thymus is discussed in the chapter on the anterior mediastinum (chapter 5).

The left innominate (brachiocephalic) vein, formed by the confluence of the left internal jugular vein and the left subclavian vein, courses to the right in front of the arterial trunks (Fig. 4.1). It meets the similarly formed right innominate (brachiocephalic) vein behind the right side of the manubrium of the sternum where the two vessels become the superior vena cava (Fig. 4.1).

At either side of the trachea, the subclavian arteries diverge in the thoracic inlet to course laterally over the anterior aspect of each upper lobe behind the scalenus anterior muscles (Fig. 4.2). The scalenus anterior muscle is the anatomic landmark that divides the subclavian artery into its three parts. The first part runs from the aortic arch to the medial border of the scalenus anterior, the second part lies behind the muscle, and the third part extends from its lateral border to the outer edge of the first rib where the vessel becomes the axillary artery. The second part of the artery lies on the suprapleural membrane (Sibson's fascia) before entering the subclavian groove in the superior surface of the first rib. Here the artery is located behind the subclavian vein, separated from it by the scalene tubercle that receives the insertion of the scalenus anterior muscle (Figs. 4.2 and 4.9). In the thoracic inlet the common carotid arteries are found anterior to the subclavian arteries and posterior and medial to the subclavian veins, running along the anterolateral aspect of the trachea (Fig. 4.2).

The anterior rami of C-8 and T-1 form the lower trunk of the brachial plexus, which traverses the first rib behind the subclavian artery.

The vagus and phrenic nerves pass from the neck into the thorax in front of the subclavian arteries and behind the great veins. The phrenic nerves lie lateral to the vagi. Rarely, tumors will involve the phrenic or vagus nerves as they pass through the thoracic inlet. At this point in their course the two nerves on each side lie between the innominate veins and the subclavian arteries. Computed tomographic studies, magnetic resonance imaging examinations, or angiograms, which demonstrate separation of the arteries and veins in the thoracic inlet, should for this reason strongly suggest the likelihood of neurogenic tumor [78].

In the plane of the thoracic inlet, the trachea is situated in the midline behind the great vessels and in front of the esophagus (Fig. 4.1). The

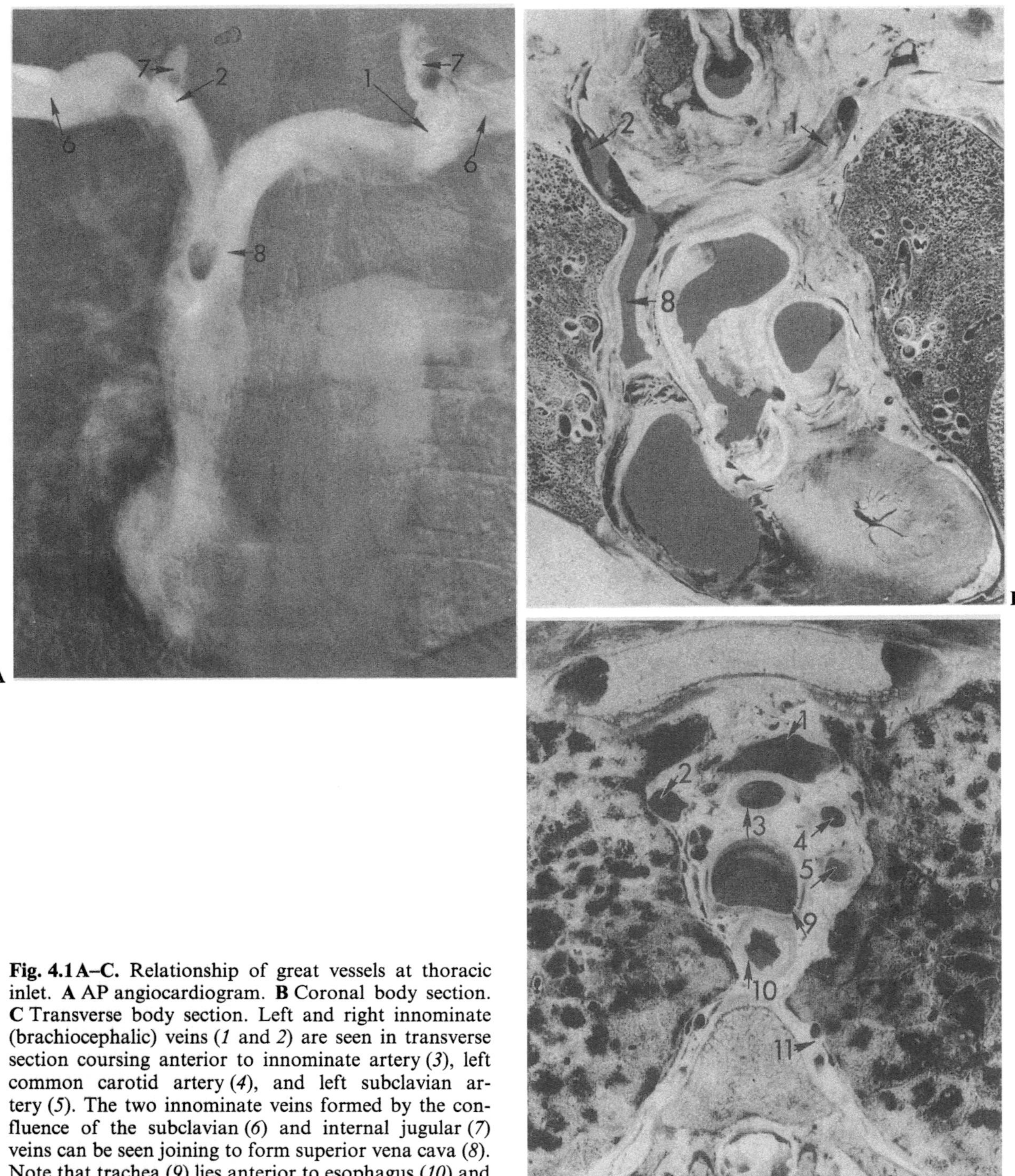

Fig. 4.1A–C. Relationship of great vessels at thoracic inlet. **A** AP angiocardiogram. **B** Coronal body section. **C** Transverse body section. Left and right innominate (brachiocephalic) veins (*1* and *2*) are seen in transverse section coursing anterior to innominate artery (*3*), left common carotid artery (*4*), and left subclavian artery (*5*). The two innominate veins formed by the confluence of the subclavian (*6*) and internal jugular (*7*) veins can be seen joining to form superior vena cava (*8*). Note that trachea (*9*) lies anterior to esophagus (*10*) and that esophagus lies slightly to left of midline at this level. Intercostal arteries and veins are also demonstrated (*11*). (**A** Courtesy G. Weinberger, Syracuse, N.Y.)

Fig. 4.2 A–C. Anatomy of subclavian arteries at thoracic inlet. Coronal (**A**) and transverse (**B**) body sections. **C** Is a radiograph of section shown in **B**. Left subclavian artery (*1*) is seen passing over left apex and grooving anterior aspect of left upper lobe (*2*). Scalenus anterior muscle (*3*) courses downward to its insertion into the first rib (*4*). Note position of subclavian artery between first rib and clavicle (*6*) above. Observe also position of left subclavian vein (*7*) anterior to left subclavian artery. Common carotid arteries (*8*) are shown at anterolateral aspect of trachea (*5*)

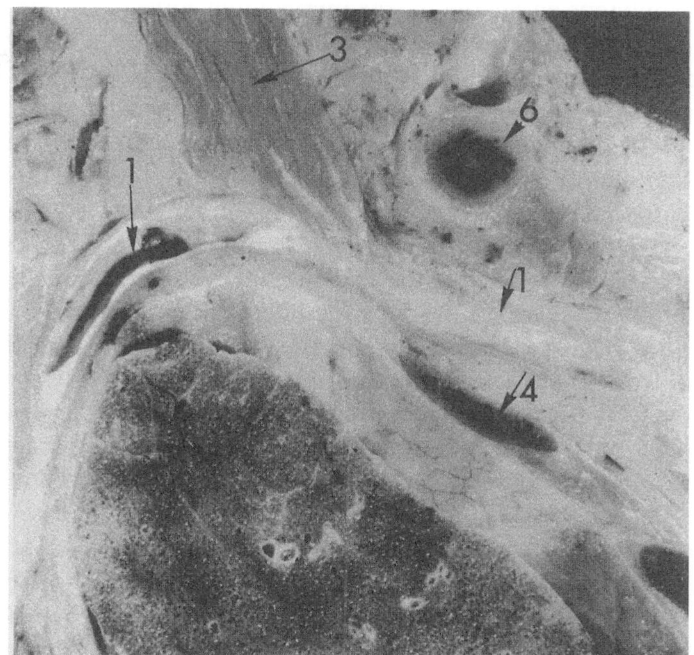

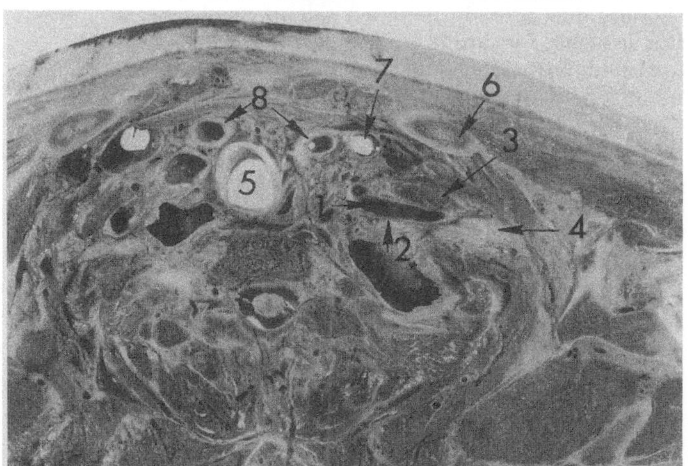

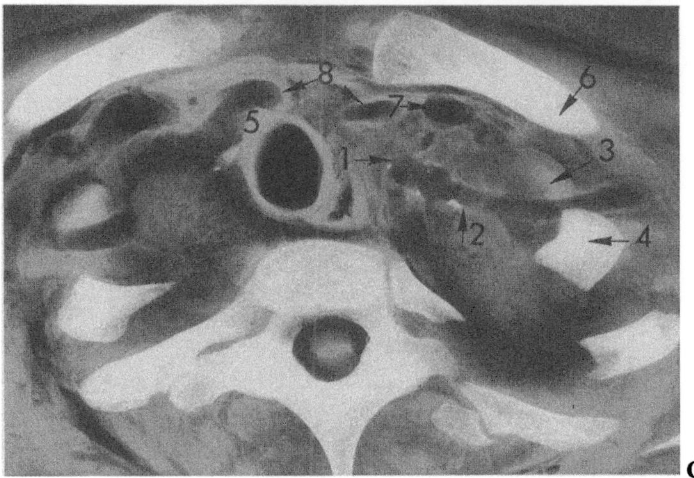

esophagus enters the thorax immediately anterior to the spine and slightly to the left of the midline (Fig. 4.1). The trachea and the esophagus are enveloped in the perivisceral fascia, as discussed in chapter 3 (see Fig. 3.14). The recurrent laryngeal nerves on each side lie in the groove between the trachea and the esophagus.

The thoracic duct also courses along the left side of the esophagus behind the left recurrent laryngeal nerve. In the neck the duct swings forward from its paraesophageal position, passing in front of the left subclavian artery and behind the left internal jugular vein to terminate at the junction of the left internal jugular and subclavian veins (Fig. 4.3). In the upper mediastinum and neck it is particularly vulnerable to the injury from wounds of a penetrating type. Its prox-

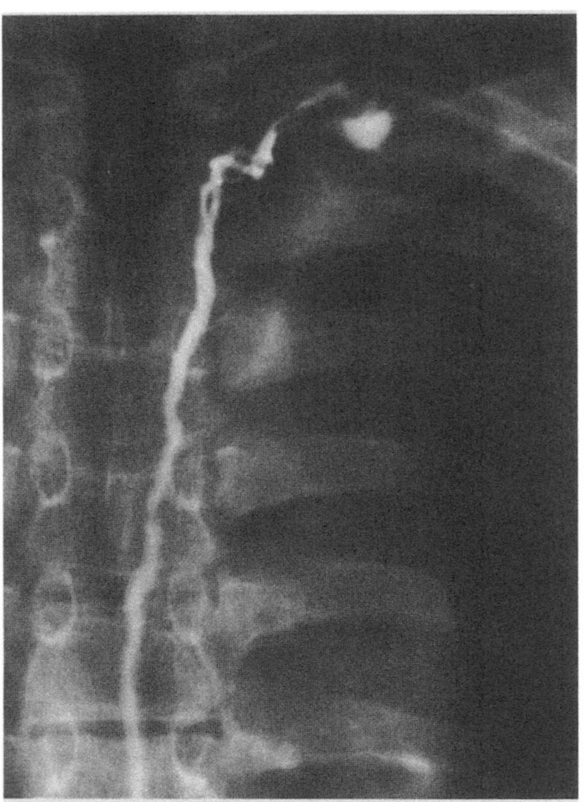

Fig. 4.3. Thoracic duct in thoracic inlet (AP radiograph). Thoracic duct ascends along left side of esophagus; in neck it swings forward in front of left subclavian artery and behind left internal jugular vein to terminate at junction of left internal jugular and subclavian artery. (Courtesy E.M. Levinsohn, Syracuse, N.Y.)

imity to the left pleura explains the occurrence of left chylothorax following trauma to the left upper chest or neck [57]. The correlated radiologic anatomy of thoracic duct is discussed further in the chapter on the infra-aortic area (chapter 7).

The posterior intercostal arteries, veins, and nerves lie extrapleurally along the paraspinal musculature (Fig. 4.1) and are crossed anteriorly and laterally by the sympathetic trunks (see Fig. 8.4). The superior intercostal veins drain the second, third, and fourth posterior intercostal spaces as they pass forward over the paraspinal soft tissues. The right superior intercostal vein terminates in the azygos vein as that vessel turns forward from its prespinal location; the left passes around the lateral aspect of the aortic arch and then runs upward and forward between the left phrenic and vagus nerves to terminate in the left innominate vein (see Figs. 6.20, 6.21, 8.4). The correlated radiographic anatomy of the superior intercostal veins will be discussed in the chapters on the supra-aortic and supra-azygos areas (chapters 6 and 8).

The cupola of the pleura contains the lung apex, reaching as high as the posterior aspect of the first rib (Figs. 4.2 and 4.28). From the cupola the superior reflections of the pleura extend obliquely downward and meet at the level of the sternal notch. Superiorly and laterally, the cupola of the pleura is reinforced by the suprapleural membrane. This sickle-shaped membrane is attached behind to the anterior edge of the transverse process of the seventh cervical vertebra and anteriorly to the inner margin of the first rib from the scalene tubercle to the manubrium of the sternum. According to Arnold [3], the membrane is adherent to the cupola of the pleura and serves to strengthen it. Medially and posteriorly, the membrane is continuous with the dense prevertebral fascia which helps to form the sheaths of the great vessels and nerves. Anteriorly, the suprapleural membrane fuses with the perivisceral fascia. Together, the membrane and perivisceral fascia tend, to some extent, to "wall off" the anterior (pretracheal) perivisceral space from the anterior mediastinum. Nevertheless, the pretracheal space is used by the mediastinoscopist to enter the mediastinoscope from the neck into the mediastinum. Anterior goiters in their descent into the thorax use the same route. Posterior to the coronal plane of the trachea, the neck and mediastinum are in free communication through the visceral compartment within perivisceral fascial sheath. Each of the anatomic points just made has considerable significance to the interpretation of shadows seen at the thoracic inlet on chest radiographs.

4.2 Radiologic Correlations with Anatomy and Pathology

4.2.1 Radiographic Anatomy at the Thoracic Inlet

4.2.1.1 Frontal Projection

The normal radiographic appearance of the thoracic inlet is influenced in a major way by the anatomy of the major blood vessels. As the innominate veins cross anterior to the carotid and subclavian arteries to meet behind the manubrium of the sternum, their entire course can at times be seen on frontal radiographs and especially on AP tomograms due to their impingement against the anterior portions of the upper lobes. Their configuration is like a widely angled letter V as they cause the characteristic separation of the pleurae at the upper end of the anterior junction line (Fig. 4.4).

It is worthy of emphasis that the innominate veins are very mobile structures. At surgery, they can easily be retracted for a distance of 2–3 cm. On PA or AP radiographs this mobility is often demonstrated when a central venous catheter traverses the vessels. The course of the catheter may change from film to film as the vessel adapts to buckling or straightening of the catheter (Fig. 4.5).

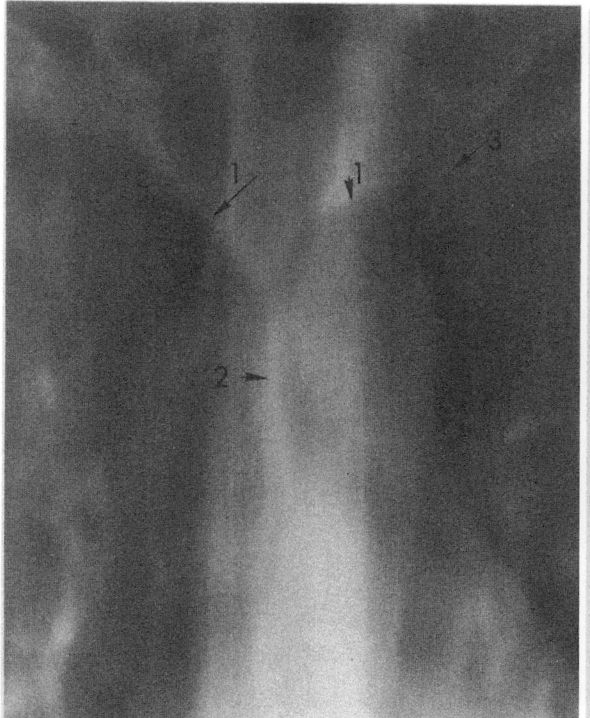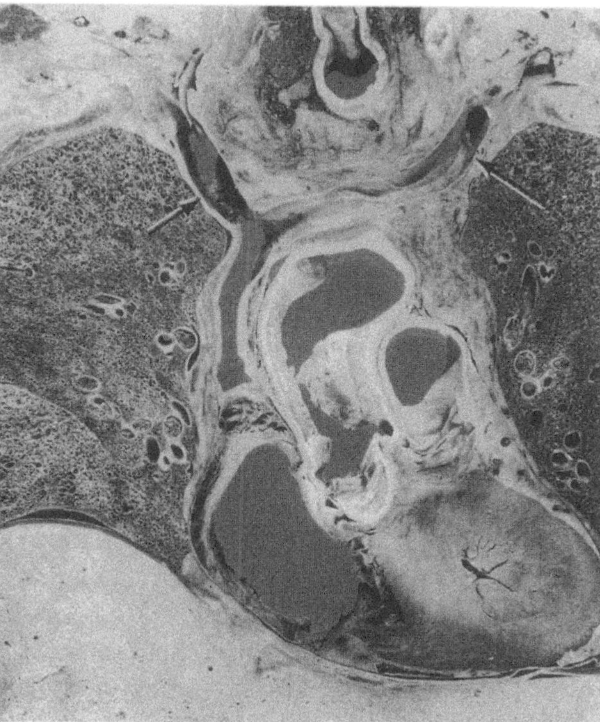

Fig. 4.4A, B. Reflections of anterior lung margins over brachiocephalic veins. **A** AP tomogram and **B** coronal body section. In the tomogram the reflection of anterior lung margins off brachiocephalic veins (*1*) to form anterior junction line (*2*) is clearly shown. Manubrium of sternum can also be identified (*3*). The coronal body section also demonstrates the contact of each lung with the brachiocephalic veins

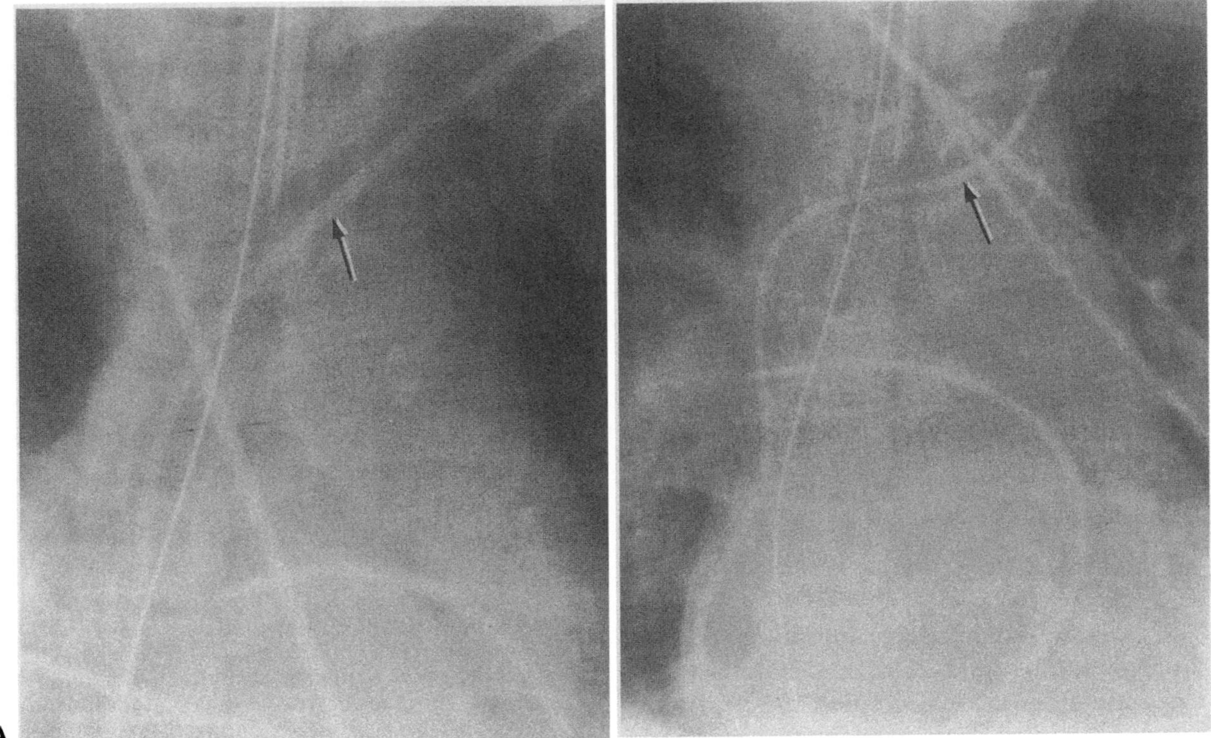

A   B

Fig. 4.5A, B. Mobility of the left innominate vein. **A** and **B** portable radiographs made 10 days apart. Note the distinctly different course taken by the Swan-Ganz catheter (*arrow*) as it passes through the left subclavian vein, due to greater bucking of the catheter in **B**. At surgery, the vein can be moved or retracted 2–3 cm

The subclavian arteries are identified in the thoracic inlet on frontal radiographs somewhat more frequently than are the innominate veins. Gondos [31] credits Assman as being the first to identify the subclavian artery-lung interface on normal radiographs. The portion of the vessel seen in the inlet is its second part, lying behind the scalenus anterior muscle (Figs. 4.2 and 4.6). Gondos [31] was able to identify the subclavian artery in the pulmonary apex in 40% of 300 patients studied by him; it was seen twice as often on the left as on the right. This part of the subclavian artery is easy to recognize when it is calcified (Fig. 4.6). Even when not calcified, it can often be identified in the second or third anterior interspace as a tubular shadow of increased density with a convexity directed upward (Fig. 4.6). Many times this part of the

vessel can be traced proximally to the shadow of the first part of the subclavian artery thus permitting its precise identification (Fig. 4.6). Lordotic films will frequently demonstrate this continuity clearly when PA radiographs fail to do so (Fig. 4.21). Proto and Chaliff [59], in a recent article, pointed out that the second portion of the subclavian arteries can produce a poorly defined round or oval opacity projected in the second or third anterior interspace on PA radiographs in about 15% of normal patients (Fig. 4.7). The appearance of the density is variable from patient to patient dependent upon beam angle and the degree to which the vessel impinges on anterior lung. Computed tomography may be required to distinguish this anatomic variant from a true apical lesion in the pulmonary parenchyma.

In some instances, the brachiocephalic veins and the subclavian artery shadows are visible on the same frontal radiograph (Fig. 4.8).

Masses situated in the root of the neck cross the thoracic inlet into the upper mediastinum either in front of the innominate (brachiocephalic) veins and subclavian arteries or behind

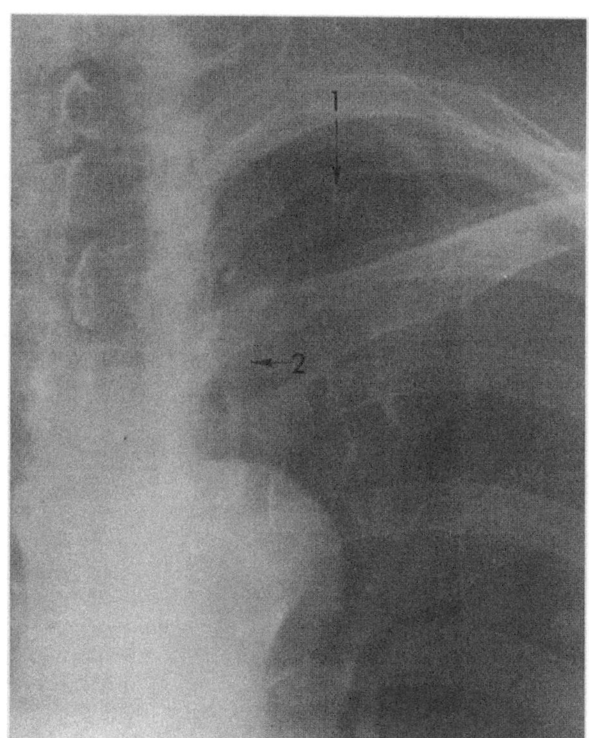

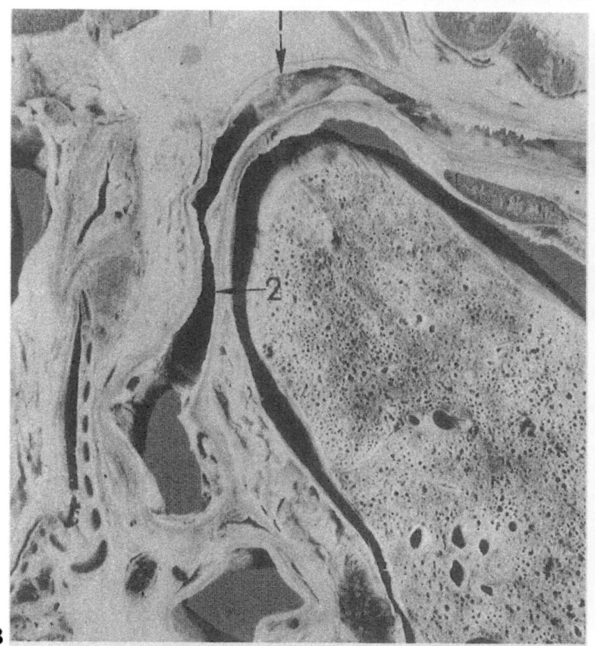

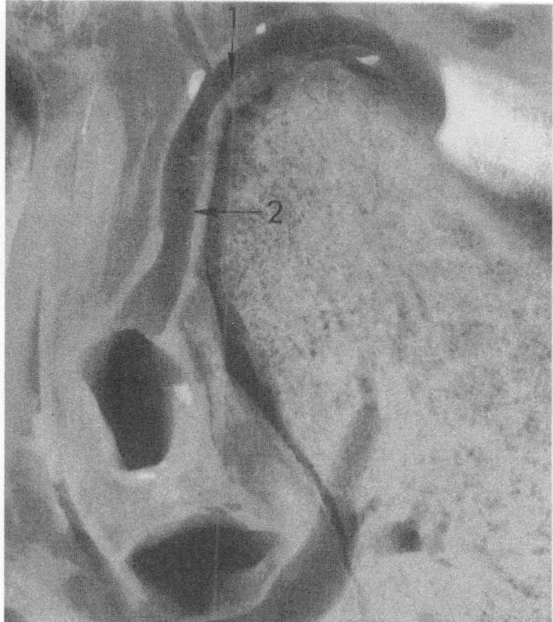

Fig. 4.6A–C. Second portion of subclavian artery. **A** PA radiograph. **B** Coronal body section. **C** Is radiograph of section shown in **B**. Second portion of the subclavian artery, here shown on the left side, is that portion lying behind the scalenus anterior muscle. It is seen as an arcuate structure with convexity directed cephalad overlying lung apex (*1*). Note that shadow can be followed proximally to shadow of first part of subclavian artery (*2*), permitting its precise identification

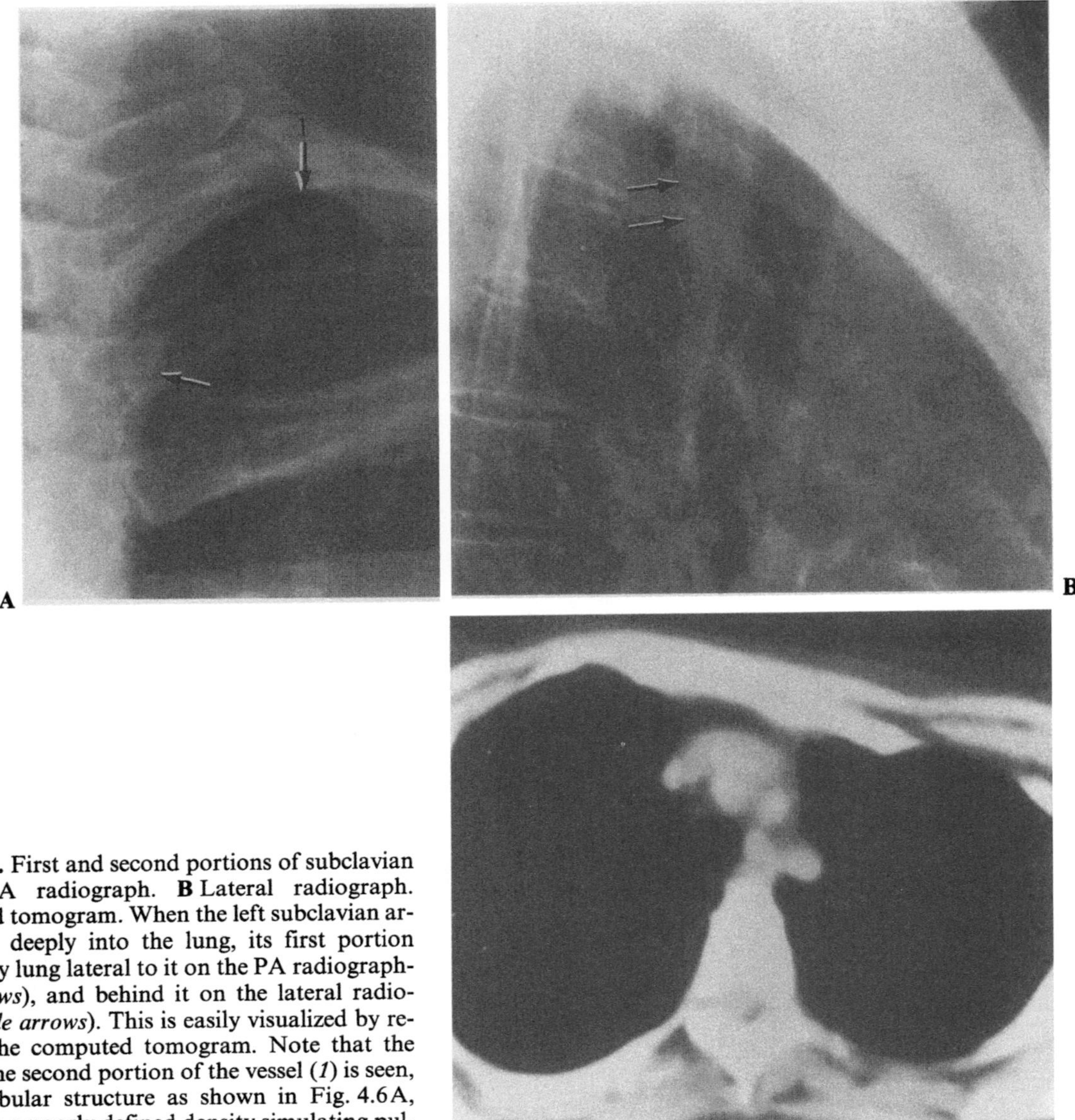

Fig. 4.7 A–C. First and second portions of subclavian artery. **A** PA radiograph. **B** Lateral radiograph. **C** Computed tomogram. When the left subclavian artery indents deeply into the lung, its first portion is outlined by lung lateral to it on the PA radiograph (*single arrows*), and behind it on the lateral radiograph (*double arrows*). This is easily visualized by reference to the computed tomogram. Note that the shadow of the second portion of the vessel (*1*) is seen, not as a tubular structure as shown in Fig. 4.6A, but rather as a poorly defined density simulating pulmonary parenchymal disease [59] (see text)

them. If they descend anteriorly, they separate and distort the upper end of the anterior junction line and displace the anterior extrapleural line (see chapter 5). Masses crossing the thoracic inlet anterior to the great vessels are most often of thyroid or thymic origin. Thyroid masses may also cross the thoracic inlet posterior to the great vessels. The changes caused by thyroid masses are considered subsequently in this chapter. The radiographic appearances of thymic lesions are discussed in the chapter on the anterior mediastinum (chapter 5). Poker et al. [58] have provided an excellent review of the radiologic anatomy of the subclavian arteries, as well as a comprehensive discussion of the changes in the appearance of the vessels caused by disease.

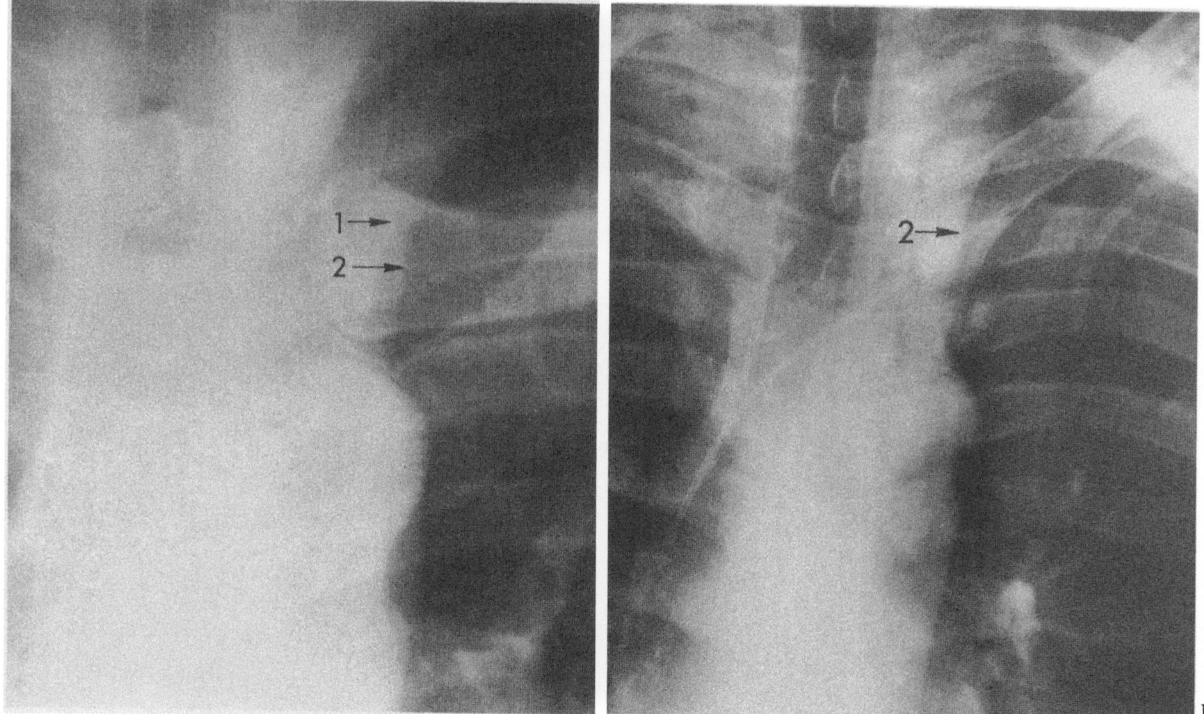

Fig. 4.8A, B. Relationship of subclavian arteries and innominate veins as seen on frontal radiographs. A PA radiograph. B PA radiograph with a catheter in left innominate vein. Sometimes shadows of subclavian arteries and innominate veins can be identified on same frontal radiograph. Shadow of innominate vein (1) assumes more horizontal course, and its caudal extent progresses more medially than does lower edge of subclavian artery (2). (A Courtesy M. Bein, Los Angeles, California)

4.2.1.2 Lateral Projection

The innominate veins produce an impression on the lung anterior and inferior to the point where the arteries, primarily the subclavian arteries but apparently sometimes the distal innominate artery as well, make their major imprint into the anterior aspect of the lung apex. Therefore, on lateral radiographs two impressions can be seen – a lower one behind the manubrium caused by the veins and a second higher and more posterior one produced by the arteries (Figs. 4.2 and 4.9). This gently undulating appearance has been termed the "vascular incisura" by Whalen et al. [78].

In discussing venous anatomy at the thoracic inlet, Proto and Speckman [61] have pointed out that the right brachiocephalic vein adopts a vertical course on its way to the vena cava while the left brachiocephalic vein arcs forward in a retrosternal position in its left to right course across the mediastinum (Fig. 4.10). In fact, failure of a left-sided venous catheter to assume this configuration should be used as evidence that it is improperly positioned. Proto and Speckman [61] feel therefore that the lowermost of the bulges of the vascular incisura is produced by the left brachiocephalic vein. Godwin and Chen [28], however, state that, "...the main sweep of the left brachiocephalic vein, where it arcs anteriorly and downward across the mediastinum, does not contribute to the posteriorly marginated retrosternal opacity because, where it crosses the mediastinum, the brachiocephalic vein has no lung behind it that could create a visible margin."

Our anatomic material suggests that either brachiocephalic vein may abut lung – on the right before the vessel adopts a downward course and on the left before the vessel becomes

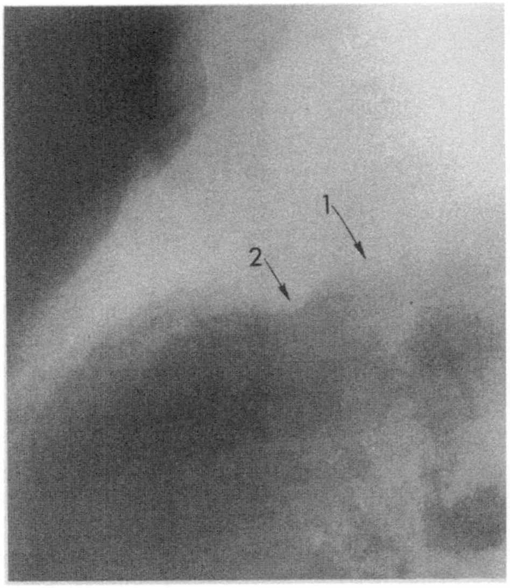

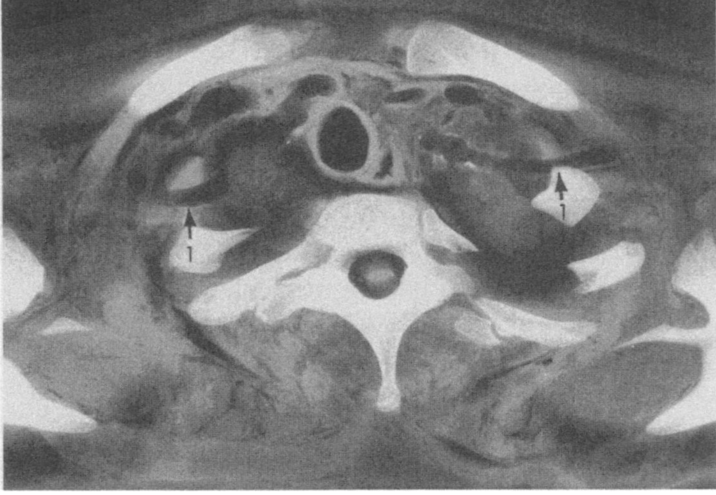

Fig. 4.9 A–D. Relationship of subclavian arteries to innominate veins at thoracic inlet – lateral projection – the "vascular incisura." A Lateral radiograph. B Transverse body section. C Is a radiograph of B. D Is a radiograph of a contiguous slice 1 cm cephalad from the same cadaver. Lateral films often show two impressions on anterior and superior aspects of lung at thoracic inlet. The higher and more posterior of the two is produced by subclavian arteries (1), whereas lower and more anterior impression is produced by innominate veins (2). Transverse body section (B) and radiograph made on same cadaver at same level (C) clearly show impressions made by innominate veins (2) anteriorly and impressions made more posteriorly by subclavian arteries (1). In D it can be appreciated that impressions made by the arteries are at higher level. See also Fig. 4.2

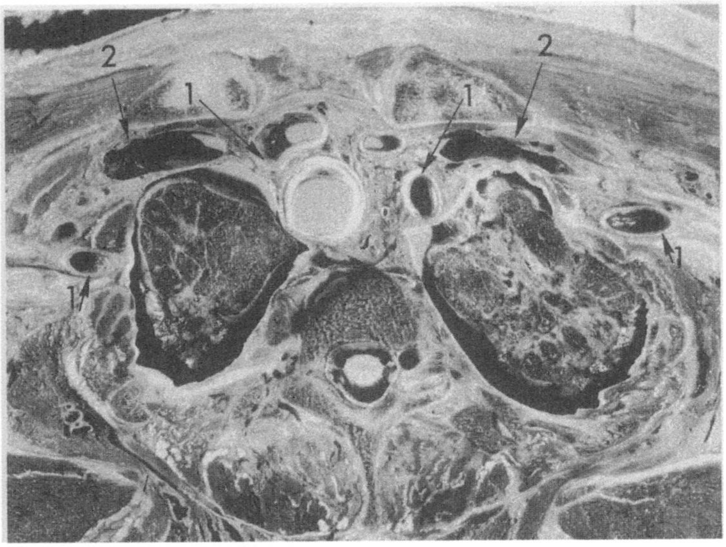

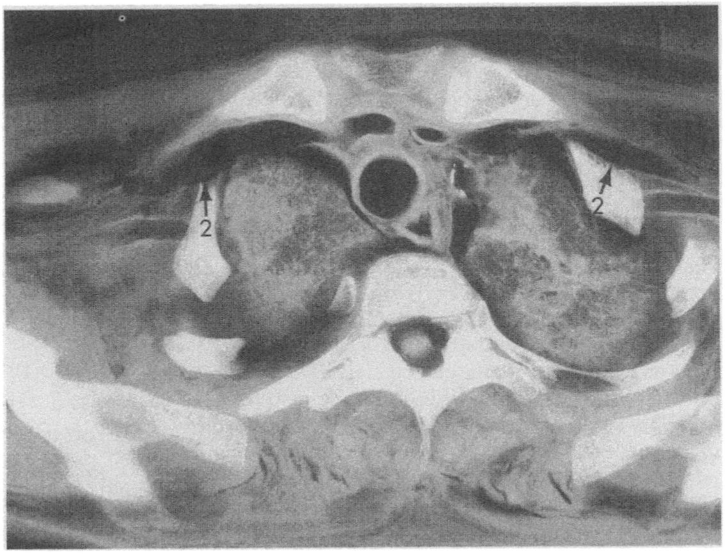

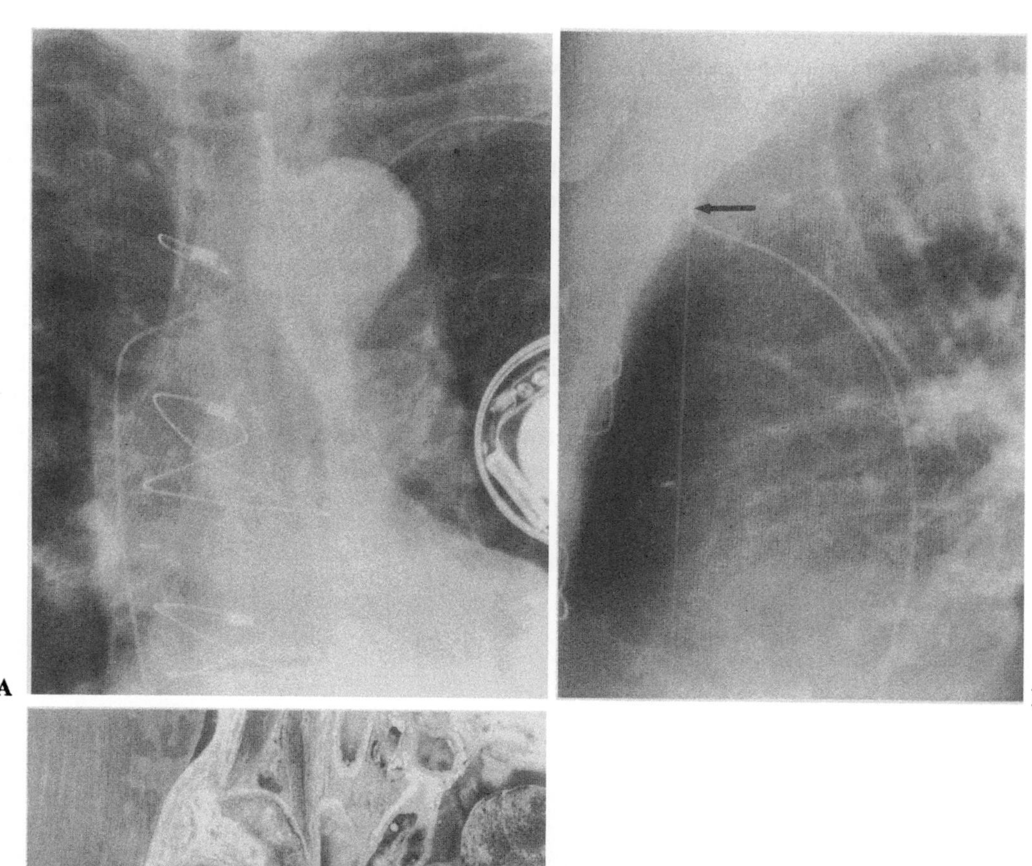

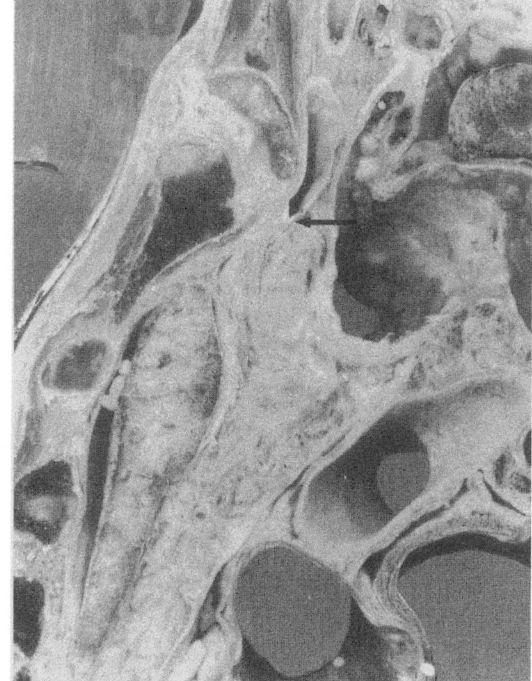

Fig. 4.10 A–C. Anterior substernal course of the left brachiocephalic vein. Lateral perspective. **A** PA radiograph. **B** Lateral radiograph. **C** Sagittal body section through the aortic arch. Note the anterior substernal course of the left brachiocephalic vein (*arrow*) identified by the pacing lead as it crosses the mediastinum. Failure of a catheter to adopt this retrosternal position in its course strongly suggests malposition. Either brachiocephalic vein can produce the lowermost bulge of the vascular incisura (see text)

mediastinal. On either side, the portion of the vein in question accompanies the second portion of the corresponding subclavian artery (Fig. 4.9).

Recognition of the vascular incisura as a reflection of normal radiographic anatomy will prevent misinterpretation of these shadows as nodes or masses.

Whalen et al. [78] have pointed out a third protrusion into lung, which may be identified below the venous imprint on lateral radiographs. This is produced by the costochondral junction of the first rib; it may become a very prominent shadow if hypertrophic changes, or less frequently an osteochondroma, arise from the costochondral junction (Figs. 4.11 and 4.18).

It should be reemphasized that the arterial impression at the thoracic inlet on the lateral radiographs is caused primarily by the second part of the subclavian artery grooving the anterior aspect of the lung apex. If lung inserts itself against the mediastinum behind the first or ascending portion of the left subclavian artery, an arcuate shadow with either convexity or concavity directed posteriorly or a gently undulating shadow can be seen on lateral radiographs extending downward from the thoracic inlet to the aortic arch (Fig. 4.7, see also Figs. 6.10 and 6.11). A review of venous anatomy as seen on PA and lateral radiographs has recently been provided by Godwin and Chen [28].

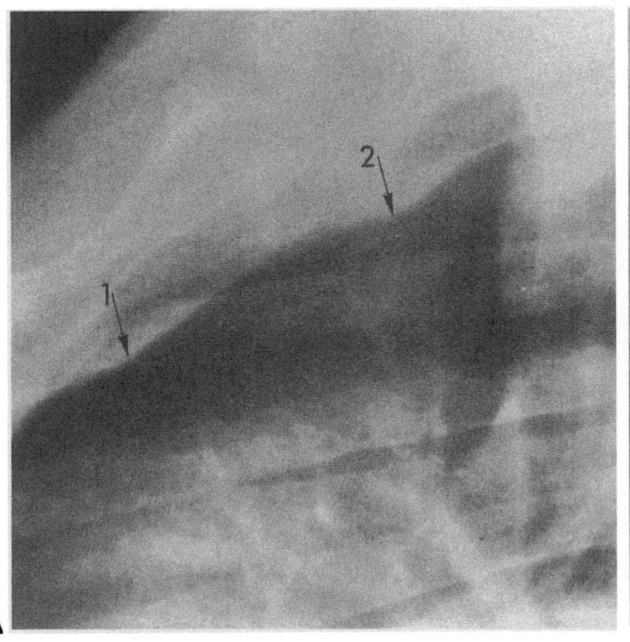

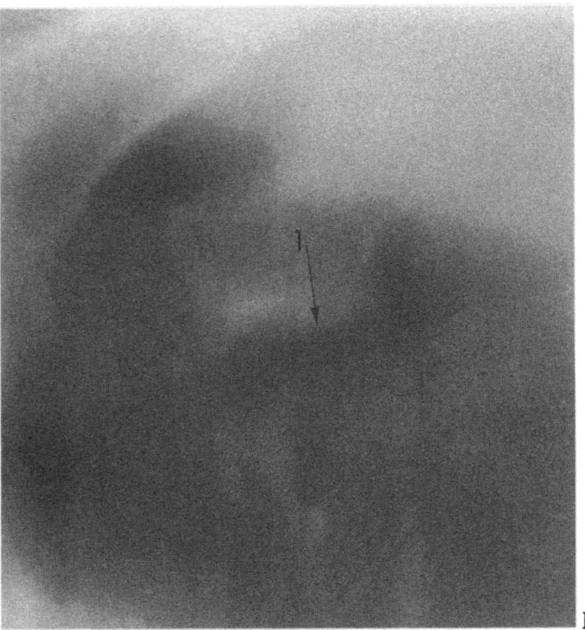

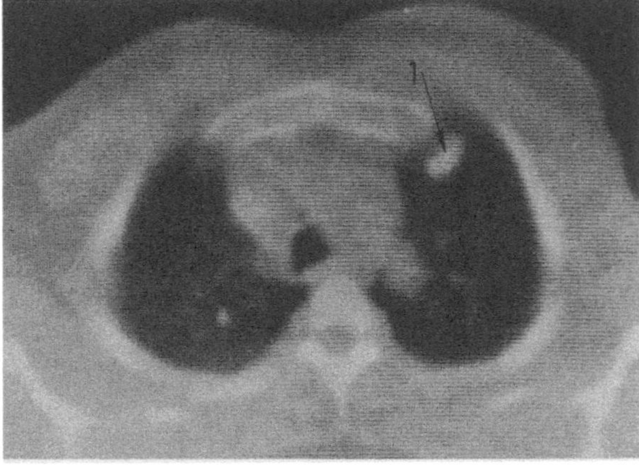

Fig. 4.11 A–C. Impressions made on anterior lung by first costochondral junction. A Lateral radiograph. B PA radiograph. C Computed tomogram. Hypertrophic changes or osteochondromas of first rib can produce impression on anterior lung (1) inferior to that produced by brachiocephalic veins (2). Intrusion made by hypertrophic changes on anterior surface of left lung (1) is clearly shown on computed tomogram of this patient

4.2.1.3 Axial Projection

Computed tomographic examinations and magnetic resonance studies demonstrate the vascular anatomy at the thoracic inlet with great clarity [4, 28]. Sagel [68], Vock and Owens [76], and Zylak et al. [80] have provided general reviews of the anatomy of the inlet as shown on computed tomograms.

The appearance of the right and left innominate veins in axial projection is markedly different. The vein on the right side is imaged as a round or oval shadow due to its vertical orientation (Figs. 4.12 and 4.13). Its upper extremity lies somewhat lateral to its lower portion. The left innominate vein is seen as a tubular (Figs. 4.12 and 4.13) or sometimes elliptical

(Figs. 4.14 and 4.15) shadow due to its more horizontal and often undulating course through the plane of the thoracic inlet. Its more cephalad portion will be seen laterally while its more caudal part will be found medially (Figs. 4.12 and 4.13). In higher images, the more oblique course of the vessel through the plane of section may cause it to be imaged as an oval density simulating a node or mass [60] (Fig. 4.14). The position of the left innominate vein is somewhat variable; although in many patients it can be seen passing anterior to the innominate artery on its way to meet the right innominate vein (Figs. 4.12, 4.13, and 4.14), sometimes it passes anterior to the ascending aorta (Fig. 4.15). The left innominate vein arches anteriorly and then posteriorly as it swings around the innominate

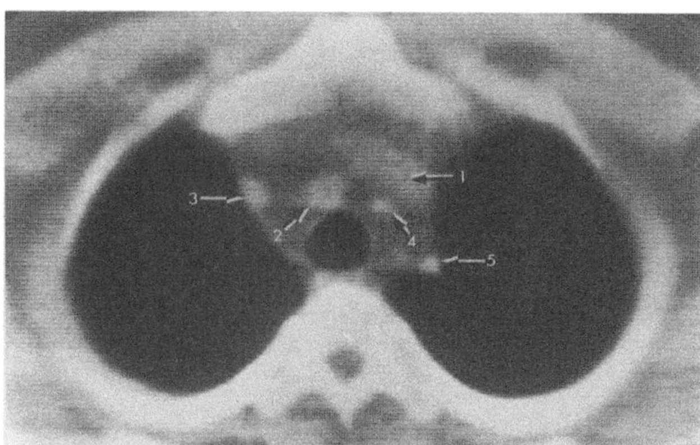

A

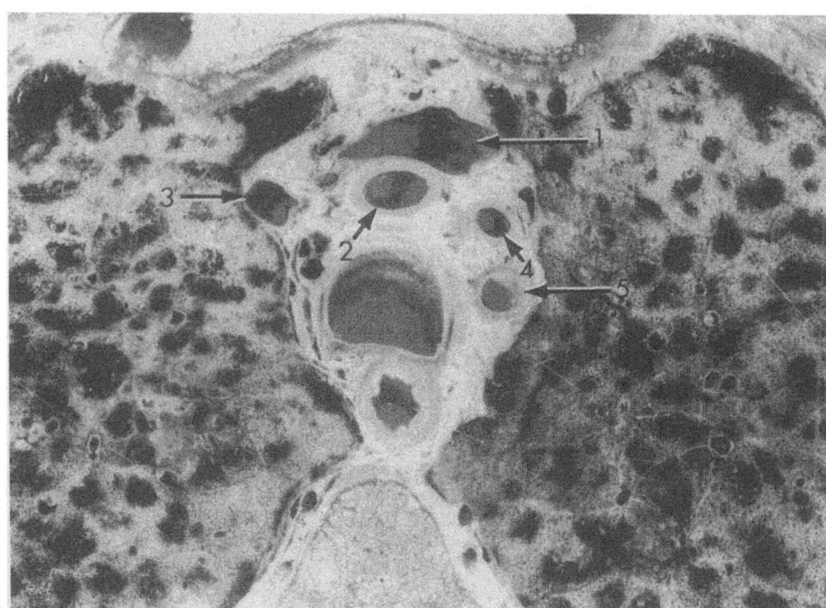

B

Fig. 4.12 A, B. Anatomy at the thoracic inlet as demonstrated at computed tomography.
A Computed tomogram. **B** Transverse body section at same level. The left brachiocephalic vein (*1*) is imaged to the left side of the anterior mediastinum as a tubular structure crossing anterior to the innominate artery (*2*). The right brachiocephalic vein (*3*) adopts a more vertical course and is seen as a round or oval density. The left common carotid artery (*4*) and the first part of the left subclavian artery (*5*) are also shown

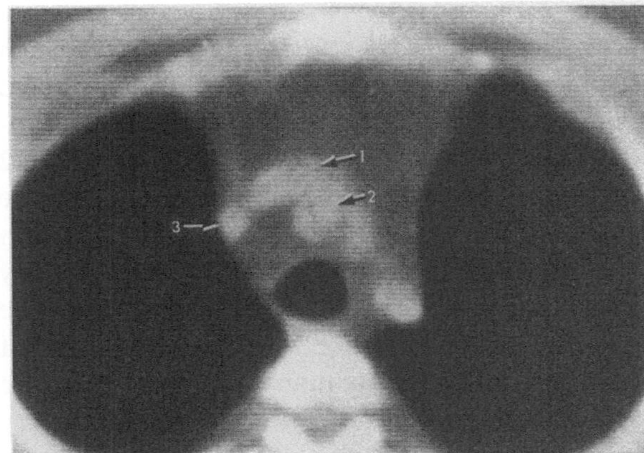

A

Fig. 4.14A, B. Variant appearance of the left innominate ▷ vein at computed tomography. **A** Computed tomogram. **B** Transverse body section at same level. Sometimes the left innominate vein may be imaged as a rounded or oval shadow simulating a mass (*arrow*). Note that the vessel arcs anteriorly in a retrosternal position in its passage across the mediastinum. See Fig. 4.10. A contrast-enhanced study will prove the density to be vascular

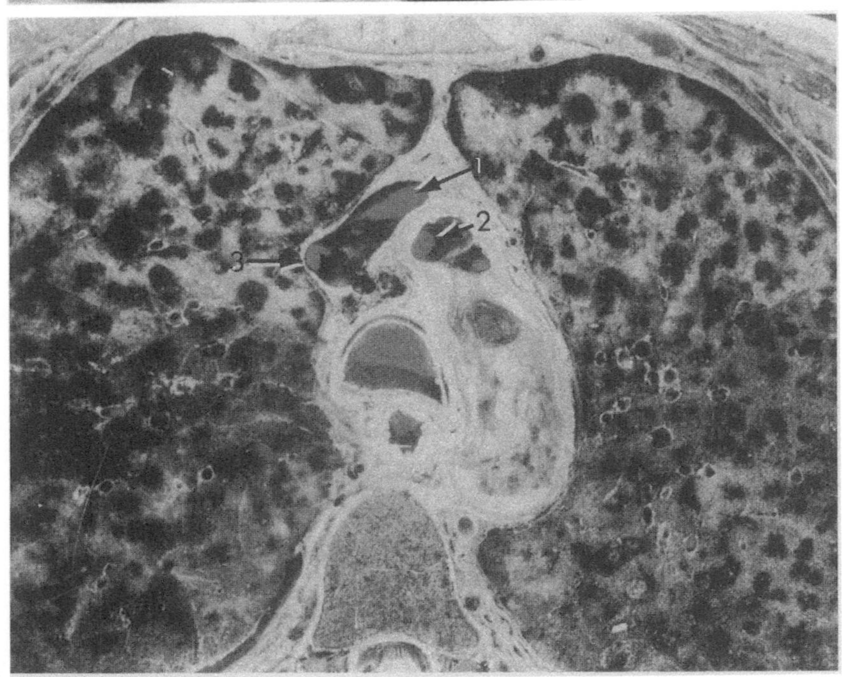

B

△
Fig. 4.13A, B. Anatomy of the thoracic inlet as demonstrated at computed tomography. Level slightly below that in Fig. 4.12. **A** Computed tomogram. **B** Transverse body section at same level. The left brachiocephalic vein (*1*) is imaged to the right side of the mediastinum. It is again seen as a tubular structure crossing anterior to the innominate artery (*2*) on its way to join the right brachiocephalic vein (*3*). The latter is again imaged as a round or oval shadow

Fig. 4.15A, B. Variant appearance of the left subclavian ▷ vein at computed tomography. **A** Computed tomogram. **B** Transverse body section at same level. Sometimes the left brachiocephalic vein (*single arrow*) can simulate a mass as it approaches its junction with the right innominate vein. In this location, fat and areolar tissue lying between the vein and the anterior aspect of the ascending aorta can simulate the intimal flap of an aortic dissection (*double arrows*)

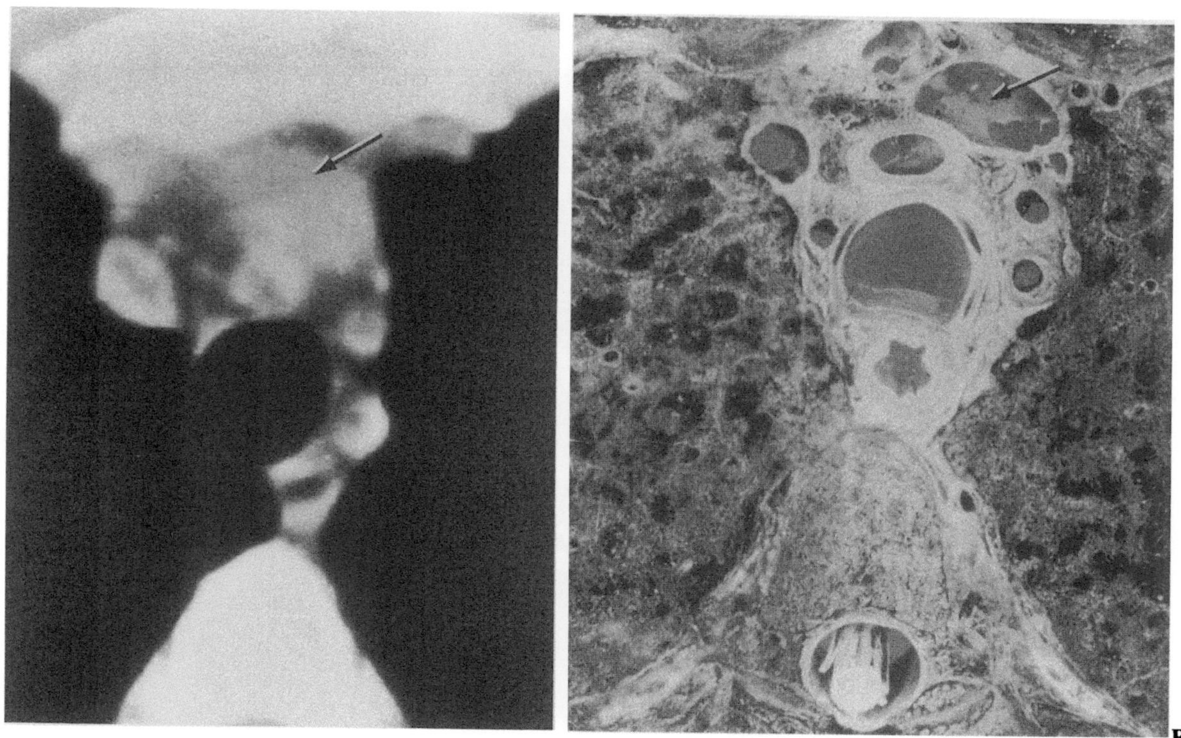

Fig. 14
A
B

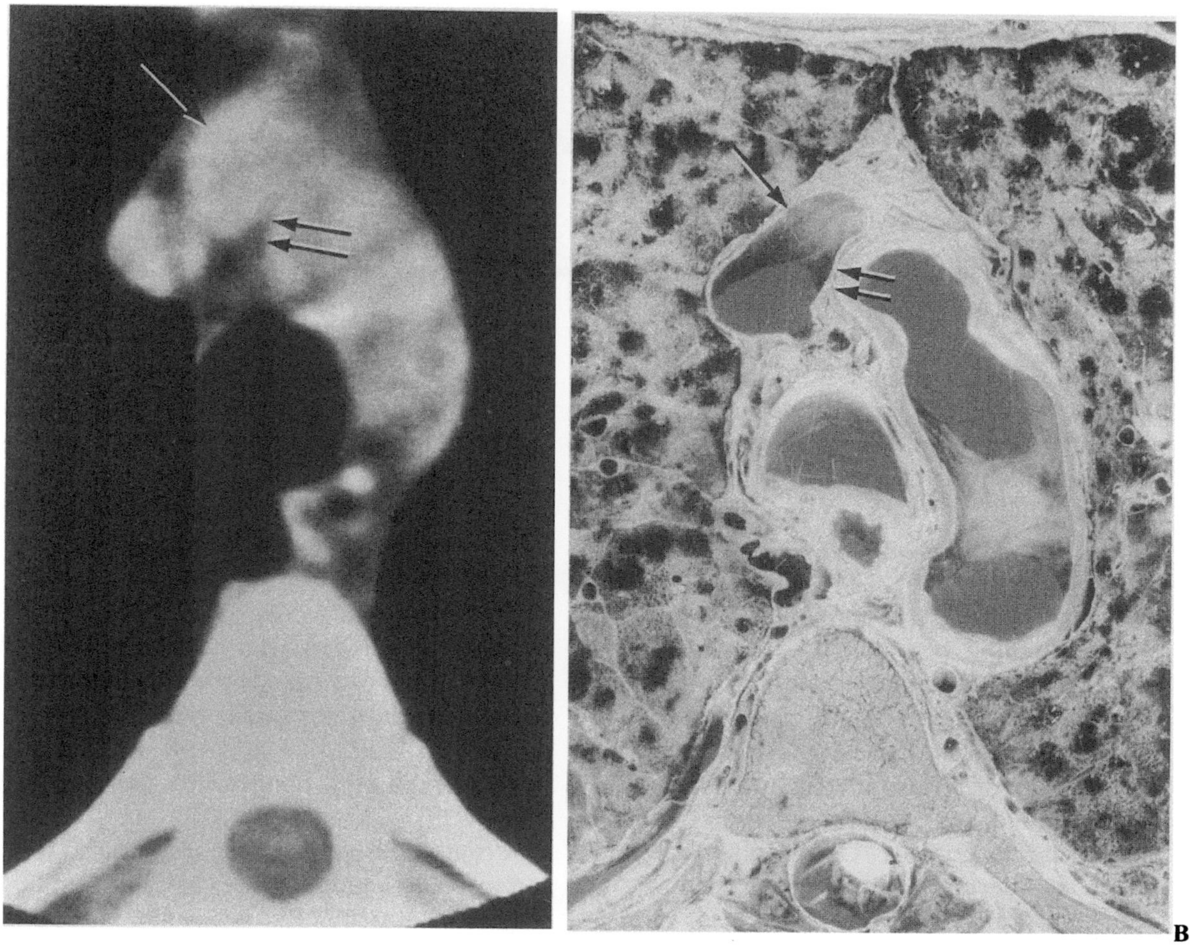

Fig. 15
A
B

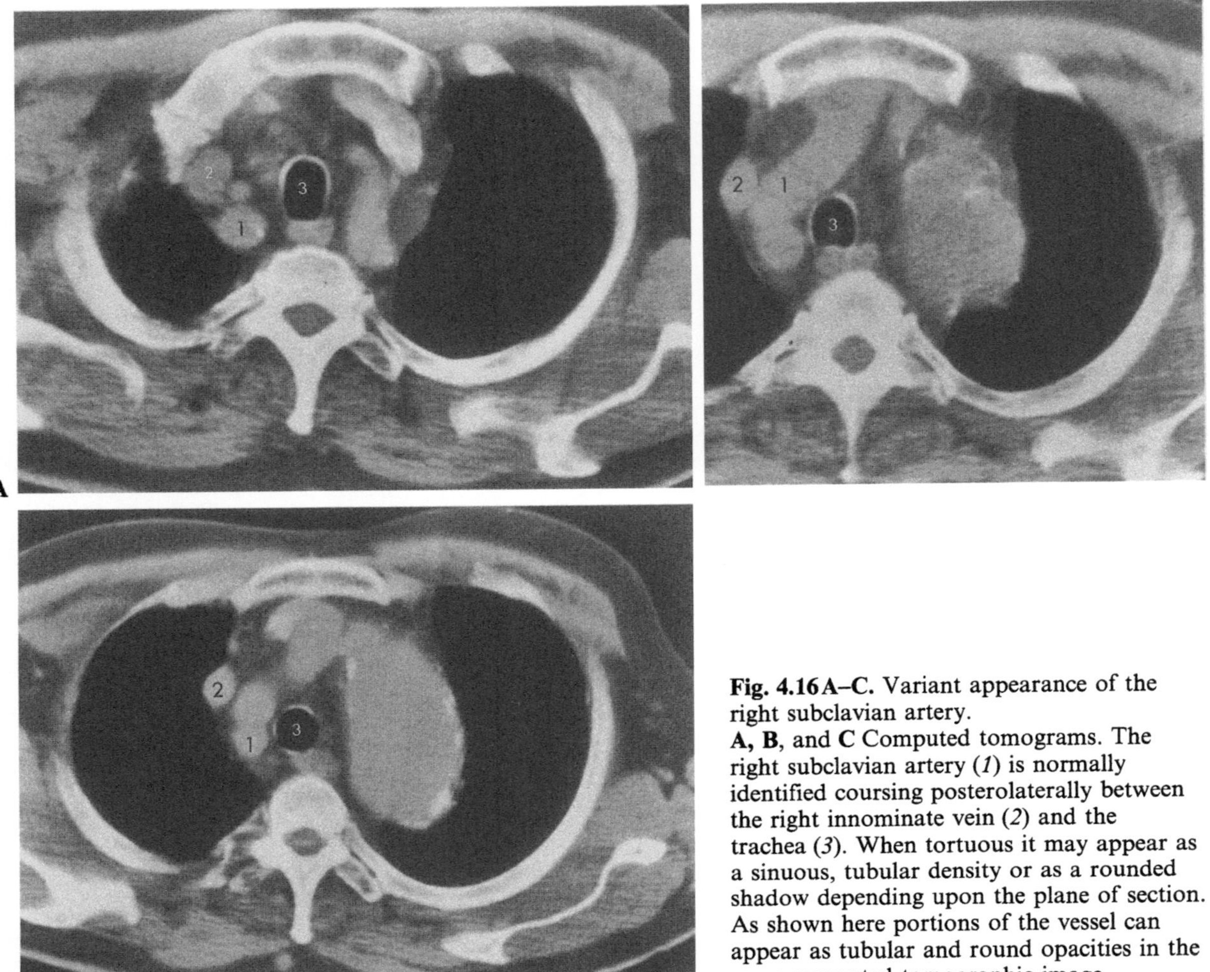

Fig. 4.16A–C. Variant appearance of the right subclavian artery.
A, B, and **C** Computed tomograms. The right subclavian artery (*1*) is normally identified coursing posterolaterally between the right innominate vein (*2*) and the trachea (*3*). When tortuous it may appear as a sinuous, tubular density or as a rounded shadow depending upon the plane of section. As shown here portions of the vessel can appear as tubular and round opacities in the same computed tomographic image

artery or the ascending aorta (Figs. 4.10 and 4.14). When the left innominate artery crosses anterior to the ascending aorta, the plane between the two vessels can simulate the intimal flap of an aortic dissection [60] (Fig. 4.15). The right subclavian artery, arising from the innominate artery anterior to the trachea, adopts a lateral and somewhat posterior course running between the right innominate vein and the right anterolateral aspect of the trachea. Depending upon its course through the plane of section, it can be imaged as a tubular structure, or as a tubular structure in continuity with a round opacity either at its proximal or distal end (Fig. 4.16). Occasionally the right subclavian artery may be imaged as two rounded densities. These variant appearances are particularly evident, and may cause significant problems in interpretation when the innominate artery is tortuous and buckled [60] (see chapter 8).

The subclavian arteries can then often be identified in company with the innominate veins as they extend across the anterior aspect of the upper lobe on their way to the axilla (Fig. 4.17). The left subclavian artery in the inlet is sometimes imaged as a round structure in the mediastinum lateral or somewhat posterior to the trachea (Figs. 4.12, 4.13, and 4.14) or as a tubular structure passing anterior to the upper lobe (Fig. 4.17).

Proto and Rost [60] have emphasized that, on occasion, imaging of the clavicular head and adjacent musculature (sternohyoid and ster-

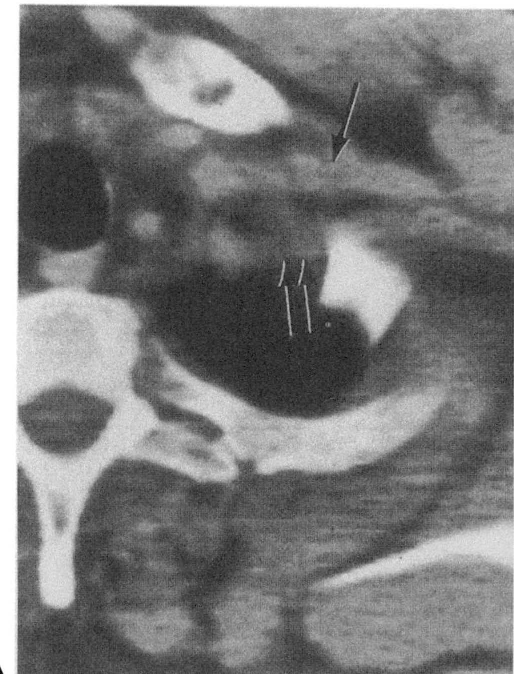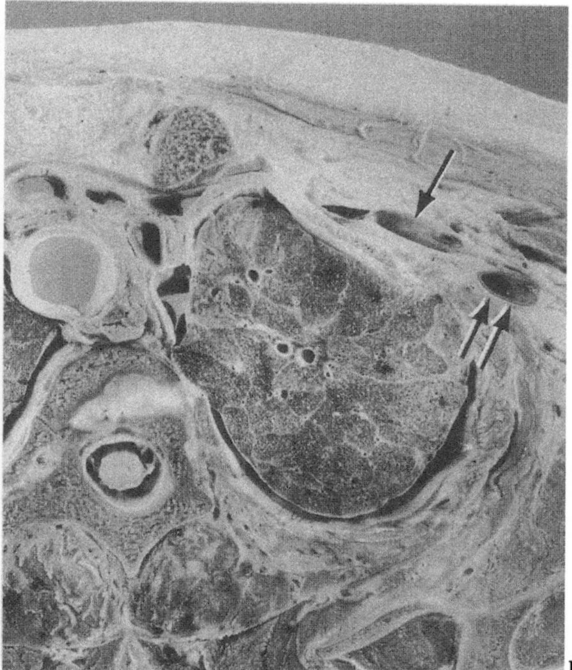

Fig. 4.17A, B. Course of the innominate vein and subclavian artery to the axilla. **A** Computed tomogram. **B** Transverse body section at same level. The brachiocephalic vein (*single arrow*) and subclavian artery (*double arrows*) pass behind the scalenus anterior muscle lying on the upper surface of the first rib, the artery is posterior behind the tubercle. Lateral to the lateral aspect of the first rib the vessels are termed the axillary vein and artery

nothyroid muscles) may stimulate a mass anterior to the innominate vein on that side. The shadow may mimic a vascular structure.

In the plane of the thoracic inlet the common carotid arteries can be seen coursing through the carotid sheath anterolateral to the trachea and medial to the upper portions of the innominate veins.

In the discussion of the radiographic anatomy at the thoracic inlet as shown in lateral projection it was emphasized that the costochondral junction of the first rib may, when prominent, impinge on the anterior aspect of the lung below the vascular impressions. This impingement can be seen on computed tomograms and, if the impression is deep enough, the junction can be imaged with lung completely surrounding it [53, 60] (Fig. 4.18). Under these circumstances, a pulmonary nodule may be simulated. Often this spurious nodule appears to be calcified but if a cartilaginous cap over the junction is primarily in the plane of section, the process will appear less dense. Usually fine sections through the area resolve the problem.

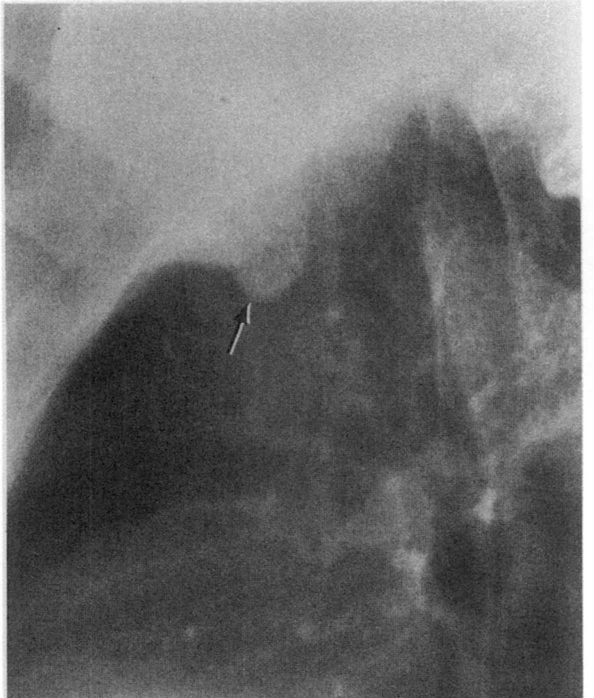

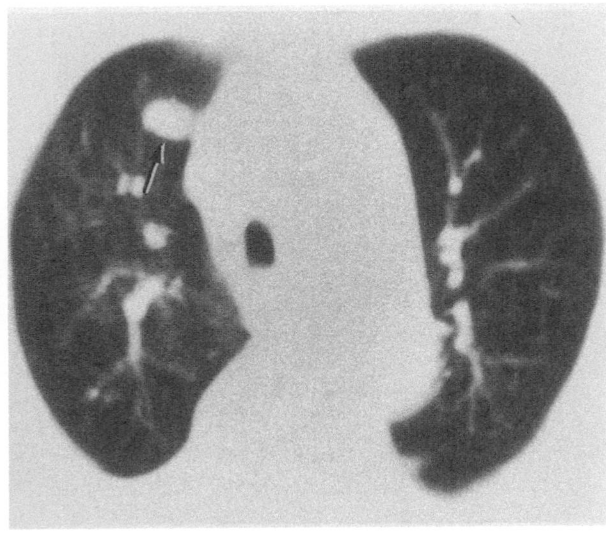

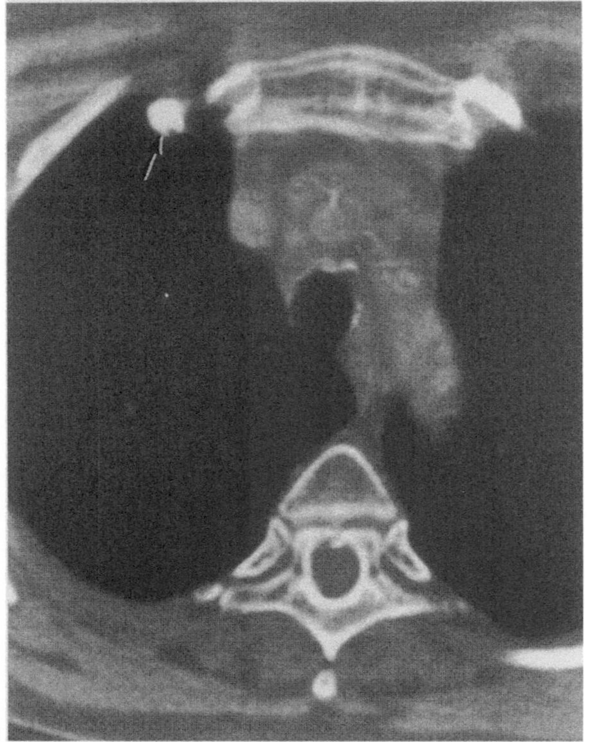

Fig. 4.18 A–C. Prominent costochondral junction of first rib simulating a pulmonary nodule at computed tomography. **A** Lateral radiograph. **B** and **C** Computed tomograms. A prominent costochondral junction of the first rib can intrude deeply into the lung (*arrow*). Computed tomograms may image the tip of the costochondral junction totally surrounded by lung. A pulmonary nodule may be simulated. Usually, as in **C**, mediastinal or bone window settings prove the calcified nature of the mass. If only a cartilaginous cap is imaged, calcium in the shadow will not be seen. Thin sections may be necessary to establish continuity of the density with the first rib

4.2.2 The Thoracic Outlet Compression Syndrome

The thoracic outlet compression syndrome is a term coined by Rob and Standeven [66] to supplant such terms as the "scalenus anticus syndrome," the "shoulder-arm syndrome," and the "hyperabduction syndrome," all of which were thought by them to be not sufficiently inclusive. This volume has used the term "thoracic inlet" rather than "outlet," but the terms are clearly synonymous.

The thoracic outlet compression syndrome is "a symptom complex consisting of neural, arterial, and venous disorders of the upper extremity which are caused by compression of the neurovascular structures between the clavicle and the first rib" [50]. A large experience with the condition has been reported by Stallworth and Horne [72].

The syndrome is considered briefly here to emphasize the importance of the radiologic evaluation of patients with this condition and to point out the dependence of correct evaluation on the correlated radiographic anatomy of this portion of the thoracic inlet (or outlet).

The subclavian vein traverses the upper surface of the first rib anterior to the scalene tubercle; the subclavian artery and the lower trunk of the brachial plexus derived from C-8 and T-1 are located behind the tubercle (Figs. 4.2 and 4.9). The clavicle lies immediately above these neurovascular structures (Fig. 4.19).

The symptoms resulting from compression of the lower trunk of the brachial plexus are pain, weakness, and paresthesias, usually in the distribution of the ulnar nerve (Fig. 4.19). Arterial compromise produces pain, numbness, pallor, and sensitivity to cold with aggravation of these findings upon elevation of the arm (Fig. 4.19).

Fig. 4.19 A, B. Thoracic outlet compression syndrome. **A** Coronal body section. **B** Subclavian arteriogram. Coronal body section shows subclavian artery (*1*) as it courses posterior to scalenus anterior muscle (*2*), inferior to the clavicle (*3*), and superior to the first rib (*4*). Compression of subclavian artery as shown in **B** (*5*) constitutes one of causes of thoracic outlet compression syndrome. This 21-year-old woman had a 10-year history of left shoulder pain, radiating down arm in an ulnar distribution. Occasional paresthesias were experienced. Eighty degrees of abduction caused subclavian murmur and loss of radial pulse. (**B** Courtesy P. Randall, Syracuse, N.Y.)

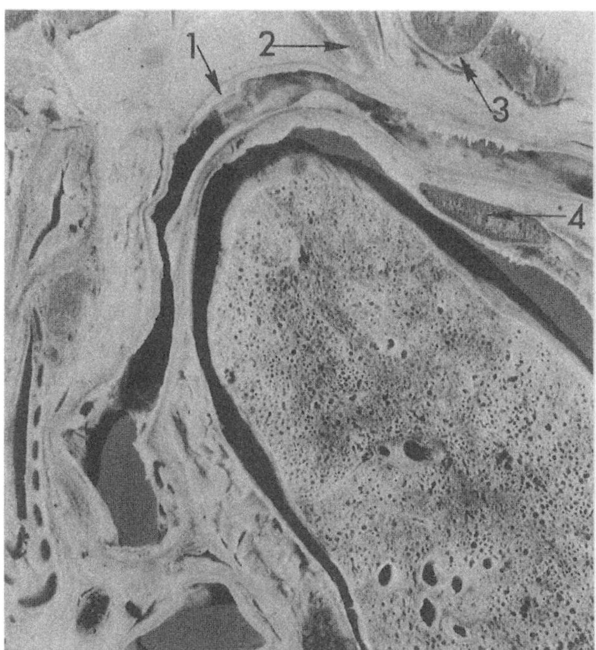

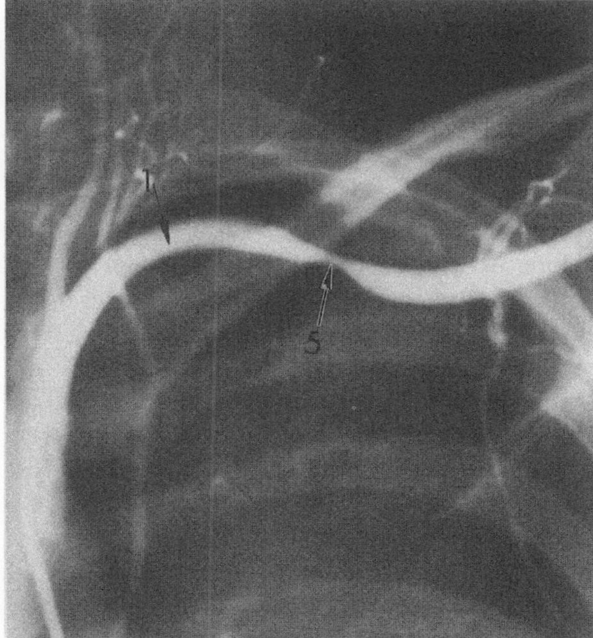

A   B

Venous compression results in swelling and cyanosis.

Although the thoracic outlet compression syndrome may be initiated by trauma such as whiplash injury or may be of idiopathic cause, many cases are the result of pathologic processes that can be identified on plain chest radiographs. Plain film findings of significance are fracture, osteochondroma, or other process increasing the bony mass of the first rib or clavicle [50, 51]. Bony compression can also result from cervical ribs [74]. Cervical ribs are present in 1% of the population [14], but apparently cause symptoms in only one patient out of ten [33]. In the series of 31 patients with the thoracic outlet syndrome reported by Lascelles [42], 14 had bilateral cervical ribs and another four had a unilateral cervical rib on the affected side. A long first rib, especially one fused with the second rib, is particularly likely to cause symptoms and should be looked for and reported in all patients with the syndrome [50].

In those cases demonstrating equivocal clinical findings, arteriography and venography may be helpful in clarifying the diagnosis [41, 50] (Fig. 4.19). It may be the only means by which compression of more than one of the neurovascular structures at the thoracic outlet can be proven [41]. In our experience, computed tomography has been disappointing as a diagnostic tool in this condition.

4.2.3 Intrathoracic Goiter

According to Sweet [73], an intrathoracic goiter is one in which "the greatest diameter of the tumor lies in the mediastinum below the thoracic inlet." He points out that the terms "substernal goiter" and "intrathoracic goiter" are sometimes used synonymously and states that the use of the terms in this manner is an error because although some intrathoracic goiters lie anteriorly and are truly substernal, others are found to lie far posteriorly. In fact, intrathoracic goiters are usually divided into two groups, anterior and posterior, on the basis of their relationship to the recurrent laryngeal nerves and

great vessels in the thoracic inlet; anterior goiters lie in front of the nerves, subclavian arteries, and innominate veins; posterior goiters lie behind them [73].

Most intrathoracic goiters are situated substernally. These anteriorly placed goiters arise from lateral thyroid lobes or isthmus and descend in front of the great veins and the recurrent laryngeal nerve. Older anatomic literature cited by Leszczynski [43] describes an anterior fascial membrane separating the neck and the mediastinum. He states that this membrane is not equally competent in all individuals and allows an anterior descent of the goiter in these patients. However, it seems equally likely that the suprapleural membranes, which are attached to the first rib forward to the sternum but are not attached to the manubrium, leave an unprotected pathway anterior to the veins in the midline.

Substernal goiters, if sufficiently large, will displace the trachea and the esophagus posteriorly (Fig. 4.20). They separate the pleurae forming the upper end of the anterior junction line backward in a manner characteristic of an extrapleural mass. They are usually found to lie above and below the thoracic inlet and demonstrate a cervicothoracic sign indicative of an anteriorly situated mass on radiographs (Fig. 4.20).

Radioisotopic studies are often definitive in the diagnosis of mediastinal thyroid [35, 46], but computed tomography is also of considerable value [26, 71] (Fig. 4.23). Glazer et al. [26] have commented on the findings at computed tomography that suggest a mediastinal mass may be of thyroid origin. These are: (a) anatomic continuity with the cervical thyroid; (b) focal calcifications; (c) relatively high CT number (in the range of 100 Hounsfield units); (d) rise in CT number after bolus injection of contrast material; and (e) prolonged enhancement after contrast administration.

Posterior goiters arise from the posterior and lateral aspects of the thyroid gland and descend into the thorax behind the great vessels and the recurrent laryngeal nerve. They are not rare; 25% of substernal goiters in one series were posterior [65]. Their path of descent is along the

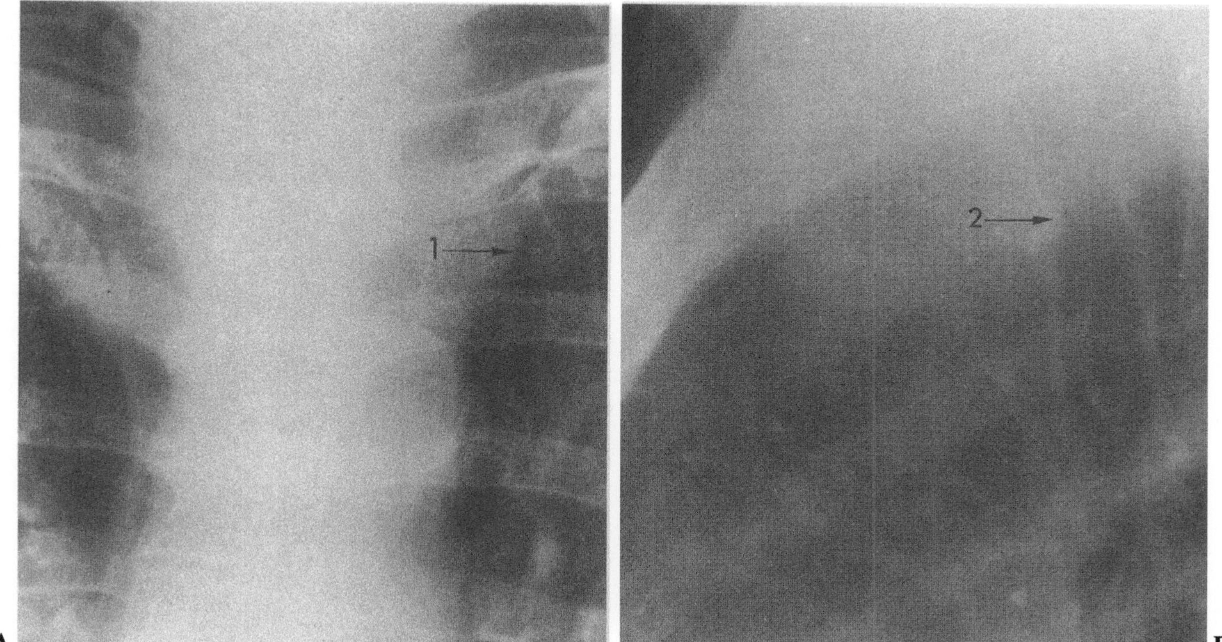

Fig. 4.20 A, B. Substernal goiter. PA (**A**) and lateral (**B**) radiographs. Substernal thyroid masses characteristically cross thoracic inlet and, as demonstrated in this patient, demonstrate cervicothoracic sign indicative of anteriorly placed mass (*1*). Note that entire right side of mass is outlined by tracheal air rather than air in lung. Trachea is also displaced posteriorly (*2*)

perivisceral fascia about the trachea and esophagus. Although Sweet [73] has reported posterior goiters situated to the left side, Negre and Balmes [49] reported 16 cases of posterior goiter all of which were right sided and intruded into the supra-azygos area. All 12 of the posterior goiters reported by Rietz and Werner were on the right [65]. Rietz and Werner contend that the predominant right-sided position of posterior goiters is related to the position of the left innominate vein, the left common carotid artery, and the left subclavian artery, which they feel deflect the mass to the right side in its descent.

Posterior goiters are usually connected to the thyroid gland by a pedicle and classically are seen to lie totally below the plane of the thoracic inlet on radiographs (Fig. 4.21). The impression of posterior goiters on lung is often marked, and commonly they are confined at their lower margin by the azygos arch (Figs. 4.22 and 4.23). Most posterior goiters are found immediately in front of the spine and therefore tend to displace the esophagus more than the trachea. The trachea is sometimes pushed forward, however, and occasionally the mass separates the trachea and esophagus. Sweet [73] has pointed out that posterior goiters are often misdiagnosed as other lesions. He states further that radiologic studies should always be made to determine whether an upper mediastinal mass lesion is anterior or posterior to the great vessels, since anterior masses can be removed through a standard thyroidectomy incision, whereas posterior lesions, including goiters, commonly require thoracotomy for removal. Today, many surgeons feel that virtually all posterior goiters can be removed through a neck incision. Determination of the relationship of a mass to the great vessels at the thoracic inlet usually requires only an assessment of whether the trachea, the esophagus, or both are displaced anteriorly or posteriorly. Computed tomography is an ideal study to make this determination [7]. In all doubtful cases, Rietz and Werner [65] feel that angiography should be performed, but with computed tomography this should rarely be required.

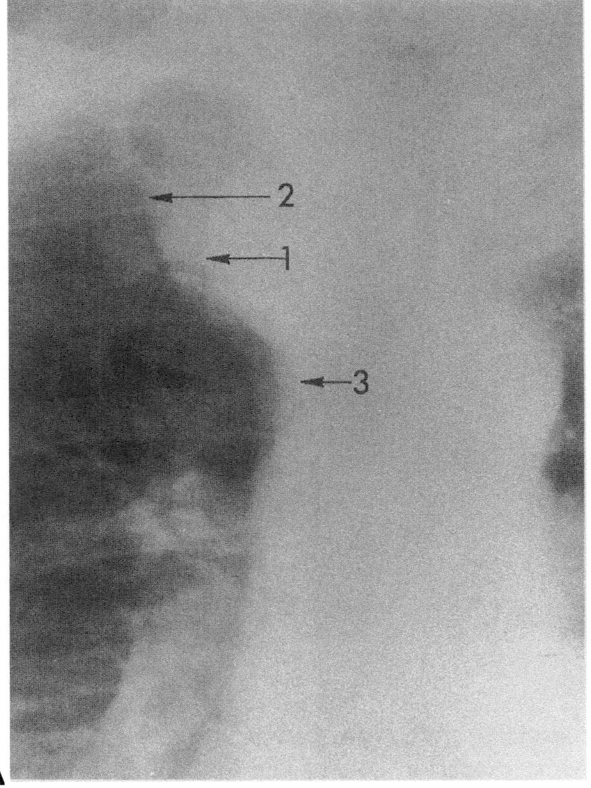

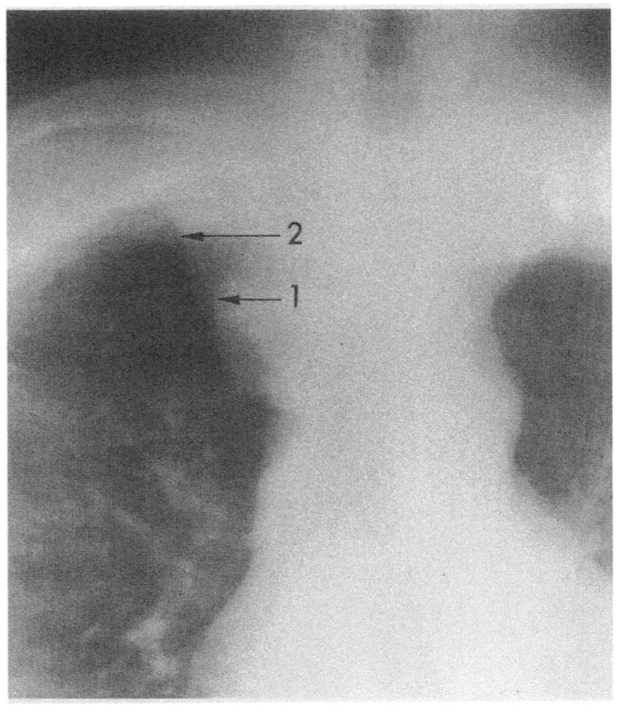

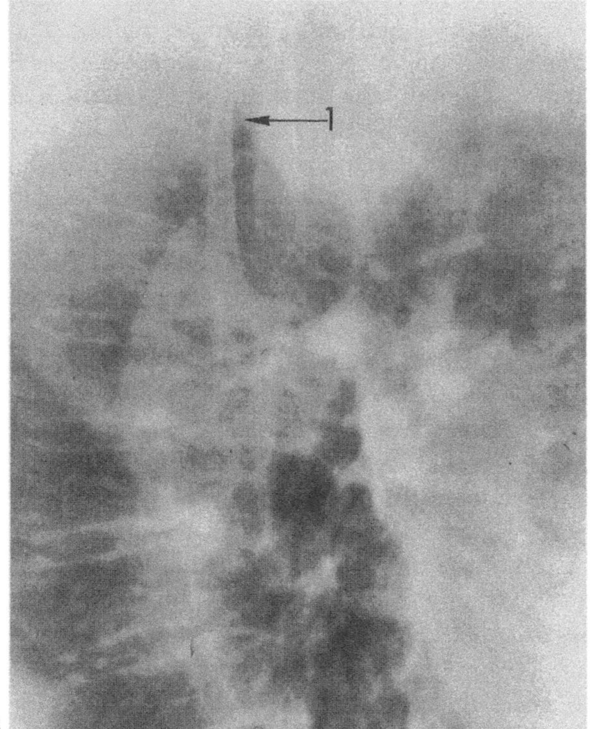

Fig. 4.21 A–C. Posterior goiter. PA (**A**), lateral (**B**), and lordotic (**C**) radiographs. Lateral film clearly shows posterior, prespinal position of this thyroid mass (*1*). Mass is totally intrathoracic. Note that it is large enough so that its anterior aspect lies medial to innominate and right subclavian arteries, displacing them laterally into lung (*2*). Inferior pole of goiter reaches to level of azygos arch (*3*). Mass overlies medial end of clavicle on frontal view but is widely separated from it on lordotic view, a finding indicative of its posterior position. Note also characteristic appearance of great vessels at thoracic inlet on lordotic view. This projection brings vascular shadows into greater profile against anterior portions of lung. On lordotic radiographs shadows of great vessels can usually be followed laterally in arcuate sweep across lung to lateral chest wall

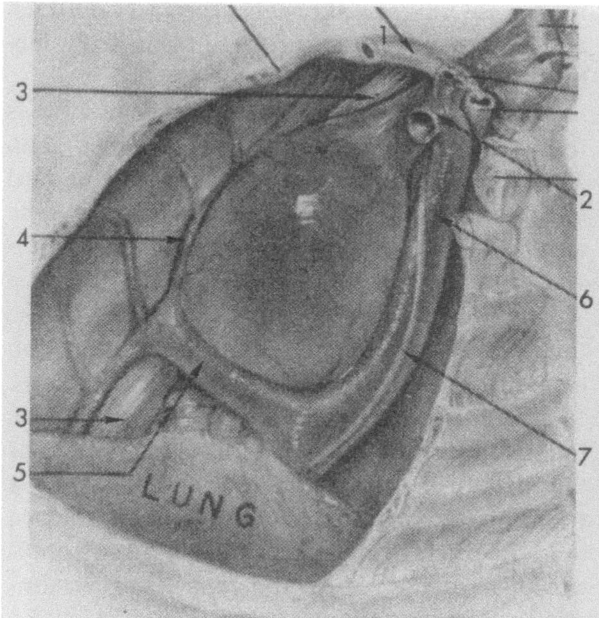

Fig. 4.22. Posterior goiter. Drawing made at operation. A posterior goiter is shown extending into right side of mediastinum behind subclavian artery (*1*) and subclavian vein (*2*). Mass lies to right side of esophagus (*3*) and is confined posteriorly by right superior intercostal vein (*4*), inferiorly by azygos arch (*5*), and anteriorly by superior vena cava (*6*). Right phrenic nerve (*7*) is seen passing inferiorly along superior vena cava. (Modified from [73])

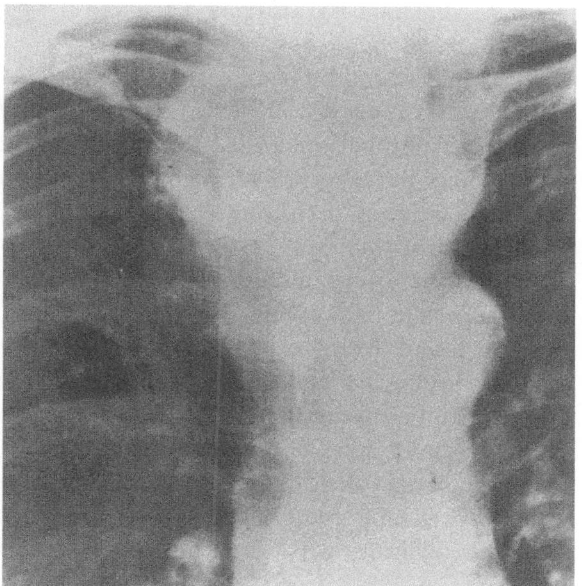

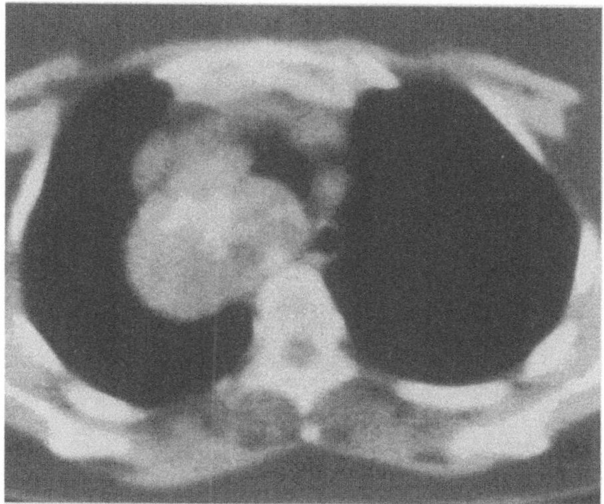

A tracheal tug or movement of the mass during swallowing under fluoroscopy supports the diagnosis of a thyroid origin of the tumor. Often, however, the lesions are large and are wedged in the thoracic inlet so that motion is impossible.

Fig. 4.23 A, B. Posterior goiter. **A** PA radiograph. **B** Computed tomogram. A large, right-sided posterior goiter is shown extending downward to the level of the azygos arch. The mass has followed the perivisceral space from the neck into the mediastinum. The mass is shown to be calcified and it displaces the trachea forward and the esophagus to the left

4.2.4 Mediastinal Parathyroid Adenoma

Parathyroid adenoma is an uncommon mediastinal lesion [17, 40, 48, 77]. In a literature review of a large number of cases, Wang [77] found only 19% of parathyroid adenomas to be within the mediastinum. Although mediastinal adenomas constitute only a small percentage of all hyperfunctioning glands, they remain a serious concern in patients in whom initial exploration has failed. Many intramediastinal parathyroid adenomas are enclosed within the thymus anterior to the innominate veins [77] (Fig. 4.24). Wang [77] and Edis [17] comment that many of the mediastinal adenomas lie in the thoracic inlet and are usually readily accessible from a cervical approach. In Edis' series, 15 of 21 inlet tumors were removed through a cervical approach and were thus not classified as being truly mediastinal.

The vast majority of parathyroid adenomas found in the mediastinum are smaller than 3 cm [40] and are not demonstrable on standard radiographs. Computed tomography is the ideal, noninvasive modality to make the diagnosis [16, 40] (Fig. 4.24).

Doppman et al. [16] noted that many of the tumors overlooked at initial cervical exploration lie at the inlet in the tracheoesophageal groove caudad to the thyroid gland. He developed the following computed tomographic criteria for the diagnosis of parathyroid adenoma: (a) a round mass lying against the posterior trachea or in the tracheoesophageal groove; (b) a homogeneously dense mass; and (c) a mass demonstrating contrast enhancement (Fig. 4.24).

Other modalities, including angiography, can be successfully employed for detecting parathyroid adenoma but computed tomography remains the initial screening tool to identify tumors not identified at initial exploration. Recently, magnetic resonance imaging has emerged as an effective modality for the detection of parathyroid adenoma, competing favorably with computed tomography [39].

4.2.5 Spread of Infection Through the Thoracic Inlet

The pathways by which phlegmonous processes pass through the thoracic inlet are also dependent upon the anatomy of the area; the radiologic findings caused by such localized or diffuse inflammatory processes are similarly influenced [2, 13, 15, 19, 34, 52]. The spread of infection through the thoracic inlet is considered by Leszczynski to be rare [43]. Nonetheless,

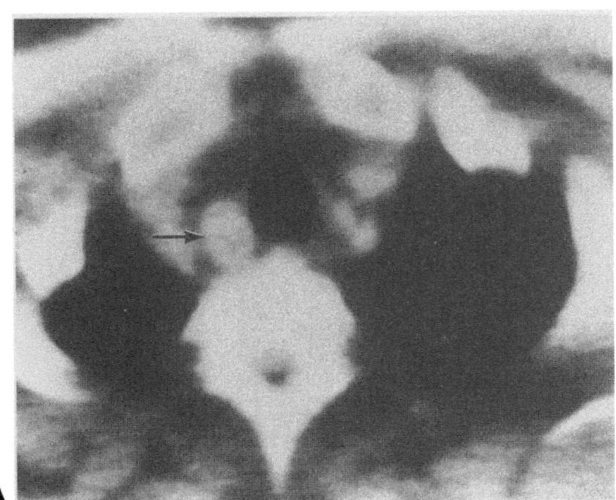

A

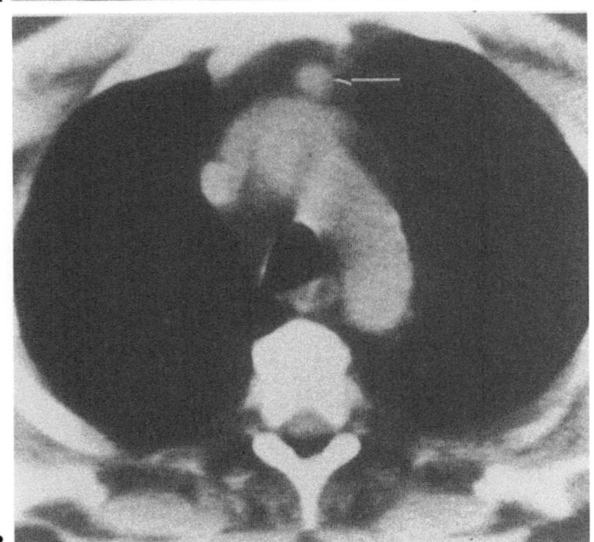

B

Fig. 4.24A, B. Parathyroid adenoma. **A** and **B** Computed tomograms on different patients. Ectopic parathyroid adenomas (*arrow*) commonly lie in the plane of the thoracic inlet often anterior to the innominate veins. Note that in **B** the adenoma might be mistaken for the subclavian artery. Study of serial sections and/or contrast enhancement should prevent this pitfall most large institutions see a few cases each year. Descending spread of the inflammatory process usually results from pharyngeal infection or dental disease [2, 13, 15, 19, 23, 34, 52] (Fig. 4.25), although interestingly, in Leszczynski's series of 58 cases none stemmed from the latter source [43]. Ascending dissemination of infection is most often the result of esophageal perforation [8, 11, 12, 54, 67]. Since most spontaneous perforations of the esophagus produce radiologic findings in the lower mediastinum on the left, this entity has been discussed more completely in the chapter on the infra-aortic area (chapter 7).

The principal pathways of spread across the thoracic inlet are dependent upon the distribution of the cervical and mediastinal fascia [44, 45, 64], as discussed in chapter 3. These are as follows:

1. Along the visceral compartment within the perivisceral sheath and along the danger space between the alar and prevertebral layers of the deep cervical fascia.
   - About the trachea and esophagus. This route is commonly involved in the extension of inflammation from the retropharyngeal space and by the cephalad dissection of purulent fluid following spontaneous esophageal rupture.
   - Along the great vessels. This pathway is involved in the extremely rare spread of infection to the mediastinum from the mastoid [43].
2. Behind the prevertebral fascia [52]. Spread along this compartment may also result from retropharyngeal disease, especially in children, due to secondary involvement of lymph nodes lying in front of the second cervical vertebra [34].

Extension of the inflammatory process anterior to the great vessels is uncommon; involvement of the anterior mediastinum is said to be five to ten times less frequent than is localization of disease in the more posterior compartments. This is probably due to the fact that infection involving the cervical space anterior to the pretracheal fascia (the anterior aspect of the middle layer of the deep cervical fascia) is rare. It should be understood that cervical and mediastinal infection does not necessarily respect fascial planes; tissue necrosis may result in complete dissolution of such boundaries [55].

On radiographs, the spread of infection across the thoracic inlet causes diffuse or localized mediastinal widening (Figs. 4.25 and 4.26) often accompanied by mediastinal emphysema (Fig. 4.25). If the route of spread has been along the perivisceral fascia, the process may become so extensive as to fill this fascial space and then may track along the major bronchi into the lung, producing significant accentuation of bronchovascular markings on radiographs [43] (Fig. 4.25). Sometimes the spread of infection from the neck may produce a relatively localized abscess in the upper mediastinum (Fig. 4.26). These more confined infectious processes occur more often on the right than they do on the left [43]. No anatomic explanation for this predilection is known, although the position of the left innominate vein, the left common carotid artery, and the left subclavian artery may play a role in deflecting infected material to the right. Inflammation localized primarily to the upper mediastinum is often confined inferiorly by the azygos arch on the right and the aortic arch on the left [43]. Bulging of the supra-azygos recess may simulate a solid mediastinal mass (Fig. 4.26). Localized upper mediastinal abscess is similar to posterior goiter in that both tend to localize on the right side and both tend to be confined inferiorly by the azygos arch. If the pathway by which the process is extending is behind the prevertebral fascia – a rare event [52] – widening of the paraspinal line is the upper thorax may be an early radiographic finding [43], Ramilo et al. [62] have reported empyema as a complication of retropharyngeal and other neck abscesses in children.

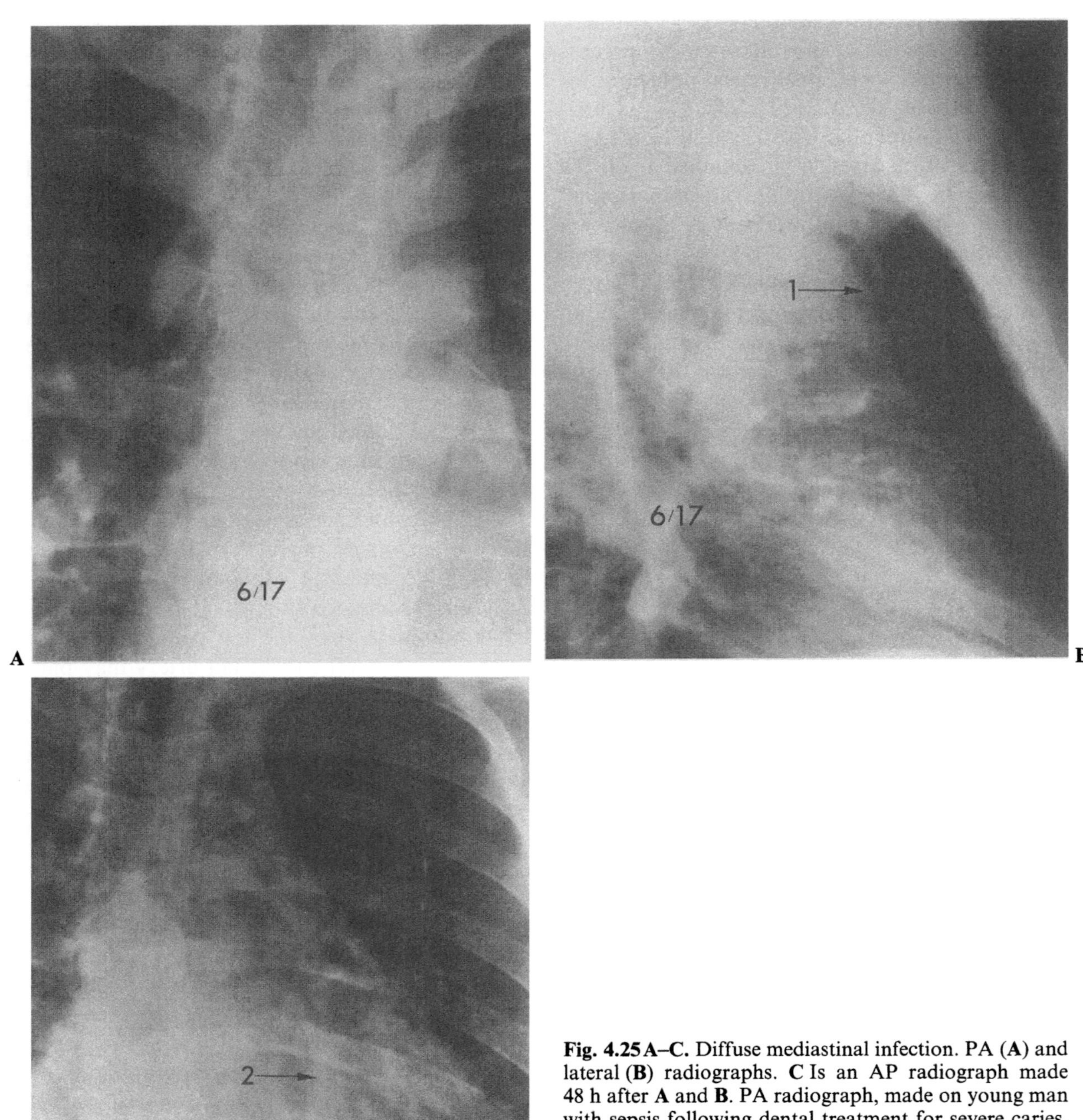

Fig. 4.25 A–C. Diffuse mediastinal infection. PA (**A**) and lateral (**B**) radiographs. **C** Is an AP radiograph made 48 h after **A** and **B**. PA radiograph, made on young man with sepsis following dental treatment for severe caries, was thought to be normal, but lateral film demonstrated gas in mediastinum outlining the ascending aorta (*1*). Patient's condition rapidly deteriorated, and film 48 h later (**C**) showed diffuse mediastinal widening with extensive mediastinal emphysema. Infectious material within mediastinum has extended along central bronchovascular trunks into lung parenchyma (*2*)

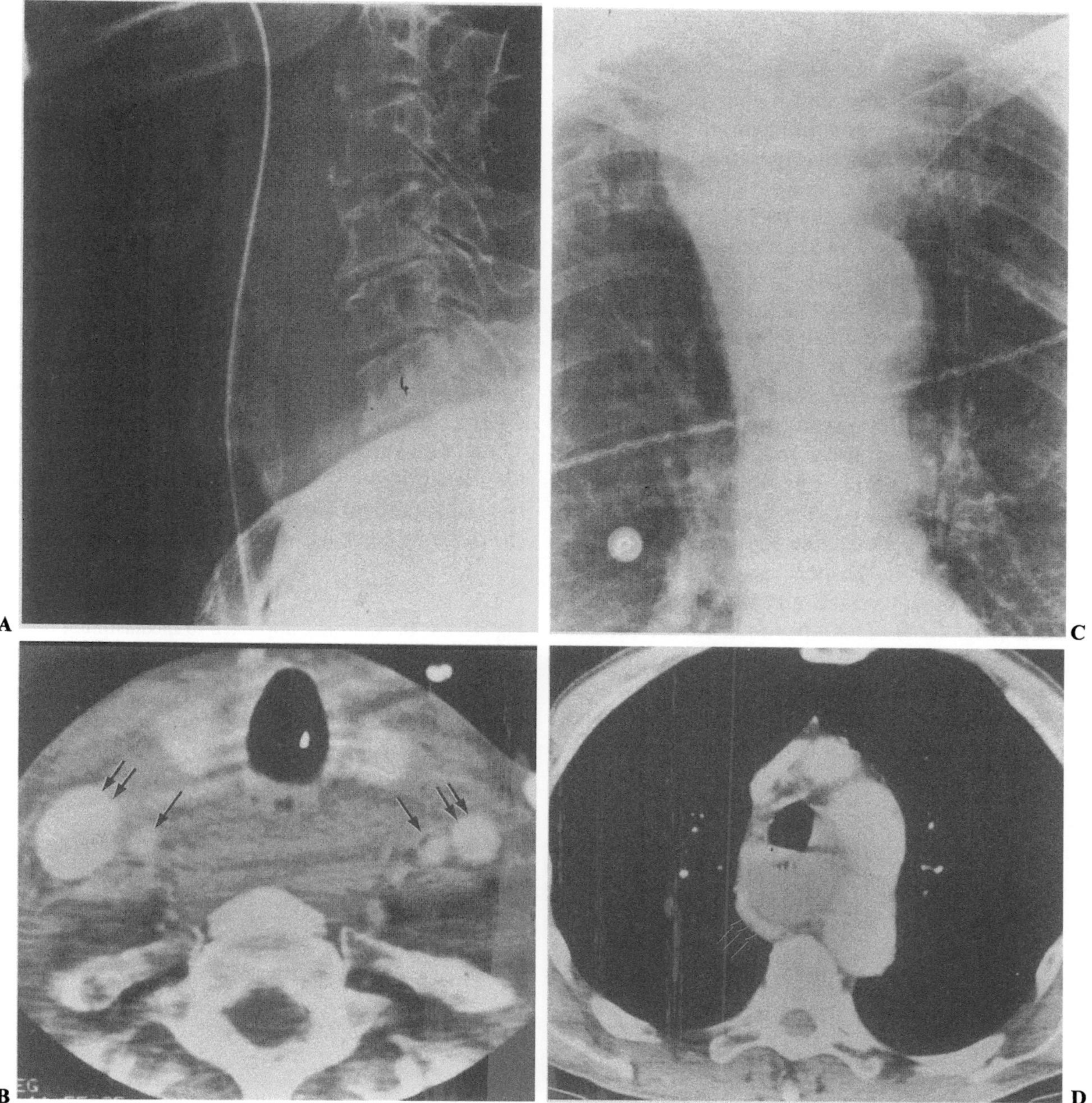

Fig. 4.26A–D. Localized mediastinal infection. **A** Lateral radiograph of neck. **B** Computed tomogram of neck. **C** PA chest radiograph. **D** Computed tomogram through level of azygos arch. This patient developed neck fullness and fever after attempted esophagoscopy. The lateral neck radiograph and computed tomogram of the neck show a diffuse soft tissue mass which, on the computed tomographic study, displaces the carotid arteries (*single arrow*) and internal jugular veins (*double arrows*) laterally. The mass proved to be an abscess which dissected downward through the perivisceral space to produce the supra-azygous mass shown in **C**. In **D** the process is seen in the posterior perivisceral space and is partially confined by the azygos arch (*triple arrows*)

4.2.6 Mediastinoscopy

Mediastinoscopy has become an important diagnostic tool to view and biopsy accessible mediastinal mass lesions and lymph nodes [1, 24, 36, 37, 56, 70, 75]. This operative procedure is being discussed in a radiologic book because mediastinoscopy and the roentgen examination are complementary procedures in the study of mediastinal disease. The advantages and disadvantages of each approach should be understood to effect the most satisfactory diagnostic results. The major advantage of mediastinoscopy is that it enables one to view pathology directly and to biopsy it. Its drawback lies in the fact that the areas that can be inspected are somewhat limited. The technique of mediastinoscopy employs a transverse suprasternal incision through which the instrument is passed downward along the perivisceral fascial sheath behind the great vessels and in front of the trachea (Fig. 4.27). This approach to the mediastinal contents predicates which structures can be visualized and which ones cannot be seen. Simply stated, the anatomy of the supra-azygos and supra-aortic areas is presented to view; the

anterior mediastinum, the infra-azygos and infra-aortic areas are not accessible, although in some cases the immediate subcarinal area can be seen. Usually, it is possible to visualize the trachea and the paratracheal areas, the carina, both main bronchi, and the right upper lobe bronchus, the aortic arch, the innominate artery, the right pulmonary artery, the left recurrent laryngeal nerve, and the esophagus down to the carina [29].

Since the structures of the anterior mediastinum and the aortic-pulmonic window are not within range of view, the internal mammary nodes, inferior left paratracheal nodes, and the ductus nodes cannot be evaluated [37, 56]. These nodal groups are readily studied by radiologic examination, a definite advantage of this type of investigation over mediastinoscopy. On the other hand, a significant limitation of radio-

Fig. 4.27 A, B. Anatomic approach to mediastinum used at mediastinoscopy. Frontal (**A**) and lateral (**B**) photographs of model. Following transverse suprasternal incision, instrument is passed downward along perivisceral fascial sheath behind great vessels and in front of trachea. (From [29])

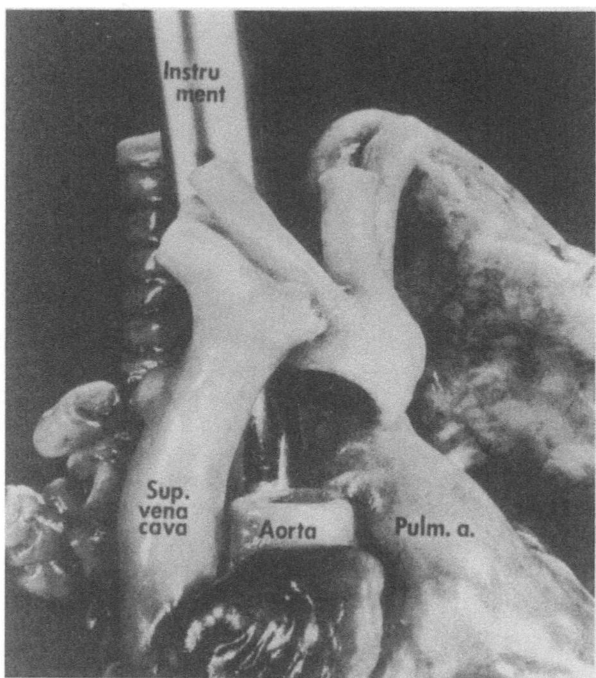

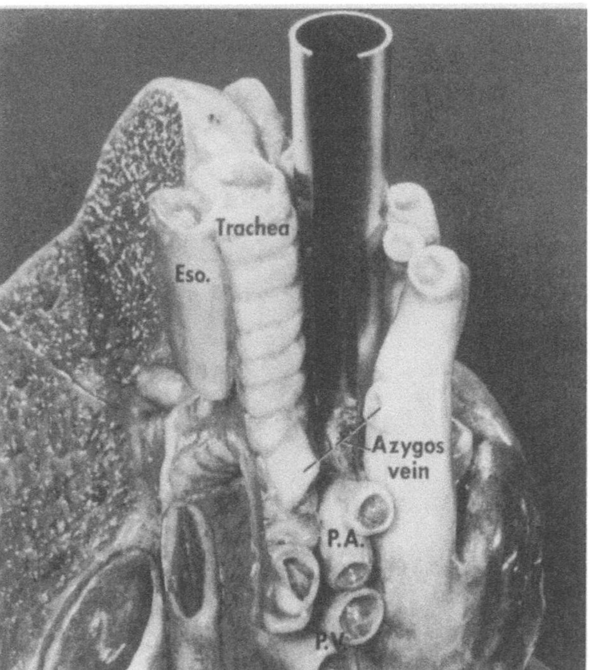

A   B

logic examination is that some diseased nodes are not enlarged and of course pathology within them cannot be appreciated on the X-ray study. A review by Whitcomb et al. [79] pointed out that plain film radiologic evaluation was negative in 50% of patients proven to have pathology by mediastinoscopy. A similar figure was reported by Schlorf [69]. The latter article makes an additional interesting point: when the radiographs in this series were reviewed in retrospect, 83% of cases were found to show mediastinal disease, although at original reading only one-half were considered abnormal. Although a part of this discrepancy might be accounted for by the retrospective nature of the film analysis, which very likely caused great attention to be focused on the mediastinum, the findings of this study point out that mediastinal abnormality is often overlooked in the routine interpretation of radiographs. Undoubtedly, a skilled observer carefully studying the mediastinum with adequate plain radiographs will detect far more than 50% of the abnormal nodes subsequently identified at mediastinoscopy.

Computed tomography has, of course, greatly increased our ability to detect mediastinal lymphadenopathy [10]. This topic is addressed in detail in chapter 3. Studies comparing mediastinoscopy and computed tomography indicate that computed tomography has greater sensitivity than mediastinoscopy; however, its specificity and predictive value are low [10]. Negative computed tomography is thought to make mediastinoscopy unnecessary whether 5-mm [10] or 10-mm node size [27] is used as the upper limit of normal size.

In the final analysis these two diagnostic approaches should not be viewed as competitors but as complementary methods to evaluate patients with known or suspect mediastinal disease.

4.2.7 The Cervicothoracic Sign

The thoracic inlet is an inclined plane parallel to the first rib; it is higher in back than it is in front (Fig. 4.28). The extreme anterior portions of the lungs do not extend above the clavicle; the higher lung apices are more posterior and do project above the clavicle. Since the cephalic border of the anterior portion of the mediastinum ends at the level of the clavicles, whereas that of the posterior portion extends much higher, a lesion clearly visible above the clavicles on the frontal view as the result of its contact with lung must lie entirely within the thorax (Figs. 4.20, 4.28, and 5.6). According to Felson: "the trachea is the dividing line: a mediastinal mass anterior to the trachea loses its lateral margins as it reaches the lower border of the clavicles since the neck is above this area, but a lesion behind the trachea is visible above the clavicles" [20]. He has called this diagnostic clue the "cervicothoracic sign" [20, 21].

Figure 4.28B shows the application of the cervicothoracic sign to a substernal goiter, an anteriorly situated mass. The lesion shown at the medial aspect of the left apex in Fig. 4.28C proved to be a neurofibroma. The fact that air-filled lung outlines the lesion, which extends to the apex of the pleural cavity, indicates that the lesion must be posteriorly situated. Certainly in this case esophageal duplication or other posterior mediastinal masses could not be excluded, but neurogenic tumor should be the preferred diagnosis on a statistical basis.

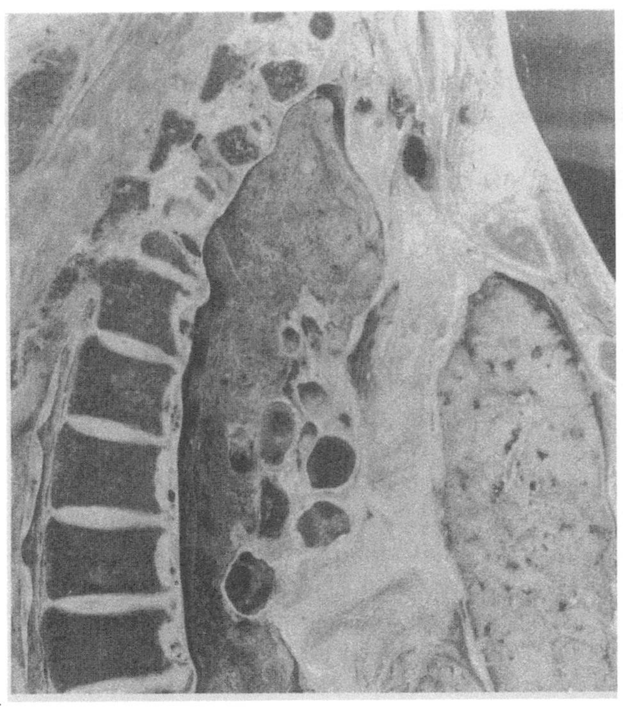

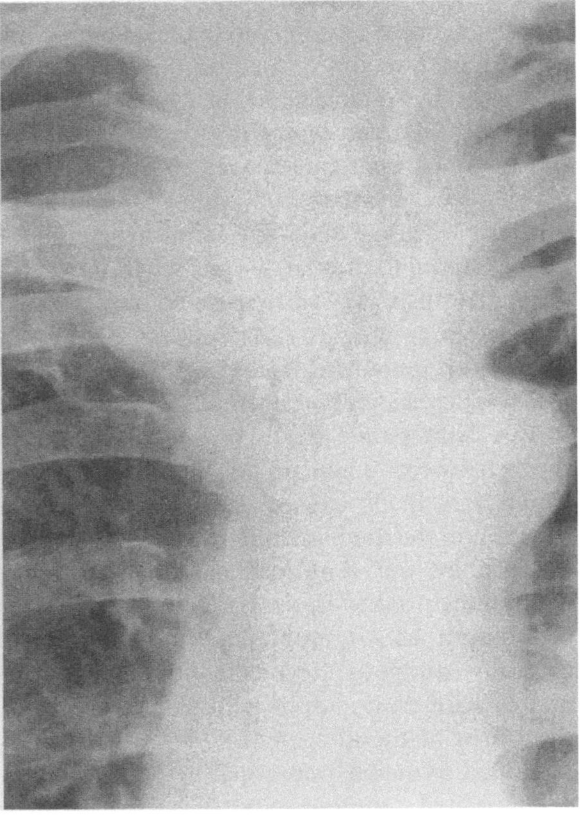

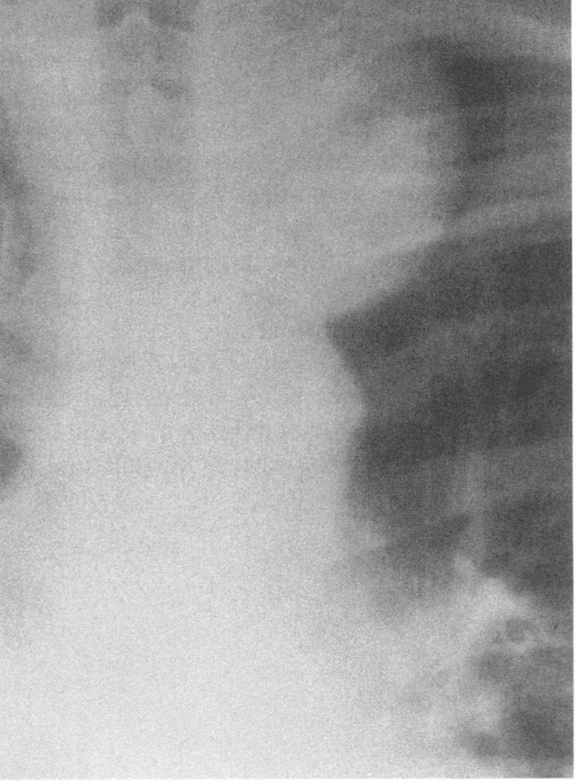

Fig. 4.28 A–C. The cervicothoracic sign. **A** Sagittal body section. **B** and **C** PA radiographs. The sagittal body section shows that anterior aspect of lung does not reach as high as posterior aspect. Cephalic border of anterior portion of mediastinum ends at level of clavicles, whereas that of posterior mediastinum extends much higher. Therefore, a lesion clearly visible above clavicles on frontal radiograph as a result of its contact with lung must lie entirely within thorax and must be posteriorly situated. Mass shown in **B** is anteriorly situated and is a substernal goiter. Lesion shown in **C** is posteriorly situated and is a neurofibroma

References

1. Acosta JL, Manfredi F (1977) Selective mediastinoscopy. Chest 71:150–154
2. Archer WH (1975) Oral, face and neck infections. In: Archer WA (ed) Oral and maxillofacial surgery, edn 5. Saunders, Philadelphia, pp 438–517
3. Arnold M (1968) Reconstructive anatomy: a method for the study of human structure. Saunders, Philadelphia
4. Baron RL, Gutierrez FR, Sagel SS, Levitt RG, McKnight RC (1981) CT of anomalies of the mediastinal vessels. AJR 137:571–576
5. Baron RL, Lee JKT, Sagel SS, Peterson RR (1982) Computed tomography of the normal thymus. Radiology 142:121–125
6. Baron RL, Lee JKT, Sagel SS, Levitt RG (1982) Computed tomography of the abnormal thymus. Radiology 142:127–134
7. Binder RE, Pugatch RD, Faling LJ, Kanter RA, Sawin CT (1980) Diagnosis of posterior mediastinal goiter by computed tomography. J Comput Assist Tomogr 4:550–552
8. Bobo WO, Billups WA, Hardy JB (1970) Boerhaave's syndrome: a review of six cases of spontaneous rupture of the esophagus secondary to vomiting. Ann Surg 172:1034–1038
9. Boyd E (1932) Weight of the thymus gland in health and disease. Am J Dis Child 43:1162–1214
10. Brion JP, Depauw L, Kuhn G, deFrancquen P, Friberg J, Rocmans P, Struyven J (1985) Role of computed tomography and mediastinoscopy in preoperative staging of lung carcinoma. J Comput Assist Tomogr 9:480–484
11. Brownstein EG (1969) Spontaneous rupture of the distal thoracic esophagus. Med J Aust 1:849–852
12. Christoforidis A, Nelson SW (1957) Spontaneous rupture of the esophagus with emphasis of roentgenologic diagnosis. Am J Roentgenol 78:574–580
13. Cogan M (1973) Necrotizing mediastinitis secondary to descending cervical cellulitis. Oral Surg 36:307–320
14. Davis DB, King JC (1938) Cervical rib in early life. Am J Dis Child 56:744–755
15. deLorimier AA, Haskin D, Massie FS (1966) Mediastinal mass caused by vertebral osteomyelitis. Am J Dis Child 111:639–643
16. Doppman JL, Krudy AG, Brennan MF, Schneider P, Lasker RD, Marx SJ (1982) CT appearance of enlarged parathyroid glands in the posterior superior mediastinum. J Comput Assist Tomogr 6:1099–1102
17. Edis AJ, Sheedy PF, Beahrs OH, Van Heerden JA (1978) Results of reoperation for hyperparathyroidism with evaluation of preoperative studies. Surgery 84:384–393
18. Ellis K, Gregg HG (1964) Thymomas – roentgen considerations. Am J Roentgenol 91:105–119
19. Enquist RW, Blanck RR, Butler RH (1976) Nontraumatic mediastinitis. JAMA 236:1048–1049
20. Felson B (1969) The mediastinum. Semin Roentgenol 4:41–58
21. Felson B (1973) Chest roentgenology. Saunders, Philadelphia
22. Fisher ER (1964) Pathology of the thymus and its relation to human disease. In: Good RA, Gabrielson AE (eds) The thymus in immunology. Harper and Row, New York
23. Forrest JV, Schackleford GD, Bramson RT, Anderson LS (1973) Acute mediastinal widening. Am J Roentgenol 117:881–885
24. Fosburg RG, O'Sullivan JJ, Ah-Tye P, Gibbons JA, Oury JH (1974) Positive mediastinoscopy; an ominous finding. Ann Thorac Surg 18:346–356
25. Francis IR, Glazer GM, Bookstein FL, Gross BH (1985) Thymus: reexamination of age related changes in size and shape. AJR 145:249–254
26. Glazer GM, Axel L, Moss AA (1982) CT diagnosis of mediastinal thyroid. AJR 138:495–498
27. Glazer GM, Orringer MB, Gross BH, Quint LE (1984) The mediastinum in non-small cell lung cancer: CT-surgical correlation. AJR 142:1101–1105
28. Godwin JD, Chen JTT (1986) Thoracic venous anatomy. AJR 147:674–684
29. Goldberg EM, Shapiro CM, Glicksman HS (1974) Mediastinoscopy for assessing mediastinal spread in clinical staging of lung carcinoma. Semin Oncol 1:205–215
30. Goldstein G, McKay IR (1969) The human thymus. Green, St. Louis
31. Gondos B (1961) Roentgen image of the subclavian artery in the pulmonary apex. Am J Roentgenol 86:1058–1060
32. Heiberg E, Wolverson MK, Sundaram M, Nouri S (1982) Normal thymus: CT characteristics in subjects under age 20. AJR 138:491–494
33. Hill RM (1939) Vascular anomalies of the upper limb associated with cervical ribs. Br J Surg 27:100–139
34. Hora JF (1963) Deep neck infections. Arch Otolaryngol 77:129–136
35. Irwin RS, Braman SS, Arvanitidis AN, Hamolsky MW (1978) I^{131} thyroid scanning in the preoperative diagnosis of mediastinal goiter. Ann Intern Med 89:73–74
36. James EC, Ellwood RA (1974) Mediastinoscopy and mediastinal roentgenology: clinical correlation. Ann Thorac Surg 18:531–538
37. Jolly PC, Hill LD, Lawless PA, West TL (1973) Parasternal mediastinotomy and mediastinoscopy. Adjuncts in the diagnosis of chest disease. J Thorac Cardiovasc Surg 66:549–556
38. Keynes G (1954) Physiology of the thymus gland. Br Med J 2:659–663
39. Kier R, Herfkens RJ, Blinder RA, Leight GS, Utz JA, Silverman PM (1986) MRI with surface coils for parathyroid tumors: preliminary investigation. AJR 147:497–500
40. Krudy AG, Doppman JL, Brennan MF, Marx SJ, Spiegel AM, Stock JL, Aurbach GD (1981) The detection of mediastinal parathyroid glands by com-

puted tomography, selective arteriography and venous sampling. Radiology 140:739–744
41. Lang EK (1965) Arteriographic diagnosis of the thoracic outlet syndrome. Radiology 84:296–303
42. Lascelles RG, Mohr PD, Neary D, Bloor K (1977) Thoracic outlet syndrome. Brain 100:601–612
43. Leszcynski SZ (1972) Purulent and fibrous mediastinitis: radiological diagnosis. Polish Medical Publishers, Warsaw
44. Levitt GW (1970) Cervical fascia and deep neck infections. Laryngoscope 80:409–435
45. Levitt GW (1976) Cervical fascia and deep neck infections. Otolaryngol Clin North Am 9:701–716
46. Lin DS (1983) Thyroid imaging: mediastinal uptake in thyroid imaging. Semin Nucl Med 13:395
47. Moore AV Jr, Korobkin M, Olanow W, Heaston DK, Ram PC, Dunnick NR, Silverman PM (1983) Age related changes in the thymus gland: CT pathologic correlation. AJR 141:241–246
48. Nathaniels ER, Nathaniels AM, Wang CA (1970) Mediastinal parathyroid tumors: a clinical and pathological study of 84 cases. Ann Surg 171:165–170
49. Negre E, Balmes A (1950) Les goitres du mediastin postérieur. J Chir (Paris) 66:190
50. Nelson RM, Davis RW (1969) Thoracic outlet compression syndrome. Ann Thorac Surg 8:437–451
51. Nelson RM, Hess WE, Lyman JH (1963) Venous obstruction with hypertrophy of an upper extremity due to osteochondroma. Surgery 54:871–875
52. Oliphant M, Wiot JF, Whalen JP (1976) The cervicothoracic continuum. Radiology 120:257–262
53. Paling MR, Dwyer AJ (1980) First rib as the cause of a "pulmonary nodule" on chest computed tomography. J Comput Assist Tomogr 4:847–848
54. Panaro VA, Leslie ES (1965) Spontaneous rupture of the esophagus. Radiology 84:252–258
55. Payne WS, Larson RH (1969) Acute mediastinitis. Surg Clin North Am 49:999–1009
56. Pearson FG, Nelems JM, Henderson RD, DeLarue NC (1972) The role of mediastinoscopy in the selection of treatment for bronchial carcinoma with involvement of superior mediastinal lymph nodes. J Thorac Cardiovasc Surg 64:382–390
57. Penn I (1962) Injuries of the cervical portion of the thoracic duct. Br J Surg 50:19–23
58. Poker N, Finby N, Steinberg I (1958) Subclavian arteries: study in health and disease. Am J Roentgenol 80:193–216
59. Proto AV, Chaliff MI (1986) Apical opacity: a normal finding on PA chest radiographs. Radiology 161:429–432
60. Proto AV, Rost RC Jr (1985) CT of the thorax: pitfalls in interpretation. Radiographics 5:693–812
61. Proto AV, Speckman JM (1979) The left lateral radiograph of the chest. Medical radiography and photography.
62. Ramilo J, Harris JV, White H (1978) Empyema as a complication of retropharyngeal and neck abscesses in children. Radiology 126:743–746
63. Reede DL, Whelan MA, Bergeron RT (1982) Computed tomography of the infrahyoid neck. I. Normal anatomy. Radiology 145:389–395
64. Reede DL, Whelan MA, Bergeron RT (1982) Computed tomography of the infrahyoid neck. II. Pathology. Radiology 145:397–402
65. Rietz KA, Werner B (1960) Intrathoracic goitre. Acta Chir Scand 119:379–388
66. Rob CG, Standeven A (1958) Arterial occlusion complicating thoracic outlet compression syndrome. Br Med J 2:709–712
67. Rogers LF, Puig AW, Dooley BN, Cvello L (1972) Diagnostic considerations in mediastinal emphysema: a pathophysiologic-roentgenologic approach to Boerhaave's syndrome and spontaneous pneumomediastinum. Am J Roentgenol 115:495–511
68. Sagel SS (1983) Thoracic anatomy and mediastinum. In: Lee JKT (ed) Computed body tomography. Raven, New York, pp 55–97
69. Schlorf RA, L'Heureux P, Duvall AJ (1971) Value of chest roentgenograms in mediastinoscopy: a retrospective study. Arch Otolaryngol 94:486–489
70. Sealy WC (1974) Mediastinoscopy – does it have a place in the management of carcinoma of the lung? Ann Thorac Surg 18:433–436
71. Silverman PM, Newman GE, Korobkin M, Workman JB, Moore AV, Coleman RE (1984) Computed tomography in the evaluation of thyroid disease. AJR 142:897–902
72. Stallworth JM, Horne JB (1984) Diagnosis and management of thoracic outlet syndrome. Arch Surg 119:1149–1151
73. Sweet RH (1949) Intrathoracic goiter located in the posterior mediastinum. Surg Gynecol Obstet 89:57–66
74. Telford ED, Stopford JSB (1930–1931) The vascular complications of the cervical rib. Br J Surg 18:557–564
75. Thermann M, Poser H, Muller-Hermelink KH, Troidl H, Brieler S, Amend V, Schroder D (1984) Evaluation of tomography and mediastinoscopy for the detection of mediastinal lymph node metastases. Ann Thorac Surg 37:443–447
76. Vock P, Owens A (1982) Computed tomography of the normal and pathological thoracic inlet. Eur J Radiol 2:187–193
77. Wang CA (1977) Parathyroid reexploration: a clinical and pathological study of 112 cases. Ann Surg 186:140–145
78. Whalen JP, Oliphant M, Evans JA (1975) Anterior extrapleural line: superior extension. Radiology 115:525–531
79. Whitcomb ME, Barham E, Goldman AL, Green DC (1976) Indications for mediastinoscopy in bronchogenic carcinoma. Am Rev Respir Dis 113:189–195
80. Zylak CJ, Pallie W, Pirani M, Wandtke JC, Kothari K (1983) Anatomy and computed tomography: a correlative module on the cervicothoracic junction. Radiographics 3:478–533

5 The Anterior Mediastinum

5.1 General Anatomic Considerations

The anterior mediastinum is situated behind the sternum and in front of the great vessels and the pericardium. Its lateral margins are the mediastinal pleurae in contact with the anteromedial aspect of each lung (Figs. 5.1, 5.2, 5.8). Inferiorly, it reaches the diaphragm, while its upper limit is arbitrarily stated in most textbooks of anatomy as a line extending from the lower end of the manubrium of the sternum posteriorly to the inferior margin of the body of the fourth thoracic vertebra [18, 128]. For the purposes of this discussion, the anterior mediastinum can be considered to merge at its upper end with the thoracic inlet and to lie in front of the supra-azygos and infra-azygos areas on the right and the supra-aortic and infra-aortic areas on the left.

Bordering the anterior mediastinum in front is the transverse thoracic (transversus thoracis)

Fig. 5.1A, B. Boundaries of anterior mediastinum. **A** Transverse body section through level of aortic arch. **B** Transverse body section through level of left atrium. Anterior mediastinum is seen to lie between anterior aspects of two lungs immediately behind sternum. It is bounded posteriorly by great vessels above (2) and pericardium below (3). When two lungs meet to form anterior junction line (4), anterior mediastinum between them is potential space only. Anterior mediastinum is triangular in shape with apex directed toward sternum (1). Its lateral margins are concave or straight. Left internal mammary artery is clearly shown (5). Artery is accompanied by internal mammary vein; internal mammary lymph nodes are found in close proximity to internal mammary vessels

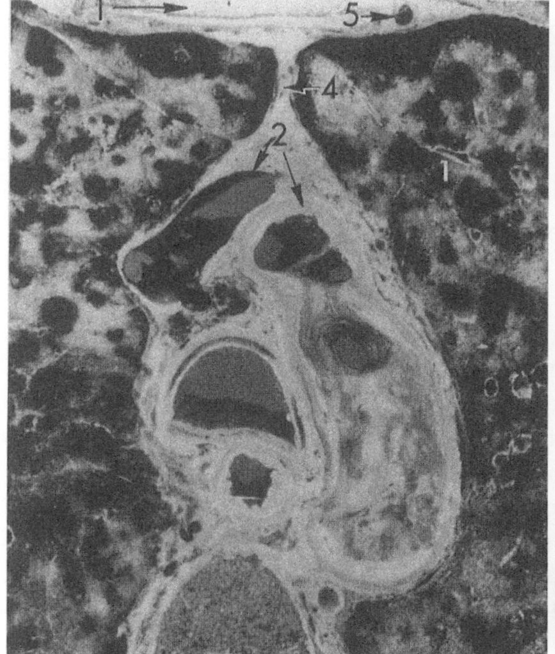

A

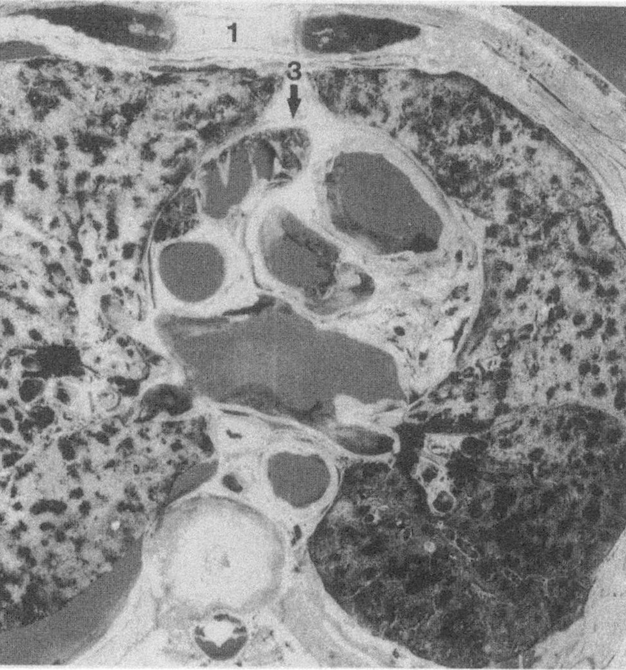

B

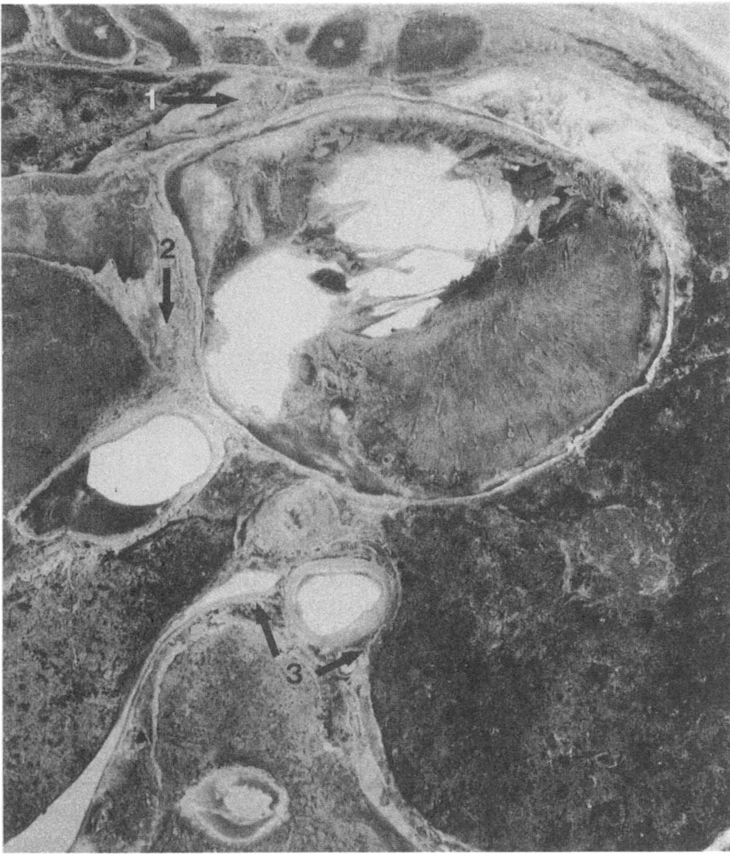

Fig. 5.2. Cardiophrenic angle nodes. (Anterior and middle diaphragmatic nodes.) Transverse body section. Anterior diaphragmatic nodes are situated behind xiphoid process and costal cartilage of seventh rib on either side (*1*). Middle group of diaphragmatic nodes are found close to point of entry of phrenic nerves into diaphragm. On right side, they lie anterior to inferior vena cava (*2*). They are often absent on left. Posterior group of diaphragmatic nodes lie in back of diaphragmatic crura (*3*)

muscle. This thin muscle plane originates from the lower third of the sternum, from the xiphoid, and from the costal cartilages of the lower three or four true ribs on either side. Its fibers spread out in fan-like fashion to be inserted into the medial ends of the second to the sixth ribs and into their costal cartilages [128].

The internal mammary artery (Figs. 5.1, 5.28) arises from the first part of the subclavian artery on each side just before that vessel passes under the scalenus anterior muscle. It courses forward and then downward behind the sternal end of the clavicle and behind the costal cartilages where it lies between the transverse thoracic muscle and the parietal pleura. It is accompanied by the internal mammary vein.

The internal mammary lymph nodes are situated medially in the intercostal spaces adjacent to the internal mammary vessels, lying as often medial to these vessels as lateral to them [125].

Urban and Marjani state that lymph nodes are found in the intercostal spaces with the following frequency: first intercostal space, 88%; second, 84%; third, 73%; fourth, 46%; and fifth, 12% [125]. These lymphatic channels drain the breast, the upper portion of the liver, the anterior abdominal wall above the umbilicus, and the anterior chest wall. They course cephalad to empty into the thoracic duct or its tributaries.

The anterior mediastinum also contains, at its lower limit, the anterior and middle diaphragmatic nodes [128], sometimes called the "nodes of the cardiophrenic angle" [16]. The anterior group is situated behind the xiphoid process and the costal cartilage of the seventh rib (Fig. 5.2). These nodes receive drainage from the anterior portion of the diaphragm and the liver; their efferent vessels pass to the internal mammary lymph nodes [16, 128]. The middle set of nodes is found close to the point of entry of the phrenic nerves into the diaphragm. They are often absent on the left side [16]. On the right side, some of these nodes lie within the pericardium in front of the inferior vena cava [128] (Fig. 5.2). These nodes also receive drainage from the diaphragm and the liver; their efferents pass into posteriorly situated nodes about the esophagus.

The posterior group of diaphragmatic nodes lies on the back of the diaphragmatic crura and is connected with the middle cardiophrenic angle nodes and the posterior mediastinal nodes [128]. They are discussed further in chapter 7. The anterior mediastinum is otherwise filled with areolar tissue and fat (Figs. 5.1, 5.2, 5.7).

5.1.1 Pleural Reflections of the Anterior Mediastinum

5.1.1.1 The Anterior Junction Line

The pleural reflections bordering the anterior mediastinum can often be identified on plain frontal radiographs, are very commonly seen on frontal tomograms made through the anterior part of the chest and are always identified on computed tomographic scans.

At their cephalad limit, the pleurae reflect off the great vessels, especially the more anteriorly situated innominate (brachiocephalic) veins, and progress inferiorly and medially (see Figs. 4.1, 4.4, 5.3, 5.4, and 5.5). They often contact one another, forming the anterior junction line (Figs. 5.3 and 5.4).

Since the extreme anterior portions of the lungs contact each other only from the manubrium downward, the anterior junction line has, as its upper limit, the sternal notch (Figs. 5.3, 5.4). Below, it extends to the point of contact of the heart with the retrosternal soft tissues (Fig. 5.3). In emphysematous and kyphotic individuals, the anterior junction line is usually prolonged further caudad than it is in normal subjects due to the larger volume of the lung in front of the heart. In fact, the length of the normal anterior junction line is quite variable. It usually runs downward to the left in a slightly oblique course (Figs. 5.3 and 5.4), in contrast to the posterior junction line, which almost al-

ways has a straight vertical orientation (Fig. 5.4). The deviation of the lower end of the anterior junction line to the left is apparently related to the left-sided position of the heart. The two leaves of the pleura that form the line diverge at their lower end to pass around the heart (Fig. 5.3). Many years ago, Knutsson noted this configuration of the anterior pleurae at the cardiac level and equated it with the "area of absolute cardiac dullness" [69]. Although the anterior junction line deviates to the left as it descends, computed tomographic studies show that its anterior limit may lie to the left or to the right of its posterior extent (Fig. 5.4). For this reason, the anterior junction line is not infrequently seen better on oblique radiographs than it is on frontal views.

The anterior junction line can be distinguished easily from the posterior junction line on frontal radiographs in most instances (see Table 5.1). The anterior junction line does not extend above the sternal notch, whereas the posterior junction line does. The anterior junction line deflects to the left at its lower end; the posterior junction line has a straight vertical orientation or shows a gentle convexity directed to the left as it extends caudally. The upper end of the anterior junction line often presents a highly characteristic radiographic appearance where it meets the pleural reflections over the innominate veins, forming an anterior triangle on PA and AP radiographs (Figs. 5.3, 5.4, and

Table 5.1. Radiographic characteristics of the anterior and posterior junction lines

Anterior
1. Reflects superiorly off innominate veins (does not extend above sternoclavicular notch)
2. Reflects inferiorly over heart
3. Inclines to the left as it progresses caudally
4. Anterior aspect may lie to right or left of posterior portion; may be better seen on oblique radiographs

Posterior
1. Reflects superiorly off lung apices (extends above sternoclavicular notch)
2. Reflects inferiorly over superior intercostal veins and azygos vein on the right and the aortic arch on the left.
3. Does not incline to right or left as it progresses caudally

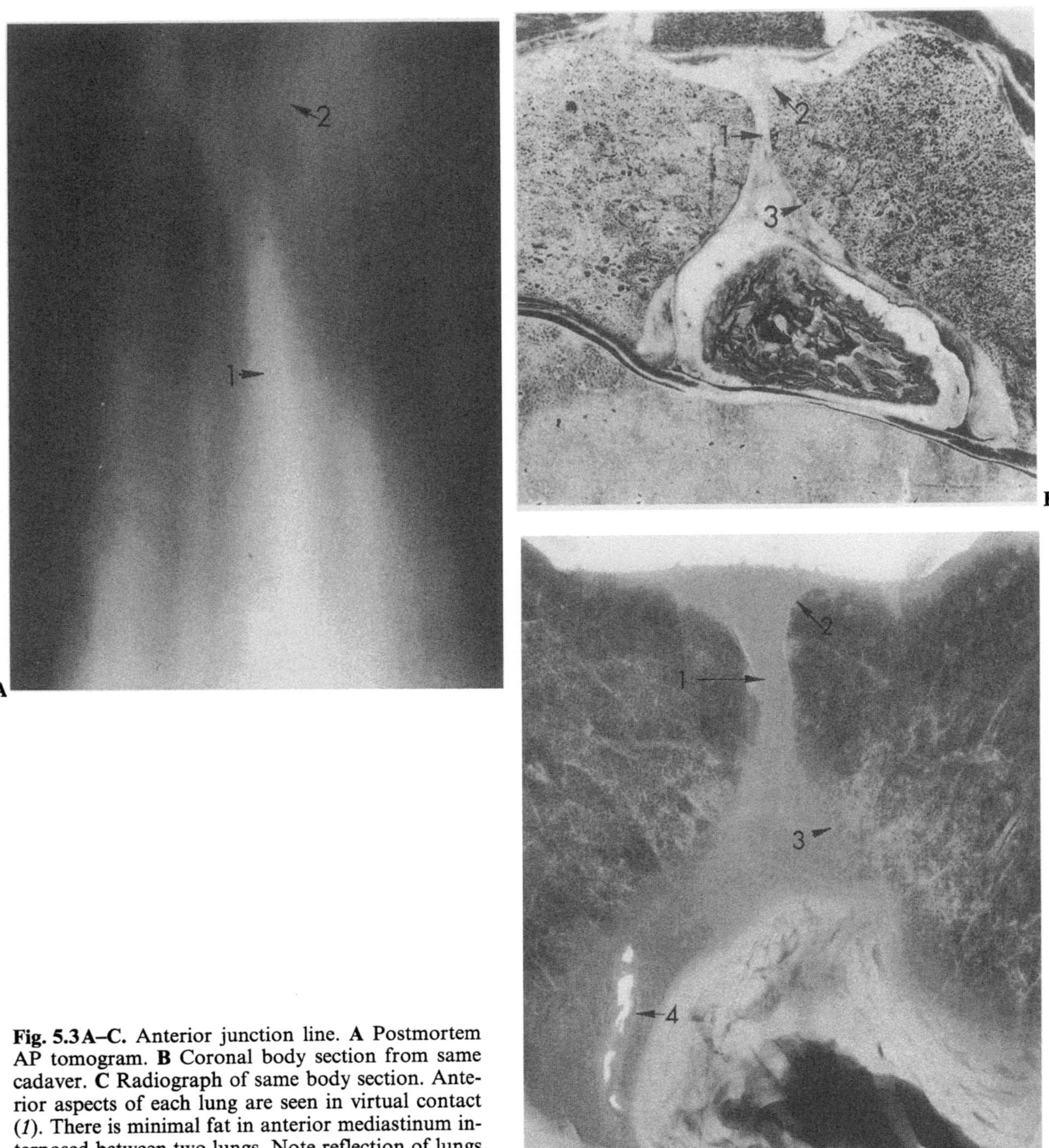

Fig. 5.3A–C. Anterior junction line. **A** Postmortem AP tomogram. **B** Coronal body section from same cadaver. **C** Radiograph of same body section. Anterior aspects of each lung are seen in virtual contact (*1*). There is minimal fat in anterior mediastinum interposed between two lungs. Note reflection of lungs cephalad over fat that lies in front of great vessels (*2*), and reflection of two lungs caudad over fat about heart (*3*). Calcification of right coronary artery is shown in **C** (*4*)

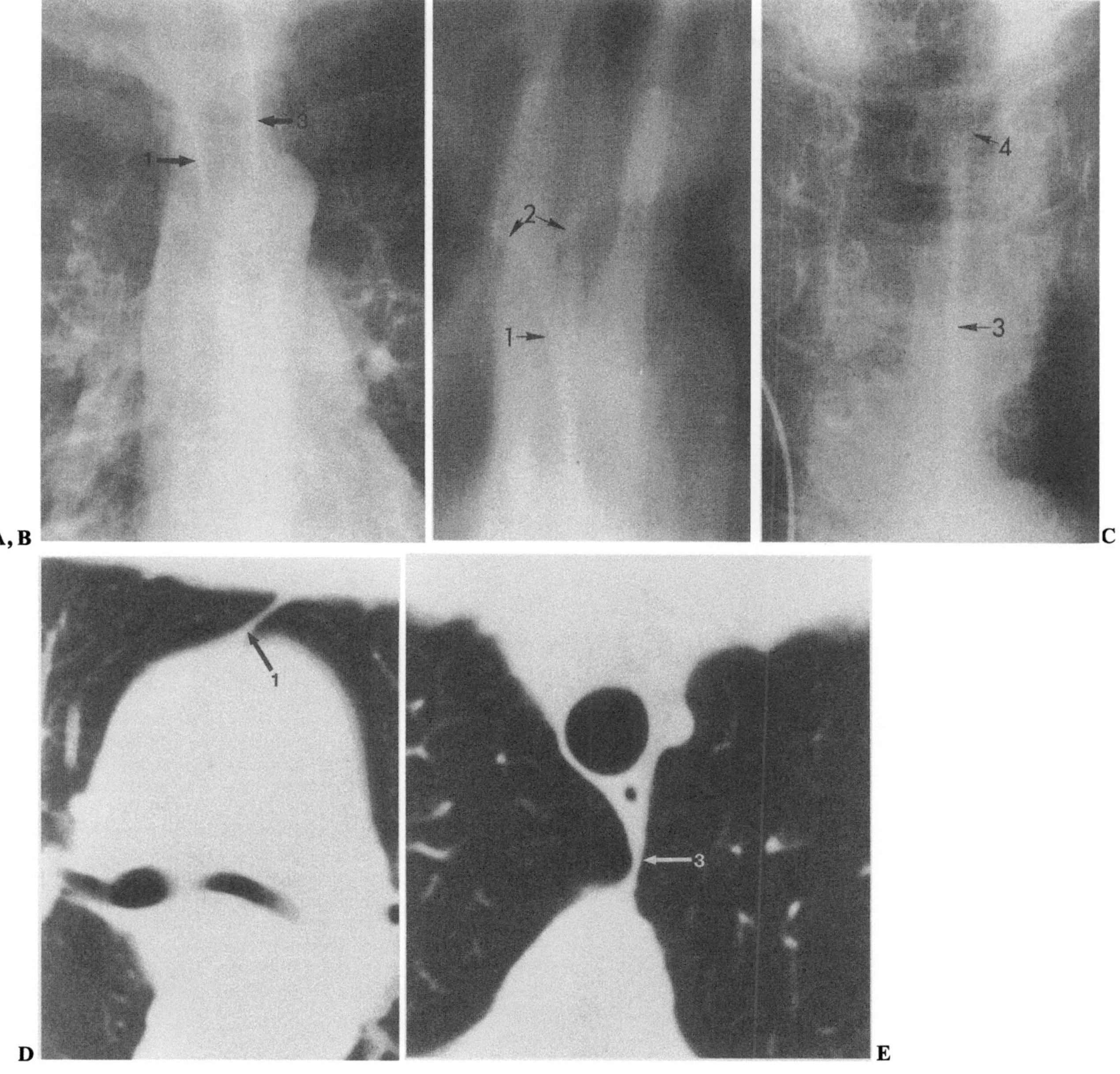

Fig. 5.4 A–E. Anterior and posterior junction line contrasted. **A** PA radiograph. **B** AP tomogram. **C** PA radiograph. **D** and **E** Computed tomogram. Anterior junction line (*1*) can be seen reflecting off shadows of innominate veins (*2*) and extending obliquely downward to left. Posterior junction line (*3*) can be seen reflecting off pulmonary apices (*4*) and descending in straight vertical direction behind the esophagus to diverge over azygos arch and aortic arch

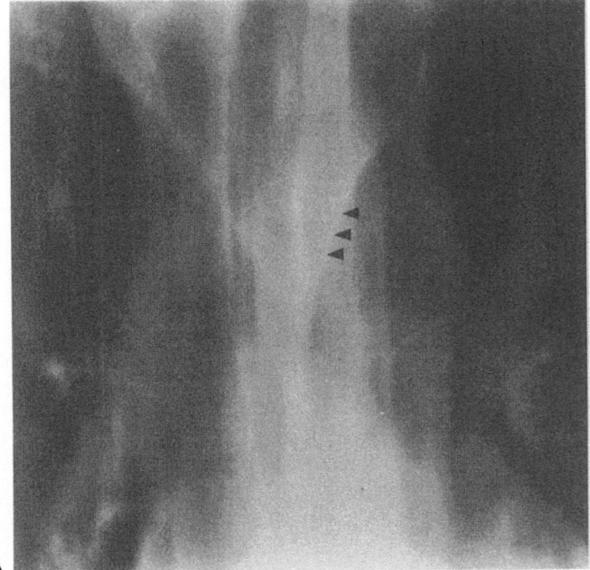

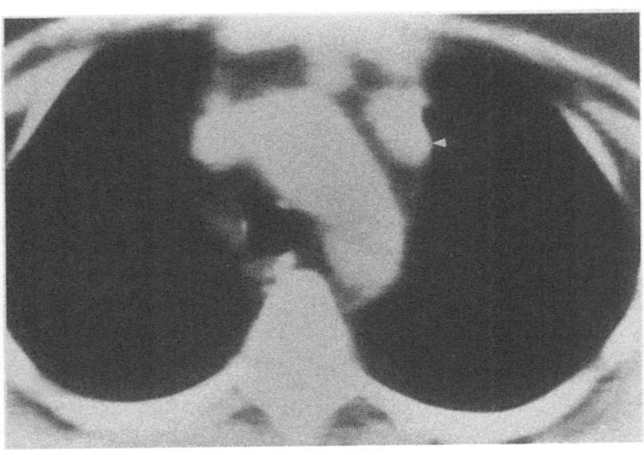

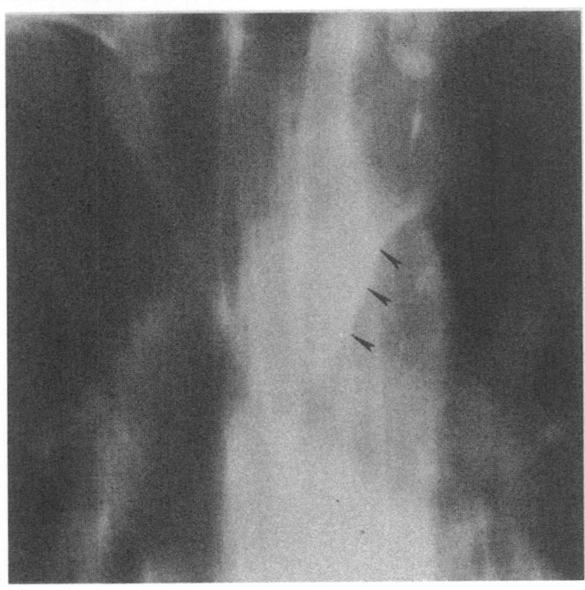

Fig. 5.5 A–C. Distortion of anterior mediastinal contours by mass. **A** and **B** AP tomograms. **C** Computed tomogram, **B** and **C** made 13 months after **A**. The anterior lung margins reflect off the brachiocephalic veins to produce an anterior triangle on PA and AP radiographs. When the lungs meet below the triangle, the anterior junction line is formed. In this case, subtle distortion of the anterior triangle in **B** (*triple arrows*) was not present on the AP tomogram (**A**), made 13 months earlier. The mass which produced the distortion is demonstrated in **C** (*single arrow*) and was a thymic carcinoid. (**A** and **B** From [37])

5.5), while the posterior junction line can be recognized due to its reflection over the azygos arch in front of the right superior intercostal vein and over the posterior aortic arch (Fig. 5.4). Differentiation of the anterior junction line from the posterior can be important. "Silhouetting out" of the lines or their distortion by pathology can serve to localize the process anteriorly or posteriorly on frontal radiographs (Fig. 5.5).

The interposition of pathologic processes between the anterior margins of the two lungs sep-arates them an thus causes the anterior triangle and/or the posterior junction line to be obliterated. A widened anterior or "superior" mediastinum is the result (Fig. 5.5, 5.6); sometimes widening of the anterior mediastinum may be considered questionable on frontal radiographs, and abnormalities in this area may be equally difficult to see on lateral films. Another problem frequently encountered is that of the widened upper mediastinum discovered as an incidental finding. Often, one is tempted to consider that the finding is an anatomic variant and to pursue

Fig. 5.6. Widening of anterior mediastinum PA radiograph. Anterior margins of each lung can be seen to be displaced laterally (*1*). These interfaces can be recognized as being anterior because their upper ends are lost at level of clavicle (the cervicothoracic sign, see chapter 4). Interface between anterior mediastinum and left lung is projected farther lateral than aortic knob (*2*), a finding strongly suggestive of a widened left anterior mediastinum (see chapter 6). On left side, process extends cephalad over lung apex (*3*). At this point pathologic process is posteriorly situated

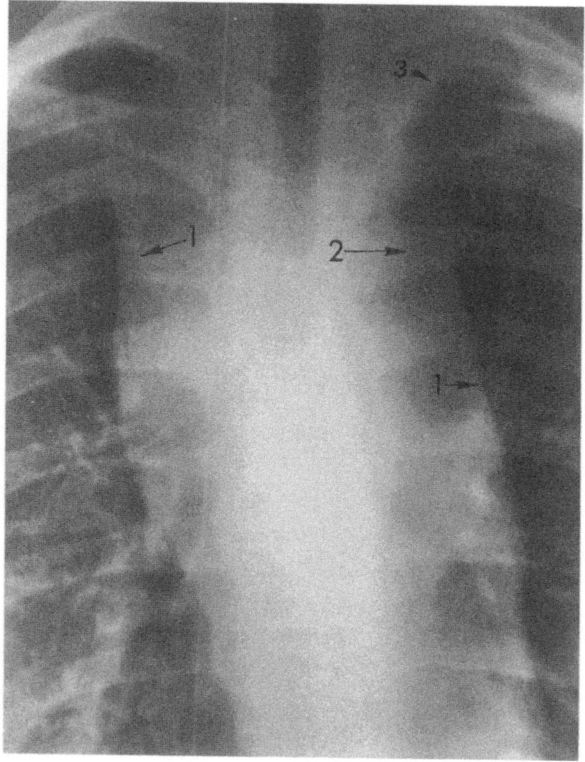

Fig. 5.7A, B. Anterior mediastinal fat. **A** Coronal body section. **B** Computed tomogram. Anterior mediastinum is widened by fat (*1*) more commonly than is generally appreciated. Although such a situation may cause conventional radiographs to appear abnormal, the innocent nature of mediastinum so infiltrated can be readily determined by computed tomography (*arrow*)
▽

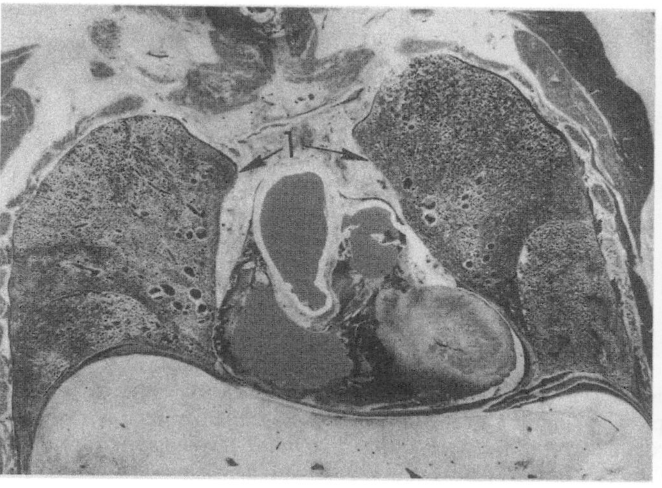

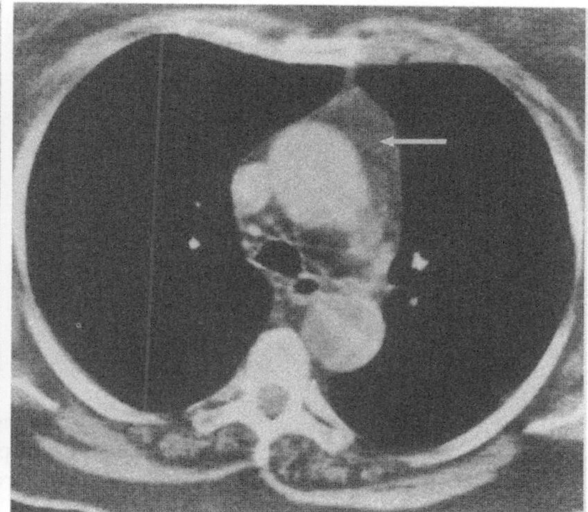

A   B

it no further. However, there is always a nagging doubt that disease may be overlooked. Computed tomography is an ideal modality to solve these dilemmas [2, 127]. In a study by Baron et al. [2], computed tomograms identified 92% of the normal variants responsible for the widening. Since this was a report relatively early in the utilization of computed tomography, it is likely that better results would be achieved today.

The mediastinum in its upper portion is often widened by normal fat accumulations (Fig. 5.7). Computed tomograms are very helpful in resolving this problem as they readily show the widening to be caused by lucent adipose tissue (see Figs. 4.12, 4.13, and 5.7). They also prove

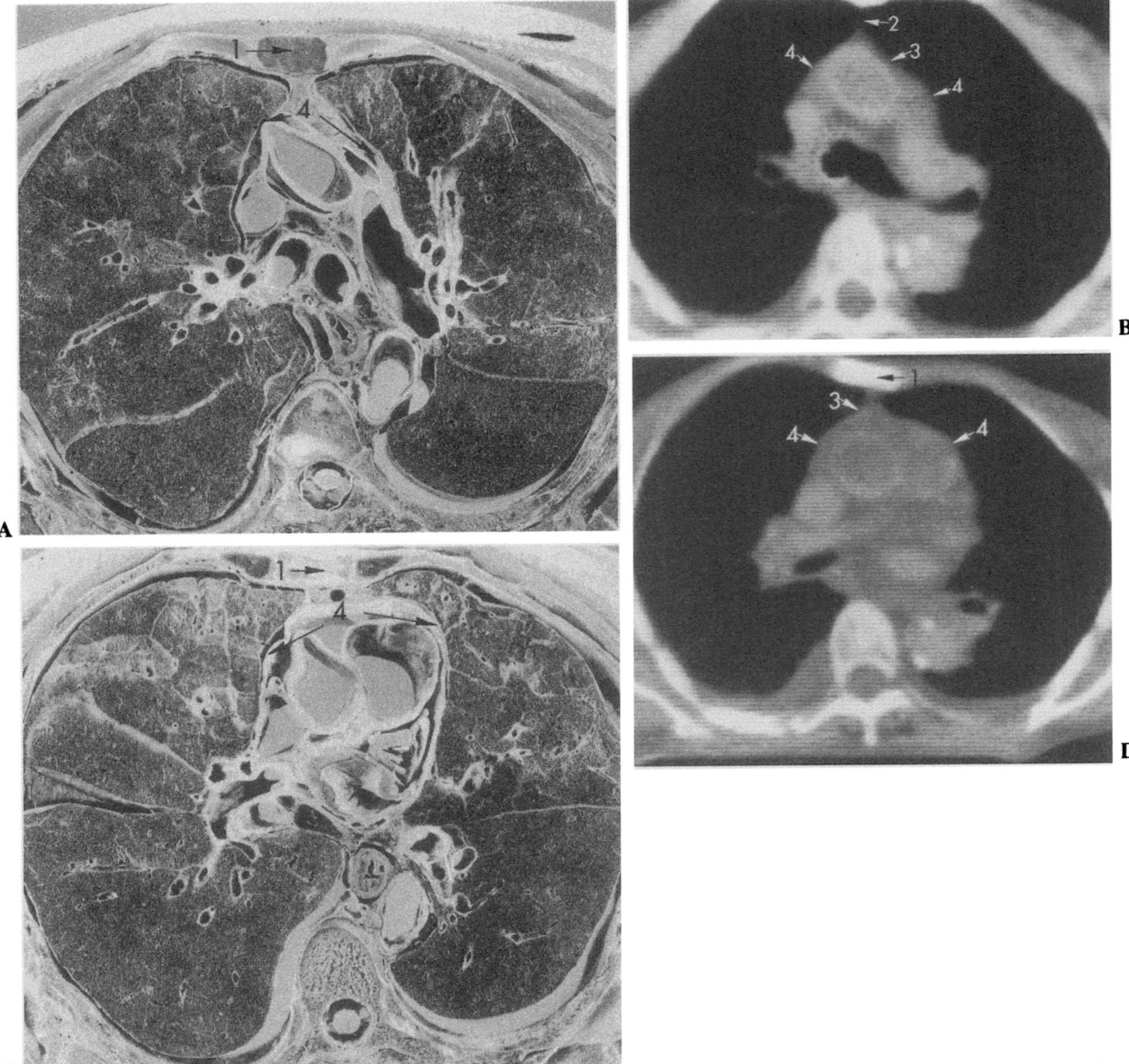

Fig. 5.8A–D. The shape of mediastinum in transverse projection. Transverse body section (**A**) and computed tomogram (**B**) of the same cadaver at same level through left pulmonary artery. Transverse body section (**C**) and computed body tomogram (**D**) of same cadaver at same level through right pulmonary artery. Characteristic triangular configuration of anterior mediastinum in axial sections is demonstrated. Apex is directed at sternum (*1*) and may become confluent with anterior junction line (*2*). Between apposed pleurae forming anterior junction line, anterior mediastinum exists as potential space only. Lateral margins of mediastinum are concave or straight (*3*), except for convex bulges produced by impressions of aorta and main pulmonary artery (*4*). Presence of anterior junction line effectively precludes anterior mediastinal disease at level of section

the innocence of the mediastinum widened by prominent great vessels. Computed tomograms show the upper portion of the anterior mediastinum to be triangular in shape with its base against the pericardium; except for the convex bulges representing the aorta, pulmonary artery, and the superior vena cava, its lateral margins are straight or show a concavity directed laterally (Figs. 5.1, 5.8); convex lateral margins generally suggest disease (Fig. 5.5). Total apposition of the pleurae marginating the anterior mediastinum produces the anterior junction line and effectively excludes gross disease at the level of the scan (Fig. 5.8). Failure to visualize an anterior junction line formerly present on serial radiographic examinations suggests that something has been interposed between the two lungs and should be considered as a sign of probable mediastinal disease.

5.1.1.2 The Anterior Extrapleural Line and the Cardiac Incisura

At the forward limit of the anterior junction line behind the sternum, the pleural interfaces diverge over the anterior aspect of each pleural cavity (Fig. 5.9). In normal individuals the anterior lungs reach the anterior chest wall, and the retrosternal area above the heart is entirely radiolucent. No significant stripe of increased density is seen posterior to the sternum on films made in a true lateral projection (Fig. 5.9). Disease processes may separate the anterior lung surfaces from the anterior chest wall to produce a linear or undulating line paralleling the sternum (see Figs. 5.27, 5.29, 5.32, 5.33, and 5.36). This line has been termed the "anterior extrapleural line" [131] or the "retrosternal line" [60, 130]. The presence of such a line on lateral radiographs is a variant of the extrapleural sign and is strong evidence in support of an extrapleural mass residing in the anterior mediastinum. However, it should be kept in mind that lateral radiographs that are not true lateral projections may demonstrate a line behind the sternum and parallel to it (Fig. 5.9). This line merely represents the contact of lung with one side of the anterior chest wall, projected behind the

contact of the other lung with the opposite anterior chest wall. For the same reason, such a line is also seen when one hemithorax cannot be inflated to as great a degree as the other. Similarly, the line is encountered when one hemithorax is smaller than the other, as in hypogenetic lung syndrome (Fig. 5.10). Apparently, in these patients the space between the anterior lung margin and the chest wall is filled in by areolar tissue [23]. Care should be taken not to mistake these causes for a linear retrosternal shadow from true extrapleural disease. Repeat radiographs in a true lateral projection will eliminate one pitfall; inspection of the patient will sometimes remove the other.

A shadow related to the anterior extrapleural line is commonly seen overlying the cardiac silhouette on lateral radiographs. As one follows the interface of the left lung with the anterior chest wall downward on lateral films, the line of contact frequently deviates posteriorly as the diaphragm is approached (Figs. 5.11 and 5.12). This appearance is due to the presence of the heart and pericardial fat which, when interposed between lung and anterior chest wall, prevents their contact. Under these conditions, the left lung can reach the chest wall lateral to the heart only (Fig. 5.11), and in many persons this point of contact is projected behind the anterior aspect of the right lung on lateral chest radiographs. The resulting X-ray appearance is a variant of the anterior extrapleural line [130]. This exclusion of lung by the heart and pericardial fat has been called "the cardiac incisura" [95] and corresponds to the "area of absolute cardiac dullness" described by Knutsson [69]. The configuration of the radiographic counterpart of the cardiac incisura on lateral films is variable. In some individuals in whom lung extends anterior to the heart, no shadow is identified. In others, the incisura appears as a tall triangle with a narrow base against the diaphragm and with an apex that lies at the most superior point of contact of the heart against the anterior chest wall. In still other individuals, the incisura has a broad base lying against the diaphragm. Its posterior edge may be irregularly serrated or may extend downward in a curvilinear fashion with a concavity directed posterior-

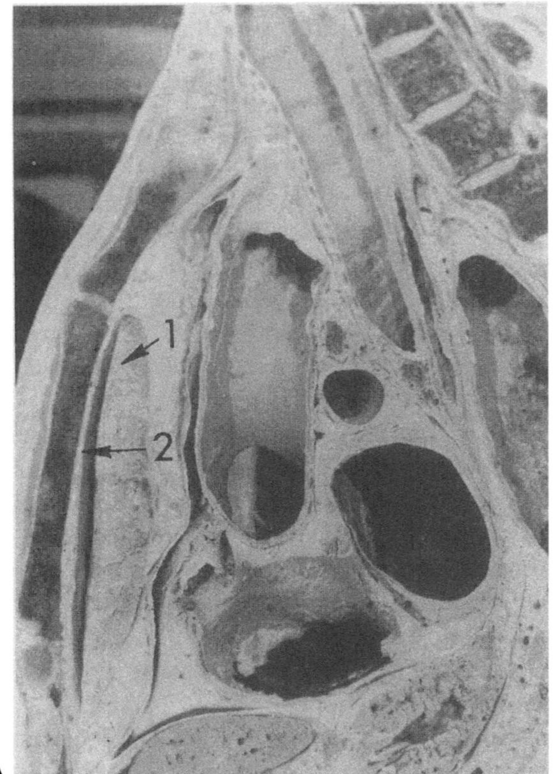

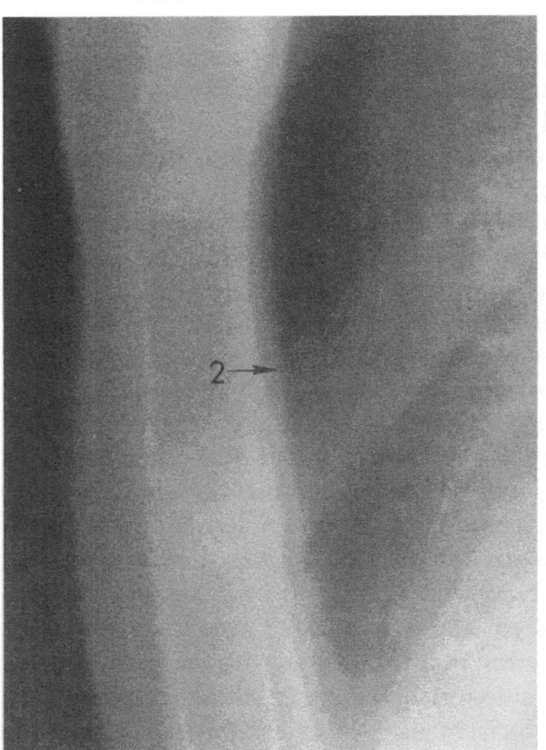

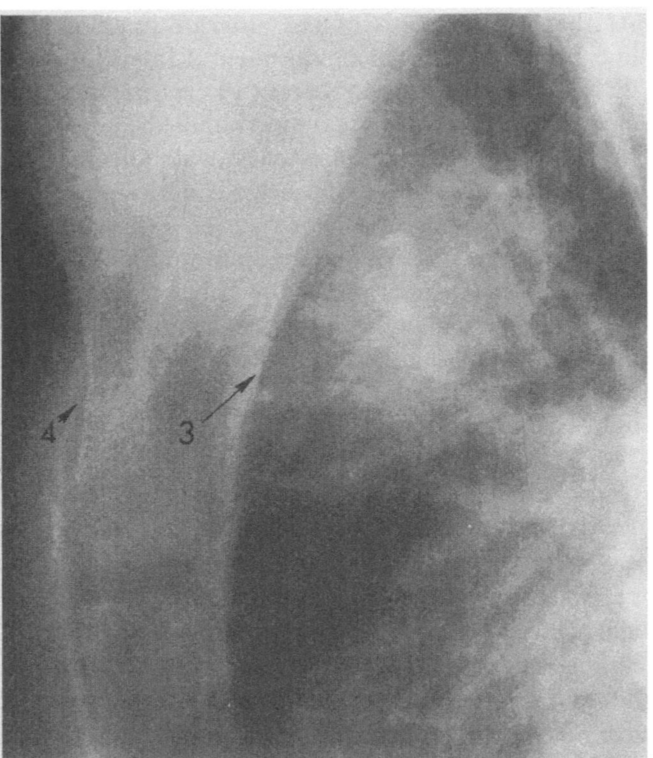

Fig. 5.9 A–C. Anterior mediastinum (lateral view).
A Sagittal body section through plane slightly to left of midline of thorax. **B** Lateral radiograph. **C** Lateral film made with moderate obliquity. Aerated lung (*1*) lies anterior to great vessels and upper portion of heart separated from sternum only by visceral and parietal pleurae and minimal retrosternal fat (*2*). Lateral film projected somewhat off true lateral suggests retrosternal abnormality (*3*). This interface, however, represents anterior surface of right lung against right anterior chest wall due to obliquity. This interface is projected behind interface of anterior aspect of left lung against left anterior chest wall (*4*)

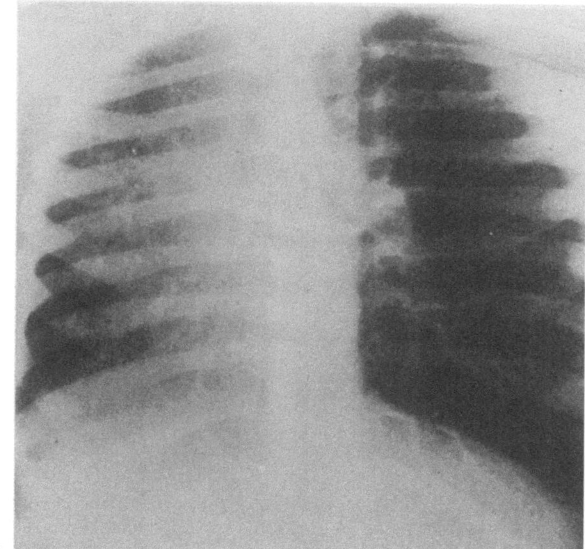

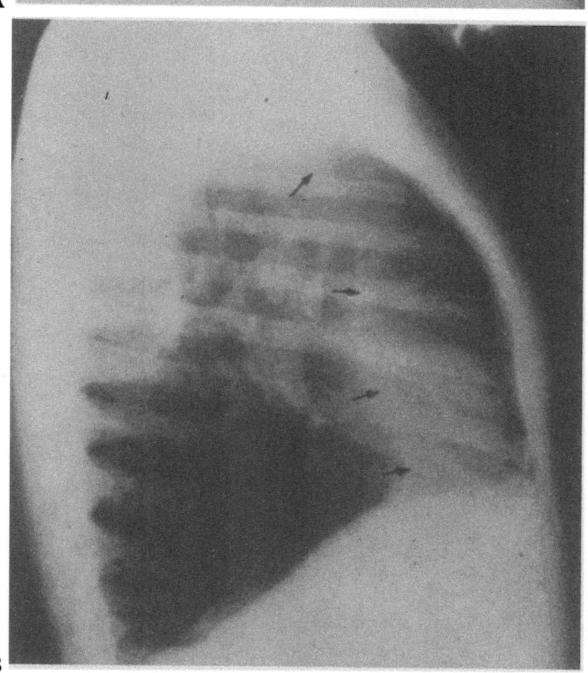

Fig. 5.10A, B. Hypogenetic lung PA (**A**) and lateral (**B**) radiographs. PA radiograph shows small right hemithorax with heart and mediastinum shifted to right side. Anterior aspect of this small right lung extends only to point well behind sternum (*arrows*). Remainder of space between anterior right lung and right chest wall is filled with alveolar tissue and fat. (From [23])

ly. Some of the different patterns of the cardiac incisura are shown in Figs. 5.11 and 5.12. Whalen et al. [130] and Shopfner et al. [113] show lateral radiographs that demonstrate a variation in the radiographic appearance of the cardiac incisura. This is a vertical stripe of increased density outlined by radiolucency in front of and behind it, superimposed over the cardiac shadow (Fig. 5.12). Whalen et al. attribute the area of density to the cardiac incisura, the anterior radiolucency to retrosternal fat, and the posterior radiolucency to the left lung [130]. At times, the line appears to represent anterior mediastinal soft tissues outlined between retrosternal fat and fat over the anterior aspect of the heart.

At times it may be difficult to distinguish the cardiac incisura from extrapleural disease in the same location. Authors who have considered the radiographic appearance of the cardiac incisura [60, 69, 130] have emphasized that the appearance of the incisura changes on lateral films made in inspiration and expiration (Fig. 5.12). The incisura is minimized in deep inspiration; if this phenomenon can be demonstrated, a cardiophrenic angle mass is less likely. One should bear in mind, however, that lesions such as pericardial cysts and even thymolipomas may change their appearance from inspiration to expiration as well. At times computed tomography will be necessary to make a definitive diagnosis.

The anatomic principles underlying the appearance of the cardiac incisura can be used to explain the gross difference in the appearance of the left heart border sometimes seen on frontal films made in various body positions. The left heart border may be clearly seen on an erect or recumbent film and not on a decubitus study made at the same time. On some decubitus films made with the left side down, the heart may drop to the left, excluding more lung from the anterior left chest than on the erect or recumbent study. If sufficient lung is displaced posteriorly so that the frontal X-ray beam is not parallel to the heart-lung interface, the left heart border may be poorly seen (Fig. 5.13).

Keats has pointed out a vertical line that he had identified in the lower mediastinum superimposed on the right side of the heart [60]

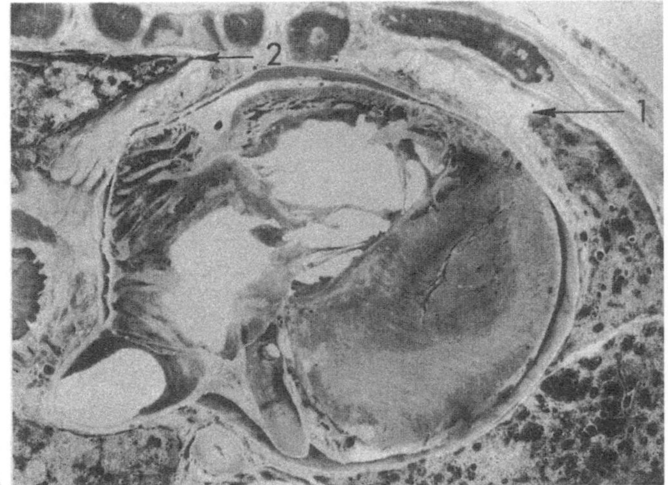

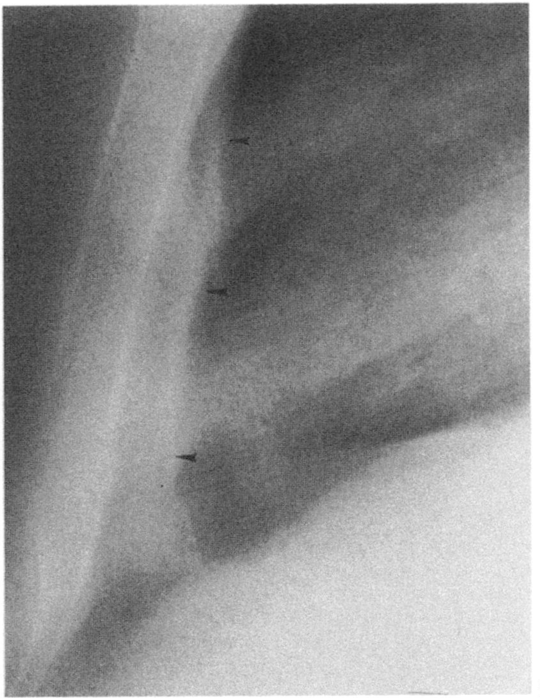

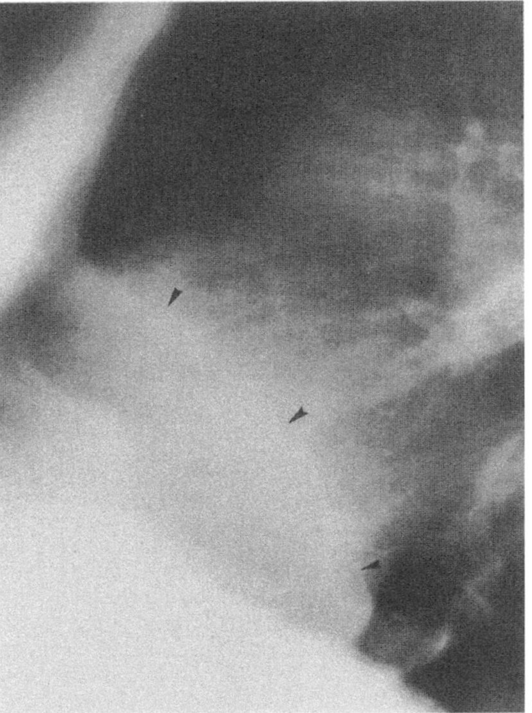

Fig. 5.11A–C. Anterior extrapleural line (the cardiac incisura). **A** Transverse body section. **B** and **C** Lateral radiograph. Due to presence of heart, left lung often cannot extend as far forward along anterior chest wall (*1*) as does right lung (*2*). Under these conditions, lateral radiographs will show anterior aspect of left lung contacting left anterior chest wall above diaphragm behind contact of right lung with right anterior chest wall (*arrows*). Resulting configurations are quite varied (see also Fig. 5.12)

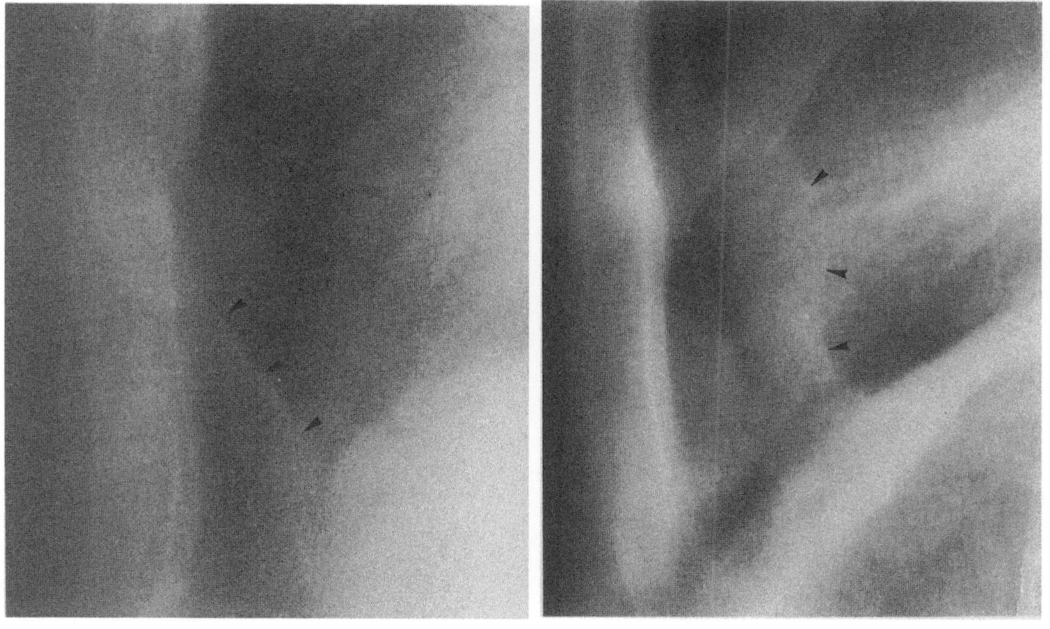

Fig. 5.12A, B. Anterior extrapleural line (the cardiac incisura). **A** Lateral radiograph made in inspiration. **B** Relative expiration. Gross change in configuration of contact of left lung with left chest wall producing cardiac incisura is clearly seen on inspiration and expiration films (*arrows*). Such a change may be helpful in distinguishing cardiac incisura from solid cardiophrenic angle mass

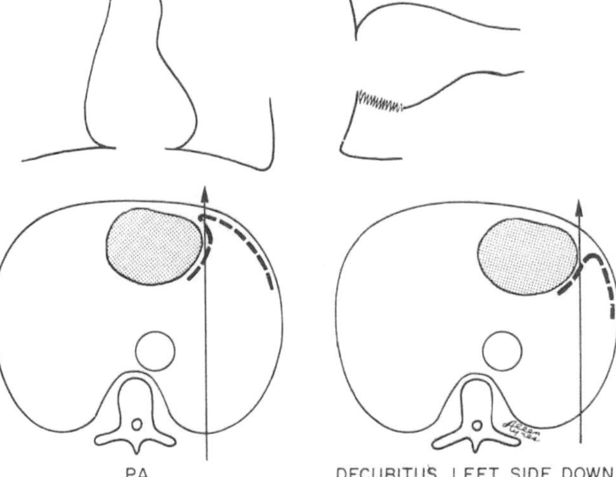

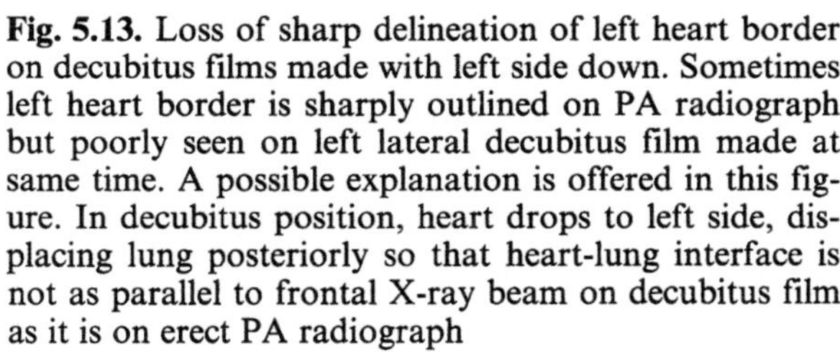

Fig. 5.13. Loss of sharp delineation of left heart border on decubitus films made with left side down. Sometimes left heart border is sharply outlined on PA radiograph but poorly seen on left lateral decubitus film made at same time. A possible explanation is offered in this figure. In decubitus position, heart drops to left side, displacing lung posteriorly so that heart-lung interface is not as parallel to frontal X-ray beam on decubitus film as it is on erect PA radiograph

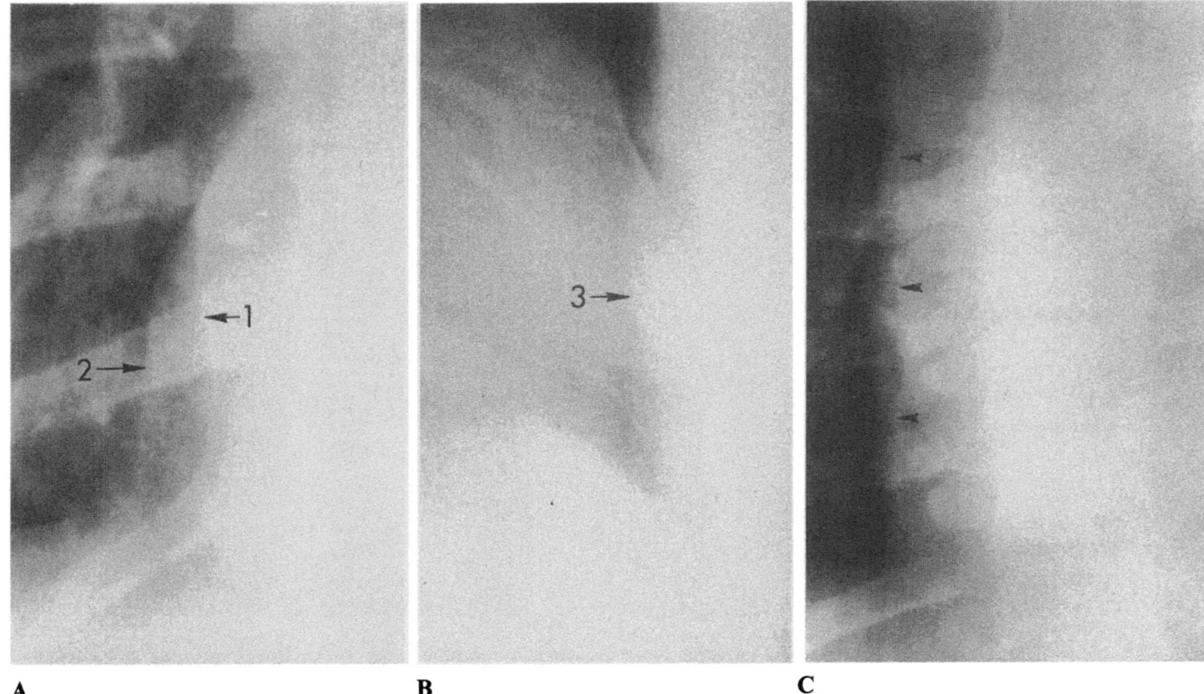

A   B   C

Fig. 5.14A–C. Right parasternal stripe. PA (**A**) and lateral (**B**) radiographs. **C** PA Radiograph. Vertical interface (*1*) is sometimes seen on frontal radiographs through shadow of right atrium (*2*). This can be shown to be anterior (*3*) and is variant of anterior extrapleural line on right side. When normal, appearance of this line is said to change from inspiration to expiration, thus allowing it to be distinguished from similar interface produced by disease. Retrosternal line shown in **C** (*arrows*) was due to involvement of anterior mediastinal nodes by Hodgkin's disease

(Fig. 5.14). He has termed this line the "right parasternal stripe" and feels that it represents the counterpart on frontal films of the inferior aspect of the anterior extrapleural line on the right side. It, too, changes its appearance on expiration and inspiration films.

In a discussion of the anterior extrapleural line some consideration should be given to the role played by the transverse thoracic muscle in the production of a linear retrosternal shadow. Although several authors have claimed that this muscle can produce such a shadow in adults and children [97, 108, 113], this fact has been contested by Whalen et al. [130]. Although we have not made a specific study of this problem, our review of adult anatomic specimens suggests that the transverse thoracic muscle is rarely, if ever, thick enough to cast a recognizable shadow on lateral radiographs of adult patients.

5.1.1.3 Pleural Reflections Over the Anterior Diaphragm

The parietal pleura over the lower anterior mediastinum and anterior chest wall reflects over the anterior diaphragmatic attachments. The anterior aspect of the diaphragm has a sternal origin represented by two fleshy strips arising from the xiphoid process (Fig. 5.15) and a costal origin from the lower anterior ribs [18] (Fig. 5.15).

Between the sternal and costal origins of the diaphragm lie small apertures sometimes referred to as the "sternocostal triangles" (foramina of Morgagni) for passage of the internal mammary (internal thoracic) artery and vein and lymphatics from the anterior abdominal wall and dome of the liver. Kleinman and Raptopoulos [67] have correlated the radiologic appearance of these diaphragmatic attachments and the potential spaces between them with the underlying anatomy. When enlarged, the sternocostal triangles may be the site of upward

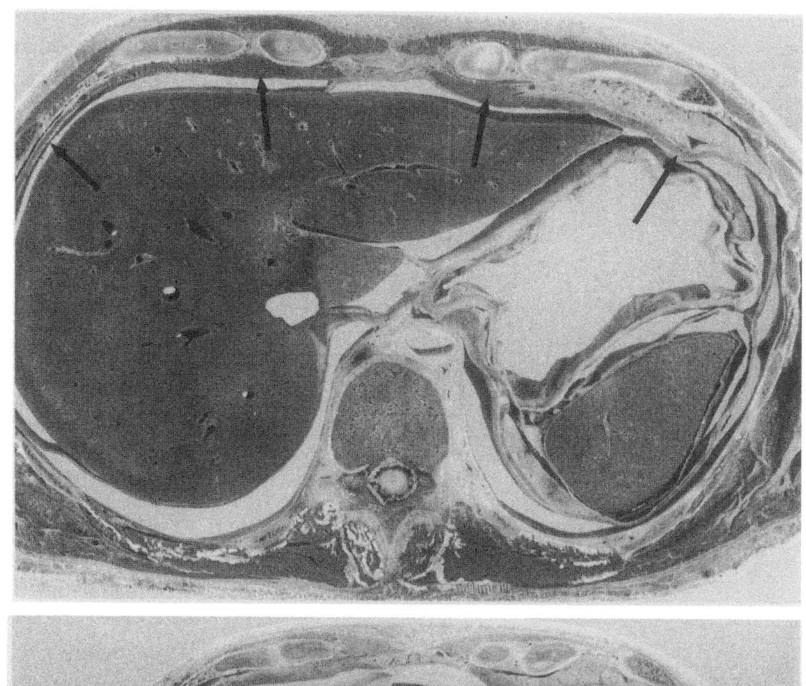

A

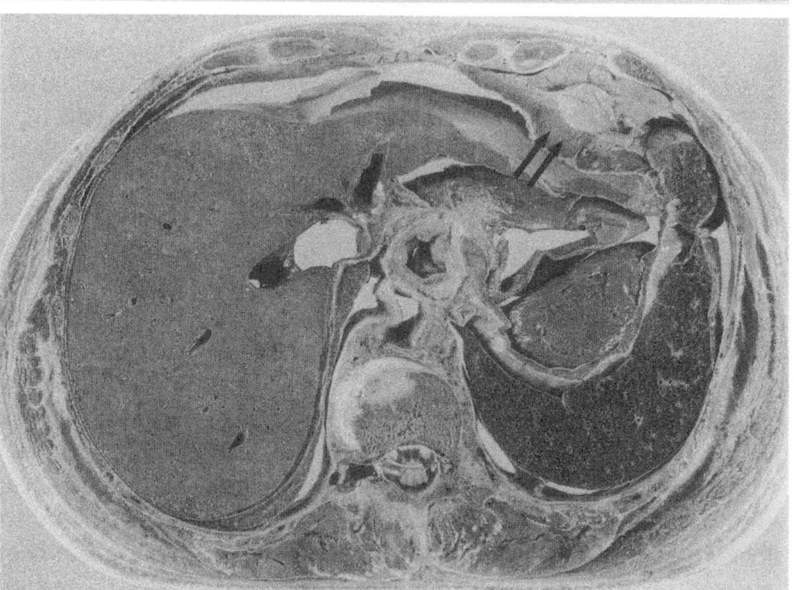

B

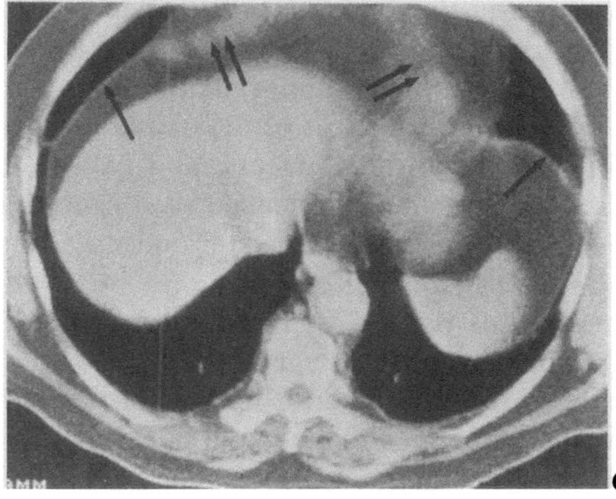

C

Fig. 5.15A–C. Anterior attachments of the diaphragm (**A** and **B**). Transverse body sections. **C** Computed tomogram. The anterior diaphragm usually crosses the midline in a continuous arc attached to the anterior ribs and sternum as seen in **A** and, on computed tomograms, is seen as a smooth or slightly undulating, continuous line as shown laterally in **C** (*single arrow*). If the central leaflet has a significantly domed characteristic, its sloping margins present broad, poorly marginated shadows on computed tomograms (**C**) (*double arrows*) closer together on more cephalad sections than on caudad ones

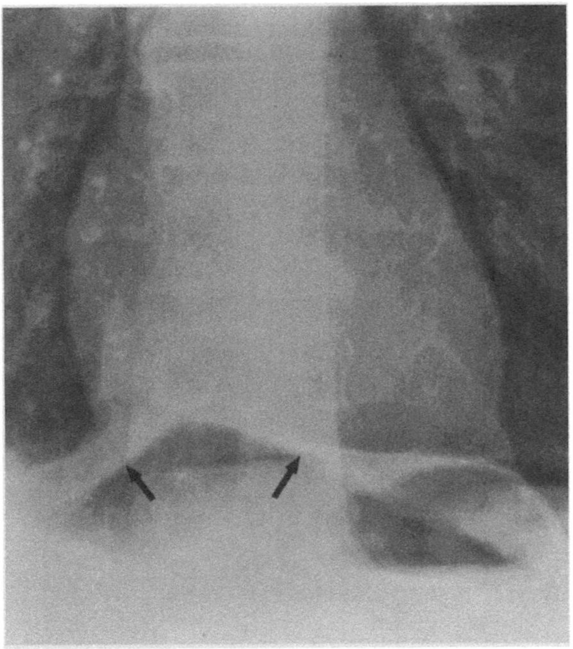

Fig. 5.16. Intraperitoneal air collected beneath the central leaflet of the diaphragm PA radiograph. Intraperitoneal air is seen below the anterior diaphragmatic attachments (*arrows*). The area under and behind these attachments is called the "central leaflet." Compare with Fig. 5.15

herniation of abdominal viscera, the so-called hernia of the foramen of Morgagni. The cephalad advance of properitoneal fat covering the herniated viscera may produce an arcuate lucency behind the lower sternum resembling an inverted letter J. This finding has been described by Lanuza [74] as the sign of the cane. It constitutes one more observation emphasizing the importance of careful attention to fat shadows as discussed in this and other chapters. Kleinman et al. [68] have shown this opening to be a pathway for mediastinal air to reach the extraperitoneal tissues of the anterior abdomen.

The anterior origins of the diaphragm are its most cephalad attachments, and behind them lies an area sometimes called the "central leaflet" [18]. Pneumoperitoneum and occasionally gas in the stomach or colon may be identified under this portion of the diaphragm and can produce unusual appearances [49, 68] (Fig. 5.16). The superior portion of this part of the diaphragm is the area outlined by air in the continuous diaphragm sign.

If the central leaflet has a significantly domed characteristic, its sloping margins may result in variant appearances on computed tomograms as recently described by Gale [49] (Fig. 5.15). The pleural reflections of the anterior mediastinum can be distorted by the normal thymus and by anterior mediastinal masses. These changes are discussed in the following sections.

5.1.2 The Normal Thymus

The thymus gland develops from the third branchial pouch; sometimes portions of the gland develop from the fourth pouch as well [128]. It consists of two almost totally distinct lateral lobes situated in the midline extending from the lower poles of the thyroid gland across the thoracic inlet to the level of the fourth costal cartilage. Below, it lies in front of the great vessels and the pericardium. Quottromani et al. [102] have reported the thymus to be enveloped by a fascial sheath anteriorly and posteriorly (see Fig. 3.15). This sheath extends downward from the thoracic inlet to merge with the anterior surface of the pericardium; it extends laterally to the mediastinal pleura (see Fig. 3.15). Quottromani et al. [102] suggest that the thymic fascia may be an extension of the perivisceral fascia and that it predicates the radiographic appearance of perithymic pneumomediastinum.

The thymus is usually a prominent structure in the radiographs of infants and young children and fills the upper mediastinum, partially obscuring the heart. The organ weighs about 15 g at birth and grows throughout early childhood, reaching a weight of about 35 g at puberty [12, 51]. The thymus achieves its maximal weight between 12 and 19 years of age; between 20 and 60 years regression in size occurs, together with replacement by adipose tissue. At age 60, the thymus is about half its weight at age 20 [4, 40].

The fact that the thymus continues to increase in size into puberty seems contrary to everyday experience with radiographs of children, which show the thymic shadow to be a relatively large one during the first 3 years of life, diminishing in size thereafter. This apparent discrepancy is easily explained: even though the thymus enlarges throughout the first decade of life, the ratio of thymic size to mediastinal size decreases with age [94]. As a result, the more capacious mediastinum easily accommodates the thymus within its confines as growth progresses. Rarely, the normal thymus is seen as a prominent anterior mediastinal structure on plain radiographs beyond the first decade of life [63] and may even be visible on plain films of adolescents and adults [30, 94]. Its normal radiographic appearance has recently been reviewed by Sone et al. [115].

The distinction of the normal thymus from a mediastinal mass lesion can be a difficult problem in pediatric radiology. Two radiographic characteristics of the normal thymus aid in this differentiation. The normal thymus may reveal a sharp inferolateral angle resembling a sail (Figs. 5.17 and 5.18). Kemp et al. [61] found this "sail shadow" to be present on the right in 6% of normal children. It was identified on the left in 2%. Rarely, the configuration was bilateral [61] (Fig. 5.18). The normal thymus is composed primarily of lymphoid tissue and is therefore soft and pliable. As a result, inspiration and expiration radiographs will often show a change in the appearance of the sail shadow.

Mulvey [91] has reported another radiographic finding that is indicative of normal thymus.

He has termed this appearance the "thymic wave sign" (Fig. 5.18). If the anterolateral margin of the mediastinal shadow in question presents an undulating configuration due to impressions produced by the overlying ribs, it can be inferred that the mass is soft and compressible and is, therefore, almost certainly thymus. The thymic wave sign also changes appearance with inspiration and expiration. According to Mulvey, the thymic wave sign is seen about as often as the sail sign [91].

The spinnaker sail sign identifies the normal thymus in cases of pneumomediastinum [36]; one or both thymic lobes may simulate a spinnaker sail as they are outlined medially by air in the mediastinum and laterally by air in the lung. This radiographic appearance of the thymus is graphic evidence of the anatomically separate nature of the two thymic lobes.

Fig. 5.17A, B. The normal thymus; the sail shadow. PA (**A**) and lateral (**B**) radiographs. PA and lateral radiographs show anterior mediastinal shadow (*1*) intruding into left lung and producing sail-like configuration. This type of appearance characteristic of normal thymus is often sharply limited at its inferior extent, producing a configuration similar to that caused by disease against a fissure (*2*). Note also that thymic shadow has inserted itself between lung and anterior chest wall to produce anterior extrapleural line (*3*)

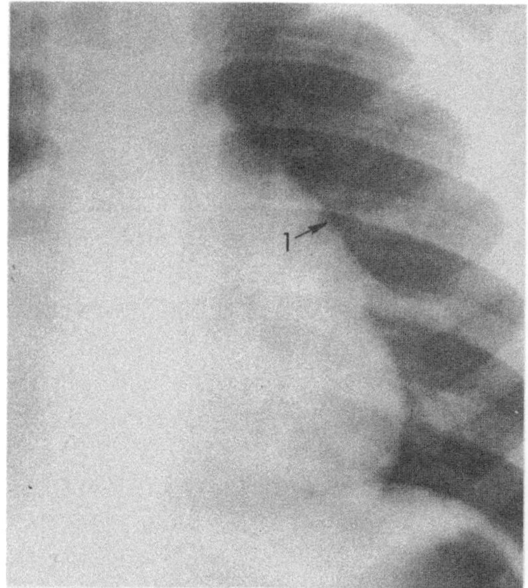
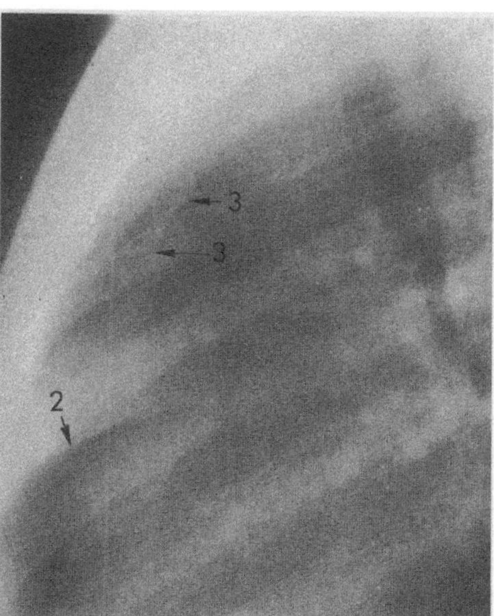

A   B

Fig. 5.18. Normal thymus. Bilateral sail shadow and thymic wave sign (PA radiograph). Bilateral sail sign is evident (*1*). Slight undulation of right lateral aspect of thymic shadow (*2*) is called thymic "wave" sign and is due to impression made by anterior ribs and costochondral junctions on very soft thymus. A striking Mach effect is seen at left margin of thymic shadow (*3*)

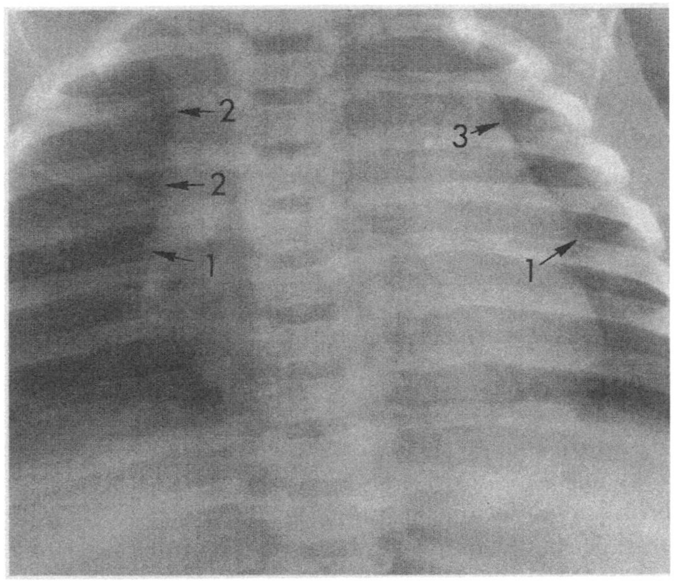

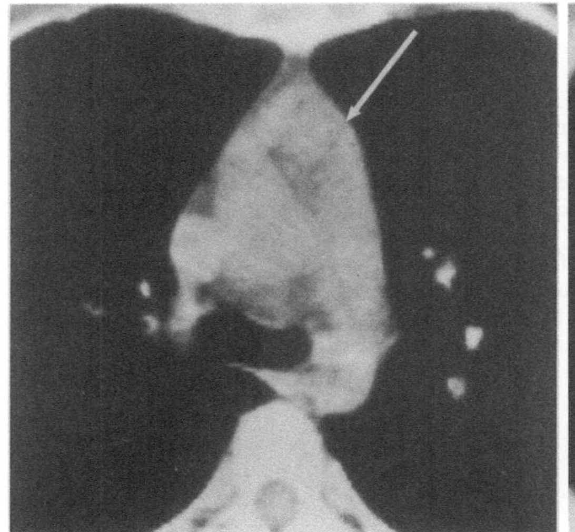

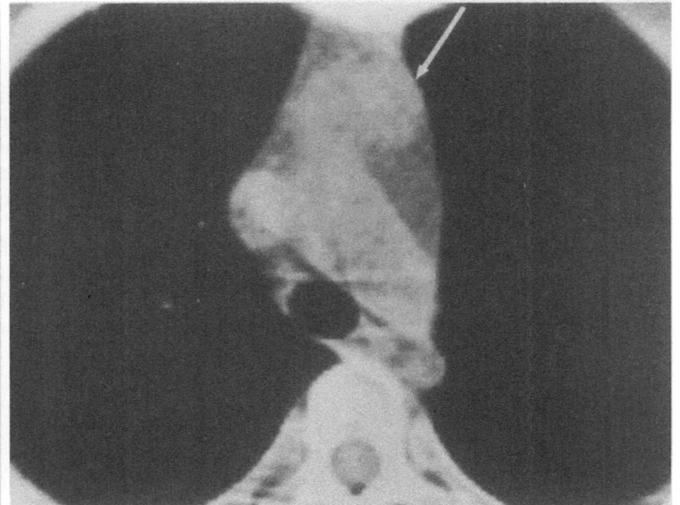

A   **B**

Fig. 5.19A, B. Normal thymus as shown on computed tomography. **A** and **B** Computed tomograms. The normal thymus is commonly identified on computed tomograms in individuals less than 50 years of age and may be seen not infrequently in older individuals. Its most common appearance is the "arrowhead" configuration shown in **A** (*arrow*). Less often, the upper poles of the thymic lobes may be seen as a round or oval density as demonstrated in **B** (*arrow*). Distinction of normal thymic tissue from diffuse thymic abnormality or from other anterior mediastinal masses can be extremely difficult. In this case serial computed tomograms showed no change in the appearance of the thymus (see text)

Computed tomography is an ideal modality to image the thymus. Several observers have studied its normal appearance on computed tomograms [4, 5, 44, 55, 90, 115, 116]. Baron et al. [4] identified the normal thymus at computed tomography in 100% of individuals less than 30 years of age, in 73% between the ages of 30 and 49 years, and in 17% of patients over age 49. Francis et al. [44], however, found that total involution of the thymus occurred in over half of the patients over the age of 40 years.

Baron et al. [4] studied the configuration of the normal thymus as shown on computed tomograms. He found an arrowhead configuration of the normal thymus in 62% of individuals (Fig. 5.19) while separate lobes were found in 32% and one lobe was identified in 6%. Characteristically, the gland has smooth, undulating margins, convex in the very young and concave in older individuals [55]. In older life, the thymus commonly adopts a small linear, round, or oval shape usually less than 7 mm in diameter [44]. When linear in appearance the involuted thymus can be confused with the pedicle of the internal mammary vessels [100]. At times the superior pole of the thymic lobes may be imaged on computed tomograms as one or two contiguous round or oval densities (Fig. 5.19). The density of the thymus on computed tomography decreases with age in keeping with its replacement by fat.

Without serial radiographic examinations, the distinction between persistence of the normal thymus and thymic disease, especially hyperplasia or diffuse involvement by lymphoma, may not be possible on plain film examinations [94]. Even with computed tomographic studies, differentation is often difficult. The computed tomographic evaluation of neoplastic involvement of the thymus is discussed further in section 5.2.7.

The thymus is an organ composed of lymphoid tissue that involutes rapidly under the influence of stress (Fig. 5.20). Systemic disease, steroid therapy, and radiation all cause the thymus to decrease in size, often with remarkable rapidity. Enlargement of the thymus to its former size following removal of stress is the rule. Increase and decrease in thymic size in children with recurrent disease, especially infection, is not rare. Thymic hyperplasia in association with thyrotoxicosis is a well-established entity [45, 54]. Absence of the thymus, associated with absence of the parathyroid glands, is known as the "DiGeorge syndrome" [26, 64].

Fig. 5.20 A, B. Involution of thymus due to stress (PA radiographs). A remarkable diminution in size of thymus in period of 10 days occurred in this patient who suffered a thermal burn. Rapid waxing and waning of size of thymus in infants and young children is commonly related to infection or other forms of stress

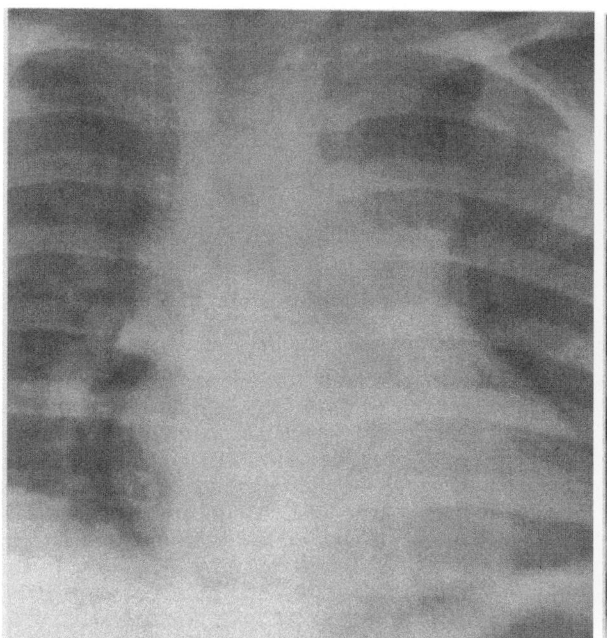

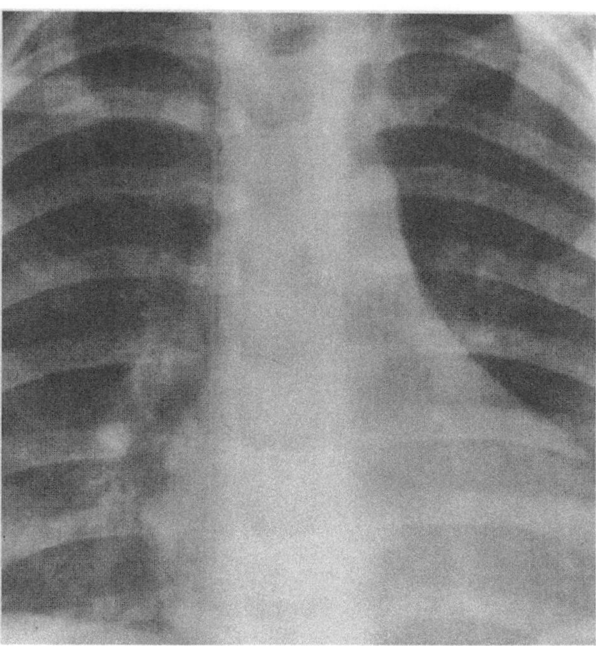

A   B

5.2 Radiologic Correlations with Anatomy and Pathology

5.2.1 Collections of Fat in the Anterior Mediastinum

5.2.1.1 The Pericardial Fat Pad

The radiologic characteristics of pericardial fat pads have received relatively little attention in the radiologic literature, particularly in recent years. Yet, as pointed out by Holt some years ago, they often produce vexing problems in differential diagnosis [57]. Fat pads are more often seen on the left side. However, in a study of 56000 photofluorograms, Holt [57] found a shadow in the right cardiophrenic angle of sufficient concern to require further investigation in 0.6%. Most of these questionably abnormal densities turned out to be pericardial fat. The incidence of atypical pericardial fat pads appears to be somewhat greater on the right side than on the left, and at times right-sided pericardial fat pads may be of a large size [57] (Fig. 5.21). Pericardial fat pads have been found in extremely obese persons [20, 57], but are not

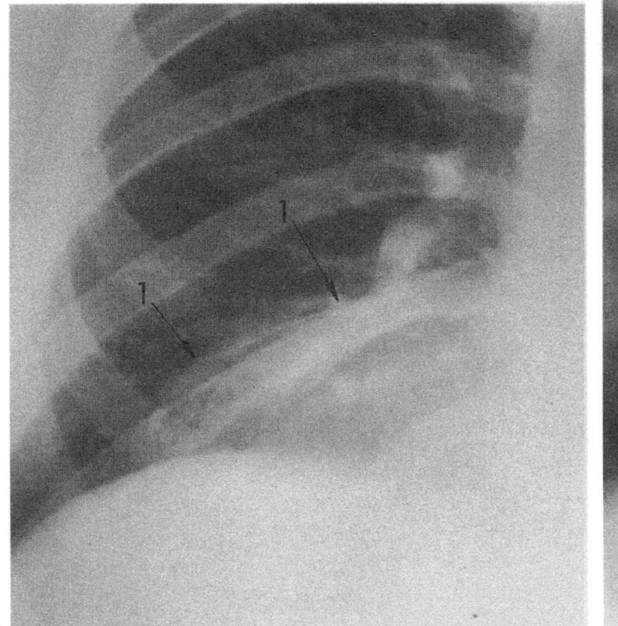

A

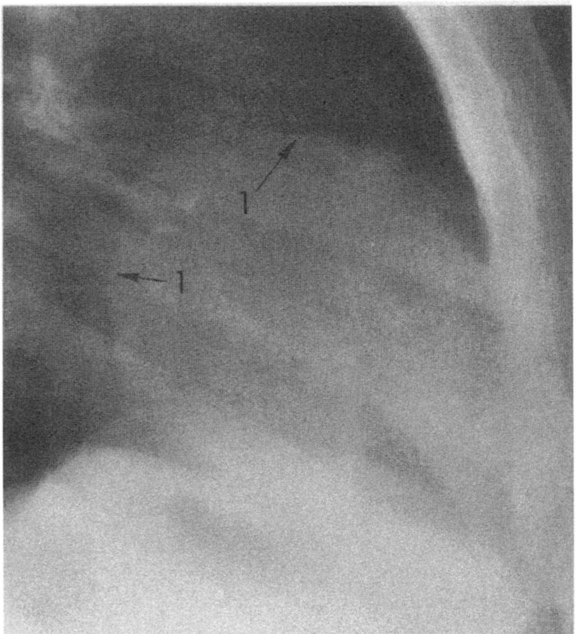

B

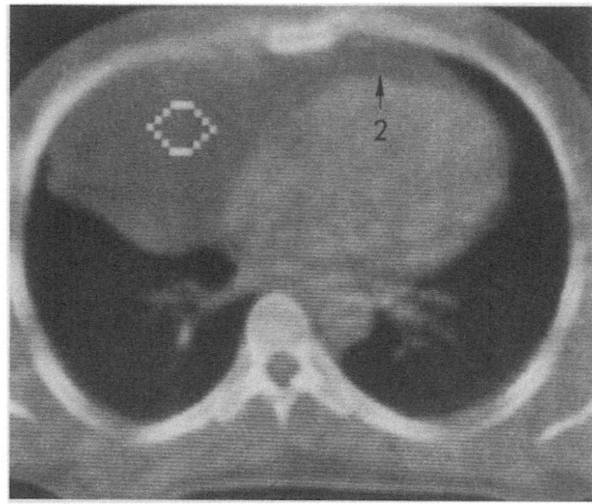

C

Fig. 5.21 A–C. Right pericardial fat pad. PA (A) and lateral (B) radiographs and computed tomogram (C). Collections of fat in cardiophrenic angles frequently produce prominent shadows on frontal and/or lateral radiographs (1). At times, these may be quite difficult to distinguish from more significant pathology in cardiophrenic angle. These collections of fat are not usually recognized as radiolucent, probably due to high contrast provided by adjacent lung. A pericardial fat pad may change shape on inspiration and expiration films. Computed tomography can establish the diagnosis. In this case the cursor reading was −120 (on a scale of 1000), proving the fatty nature of mass. Note extent of fat crossing in front of heart far to left side (2) rare in nonobese individuals [92]. Fat pads have been reported to increase in size with steroid administration [98]. The configuration of pericardial fat pads is variable. In general, their shape is triangular on both frontal and lateral radiographs, but their interface with contiguous lung may be convex or concave (see Figs. 3.22, 5.21, 5.37). The appearance on the lateral film is that of an extrapleural triangular shadow in the anterior cardiophrenic angle. The appearance previously referred to in this chapter as the "cardiac incisura" is similar to that caused by a left-sided pericardial fat pad since both the heart and the fat are extrapleural masses. In fact, the cardiac incisura and a left-sided pericardial fat pad commonly coexist. A pericardial fat pad is visible on frontal and lateral radiographs; however, the cardiac incisura is seen only on the lateral film unless it is associated with a prominent fat pad. Often the fatty nature of pericardial fat pads cannot be appreciated on plain radiographs due to the much greater radiolucency of the adjacent lung. It is possible in most cases to prove that a cardiophrenic angle mass is fat by the use of computed tomography (Fig. 5.21).

The differential diagnosis of right cardiophrenic angle masses includes pericardial cyst [66] and hernia through the foramen of Morgagni as well as a number of other much less common lesions [104]. Among the last group is thymolipoma. This lesion cannot be distinguished from a large pericardial fat pad, although progressive enlargement to very large size is more in keeping with the diagnosis of thymolipoma.

5.2.1.2 Epicardial Fat

In many individuals, a considerable quantity of fat accumulates over the epicardium anteriorly and occasionally laterally on each side [123] (see chapter 3). Not infrequently, a fine line representing the pericardium can be seen on lateral radiographs outlined by epipericardial (retrosternal) fat in front and epicardial fat behind [72] (Fig. 5.22). Jorgens et al. [59] have reported that visualization of epicardial fat some distance be-

Fig. 5.22A, B. Demonstration of pericardium on lateral radiographs. Lateral radiograph (A) and sagittal body section through plane slightly to left of midline (B). Normal pericardium (1) can occasionally be identified on lateral films outlined between retrosternal fat (2) and epicardial fat (3). (Courtesy J.A. Head, Syracuse, NY)

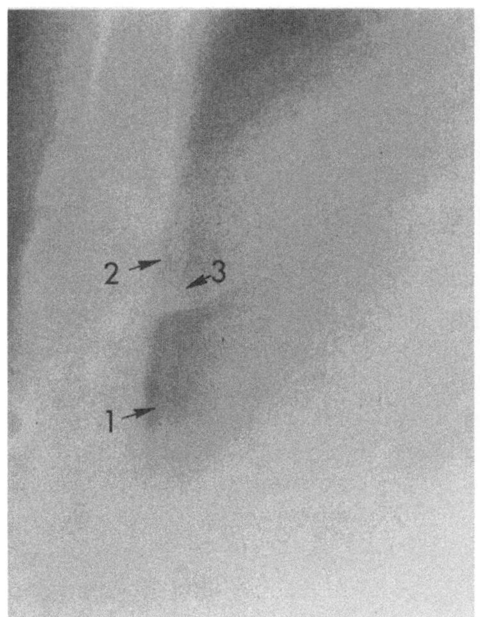

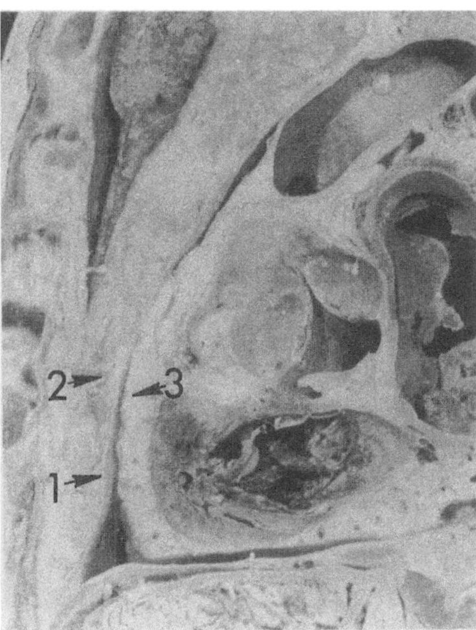

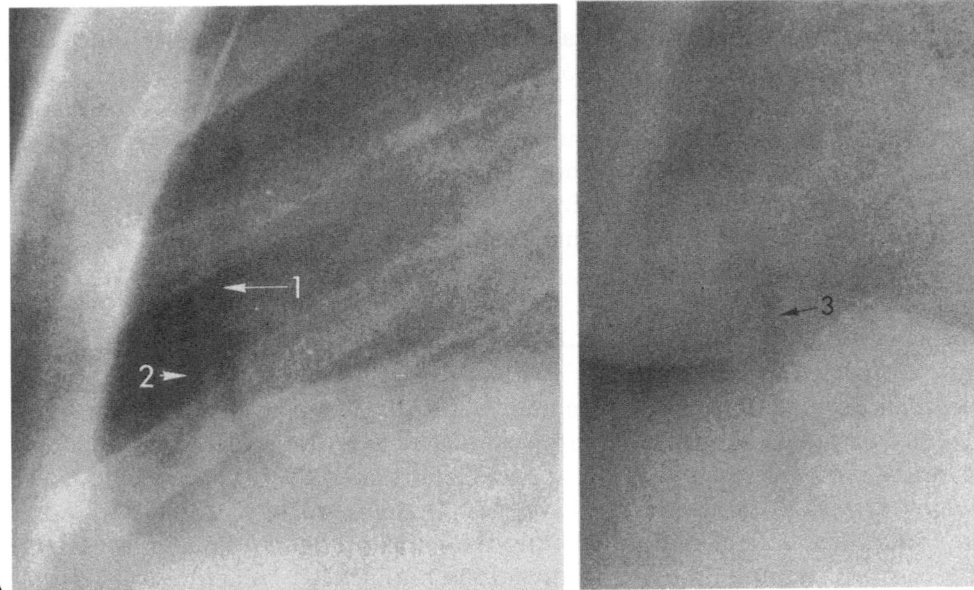

Fig. 5.23 A, B. Epicardial fat in pericardial effusion. Lateral radiographs. Epicardial fat (*1*) can be seen separated from retrosternal fat (*2*) by white stripe representing pericardial space. When this stripe exceeds 2 mm in thickness, pericardial fluid or thickening should be inferred. In **A**, minimal pericardial effusion was thought to be present. Subsequent gross displacement of epicardial fat (*3*) from sternum as result of greater accumulation of pericardial fluid

hind the sternum and well within the apparent cardiac silhouette at fluoroscopy is diagnostic of pericardial effusion. Lane and Carsky [73] and Carsky et al. [15] demonstrated the same findings on plain lateral radiographs. They concur with Kremens [72] in the opinion that separation of the epipericardial fat from the pericardial fat by 2 mm or more is highly suggestive of pericardial effusion (Fig. 5.23). Demonstration of the epicardial fat over the surface of the left ventricle on frontal radiographs has been reported as an aid in establishing cardiac size in patients with large left pleural effusions [48]. Demos et al. [25] have reported two cases of displacement of the epicardial fat pad by extrapericardial anterior mediastinal masses; one was a hematoma, the other a cyst.

5.2.1.3 Fat Deposition in Cushing's Syndrome and Following Steroid Therapy

Deposition of fat in the mediastinum in patients with an excess of circulating steroids is a recognized entity [11, 70, 99, 121] and is analogous to the unusual accumulations of fat that may develop elsewhere in the body in patients with Cushing's syndrome. Drasin et al. [28] have reported a case of mediastinal lipomatosis due to ectopic adrenocarticotropic hormone (ACTH) production.

Mediastinal fat deposition is very commonly the result of steroid therapy and only rarely is it due to Cushing's syndrome [99]. In the series reported by Price and Rigler [99] all patients were receiving prednisone at doses of 30 mg or more per day; eight of nine patients were receiving 40 mg or more per day. All patients had clinical Cushing's syndrome. Fat deposition may develop rapidly after the institution of steroid therapy. The changes are reversible if steroid dosage is lowered. The usual radiographic appearance of mediastinal lipomatosis is that of a smooth widening of the supra-aortic and supra-azygos portions of the mediastinum (Fig. 5.24). Often it is impossible on conventional radiographs to determine that the mass is of fat density. It is easy to make this determination

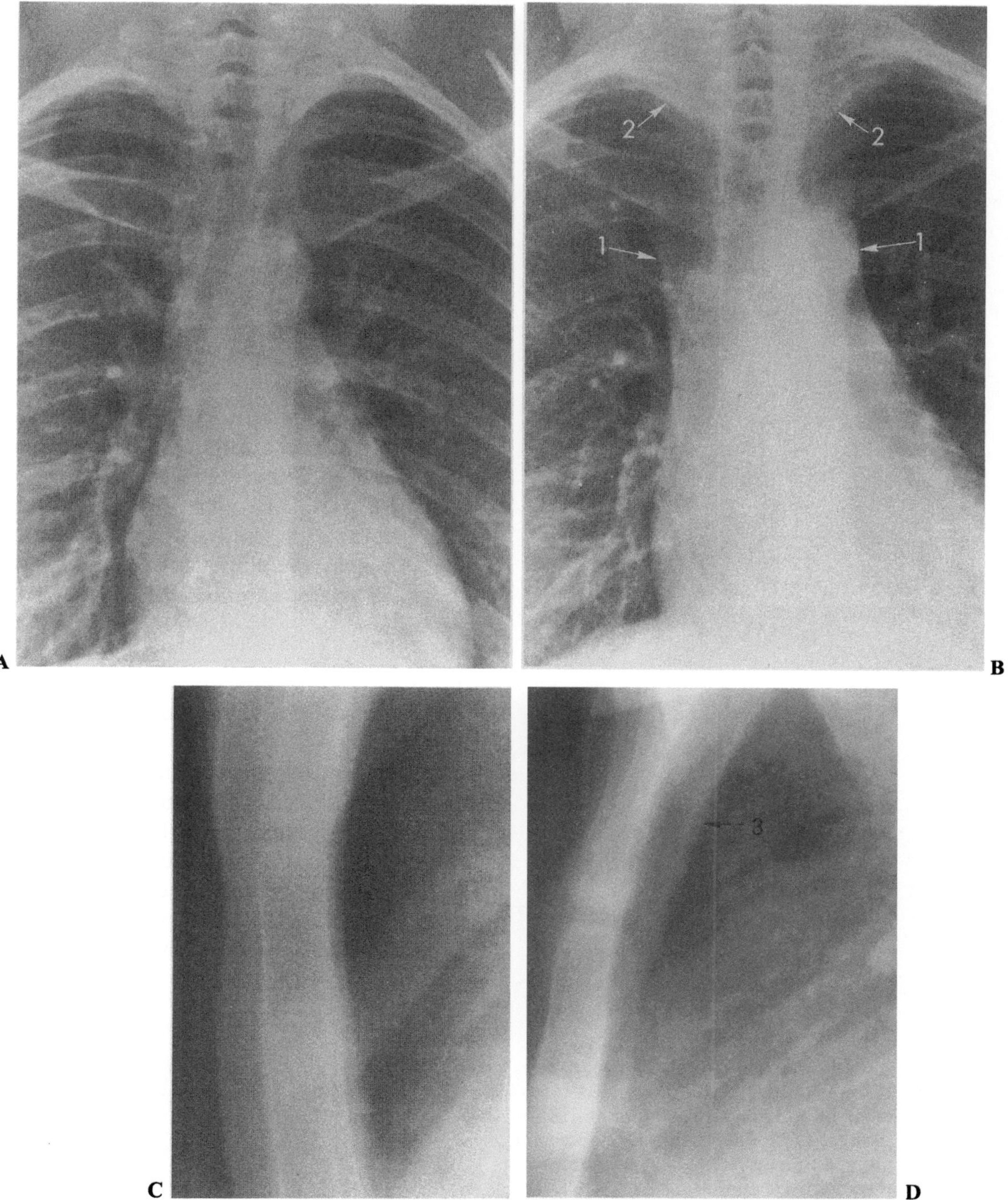

Fig. 5.24A–D. Anterior mediastinal widening due to steroid therapy. PA radiographs (**A** and **B**) and lateral radiographs (**C** and **D**). Widening of anterior mediastinum in **B** (*1*) should be compared with normal film (**A**). Note cervicothoracic sign indicative of anteriorly situated mass and that contact of left lung with anterior mediastinum is lateral to shadow of aortic knob. Fat can also be seen posteriorly over the lung apices (*2*). Comparison of two lateral radiographs shows increase in retrosternal fat following steroid therapy producing a smooth anterior extrapleural line (*3*). Presence of such associated extrapleural changes in thorax of patient on steroid therapy supports probability that widening of anterior mediastinum is due to fat

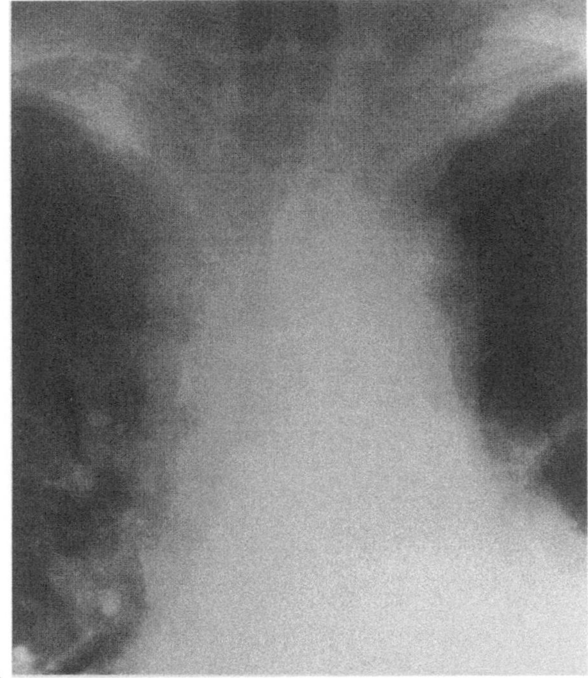

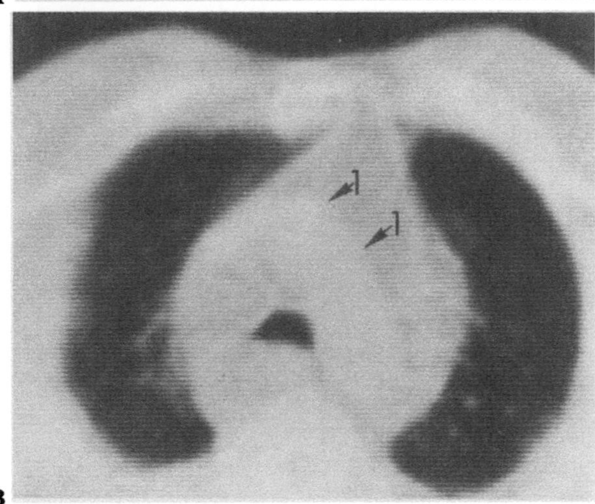

using computed axial tomography [7, 58, 101] (Fig. 5.25). Even without this diagnostic adjunct, the diagnosis of mediastinal fat deposition due to excess steroids should not pose significant problems when a supra-aortic and/or supra-azygos mass is encountered on radiographs if it is recognized that the patient is on high-dose steroid therapy. An exception to this statement may occur when large doses of steroids are being given to patients with lymphoma [99]. The development of a mediastinal mass in these individuals poses a differential diagnostic problem between mediastinal lipomatosis and lymphoma that is easily resolved by computed tomography. Price and Rigler [99] and Teates [121] have pointed out that excess steroid may cause fat to be deposited in other locations in the chest as well. The presence on radiographs of considerable pericardial fat or extrapleural fat adjacent to the rib cage or spine supports a diagnosis of steroid-induced lipomatosis [119] (Fig. 5.24).

5.2.2 Anterior "Herniation" of Lung

One of the most common forms of spatial rearrangement of thoracic anatomy following diminution of lung volume on either side is the extension of the contralateral lung to the diseased side, anterior to the heart and great vessels. A similar change occurs when one lung or upper lobe is increased in volume by disease such as

Fig. 5.25 A, B. Anterior mediastinal widening due to steroid therapy. PA radiograph (**A**) and computed tomogram (**B**). Widening of anterior mediastinum on PA radiograph was thought to be due to steroid-induced fat deposition. Computed tomogram made at level of aortic arch clearly shows arch (*1*) outlined by accumulation of fat in anterior mediastinum. In patients receiving high doses of steroid therapy for lymphoma, computed tomography is helpful to distinguish iatrogenic fat deposition from progression of tumor

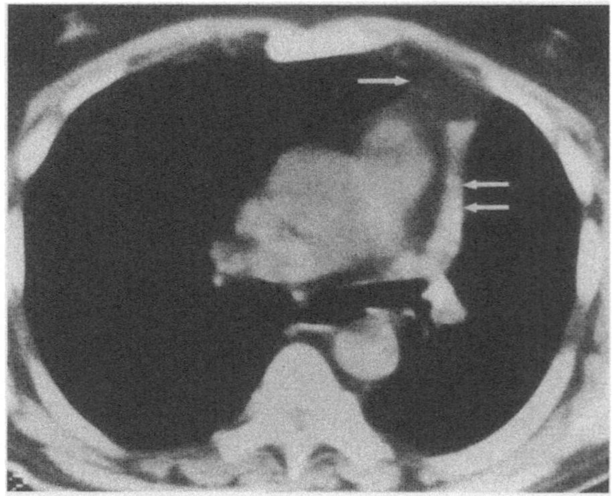

Fig. 5.26. Anterior herniation of lung. Computed tomogram shows characteristic appearance of herniated anterior portion of right lung to left in front of great vessels (*single arrow*) in a patient with a totally collapsed left upper lobe (*double arrows*)

emphysema. These projections of lung across the midline are sometimes called anterior lung "hernia" [82, 85]. The involved upper lobe crosses the midline through the anterior mediastinum, carrying the apposed visceral and parietal pleurae ahead of it. Thus, the anterior junction line is deviated in many cases. Following lung resection or complete lung collapse, the heart is displaced posteriorly and rotates into the homolateral hemithorax, permitting lung to herniate in front of it (Fig. 5.26). Anterior lung hernia is much more common than is posterior herniation of lung across the azygoesophageal recess.

5.2.3 Dilated Internal Mammary (Internal Thoracic) Arteries

Another cause for an anterior extrapleural abnormality on lateral chest films is dilatation of the internal mammary arteries. These vessels, which lie just lateral to the sternum (see Fig. 5.1), may cause the interface made between the lungs and the anterior chest wall to adopt a scalloped contour (Fig. 5.27). Dilatation of

these vessels results when they act as a pathway for collateral blood flow. The most common lesion producing dilatation of these arteries is coarctation of the aorta. Figley noted the scalloped contour of retrosternal lung in 21 of 74 patients with coarctation [38]. Bjork and Friedman [10] identified dilated internal mammary arteries in 26% of patients aged 6–10 years with coarctation and found them in 50% of patients 11–15 years of age with this lesion [10]. Following surgical correction of coarctation of the aorta, the prominent internal mammary arteries often gradually decrease in size over the ensuing year; sometimes they remain unchanged in size [93].

The complex of the internal mammary artery and vein is usually readily identified at com-

Fig. 5.27 A, B. Dilatation of internal mammary arteries. Lateral radiograph (**A**) and lateral film from an arteriogram (**B**). When internal mammary arteries act as source of collateral circulation, as in this case of coarctation of the aorta, increase in blood flow results in dilatation of vessels that may be identified retrosternally on standard lateral chest radiographs (*1*). Dilatation of internal mammary arteries is another cause for lobulated anterior extrapleural line

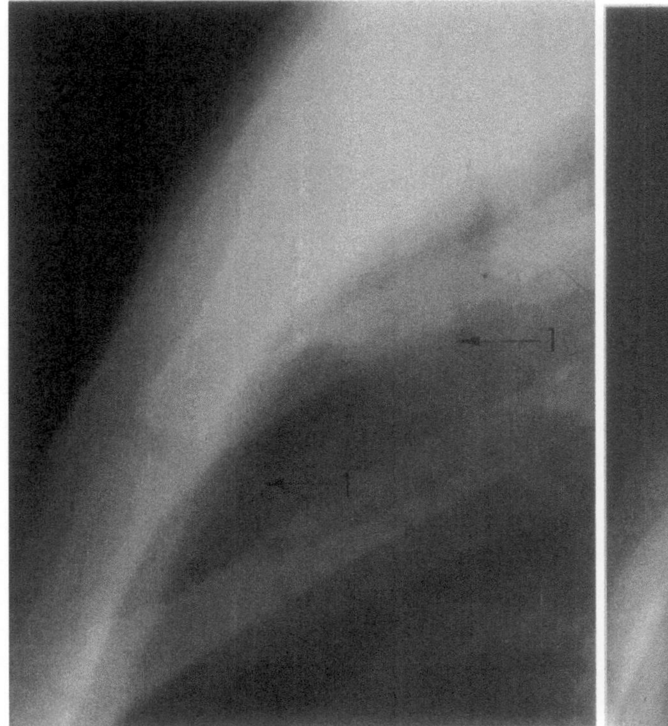

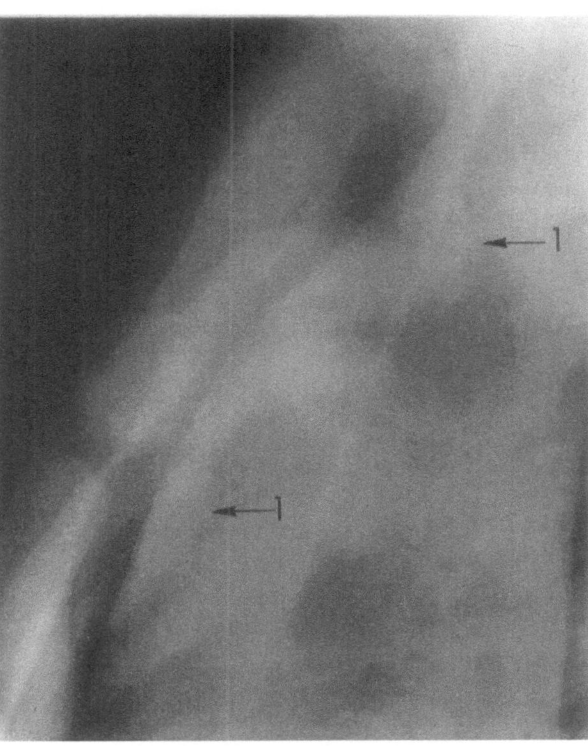

A   B

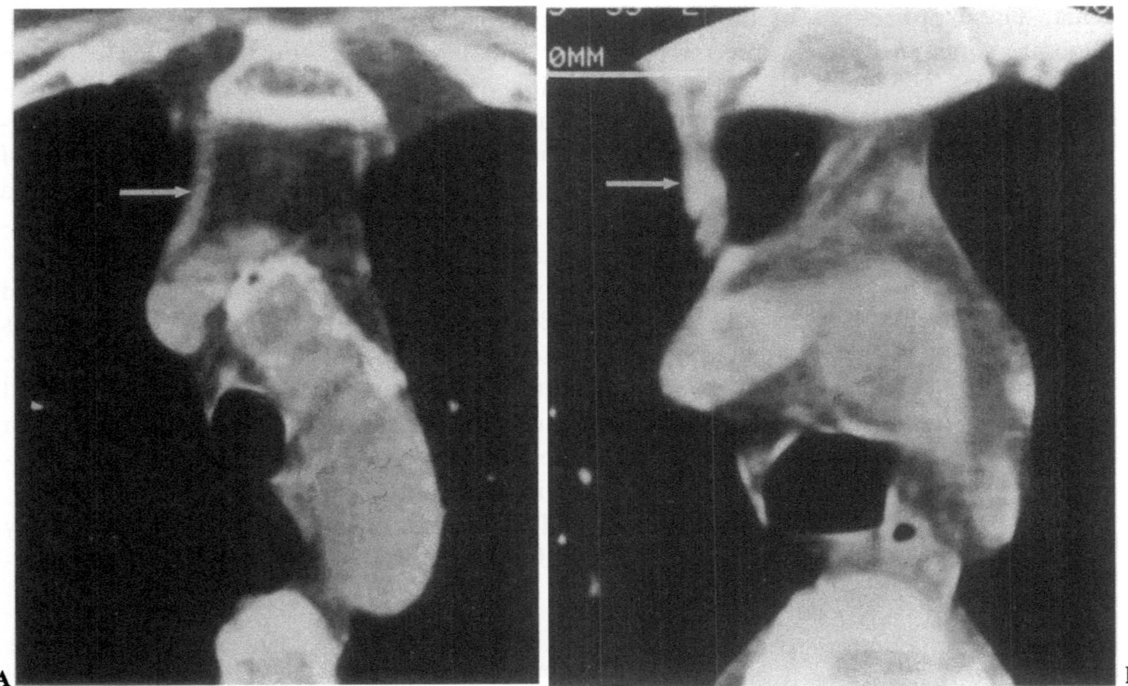

A   B

puted tomography (Fig. 5.28). Within the mediastinum they may simulate an atrophic thymic lobe [100]; retrosternally they may simulate internal mammary adenopathy on a given level of section. Demonstration of the vessels as tubular structures on contiguous scans confirms the shadows as being vascular. We have seen a case in which the internal mammary artery and vein coursed through lung on their way to the anterior chest wall creating a lobe of the internal mammary vessels analogous to an azygos lobe and the lobe of the right brachiocephalic vein, an anomaly reported by Goebel [50] (Fig. 5.28 B).

5.2.4 Anterior Mediastinal Hematoma

Anterior mediastinal hematoma is not rare and in the absence of proven arterial injury is usually ascribed to rupture of anterior mediastinal veins [43, 97, 107]. Pfister et al. [97] have emphasized that trauma to the anterior chest wall can tear the internal mammary vein to produce a hematoma. Eshaghy et al. [33] have reported mediastinal hemorrhage as a complication of cardiac catheterization. Spontaneous anterior medias-

Fig. 5.28A, B. Internal mammary vessels demonstrated crossing the anterior mediastinum on computed tomograms. At times the right internal mammary artery and vein and, less frequently, the left-sided vessels, can be identified crossing the anterior mediastinum from their origins from the brachiocephalic arteries and veins (*arrow*). They may simulate an involuted thymic lobe. In **B** the paired right vessels (*arrow*) cross through lung creating "the lobe of the internal mammary vessels" (see text)

tinal hematoma is known to occur [9, 118], especially in patients on chronic hemodialysis [31].

Raphael [103] injected the anterior mediastinal space with barium in an effort to determine the configuration of anterior mediastinal hematomas on radiographs. He concluded that hematomas were confined laterally by the mediastinal pleura, anteriorly by the loose retrosternal fascia, and posteriorly by the anterior aspect of the perivisceral fascia. His studies suggested further that dissection in a caudal direction occurred more readily on the left than on the right. Although Raphael's conclusions are in all likelihood correct, anterior mediastinal hematomas do not adopt any localization or configuration that could be said to be characteristic

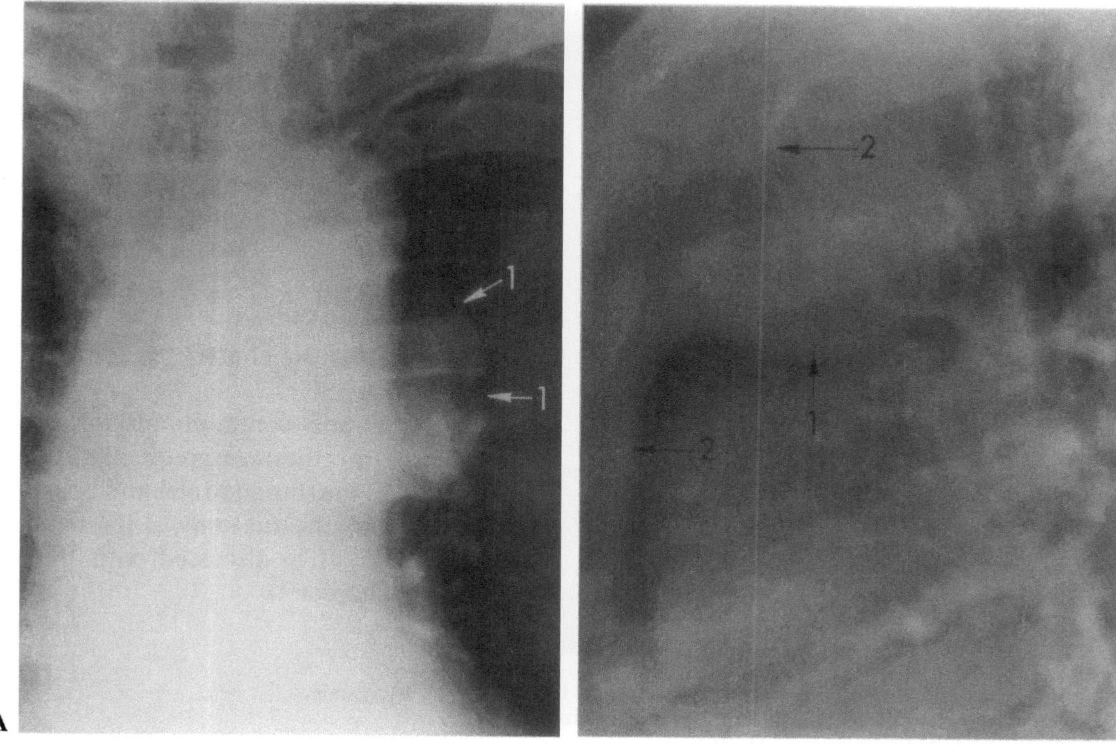

Fig. 5.29 A, B. Anterior mediastinal hematoma. PA (**A**) and lateral (**B**) radiographs. Anterior mediastinal hematoma is commonly ascribed to rupture of internal mammary veins or other smaller veins of anterior mediastinum and may be localized or diffuse. In this case, localized left anterior mediastinal mass is apparent (*1*). A clue to the fact that there is more diffuse involvement of anterior mediastinum in this case is afforded by presence of anterior extrapleural line above and below lesion (*2*)

(Fig. 5.29). Woodring et al. [133] found widening of the right paratracheal stripe after trauma to be a sensitive index of bleeding. Marnocha et al. [86] and Woodring et al. [134] found the mediastinal width/chest width ratio [109] to be an unreliable index of mediastinal hemorrhage.

5.2.5 Anterior Mediastinal Infection

Anterior mediastinal infection is uncommon. No case was encountered in Leszcynski's [79] experience. This low incidence may be due to the infrequent occurrence of infrahyoid pretracheal infection in the anterior aspect of the perivisceral space in the neck. Since infection in this

space is uncommon, dissection from it, anterior ot the great vessels at the thoracic inlet, is likewise infrequent.

There are, however, other sources from which anterior mediastinitis can arise. The most common of these is from an infected sternum following a sternal splitting incision. Obviously, not all postoperative problems associated with median sternotomy are complicated by mediastinitis, but when this occurs the fatality rate is high, reaching 70% in one series [110] and 40% in another [32].

The diagnosis of anterior mediastinitis complicating midline sternotomy can be a difficult one. Although systemic signs of sepsis are commonly present [32, 110], it may be difficult to localize the septic process to the mediastinum. Clinical signs of sternal abnormality are often not present.

Computed tomography may be helpful in the diagnosis [52] and should be performed in all suspect cases. Widening of the anterior mediastinum and the demonstration of anterior mediastinal fluid and air are telltale findings. Goodman et al. [52], however, emphasize that

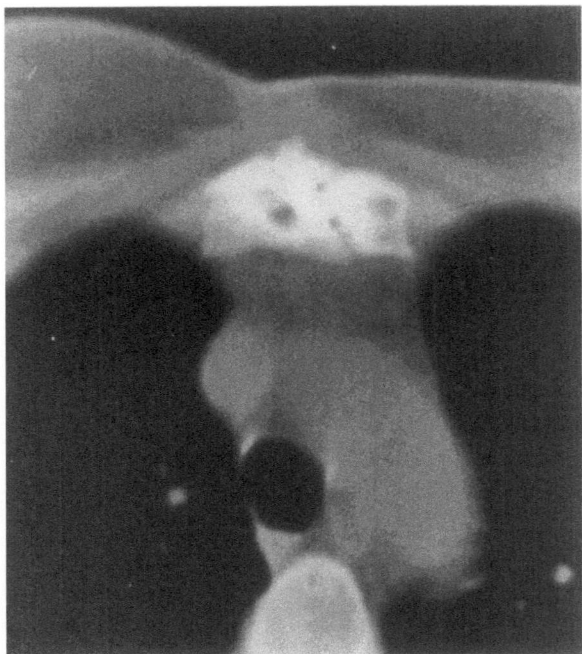

Fig. 5.30. Osteomyelitis of the sternum. Computed tomogram. Osteomyelitis of the sternum is a recognized complication of midline sternotomy. It may lead to the development of anterior mediastinal abscess, a condition with a grave prognosis. Although anterior mediastinitis may develop before radiographic signs of sternal osteomyelitis are apparent, computed tomographic study of the sternum should be performed in all suspect cases. As shown in this case of proven sternal osteomyelitis, mottled areas of sclerosis and radiolucency of the sternum are findings strongly suggestive of the diagnosis

the anterior mediastinum following sternotomy may appear abnormal due to postoperative edema or hemorrhage. The majority of cases of anterior mediastinitis following sternotomy develop before radiographic signs of sternal osteomyelitis have had a chance to develop. Nevertheless, in suspect cases, careful study of the sternum for signs of infection should be undertaken [8, 52, 138]. Goodman et al. [53] have provided a review of the computed tomographic appearance of the normal sternum. Variations from this appearance must be considered suspect; irregular, poorly marginated widening of the midline sternotomy [8, 138] and the development of mottled areas of radiolucency and sclerosis are findings of major concern (Fig. 5.30).

Proto and Rost [100] have emphasized that partial volume effect can simulate destruction

of the sternum especially at the angle of Louis on computed tomograms. Mediastinal node infection, usually by histoplasmosis, can lead to fibrosing mediastinitis. The findings of this condition as seen at computed tomography are described by Weinstein et al. [129] and include mediastinal widening and constriction of vessels and airway.

5.2.6 Intrathoracic Goiter

One of the most common anterior mediastinal masses is intrathoracic goiter. Because this lesion crosses the thoracic inlet and is significantly influenced by the anatomy of the major vessels in this area, it is discussed with the thoracic inlet (see chapter 4).

5.2.7 Thymoma

Thymoma is the most common surgical tumor of the upper anterior mediastinum [24, 30]. Of the 65 thymomas reported by Ellis and Gregg [30], all were found to lie predominantly in the anterior mediastinum. Of the thymomas in this series, 80% were located at the base of the heart, the remainder above or below this level. Only four were bilateral, and each of these was invasive.

Many interesting histologic varieties of thymic tumor occur [22, 30, 75, 83]. Hodgkin's disease involves the thymus rather commonly. Rosai and Higa [105] have pointed out that thymic carcinoids should be distinguished from thymomas and that they have ultrastructural characteristics that are typical of neuroendocrine neoplasms. Carcinoid tumors arising from the foregut (including lung and thymus) may be associated with Cushing's syndrome [37] or with the multiple endocrine neoplasia syndrome, type 1 [14] (see Fig. 5.5). Rarely, teratoid tumors of the thymus are encountered. Germ cell tumors of the mediastinum have also been shown to be of thymic origin [1, 71, 75, 80]. They occur exclusively in men, predominantly those of younger age, and carry a relatively favorable prognosis [114]. Thymolipoma is a rare variety of thymic tumor composed predominantly of fat. These tumors may reach impressive size and are often found in the cardiophrenic angle where they may insinuate themselves around the heart and along the diaphragm. The lesions are soft and may change configuration with change in body position or phase of respiration [122]. Although they are more radiolucent than adjacent soft tissues, this feature may be hard to appreciate because of the contiguous, much more radiolucent lung. Their fatty nature can be determined by computed tomographic scanning, but when this feature is confirmed, it may be difficult to distinguish thymolipoma from a large pericardial fat pad. In almost all cases thymolipoma is a self-limited condition producing no symptoms, so that its distinction from a pericardial fat pad is not ordinarily of great clinical importance. The thymus also produces cystic lesions. These masses may cross the thoracic inlet anterior to the great vessels to produce the so-called cervicothoracic form of thymic cyst [135]. They are smooth and frequently lobulated; at times calcium can be seen in their walls. They may enlarge suddenly, apparently due to hemorrhage. Because of their large size, their fluid content and their position far forward against the anterior chest wall, the diagnosis of thymic cyst can be confirmed by ultrasonography [135].

In addition of the interesting variety of pathologic forms of thymic tumor, an even more fascinating array of clinical syndromes can be associated with thymoma. Undoubtedly, the best-known of these associations is myasthenia gravis. Approximately 15% of patients with this condition have a thymoma [27]; the presence of myasthenia should require the mediastinum to be studied radiologically with meticulous care [30]. Myasthenia gravis has been reported to occur in about 25%–50% of patients with thymoma [46]. Thymomas found in association with myasthenia are less aggressive and have a better prognosis than those occurring without myasthenia [30]. The association of hypogammaglobulinemia with thymoma is a well-established entity. About 10% of patients with primary acquired hypogammaglobulinemia have a thymoma [96]; hypogammaglobulinemia has

been reported to occur in 6% of patients with thymoma [117]. Findings indicative of chronic lung infection and a sprue-like pattern in the small bowel (apparently related to decreased IgA) in association with a mediastinal mass should suggest the diagnosis [89]. Another interesting syndrome encountered in patients with thymoma is aregenerative erythroid hypoplasia [30]. Cushing's syndrome and carcinoid syndrome may be associated with thymic carcidoids; these conditions in association with thymic tumors have been reviewed in a concise manner by Ellis and Gregg [30]. Other associations are the well-established relationship of thymic hyperplasia to hyperthyroidism [45], and following treatment for hypothyroidism [136] and Addison's disease [94] in children.

The radiologic diagnosis of thymoma presents a number of interesting challenges. Ellis and Gregg [30] reported 41 thymomas found among 350 patients who were carefully studied for the presence of this tumor because they had myasthenia gravis. Eight of the tumors were identified only at autopsy. Of the remaining 33 thymomas, ten could not be seen on frontal films; in eight of these patients, the mass could be suspected on the lateral radiograph. Two tumors were not seen on lateral view but were apparent on the frontal radiograph. Although at conventional tomography no mass was found that could not be seen on plain films, the authors felt that tomograms were often helpful in making a more certain radiographic diagnosis of a mass. In general, these impressions are supported by the study of Kemp-Harper and Guyer [62]. Today, computed tomography is the ideal way to demonstrate an anterior mediastinal mass including those related to the thymus [2, 3, 37, 42, 137]. This modality has shown good reliability in the detection of thymoma in patients with myasthenia gravis and other syndromes related to thymoma. To date, magnetic resonance imaging has not proven superior to computed tomography for the detection of thymic abnormality in patients with myasthenia gravis [6].

In section 5.1.2 it was pointed out that it is not easy to distinguish normal from abnormal thymic tissue on radiographs. Computed to-

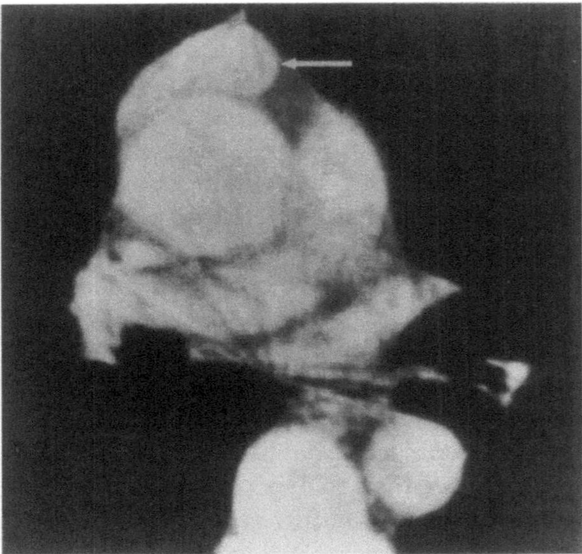

Fig. 5.31. Thymoma on computed tomogram. Thymoma presenting as an anterior mediastinal mass is easily identified on computed tomograms even when it cannot be seen on conventional roentgenograms. When thymic abnormality involves the gland diffusely, it can be very difficult to differentiate from normal thymus. As shown in this case, a localized convex bulge (*arrow*) indicates the presence of a mass

mography has improved our capability to make this differentiation but problems still exist, and it is not infrequent that uncertainty exists even after computed tomographic examination. The hallmark of abnormality is a density in the region of the thymus presenting a localized convex margin against adjacent aerated lung or mediastinal fat (Fig. 5.31). Multiple lobulations in the outline of a thymic lobe or lobes are never normal [44].

A very difficult problem is the distinction of a large normal lobe or lobes from thymic hyperplasia or diffuse involvement of the gland by tumor, particularly in patients below age 40 [42]. Without serial examinations, such a distinction is often impossible although Baron et al. [3] feel that the thickness of the gland can be a helpful criterion. Another vexing problem is thymic enlargement as a "rebound" phenomenon that is sometimes encountered after cessation of mustine, oncovin, procarbazine, and prednisone (MOPP) therapy [19] for Hodgkin's disease or following chemotherapy for testicular malignancy [65]. Under these conditions it is difficult

to determine whether the enlarging thymus is merely regenerating or whether tumor recurrence is taking place within the gland. Exceptionally, surgery is required to make the distinction.

The differential diagnosis of anteriorly situated mediastinal mass lesions can be difficult (Figs. 5.32, 5.33). The problem most frequently encountered is the distinction between thymoma and Hodgkin's disease. In the series of thymomas reported by Ellis and Gregg about one-half of the tumors were lobulated, and one-half were not [30]. Hodgkin's disease, particularly of the nodular sclerosis type, may also show gross characteristics of a lobulated mass or a smooth solitary mass. On a statistical basis, masses lying above the cardiac base are more likely to be Hodgkin's disease than thymoma. Calcification in the lesion may help. Curvilinear calcification, although uncommon, is found in thymic tumors; it is never seen in untreated Hodgkin's disease [120]. Cystic changes can be found in thymoma and in the nodular sclerosis form of Hodgkin's disease involving the thymus [35]. Whalen et al. [130] have described a radiographic finding that they feel lends support to the diagnosis of thymoma. It is based on the fact that thymic tumors are softer and more pliable than other mass lesions lying anteriorly in the mediastinum. This softer character of thymomas sometimes permits them to insinuate themselves in front of the anterior lung margins to produce an anterior extrapleural line, an appearance not usual for other solid tumors of the mediastinum (Figs. 5.32, 5.33). This finding was identified on random lateral radiographs in six of 16 thymomas studied by Whalen et al. [130]. It should be appreciated that a similar anterior extrapleural line, although not common, can at times be produced by lymphoma (see Fig. 5.36). Fleischner et al. [41] reported this appearance in Hodgkin's disease and leukemia and stated that in these conditions retrosternal abnormality may be the first sign of thoracic involvement. Fayos [34] found a retrosternal disease in eight of 414 patients with Hodgkin's disease, but all of these patients had nodes elsewhere in the chest. On a statistical basis it would seem that the presence of an anterior extra-

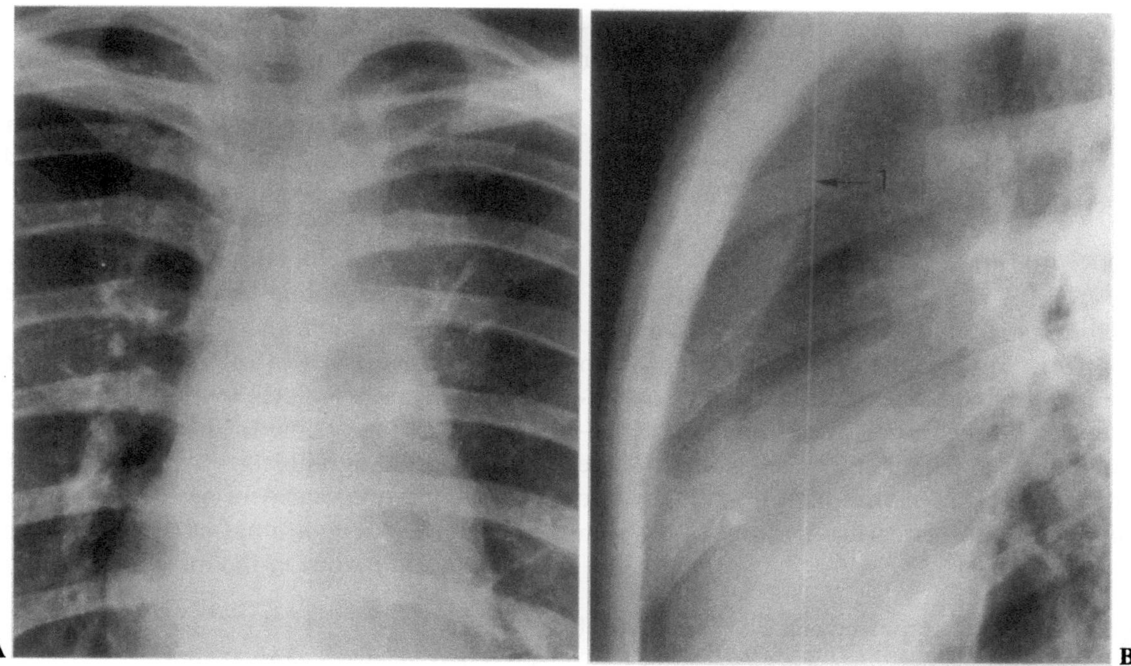

Fig. 5.32 A, B. Thymoma. PA (**A**) and lateral (**B**) radiographs. Radiographic examination demonstrates left anterior mediastinal mass, proven to be thymoma, which is producing distinct anterior extrapleural line (*1*). With exception of thymoma, solid tumors rarely produce such a smooth interface with lung. Occasionally metastatic carcinoma or lymphoma may produce such a smooth line. (From [130])

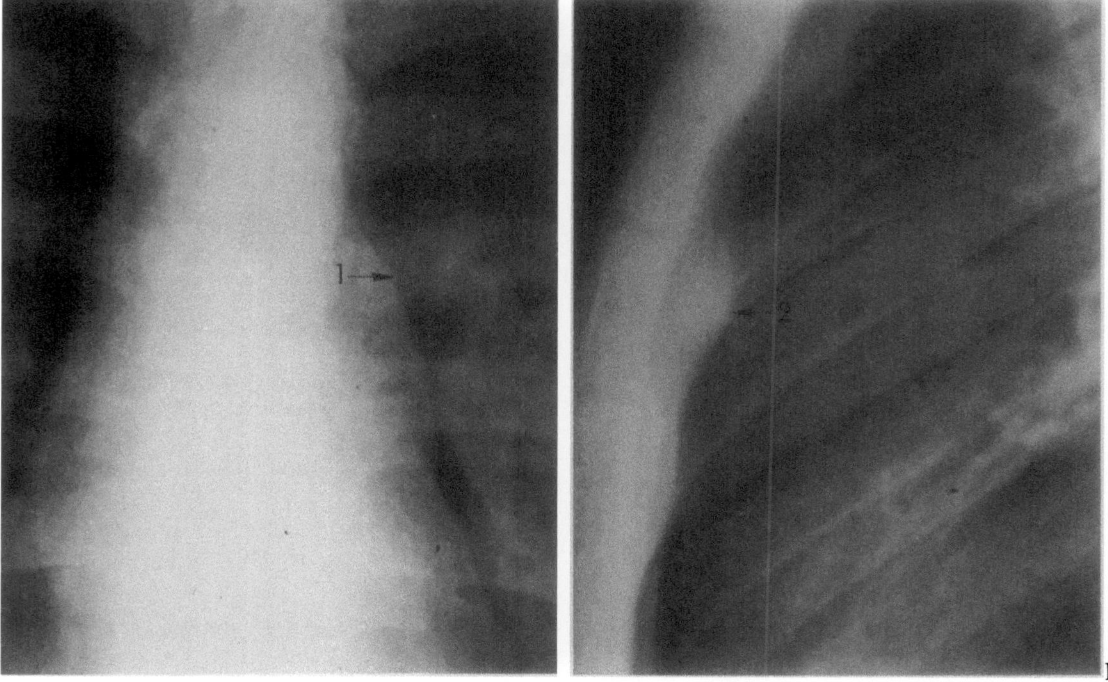

Fig. 5.33 A, B. Thymoma. PA (**A**) and lateral (**B**) radiographs of chest. PA radiograph demonstrates mass (*1*) overlying main pulmonary artery. This mass proved to be a thymoma that had extended to lie between sternum and anterior aspect of left lung to produce lobulated anterior extrapleural line (*2*)

pleural line is more often associated with thymomas than lymphoma, especially if no other disease can be found in the thorax. Thymoma rarely produces extrathoracic metastases; Brown et al. [13] reported 31 examples.

5.2.8 Mediastinal Teratoma

A teratoma is a tumor composed of tissues derived from any or all of the embryonic germ layers; these tissues are organized in an inappropriate way. In the thorax, these tumors are commonly found in the anterior mediastinum at the cardiac base [77, 78], although in children rare examples of intrapericardial teratoma have been

reported [84, 132]. Mediastinal teratomas exist in a spectrum from benign to malignant forms. The benign variety occurs in men and women with about equal frequency and can often be diagnosed on radiographs by virtue of the identification of bone, teeth, or fat within them. Peripheral calcification (Fig. 5.34) occurs, and occasionally a fat-fluid level may be seen [78]. Malignant mediastinal teratoma is encountered more often in men and usually lacks the distinguishing features of the more benign forms. Frequently, it simulates thymoma and may be difficult or impossible to distinguish from this tumor on radiographic grounds [56]. Friedman et al. [47] have recently reviewed the appearance of benign cystic teratomas at computed tomography including one in the infra-azygos area.

5.2.9 Enlargement of Internal Mammary Lymph Nodes

The internal mammary lymph nodes are found adjacent to the internal mammary arteries in the intercostal spaces. The upper three intercos-

Fig. 5.34A, B. Mediastinal teratoma. PA (**A**) and lateral (**B**) radiographs. A large left anterior mediastinal mass with peripheral calcification is shown. The presence of such calcification is not sufficient to distinguish this from thymoma since at times thymic cysts may calcify in their periphery. Note minimal anterior extrapleural line apparently due to minimal intrusion of some of mass between anterior left lung and left chest wall (*1*). (Courtesy A.S. Berne, Syracuse, NY)

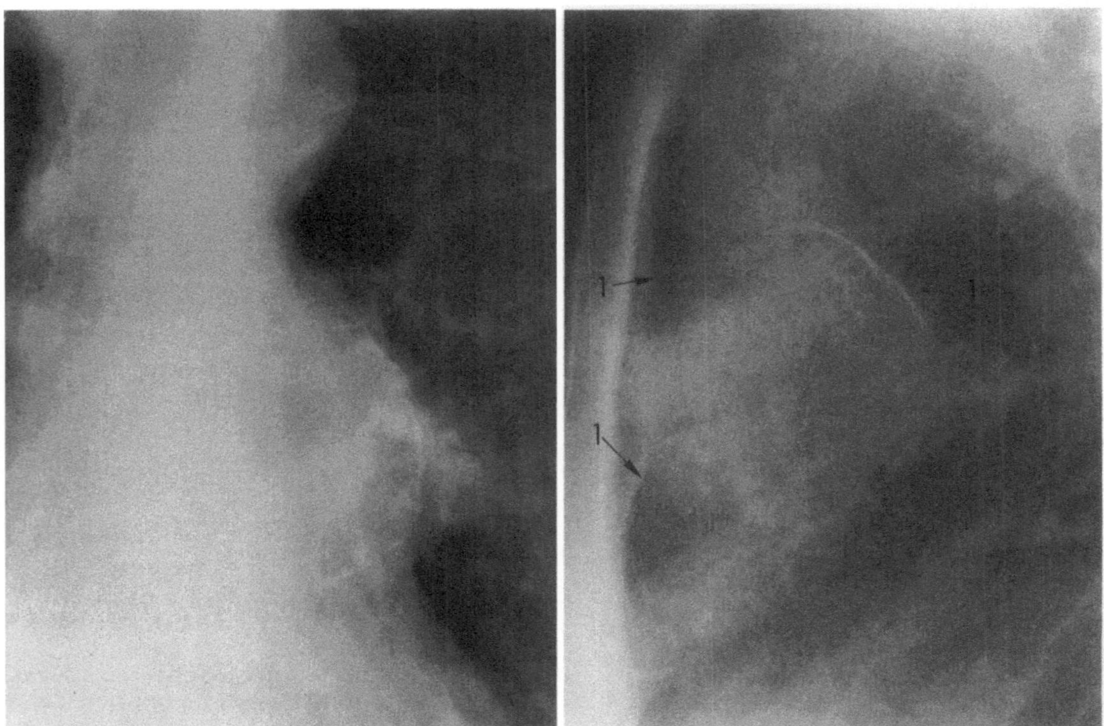

tal spaces contain nodes in a large percentage of individuals, whereas the fourth and fifth interspaces contain nodes less often [125]. These nodes drain the breast, the upper aspect of the liver, and the upper abdominal and chest wall. They are most commonly involved by tumor spread from the breast (Fig. 5.35). Urban and Marjani [125] found internal mammary metastases in 33% of their resections, although they concede that this figure may be higher than the actual incidence because of patient selection. Internal mammary nodes in the first three interspaces were most commonly involved. These nodes are also involved in patients with leukemia and lymphoma [34, 41, 97] (Fig. 5.36). Fayos found these nodes to be affected in eight of 414 patients with Hodgkin's disease [34]. Filly et al. [39] found them to be involved in about 7% of such patients and noted further that internal mammary nodes were involved ten times as frequently in patients with untreated

Hodgkin's disease as in patients with untreated non-Hodgkin's lymphoma. In Fayos' series [34], involvement of internal mammary lymph nodes by Hodgkin's disease did not occur in the absence of lymphadenopathy elsewhere in the chest.

Radiologic examination plays an important role in the detection of metastatic disease involving the internal mammary lymph nodes since this node group cannot be seen at mediastinoscopy. Patients with breast cancer, especially those who develop parasternal chest wall recurrence, should be studied with attention to the retrosternal area because such recurrences so commonly represent direct extension from internal mammary nodes [106, 124, 125]. Enlarged internal mammary nodes represent another cause for widening of the anterior extrapleural line. Most commonly, the interface made by the nodal disease with the anterior lung margins is scalloped or lobulated. Less fre-

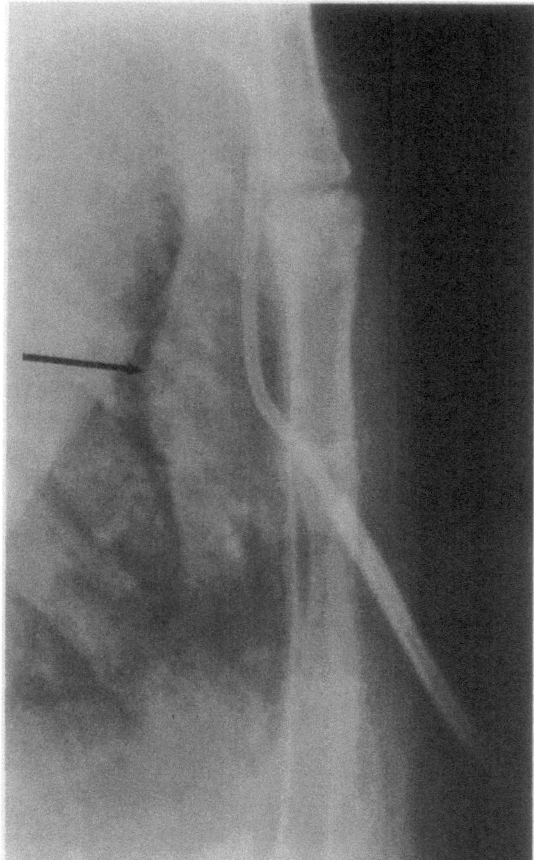

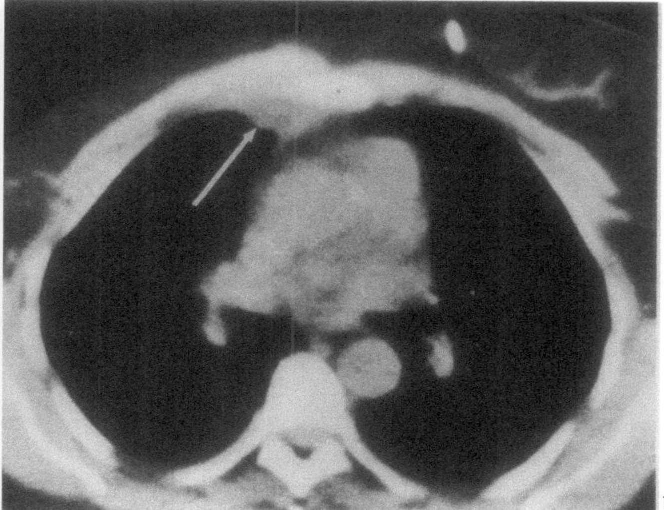

Fig. 5.35 A, B. Involvement of internal mammary lymph nodes by metastatic breast carcinoma. **A** Lateral chest radiograph. **B** Computed tomogram. Neoplastic involvement of internal mammary lymph nodes is most often secondary to carcinoma of breast, as in this patient with past history of right mammary cancer. Disease process may produce smooth or lobulated (*arrow*) anterior extrapleural line. Lymph nodes in the first, second, and third interspaces are most commonly involved. A parasternal mass is frequently noted clinically, and secondary destruction of the sternum may be visible on radiographs

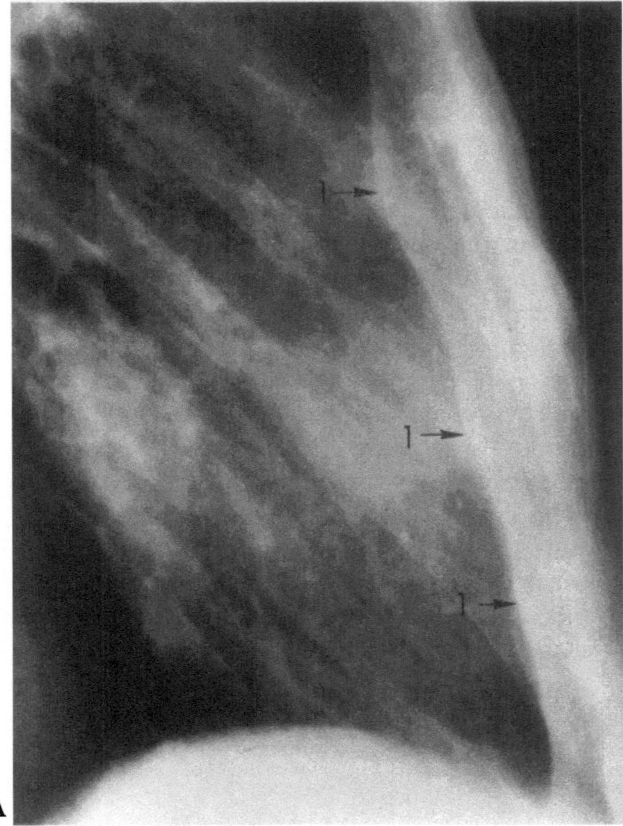

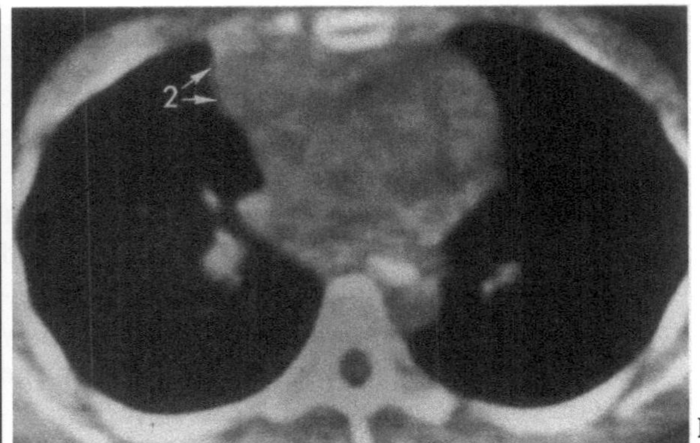

Fig. 5.36A, B. Involvement of internal mammary lymph nodes by lymphoma. Lateral radiograph (A) and computed tomogram (B). Internal mammary lymph nodes are infrequently involved by lymphoma. Hodgkin's disease is a more common cause of such enlargement than is non-Hodgkin's lymphoma. Involvement without other evidence of thoracic disease is most unusual. A smooth or lobulated anterior extrapleural line may be produced (1). Computed tomogram clearly shows involvement of anterior mediastinum retrosternally on right (2)

quently it may be smooth with the lung separated from the anterior chest wall by a stripe of increased density [41] (Figs. 5.35, 5.36). In the presence of abnormality of the anterior extrapleural line on radiographs, the mediastinal structures and hila should be studied carefully. Absence of gross disease in these regions is helpful in differential diagnosis since involvement of internal mammary nodes without involvement of the mediastinal nodes is rare in Hodgkin's disease [34]. Involvement of the internal mammary nodes as the first thoracic manifestations of this disease has, however, been reported [41]. When internal mammary nodes are enlarged by metastatic breast cancer or lymphoma, careful study of the sternum is imperative since it is so often secondarily involved.

Although PA and lateral radiographs are useful for screening patients for possible involvement of internal mammary adenopathy, computed tomography is a much more sensitive diagnostic modality [81, 87, 111, 112]. In a study

of patients with biopsy-proven breast metastases to internal mammary nodes, Meyer and Munzenrider [87] found that physical examination and plain radiographs together underestimated the extent of disease in 50% of patients. Lindfors et al. [81] also pointed out that computed tomography was much superior to physical examination for evaluation of chest wall recurrence in breast cancer. In Meyer and Munzenrider's [87] series, plain films were positive, even when studied retrospectively, in only half of the cases in which there was disease evident at computed tomography. Normal nodes were always found within 3 cm of the lateral border of the sternum and were less than 5 mm in diameter. For the evaluation study of internal mammary node involvement, Meyer and Munzenrider have stated that computed tomography assesses better, the extent of soft tissue disease of the chest wall, axillary adenopathy, sternal erosion, pleural effusion, and pulmonary or bone metastases. Ege [29] and Collier et al. [21]

have emphasized the advantages of lymphoscintigraphy in the evaluation of metastasis to internal mammary nodes.

5.2.10 Enlargement of Anterior Diaphragmatic (Cardiophrenic Angle) Lymph Nodes

The anterior and middle group of diaphragmatic lymph nodes, sometimes called the "nodes of the cardiophrenic angle", are found in the inferior portion of the anterior mediastinum [16]. The anterior group is located behind the xiphoid process and the seventh costochondral junctions. The middle group of nodes is located at the point where the phrenic nerve penetrates the diaphragm [16] (see Fig. 5.2). Castellino and Blank [16] have pointed out that these nodes are not usually identified on radiographs until they have reached a relatively large size because they are surrounded by areolar tissue and fat, which mask minimal degrees of enlargement. When they are visible in the cardiophrenic angle, they produce a mass having a convexity that is directed laterally on frontal radiographs and posteriorly on lateral films. They are difficult to distinguish from other mass lesions in the cardiophrenic angle. Enlargement of these nodes should be considered in patients with lymphoma who show the development of a cardiophrenic angle mass on serial films. In a large group of patients with lymphoma, Cho et al. [17] found cardiophrenic nodes to be involved in 7%. Filly et al. [39] have pointed out that involvement of cardiophrenic angle nodes as the sole intrathoracic site of disease occasionally occurs in non-Hodgkin's lymphoma but not in Hodgkin's disease. Interestingly, in their series, such involvement could not be correlated with disease in either upper quadrant of the abdomen [39].

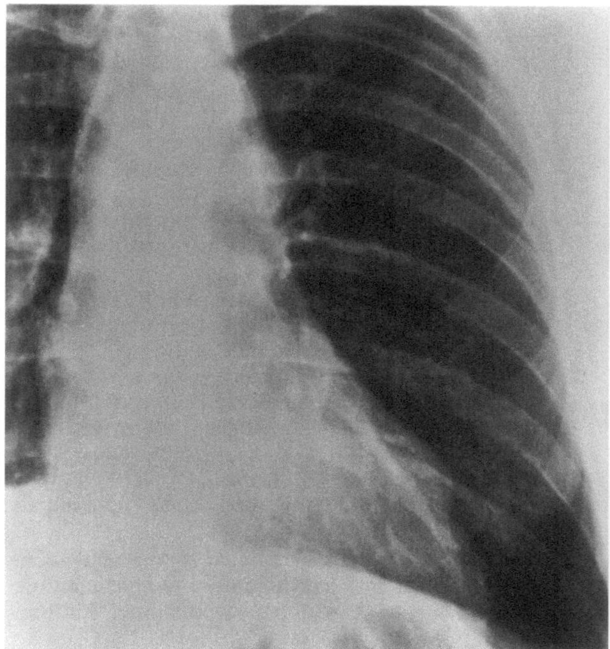

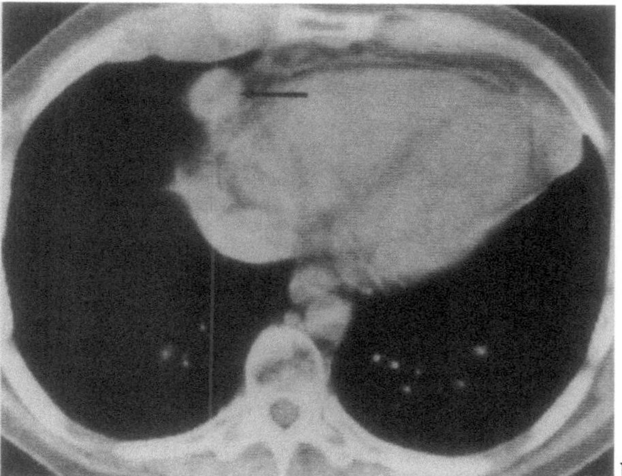

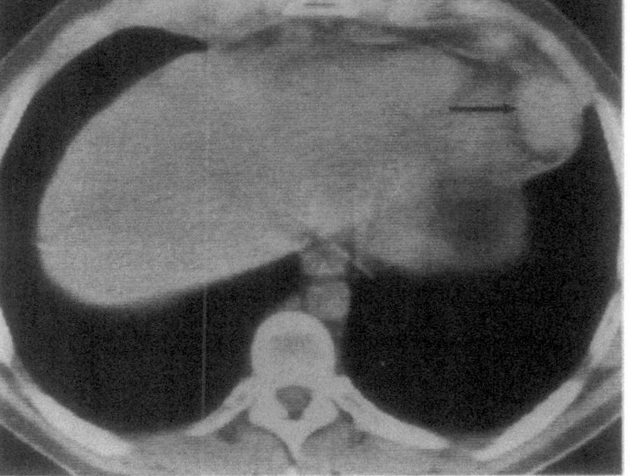

Fig. 5.37 A–C. Involvement of cardiophrenic angle nodes by lymphoma. **A** PA radiograph. **B** and **C** Computed tomograms. Involvement of cardiophrenic angle nodes can be difficult to distinguish from prominent pericardial fat pad without serial radiographs. The computed tomograms clearly show nodal masses embedded in epicardial fat (*arrow*). Compare with Figs. 5.2 and 5.21

As in other regions of the thorax, computed tomography is ideal for the study of node enlargement in the cardiophrenic angle [17, 88] (Fig. 5.37). Cho et al. [17] reported 14 patients with abnormality detected at computed tomography; only three of these patients showed evidence of disease on plain films. Computed tomography has the distinct advantage of demonstrating nodes embedded in cardiophrenic angle fat (Fig. 5.37). For this reason, it is the preferred method of following patients with lymphoma; computed tomography can detect recurrence earlier than it can be demonstrated on plain chest radiographs.

References

1. Aygun C, Slawson RG, Bajaj K, Salazar OM (1984) Primary mediastinal seminoma. Urology 23:109–117
2. Baron RL, Levitt RG, Sagel SS, Stanley RJ (1981) Computed tomography in the evaluation of mediastinal widening. Radiology 138:107–113
3. Baron RL, Lee JKT, Sagel SS, Levitt RG (1982) Computed tomography of the abnormal thymus. Radiology 142:127–134
4. Baron RL, Lee JKT, Sagel SS, Peterson RR (1982) Computed tomography of the normal thymus. Radiology 142:121–125
5. Baron RL, Lee JKT, Sagel SS, Peterson RR (1983) Standard for normal thickness of the thymus gland. Radiology 147:887
6. Batra P, Hermann C, Mulder D (1987) Mediastinal imaging in myasthenia gravis: correlation of chest radiography, CT, MR and surgical findings. AJR 148:515–519
7. Bein ME, Mancuso AA, Mink JH, Hansen GC (1978) Computed tomography in the diagnosis of mediastinal lipomatosis. J Comput Asst Tomogr 2:379–383
8. Berkow AE, Demos TE (1976) The midsternal stripe and its relationship to postoperative sternal dehiscence. Radiology 121:525
9. Bethancourt B, Pond GD, Jones SE, Grogan T, Wasserman P (1984) Mediastinal hematoma simulating recurrent Hodgkin Disease during systemic chemotherapy. AJR 142:1119–1120
10. Bjork L, Friedman R (1965) Routine roentgenographic diagnosis of coarctation of the aorta in the child. Am J Roentgenol 95:636–641
11. Bodman SF, Condemi JJ (1967) Mediastinal widening in iatrogenic Cushing's syndrome. Ann Intern Med 67:399–403
12. Boyd E (1932) Weight of the thymus gland in health and disease. Am J Dis Child 43:1162–1214
13. Brown RC, Cohen WN, Rose EF (1976) Malignant thymoma with penetration into the gastrointestinal tract. South Med J 69:409–412
14. Brown LR, Augenbaugh GL, Wick MR, Baker BA, Salassh RM (1982) Roentgenologic diagnosis of primary corticotropin producing carcinoid tumors of the mediastinum. Radiology 142:143–148
15. Carsky EW, Azimi F, Mauceri R (1980) Epicardial fat sign in the diagnosis of pericardial effusion. JAMA 244:2762–2764
16. Castellino RA, Blank N (1972) Adenopathy of the cardiophrenic angle (diaphragmatic) lymph nodes. Am J Roentgenol 114:509–515
17. Cho CS, Blank N, Castellino RA (1984) CT evaluation of cardiophrenic angle lymph nodes in patients with malignant lymphoma. AJR 143:719–721
18. Clemente CD (1985) Anatomy of the human body by Henry Gray, 30th Am edn. Lea and Febiger, Philadelphia
19. Cohen M, Hill CA, Cangir A, Sullivan MP (1980) Thymic rebound after treatment of childhood tumors. AJR 135:151–156
20. Cohen SL (1953) The right pericardial fat pad. Radiology 60:391–392
21. Collier BD, Palmer DW, Wilson JF, Greenberg M, Komaki R, Cox JD, Lawson TL, Lawlor PM (1983) Internal mammary lymphoscintigraphy in patients with breast cancer. Correlation with computed tomography and impact on radiation therapy planning. Radiology 147:845–848
22. Davis LA, McCreadle SR (1962) The enlarged thymus gland in leukemia in childhood. Am J Roentgenol 88:924–927
23. Davis WS, Allen RP (1968) Accessory diaphragm – duplication of the diaphragm. Radiol Clin North Am 6:253–263
24. del Regato JA, Spjut HJ (1977) Ackerman and del Regato's Cancer – diagnosis, treatment, and prognosis, 5th edn. Mosby, St. Louis
25. Demos TC, Cardella RG, Moncada R, Reynes CJ, Love L, Churchill RJ (1983) Epicardial fat sign due to extrapericardial disease. AJR 141:289–291
26. DiGeorge AM (1965) Discussions on new concepts of cellular basis of immunity. J Pediatr 67:907–908
27. Drachman B (1978) Myasthenia gravis. N Engl J Med 298:136–142
28. Drasin GF, Lynch T, Temes GP (1978) Ectopic ACTH production and mediastinal lipomatosis. Radiology 127:610
29. Ege GN (1982) RE: Computed tomographic demonstration of internal mammary lymph node metastasis in patients with breast carcinoma. Radiology 142:253–254
30. Ellis K, Gregg HG (1964) Thymomas – roentgen considerations. Am J Roentgenol 91:105–119
31. Ellison RT III, Corrao WM, Fox MJ, Braman SS (1981) Spontaneous mediastinal hemorrhage in patients on chronic hemodialysis. Ann Intern Med 95:704–706
32. Engleman RM, Williams D, Gouge TH, Chase RM Jr, Falk EA, Boyd AD, Reed GE (1973) Mediastinitis following open-heart surgery: review of two years' experience. Arch Surg 107:772–778

33. Eshaghy B, Loeb HS, Miller SE, Scanlon PJ, Towne WD, Gunnar RM (1973) Mediastinal and retropharyngeal hemorrhage – a complication of cardiac catheterization. JAMA 226:427–431

34. Fayos JV (1968) Extrapulmonary intrathoracic manifestations of Hodgkin's disease. Radiol Clin North Am 6:131–141

35. Federle MP, Callen PW (1979) Cystic Hodgkin's lymphoma of the thymus: computed tomographic appearance. J Comput Assist Tomogr 3:542–544

36. Felson B (1973) Chest roentgenology. Saunders, Philadelphia

37. Felson B, Castleman B, Levinsohn EM, Markarian B (1982) Radiologic-pathologic correlation conference: SUNY Health Science Center at Syracuse, New York. Cushing syndrome associated with mediastinal mass. AJR 138:815–820

38. Figley MM (1954) Accessory signs of coarctation of the aorta. Radiology 62:671–686

39. Filly R, Blank N, Castellino RA (1976) Radiographic distribution of intrathoracic disease in previously untreated patients with Hodgkin's disease and non-Hodgkin's lymphoma. Radiology 120:277–281

40. Fisher ER (1964) Pathology of the thymus and its relation to human disease. In: Good RA, Gabrielson AE (eds) The thymus in immunology. Harper and Row, New York

41. Fleischner FG, Bernstein C, Levine BE (1948) Retrosternal infiltration in malignant lymphoma. Radiology 51:350–357

42. Fon GT, Bein ME, Mancuso AA, Keesey JC, Lupetin AR, Wong WS (1982) Computed tomography of the anterior mediastinum in myasthemia gravis: a radiologic-pathologic correlative study. Radiology 142:135–141

43. Forrest JV, Schackleford GD, Bramson RT, Anderson LS (1973) Acute mediastinal widening. Am J Roentgenol 117:881–885

44. Francis IR, Glazer GM, Bookstein FL, Gross BH (1985) Thymus: reexamination of age related changes in size and shape. AJR 145:249–254

45. Franken EA (1968) Radiological evidence of thymic enlargement in Graves disease. Radiology 91:20–22

46. Fraser RG, Pare JAP (1977) Diagnosis of diseases of the chest, 2nd edn. Saunders, Philadelphia

47. Friedman AC, Pyatt RS, Hartman DS, Downey EF, Olson WB (1982) CT of benign cystic teratomas. AJR 138:659–665

48. Frolich DJ, Clements JL Jr, Weens HS (1975) Epicardial fat line in left pleural effusion. AJR 124:394–396

49. Gale ME (1986) Anterior diaphragm: variations in the CT appearance. Radiology 161:635–639

50. Goebel N (1983) The "lobe" of the right brachiocephalic vein. CT-sonographie 3:146–148

51. Goldstein G, McKay IR (1969) The human thymus. Green, St. Louis

52. Goodman LR, Kay HR, Teplick SK, Mundth ED (1983) Complications of median sternotomy: computed tomographic evaluation. AJR 141:225–230

53. Goodman LR, Teplick SK, Kay HR (1983) Computed tomography of the normal sternum. AJR 141:219–223

54. Gunn A, Michie W, Irvine WJ (1964) The thymus in thyroid disease. Lancet 2:776–778

55. Heiberg E, Wolverson MK, Sundaram M, Nouri S (1982) Normal thymus: CT characteristics in subjects under age 20. AJR 138:491–494

56. Hochholzer L, Theros EG, Rosen SH (1969) Some unusual lesions of the mediastinum: roentgenologic and pathologic features. Semin Roentgenol 4:74–90

57. Holt JF (1947) Epipericardial fat shadows in differential diagnosis. Radiology 48:472–479

58. Homer MJ, Wechsler RJ, Carter BL (1978) Mediastinal lipomatosis. CT confirmation of a normal variant. Radiology 128:657–661

59. Jorgens J, Kundel R, Lieber A (1962) Cinefluorographic approach to diagnosis of pericardial effusion. Am J Roentgenol 87:911–916

60. Keats TE (1974) Right parasternal stripe – a new mediastinal shadow and a contribution to the nature of the retrosternal line. Am J Roentgenol 120:898–900

61. Kemp FH, Morley HMC, Embrys-Roberts E (1948) A sail-like triangular projection from the mediastinum: a radiographic appearance of the thymus gland. Br J Radiol 21:618–624

62. Kemp-Harper RA, Guyer PB (1965) The radiological features of thymic tumors: a review of 65 cases. Clin Radiol 16:97–105

63. Keynes G (1954) Physiology of the thymus gland. Br Med J 2:659–663

64. Kirkpatrick JA Jr, DiGeorge AM (1968) Congenital absence of the thymus. Am J Roentgenol 103:32–37

65. Kissin CM, Husband JE, Nicholas D, Eversman W (1987) Benign thymic enlargement in adults after chemotherapy: CT demonstration. Radiology 163:67–70

66. Klatte EC, Yune HY (1972) The diagnosis and treatment of pericardial cysts. Radiology 104:541–544

67. Kleinman PK, Raptopoulos V (1985) The anterior diaphragmatic attachments: an anatomic and radiologic study with clinical correlates. Radiology 155:289–293

68. Kleinman PK, Brill PW, Whalen JP (1978) Anterior pathway for transdiaphragmatic extension of pneumomediastinum. AJR 131:271–275

69. Knuttson F (1955) Mediastinal pleura. Acta Radiol 43:265–275

70. Koerner HJ, Sun Di-C (1966) Mediastinal lipomatosis secondary to steroid therapy. Am J Roentgenol 98:461–464

71. Kountz SL, Connolly JE, Cohn R (1963) Seminoma-like (or seminomatous) tumors of the anterior mediastinum. J Thorac Cardiovasc Surg 45:289–301

72. Kremens V (1955) Demonstration of pericardial shadow on routine chest roentgenograms: new roentgen finding, preliminary report. Radiology 64:72–80

73. Lane EJ, Carsky EW (1968) Epicardial fat: lateral plain film diagnosis in normals and in pericardial effusion. Radiology 91:1–5

74. Lanuza A (1971) The sign of the cane. A new radiological sign for the diagnosis of small Morgagni hernias. Radiology 101:293–296

75. Lattes R (1962) Thymoma and other tumors of the thymus; analysis of 107 cases. Cancer 15:1224–1261

76. Lee WJ, Fattal G (1976) Mediastinal lipomatosis in simple obesity Chest 70:308–309

77. Leigh TF, Weens HS (1959) The mediastinum. Thomas, Springfield, IL

78. Leigh TF, Weens HS (1969) Roentgen aspects of mediastinal lesions. Semin Roentgenol 4:59–73

79. Leszcynski SZ (1972) Purulent and fibrous mediastinitis; radiologic diagnosis. Polish Medical Publishers, Warsaw

80. Levitt RG, Husband JE, Glazer HS (1984) CT of primary cell tumors of the mediastinum. AJR 142:73–78

81. Lindfors KK, Meyer JK, Busse PM, Kopans DB, Munzenreider JE, Sawicka JM (1985) CT evaluation of local and regional breast cancer recurrence. AJR 145:833–837

82. Lodin H (1957) Mediastinal herniation and displacement – studied by transversal tomography. Acta Radiol 48:337–350

83. Lowenhaupt E, Brown R (1951) Carcinoma of thymus of granulomatous type, clinical and pathological study. Cancer 4:1193–1209

84. Lubin BH, Friedman S, Miller WM (1967) Intrapericardial teratoma associated with pericardial effusion – an acute surgical problem in infancy. J Pediatr Surg 2:336–342

85. Maier HC (1938) Mediastinal hernia in the absence of pneumothorax. Am J Roentgenol 39:687–697

86. Marnocha KE, Maglinte DDP, Woods J, Goodman M, Peterson P (1984) Mediastinal width/chest width ratio in blunt chest trauma: a reappraisal. AJR 142:275–277

87. Meyer JE, Munzenrider JE (1981) Computed tomographic demonstration of internal mammary lymph node metastasis in patients with locally recurrent breast carcinoma. Radiology 139:661–663

88. Meyer JE, McLoud TC, Lindfors KK (1985) CT demonstration of cardiophrenic angle lymphadenopathy in Hodgkin disease. J Comput Assist Tomogr 9:485–488

89. Moffat RE (1976) Radiologic changes in the thymoma – hypogammaglobulinemia syndrome. AJR 126:1219–1222

90. Moore AV Jr, Korobkin M, Olanow H, Heaston DK, Ram PC, Dunnick NR, Silverman P (1983) Age related changes in the thymus gland: CT pathologic correlation. AJR 141:241–246

91. Mulvey RB (1963) The thymic "wave" sign. Radiology 81:834–838

92. Nahon JR (1955) Roentgenologic characteristics of the epipericardial fat pad, with a case report. Radiology 65:745–748

93. Odman P (1953) The appearance of the internal mammary arteries in coarctation of the aorta. Acta Radiol 39:47–56

94. Oh KS, Weber AL, Borden S IV (1971) Normal mediastinal mass in childhood. Radiology 101:625–628

95. Pernkopf E (1963) Atlas of topographic and applied human anatomy, vol 2. Saunders, Philadelphia

96. Peterson ROA, Cooper MD, Good RA (1965) The pathogenesis of immunologic deficiency disease. Am J Med 38:579–604

97. Pfister RC, Kook SO, Ferrucci JT (1970) Retrosternal density – a radiographic evaluation of the retrosternal – premediastinal space. Radiology 96:317–324

98. Pond GD, Bjelland JC (1980) Enlarging pericardial fat pad mimicking tumor. J Can Assoc Radiol 31:267–268

99. Price JE, Rigler LG (1970) Widening of the mediastinum resulting from fat accumulation. Radiology 96:497–500

100. Proto AV, Rost RC Jr (1985) CT of the thorax: pitfalls in interpretation. RadioGraphics 5:693–812

101. Pugatch RE, Faling LJ (1982) Computed tomography of the thorax: a status report. Chest 80:618–626

102. Quottromani FL, Foley LC, Bowen A III, Weissman L, Hernandez J (1981) Fascial relationship of the thymus; radiologic-pathologic correlation in neonatal pneumomediastinum. AJR 137:1209–1211

103. Raphael MJ (1963) Mediastinal hematoma – a description of some radiological appearances. Br J Radiol 36:921–924

104. Rogers JV, Leigh TF (1953) Differential diagnosis of right cardiophrenic angle masses. Radiology 61:871–877

105. Rosai J, Higa E (1972) Mediastinal endocrine neoplasm, of probable thymic origin, related to carcinoid tumor. Clinicopathologic study of 8 cases. Cancer 29:1061–1074

106. Rubin P, Bunyagidj S, Poulter C (1971) Internal mammary lymph node metastases in breast cancer: detection and management. Am J Roentgenol 111:588–598

107. Sandor F (1967) Incidence and significance of traumatic mediastinal hematoma. Thorax 22:43–62

108. Scheff S, LaForet EG (1966) The internal thoracic muscle and the lateral chest roentgenogram. Radiology 86:27–30

109. Seltzer SE, D'Orsi C, Kirshner R, DeWeese JA (1981) Traumatic aortic rupture: plain radiographic findings. AJR 137:1011–1014

110. Serry C, Bleck P, Javid H, Hunter JA, Goldin MD, Delaria GA, Najafi H (1980) Sternal wound complications. J Thorac Cardiovasc Surg 80:861–867

111. Shea WJ Jr, deGeer G, Webb WR (1987) Chest wall after mastectomy. I CT appearance of normal postoperative anatomy, post irradiation changes and optimal scanning techniques. Radiology 162:157–161

112. Shea WJ Jr, deGeer G, Webb WR (1987) Chest wall after mastectomy. II CT appearance after tumor recurrence. AJR 162:162–164

113. Shopfner CE, Jansen C, O'Kell RT (1968) Roentgen significance of transverse thoracic muscle. Am J Roentgenol 103:140–148

114. Slawson R, Aygun C, Carbone D, Hafiz M, Attar S, Whitley N (1983) Primary mediastinal seminoma. RadioGraphics 3:100–106

115. Sone S, Higashihara T, Morimoto S, Yokota K, Ikezoe J, Masaoka A, Monden Y, Kagotani T (1980) Normal anatomy of thymus and anterior mediastinum by pneumomediastinography. AJR 134:81–89

116. Sone S, Higashihara T, Morimoto S, Yokota K, Ikezoe J, Oomine H, Arisawa J, Monden Y, Nakahara K (1982) Potential spaces of the mediastinum: CT pneumomediastinography. AJR 138:1051–1057

117. Souadjian JV, Enriquez P, Silverstein MN, Pepin JM (1974) The spectrum of diseases associated with thymoma: coincidence or syndrome? Arch Intern Med 134:374–379

118. Stilwell ME, Weisbrod GL, Ilves R (1981) Spontaneous mediastinal hematoma. J Can Assoc Radiol 32:60–61

119. Streiter ML, Schneider HJ, Proto AV (1982) Steroid-induced thoracic lipomatosis: paraspinal involvement. AJR 139:679–681

120. Strickland B (1967) Intrathoracic Hodgkin's disease. II. Peripheral manifestations of Hodgkin's disease in the chest. Br J Radiol 40:930–938

121. Teates CD (1970) Steroid-induced mediastinal lipomatosis. Radiology 96:501–502

122. Teplick JG, Nedwich A, Haskin ME (1973) Roentgenographic features of thymolipoma. Am J Roentgenol 117:873–877

123. Torrance DJ (1955) Demonstration of subepicardial fat as an aid in diagnosis of pericardial effusion or thickening. Am J Roentgenol 74:850–855

124. Urban JA (1959) Clinical experience and results of excision of internal mammary lymph node chain in primary operable breast cancer. Cancer 12:14–22

125. Urban JA, Marjani MA (1971) Significance of internal mammary lymph node metastases in breast cancer. Am J Roentgenol 111:130–136

126. Vock P, Hodler J (1986) Cardiophrenic angle adenopathy: update of causes and significance. Radiology 159:395–399

127. Walter E, Hubener KH (1980) Computerized tomographic characteristics of space occupying lesions in the anterior mediastinum and their differential diagnosis. ROFO 133:391–400

128. Warwick R, Williams PR (1973) Gray's anatomy, 35th edn. Saunders, Philadelphia

129. Weinstein JB, Aronberg D, Sagel SS (1983) CT of fibrosing mediastinitis: findings and their utility. AJR 141:247–251

130. Whalen JP, Meyers MA, Oliphant M, Caragol WJ, Evans JA (1973) The retrosternal line: a new sign of an anterior mediastinal mass. Am J Roentgenol 117:861–872

131. Whalen JP, Oliphant M, Evans JA (1975) Anterior extrapleural line; superior extension. Radiology 115:525–531

132. White JJ, Kaback MM, Haller JA (1968) Diagnosis and excision of an intrapericardial teratoma in an infant. J Thorac Cardiovasc Surg 55:704–710

133. Woodring JH, Pulmano CM, Stevens RK (1982) Right paratracheal stripe in blunt chest trauma. Radiology 143:605–608

134. Woodring JH, Loh FK, Kryscio RJ (1984) Mediastinal hemorrhage: an evaluation of radiographic manifestations. Radiology 151:15–21

135. Young R, Pochaczevsky R, Pollak L, Bryk D (1973) Cervico-mediastinal thymic cysts. Am J Roentgenol 117:855–860

136. Yulish BS, Owens RP (1980) Thymic enlargement in a child during therapy for primary hypothyroidism. Am J Roentgenol 135:157–158

137. Zerhouni EA, Scott WW Jr, Baker RR, Wharam MP, Siegelman SS (1982) Invasive thymomas: diagnosis and evaluation by computed tomography. J Comput Assist Tomogr 6:92–100

138. Ziter FMH (1977) Major thoracic dehiscence: radiologic considerations. Radiology 122:587–590

6 The Supra-aortic Area

6.1 General Anatomic Considerations

The supra-aortic area is that portion of the left side of the mediastinum situated behind the anterior mediastinum and extending cephalad from the aortic arch to the thoracic inlet. The radiographic anatomy of the area is predicated upon the anatomy of the aorta and its major branches.

The ascending aorta begins at the level of the lower border of the third costochondral junction behind the pulmonary artery and the right atrium (Fig. 6.2) and runs upward, anteriorly and to the right (Fig. 6.1). At the level of the aortic valves the pulmonary artery is found in front of the ascending aorta (Fig. 6.2), but as it passes upward it assumes a position to the left of the aorta (Figs. 6.1 and 6.3). The ascend-

ing aorta and the main pulmonary artery lie entirely within the pericardium (Fig. 6.1). The left atrium and right pulmonary artery lie behind the ascending aorta; the superior vena cava is lateral and posterior (Figs. 6.2 and 6.3). As it courses upward, the ascending aorta is contacted by right lung (Fig. 6.3). As it ascends,

Fig. 6.1 A, B. Anatomic relationships of ascending aorta. Coronal body section (**A**) and sagittal body section (**B**). Ascending aorta (*1*) extends upward and to right from its origin from left ventricle. Pulmonary artery lies anterior to aorta at their points of origin, but as vessels progress upward, pulmonary artery (*2*) comes to lie to left side of aorta. Both vessels are situated totally within pericardium (*3*). Ascending aorta lies in front of left atrium (*4*) below and right pulmonary artery (*5*) above and is often contacted on its anterior surface by anterior mediastinal fat (*7*) and/or right lung (*8*). Trachea (*9*) lies behind upper portion of ascending aorta and aortic arch

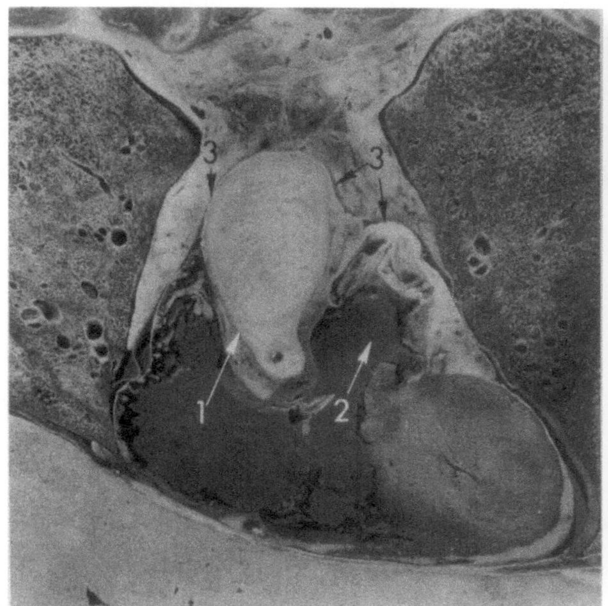

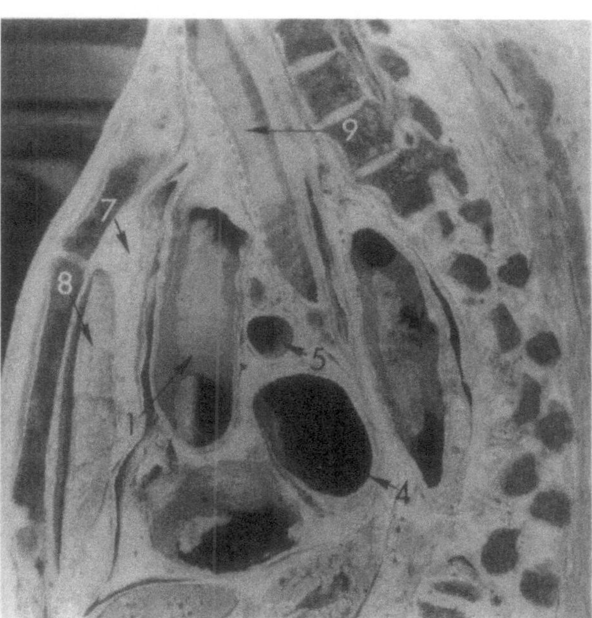

AB

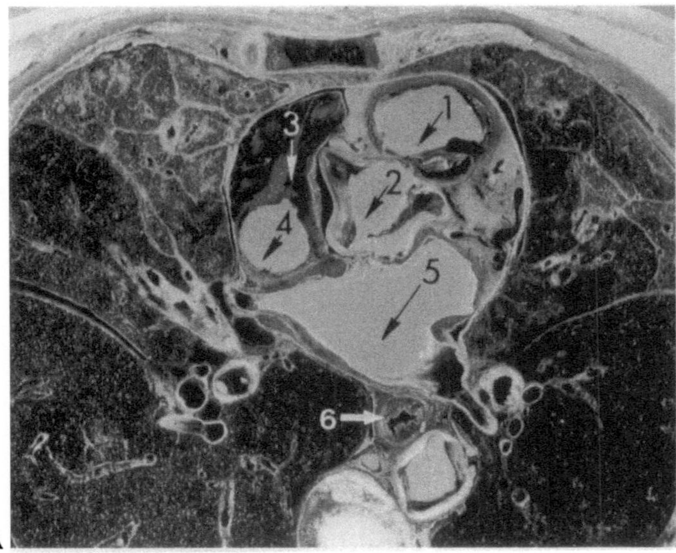

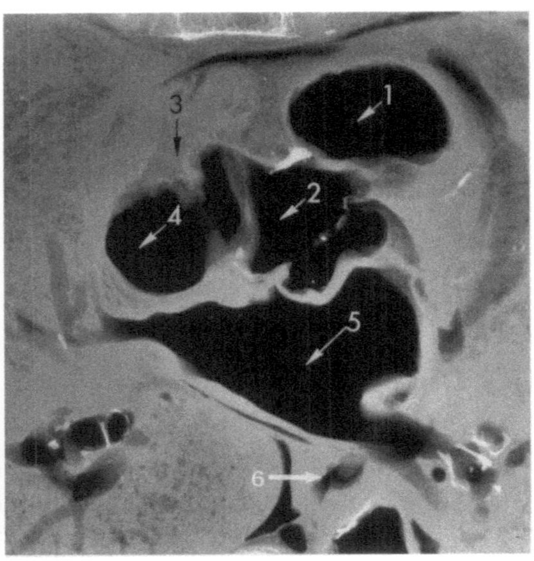

Fig. 6.2 A, B. Relationship of aorta and main pulmonary artery at their origins. Transverse body section through level of left atrium (**A**) and roentgenogram of this same transverse body slice (**B**). As aorta and main pulmonary artery arise from left and right ventricles, pulmonary artery (*1*) lies in front of aorta (*2*). Note that root of aorta is in intimate contact with upper portion of right atrium (*3*), superior vena cava (*4*) laterally, and left atrium (*5*) posteriorly. At this level, the esophagus (*6*) is anterior to the aorta

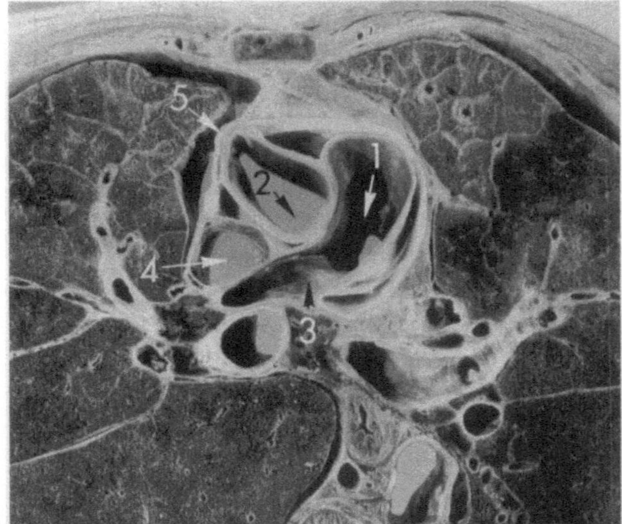

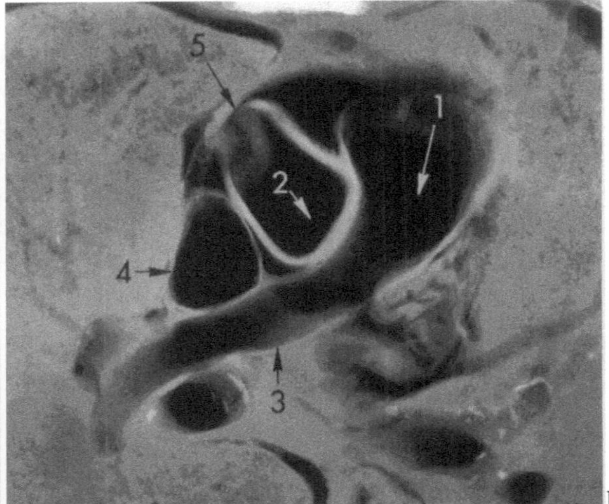

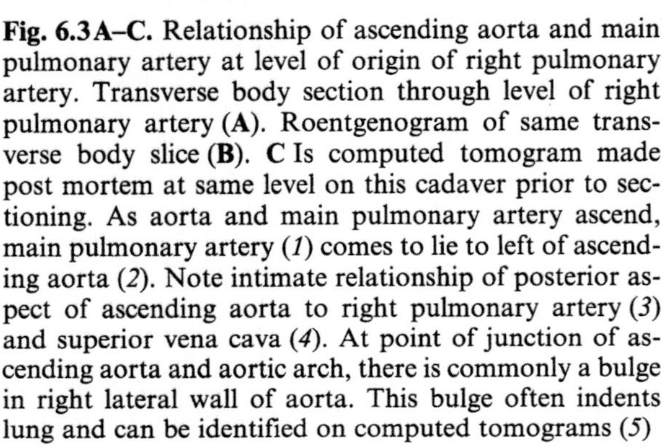

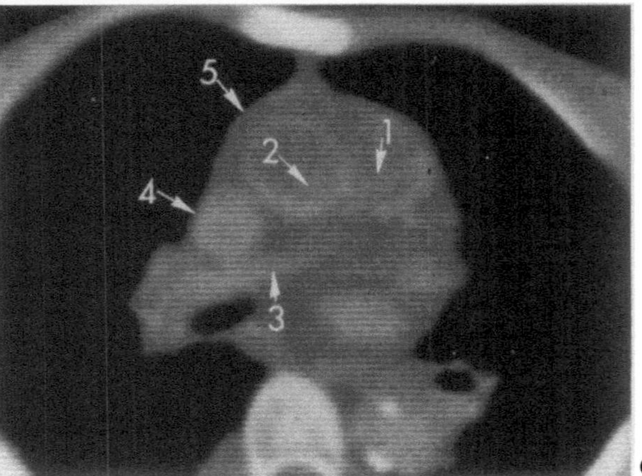

Fig. 6.3 A–C. Relationship of ascending aorta and main pulmonary artery at level of origin of right pulmonary artery. Transverse body section through level of right pulmonary artery (**A**). Roentgenogram of same transverse body slice (**B**). **C** Is computed tomogram made post mortem at same level on this cadaver prior to sectioning. As aorta and main pulmonary artery ascend, main pulmonary artery (*1*) comes to lie to left of ascending aorta (*2*). Note intimate relationship of posterior aspect of ascending aorta to right pulmonary artery (*3*) and superior vena cava (*4*). At point of junction of ascending aorta and aortic arch, there is commonly a bulge in right lateral wall of aorta. This bulge often indents lung and can be identified on computed tomograms (*5*)

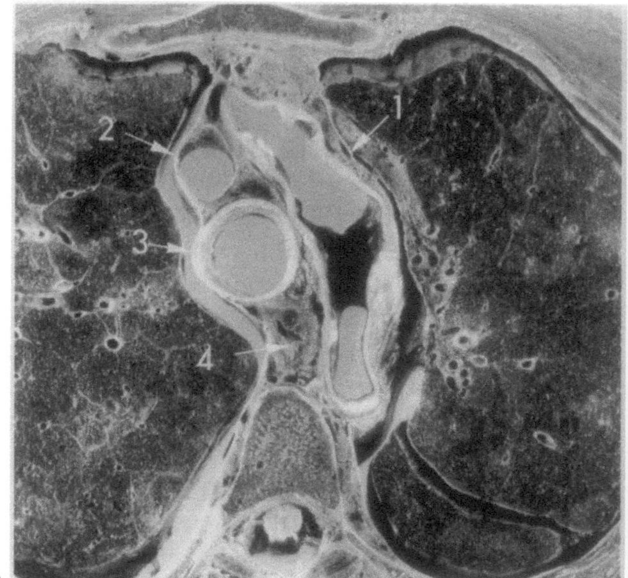

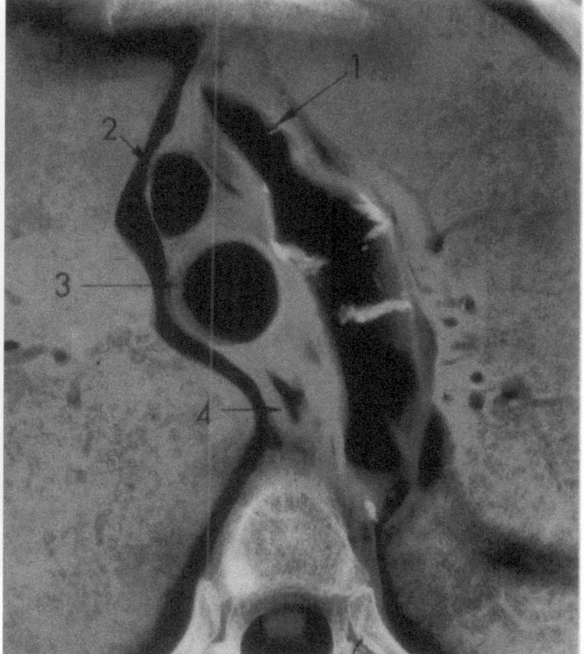

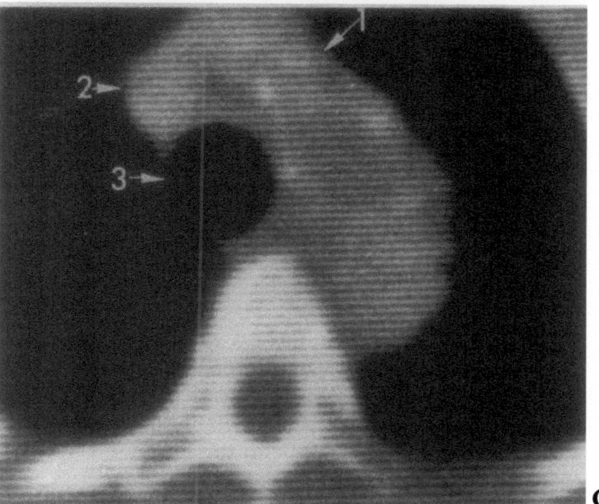

Fig. 6.4A–C. Anatomic relationships of aortic arch. Transverse body section through level of aortic arch (**A**). Roentgenogram of same body slice (**B**). **C** Is computed tomogram made post mortem at same level on this cadaver prior to sectioning. From its point of origin, aortic arch (*1*) extends posteriorly and to left. Its anterior portion lies to left of superior vena cava (*2*) and in front of trachea (*3*). As arch passes posteriorly it courses to left of trachea to become paraspinal in location. Esophagus (*4*) lies immediately to its right side

the pulmonary artery is contacted by left lung (Fig. 6.3). Rarely does the normal ascending aorta contact the left lung; the normal pulmonary artery rarely, if ever, contacts right lung.

The aortic arch begins at the level of the second sternocostal articulation on the right side and runs upward in front of the trachea (Fig. 6.1). It turns posteriorly and to the left, finally reaching the left side of the body of the fourth thoracic vertebra where it turns inferiorly to become the descending aorta (Fig. 6.4). The area above the posterior aspect of the aortic arch, behind the trachea and in front of the spine, has been called the "aortic triangle" [43], whereas the posterior turn of the aortic arch (Fig. 6.5) is commonly called the aortic "knob" in radiologic parlance. The arch gives rise to the innominate, the left common carotid, and the left subclavian arteries, which in most individuals are crossed anteriorly at their points of origin by the left innominate vein (Fig. 6.5). The first branch of the aorta, the innominate artery, courses obliquely upward and to the right in front of the trachea (Fig. 6.6A) to divide behind

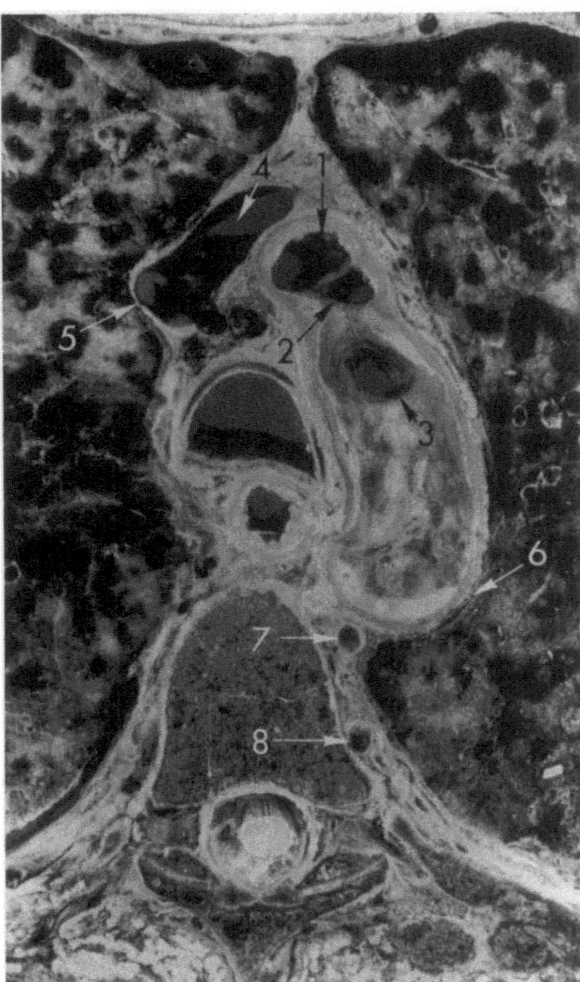

Fig. 6.5. Anatomic relationships of aortic arch (transverse body section). Origins of innominate artery (*1*), left common carotid artery (*2*), and left subclavian artery (*3*) are clearly identified. Left innominate vein (*4*) can be seen crossing anterior to these vessels on its way to meet right innominate vein to form superior vena cava (*5*). As aortic arch becomes paraspinal in location, it turns sharply inferior to level of aortic "knob" (*6*). Lung inserts itself behind aortic knob, providing contrast to allow distal aortic arch to be visible on most lateral radiographs. An intercostal artery (*7*) and hemiazygos vein (*8*) are also identified

the right sternoclavicular articulation into the right subclavian and right common carotid arteries. In a slightly more posterior coronal plane the left common carotid originates from the aorta, passing upward along the left anterolateral aspect of the trachea (Fig. 6.6). The first part of the left subclavian artery arises from the aorta behind the left common carotid artery and ascends lateral to the trachea beneath the left mediastinal pleura (see Fig. 6.11). It then arches upward and laterally across the anterior aspect of the apex of the left lung. The second part of the vessel, its highest portion, lies behind the scalenus anterior muscle. The third part continues laterally to pass through the groove for the subclavian artery in the superior surface of the first rib, there it becomes the axillary artery (see chapter 4). Before passing behind the scalenus anterior muscle, the subclavian arteries give rise to the internal mammary arteries, which pass downward behind the costal cartilages of the upper six ribs. Here they are intimately related to the internal mammary lymph nodes.

The descending aorta begins at the lower border of the fourth thoracic vertebra and descends in a curve with its convexity directed backward to terminate at the aortic hiatus (Fig. 6.7). The hemiazygos and accessory hemiazygos veins lie behind the descending aorta (Fig. 6.5). The thoracic duct lies to its right side, and further to the right is the ascending portion of the azygos vein. The esophagus coils about the aorta and is to its right in the upper part of the thorax (Fig. 6.4) and in front of the aorta lower down (Fig. 6.2). Anatomic sections and computed tomographic scans reveal that the relationship of the aorta to the esophagus at the diaphragm is somewhat variable; at times the esophagus is directly anterior to the aorta, but it may lie anteriorly and to the right or left of it (Fig. 6.2). The descending aorta gives rise to two left bronchial arteries, one at the level of the fifth thoracic vertebra and the second just below the level of the left main bronchus. The right bronchial artery, usually single, arises from the right superior intercostal artery or from the upper left bronchial artery. The descending aorta also gives off four or five esopha-

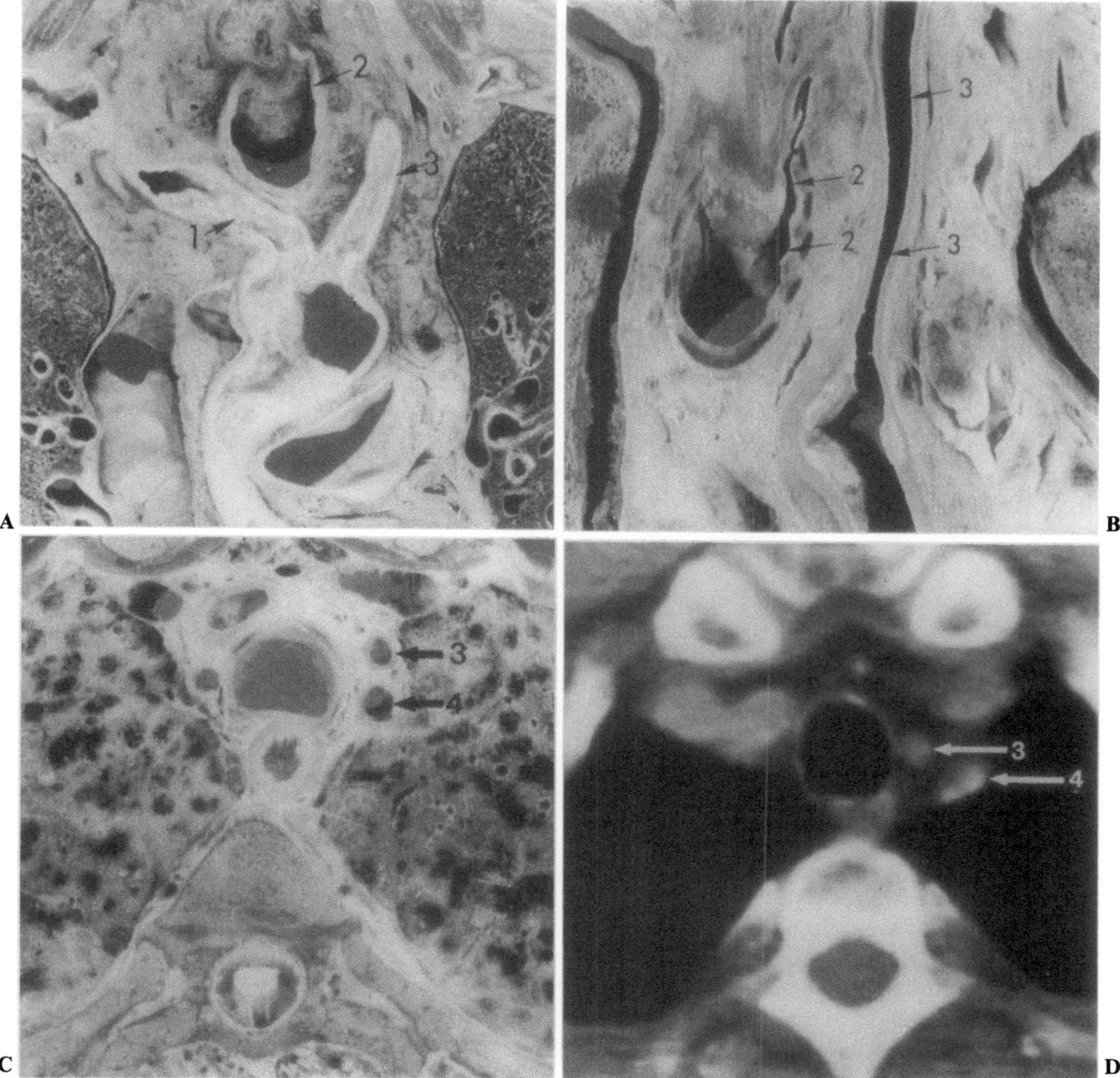

Fig. 6.6 A–D. Relationship of innominate artery and left common carotid artery to trachea. Coronal body sections (**A** and **B**), transverse body section (**C**), and computed tomogram (**D**). From its point of origin from aortic arch, innominate artery (*1*) crosses in front of trachea (*2*) in intimate contact with it. Left common carotid artery (*3*) ascends along left anterolateral margin of trachea separated from trachea and from left lung by areolar tissue and fat. Left lung abutting the mediastinum in the same coronal plane as the trachea most often contacts fat surrounding the left common carotid artery (**A**, **B**, and **D**), rarely contacts the left common carotid artery itself (**C**), and very rarely contacts the left lateral tracheal wall (see text). The first portion of the left subclavian artery (*4*) is readily identified

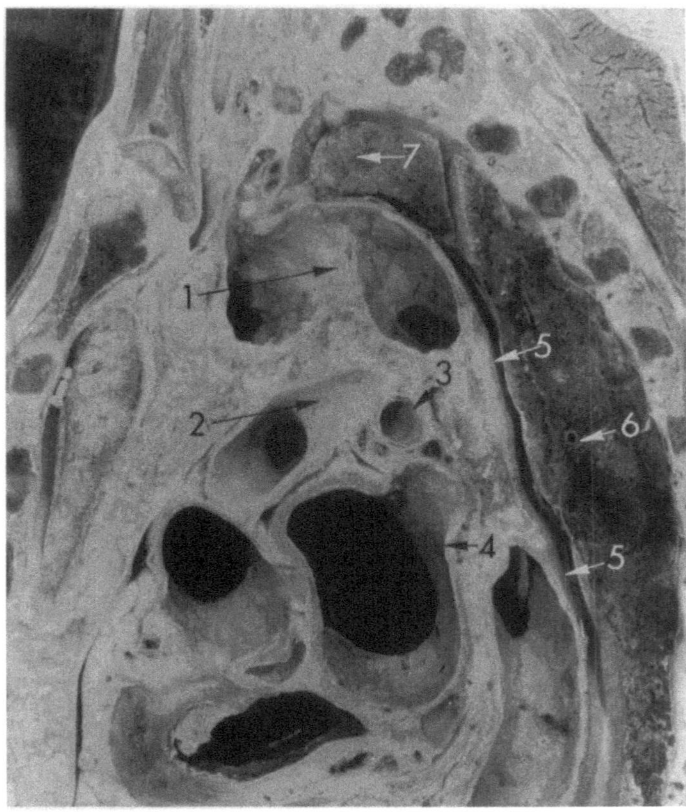

Fig. 6.7. Anatomic relationships of descending aorta. Sagittal body section through descending aorta. Aortic arch (*1*) courses posteriorly over left pulmonary artery (*2*), which, in turn, passes cephalad of the left main bronchus (*3*). The upper descending portion of the aorta lies immediately above the left atrium (*4*). Normal, slightly ectatic descending aorta (*5*) impresses against left lower lobe (*6*) and is outlined by it on lateral radiographs. Superior surface of aortic arch is outlined by left upper lobe (*7*)

geal arteries and the lower nine posterior intercostal arteries (Fig. 6.5). The first two intercostal spaces are supplied by the highest intercostal arteries, which are branches of the costocervical trunk of the subclavian artery.

The aortic bodies are aggregates of chromaffin cells derived from the neural crest. They are analogous in structure to the carotid bodies and serve to regulate the depth and rate of respiration in response to changes in blood pH and the partial pressures of oxygen and carbon dioxide in the blood [27]. They can measure up to 1 cm in their greatest dimension and are located near or along the aortic arch at four sites: (a) the pulmonary end of the ligamentum arteriosum; (b) the origin of the left common carotid artery; (c) the bifurcation of the innominate artery or lateral to the origin of the right subclavian artery; and (d) the anterolateral aspect of the left side of the aortic arch near the origin of the left subclavian artery [4].

6.2 Radiologic Correlations with Anatomy and Pathology

6.2.1 The Supra-aortic Pleural Reflections

6.2.1.1 The Anterior Junction Line

The anterior junction line is formed by the contact of the two lungs above and anterior to the aorta and in front of the structures of the upper portion of the mediastinum. Like the posterior junction line, it is formed by a double thickness of visceral and parietal pleura. Since these pleural surfaces also form the lateral margins of the anterior mediastinum, the anterior junction line is discussed in greater depth in chapter 5. It should be borne in mind, however, that behind the anterior junction line the apposed left visceral and parietal pleurae are reflected over the aorta; these reflections can be identified on radiographs as several distinct lung-soft tissue interfaces that have characteristic appearances on the left side of the mediastinum above the aorta.

6.2.1.2 The Aortic-Pulmonary Line

In 1972, Keats described a linear mediastinal shadow extending from the left upper portion of the mediastinum obliquely downward and to the left to merge at its lower end with the pleural reflections over the undivided pulmonary artery or the heart [30]. This line has been discussed by Blank and Castellino in their article on the pleural reflections of the left superior mediastinum as reflection "A" [6]. They elaborated upon the many variations in the configuration of this reflection, which is frequently superimposed on the aortic knob on frontal radiographs (Figs. 6.8 and 6.10). Keats deduced that the line represented the contact of the visceral and parietal pleurae anterior to the aorta by comparing radiographs before and after the development of pneumomediastinum as supporting evidence. It is possible to demonstrate this line on coronal sections of cadaver specimens and thus to confirm Keats' hypothesis (Fig. 6.9). Often the aortic-pulmonary line is seen as a true line rather

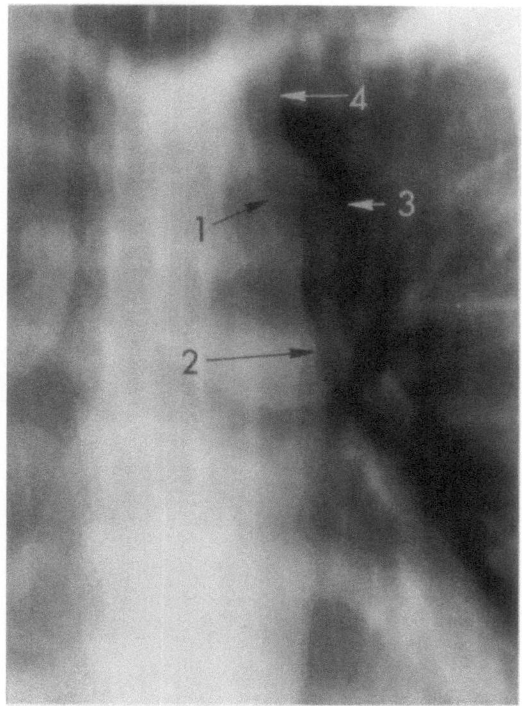

Fig. 6.8. The aortic-pulmonary line (AP tomogram). This oblique line (*1*) extending downward to merge with shadow of main pulmonary artery (*2*) is seen superimposed on aortic knob (*3*). It represents contact of lung with mediastinum anterior to interface made by lung with left subclavian artery (*4*). Sometimes it appears as interface only with no radiolucency medial to it. On other occasions, it is seen as an actual line, due either to Mach effect or to presence of mediastinal fat medial to line

than as an interface; that is, relative radiolucency can be seen on either side of it (see Fig. 3.6). The less dense tissue medial to the line is, of course, mediastinal fat. The aortic-pulmonary line represents contact of lung against the left side of the mediastinum behind the anterior junction line and in front of the pleural reflections over the great vessels arising from the aortic arch. When this zone of contact is sufficiently long from front to back and is tangential to the X-ray beam, the aortic-pulmonary line results. Lateral displacement of the line or local alterations in it, determined from serial radiographic examinations, strongly suggests mediastinal disease (see Figs. 5.6, 5.24, and 6.10). In evaluating lateral displacement of the line, the shadow of the aortic knob is a valuable reference point. If the aortic-pulmonary line projects

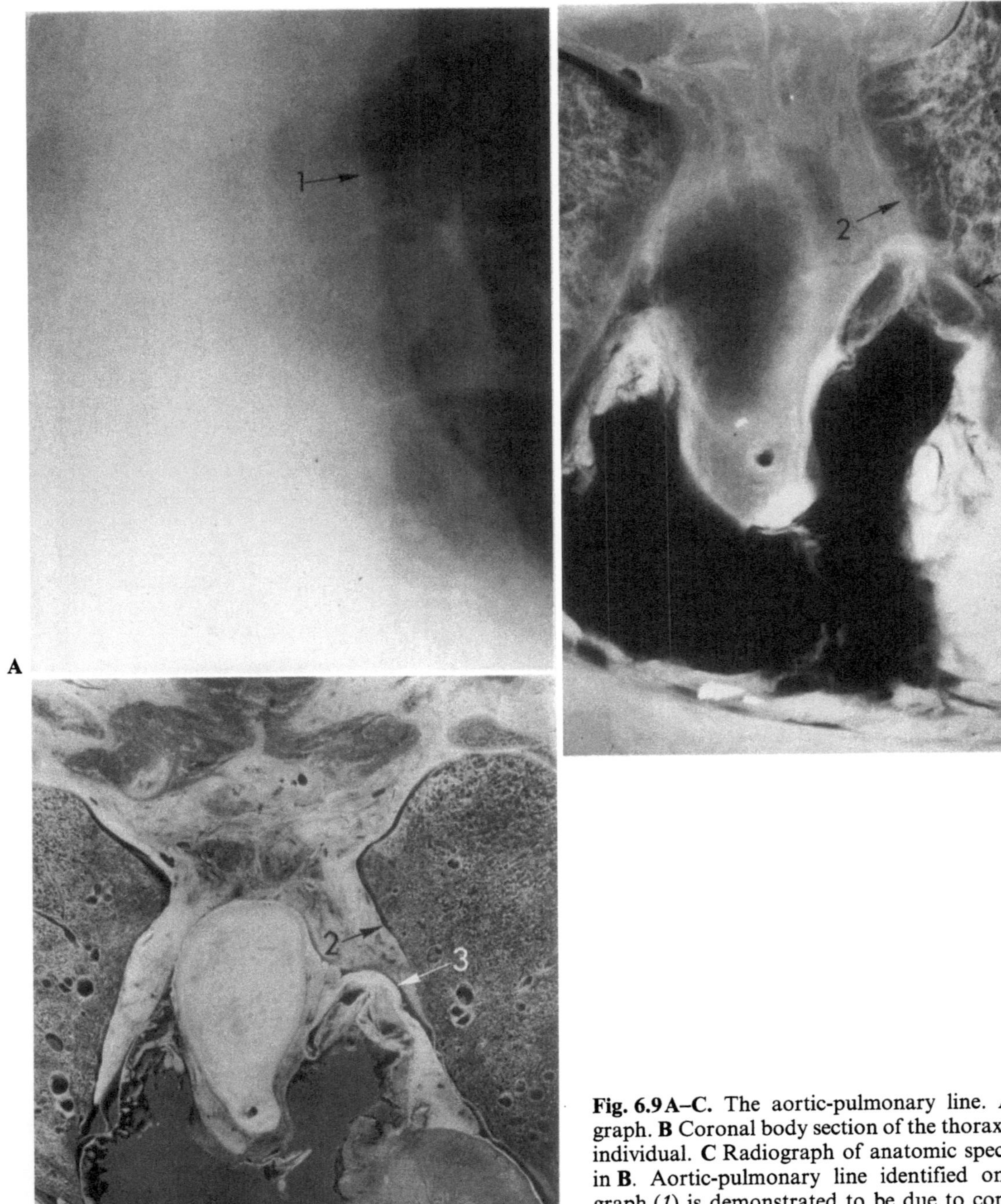

Fig. 6.9 A–C. The aortic-pulmonary line. **A** PA radiograph. **B** Coronal body section of the thorax of this same individual. **C** Radiograph of anatomic specimen shown in **B**. Aortic-pulmonary line identified on PA radiograph (*1*) is demonstrated to be due to contact of lung with mediastinum (*2*) at plane anterior to interface of lung with left subclavian artery. As line reaches its caudal extent it merges with the mediastinal pleura over main pulmonary artery (*3*)

lateral to the aortic knob, mediastinal pathology should be considered a strong possibility [6, 14]. The presence of a left superior vena cava or a left vertical vein will distort the pleural reflections behind the anterior junction line and in front of the shadows of the arteries arising from the aortic arch. These alterations will be discussed later in this chapter.

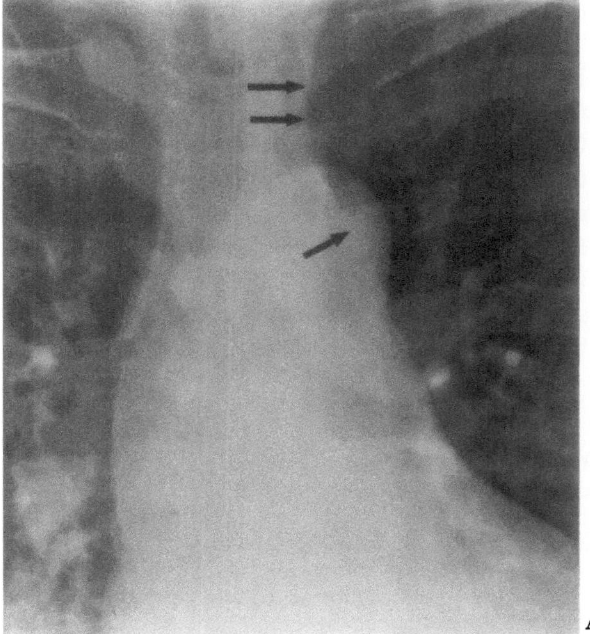

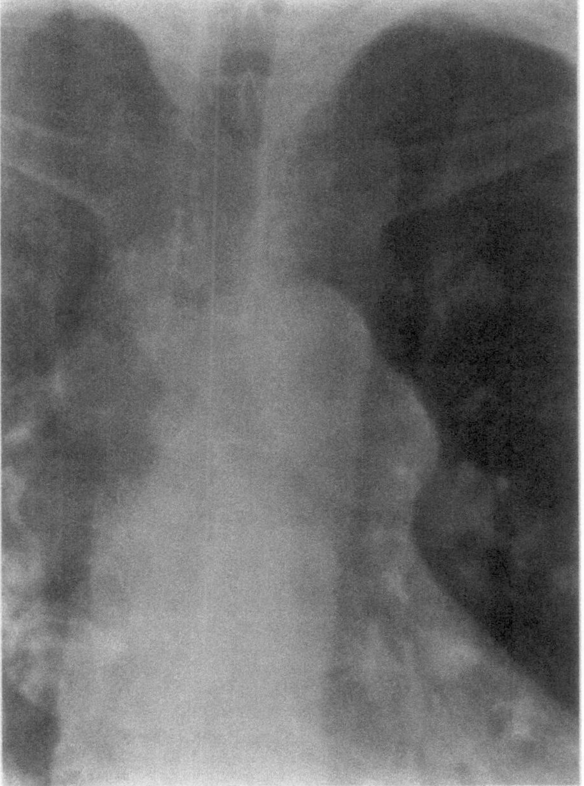

Fig. 6.10 A, B. The aortic-pulmonary line. PA radiographs made 9 months apart. The aortic-pulmonary line (*single arrow*) is commonly distorted or obliterated by mediastinal disease as in this patient with mediastinal lymph node metastases from carcinoma of the colon. Such a change in the aortic-pulmonary line places the disease process anterior to the aortic-pulmonic window. Note also obliteration of the outline of the first portion of the left subclavian artery (*double arrows*) by adenopathy surrounding the vessel. The right paratracheal line is lost as well

6.2.1.3 The Left Subclavian Artery

In many patients the first and second parts of the subclavian artery can be visualized on frontal and lateral radiographs. The first part of the vessel can be seen as it grooves the left lung in its ascent from the aortic arch (see Figs. 4.7, 6.11 and 6.12). Its lower end usually merges with the shadow of the aortic knob, but can sometimes be seen to extend below the top of the knob. In the latter circumstance the posteri-

or turn of the aortic arch (the aortic knob) lies higher in the chest than does the point of origin of the subclavian artery from the arch. On some frontal films the interface made by the lower end of the subclavian artery with lung is seen to merge with the aortic-pulmonary line anterior to it; this occurs when both interfaces are aligned parallel to the X-ray beam in the same sagittal plane (Fig. 6.13). The contact of the ascending first part of the subclavian artery with lung characteristically has a mild concavity directed to the left (Figs. 6.11 and 6.12). This is due to the fact that the first part of the subclavian artery swings laterally over the anterior aspect of the left upper lobe to become the second part, which lies behind the scalenus anterior muscle. The second part of the vessel is easily seen when it is calcified (see Fig. 4.6). Its visualization when not calcified is variable, depending upon the depth of the groove it makes in the

Fig. 6.11 A, B. First part of left subclavian artery. **A** Coronal body section. **B** Radiograph of same coronal section. First part of left subclavian artery ascends in intimate contact with medial aspect of left lung at about midcoronal plane of thorax (*1*). Its shadow is frequently visible in supra-aortic area extending upward in slightly curved fashion to become second part of subclavian artery behind scalenus anterior muscle (see chapter 4)

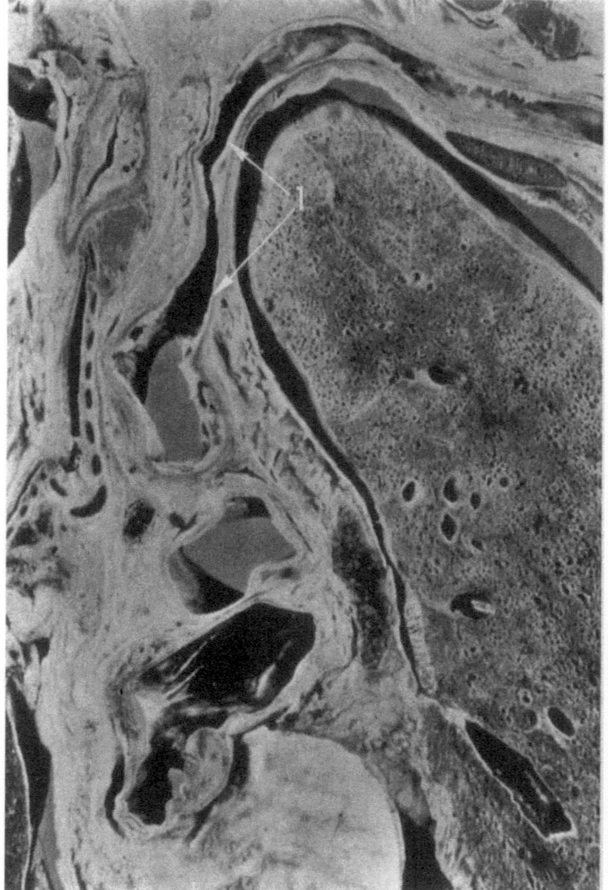
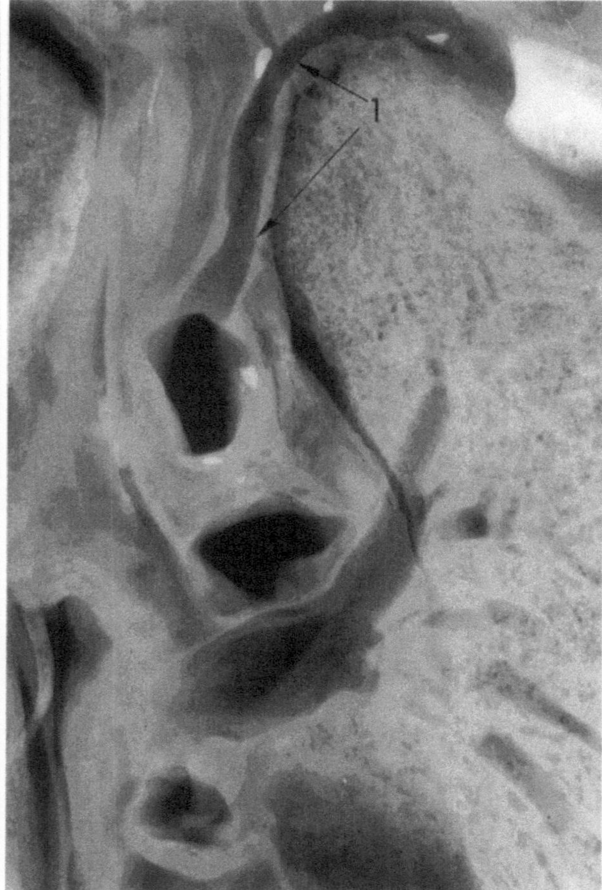

A   B

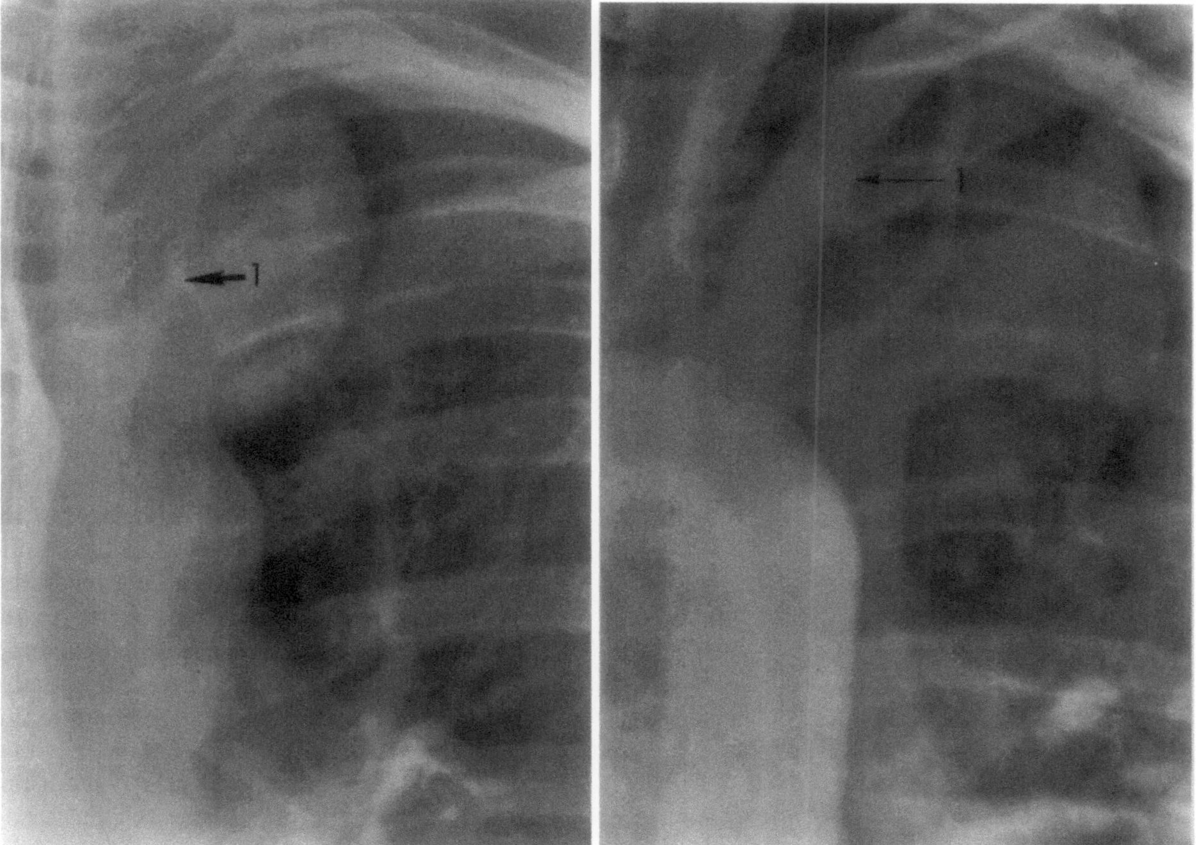

A   B

Fig. 6.12A, B. First part of left subclavian artery. **A** PA radiograph. **B** AP thoracic aortogram. In this patient with posteriorly situated supra-aortic mass, diagnosis of aneurysm of left subclavian artery was entertained. Recognition that arcuate shadow crossing left apex (*1*) could only represent contact of left lung with normal left subclavian artery should have precluded this diagnostic consideration. The first part of the left subclavian artery can sometimes be seen on lateral radiographs when lung inserts itself against the mediastinum behind the vessel (Fig. 6.14). In this projection the contact of lung with the back of the vessel can produce a convex or concave configuration seen through the shadow of the trachea or slightly posterior to it (Fig. 6.14). If the vessel is tortuous, an undulating contour may be visible from the anterior lung apex to the aortic arch (Fig. 6.14)

lung. Occasionally it produces a sharply marginated tubular shadow, usually seen in the second or third anterior interspace on PA radiographs [24] (see Fig. 4.6); sometimes a poorly defined apical opacity may result [46] (see Fig. 4.7 and chapter 4). Lordotic radiographs, which place the posterior surface of the vessel

in greater profile to the X-ray beam, often bring out this part of the lung-vessel interface to greater advantage and establish its continuity with the first part of the vessel (see Fig. 4.21). This simple expedient may be all that is required to distinguish the shadow produced by the first part of the subclavian artery from one caused by mediastinal pathology.

Recognition of the usual appearance of the subclavian artery is important; Fig. 6.12 illustrates an error in diagnosis arising from failure to appreciate this normal configuration. An interesting feature of this case is that initially the abnormality in the left superior mediastinum was thought radiographically to be consistent with an aneurysm of the left subclavian artery or ectasia of this vessel. The area was explored digitally through the root of the neck, and a similar conclusion was reached. When the lesion continued to expand, angiography was done, which excluded this possibility. In retrospect, close observation of the initial radiograph

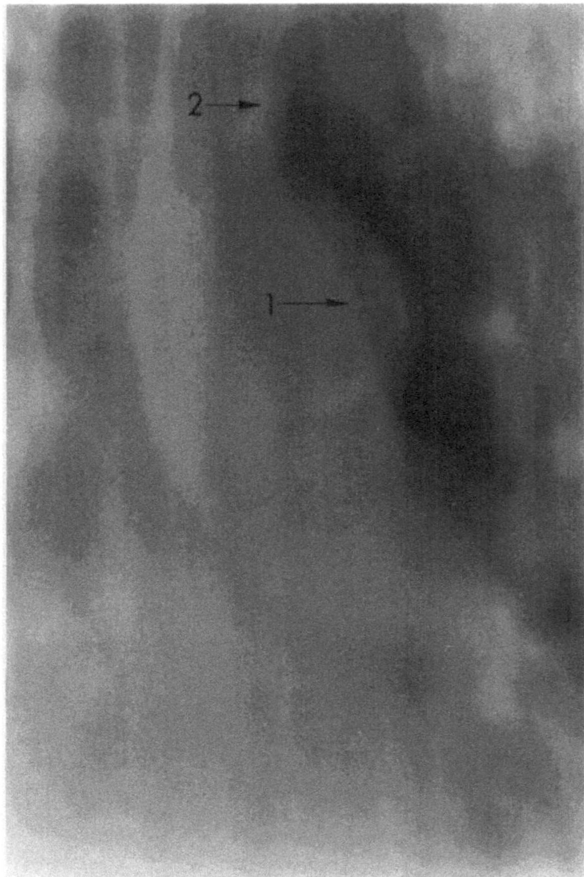

Fig. 6.13. Coincidence of aortic-pulmonary line and shadow of first part of left subclavian artery (AP tomogram). At times, contact of lung with mediastinum in front of left subclavian artery will be in identical sagittal plane with contact of lung with left subclavian artery. Under these circumstances, aortic-pulmonary line (*1*) extends cephalad to become continuous with shadow of first part of left subclavian artery (*2*)

should have made the diagnosis of such an abnormality of left subclavian artery untenable. The arcuate line crossing the shadow of the lesion is the interface of the left subclavian artery against the left lung; correct assessment of this line should have excluded dilatation of the left subclavian artery.

In a significant article, Proto and Chaliff [46] pointed out that the subclavian arteries could be responsible for a poorly marginated round or oval apical opacity usually identified in the second or third posterior interspace between the spine and the inner margin of the first rib on PA radiographs (see Fig. 4.7). The density was seen by them on the right side in 13% of patients and on the left in 17%. They theorized that the shadow represents an en face view of the second portion of the subclavian artery and is visible in some patients, but not in others due to the degree of protrusion of the vessel into lung, beam angulation and/or the effect of the scalenus anterior muscle. Computed tomographic study, of course, clarifies the problem.

The left subclavian artery is clearly identified on all computed tomograms of the chest (Fig. 6.6), sometimes throughout its entire course. The subclavian artery may be more prominent and therefore better seen when arteriosclerotic; it also enlarges in hypertension. Aneurysms of the subclavian artery are relatively rare, most commonly developing secondary to trauma. The vessel dilates and pulsates more vigorously at fluoroscopy in coarctation [45]; in pseudocoarctation it is dilated, has a longer intrathoracic course, and originates at a more caudal level [13].

Fig. 6.14A–C. First part of left subclavian artery (lateral projection). **A** Lateral radiograph. **B** Sagittal body section through left subclavian artery. **C** Lateral radiograph of patient shown in **A** with transvenous catheter entering superior vena cava by way of left innominate vein. In some patients lung inserts itself against left side of mediastinum behind first part of left subclavian artery. Shadow of left subclavian artery shown in **A** demonstrates convexity directed posteriorly (*1*). As it extends cephalad from aortic arch (*3*), interface of left subclavian artery and left upper lobe more often presents concavity directed posteriorly or is slightly undulating, as shown in **B** (*2*). Note position of left innominate vein anterior to left subclavian artery (*4*)

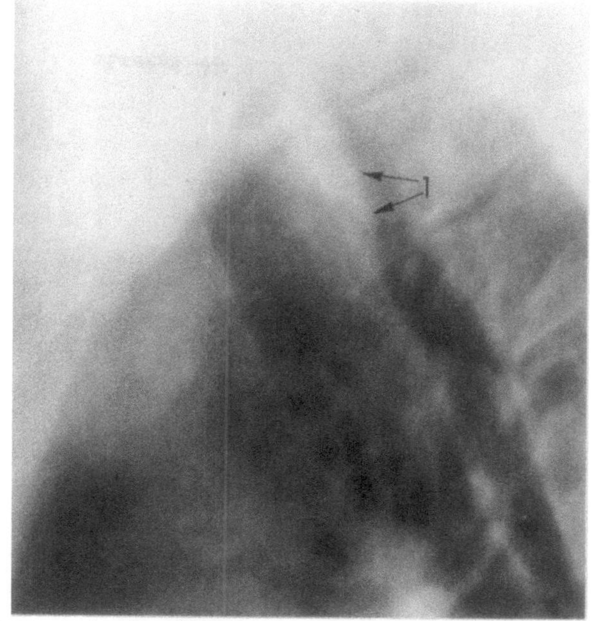

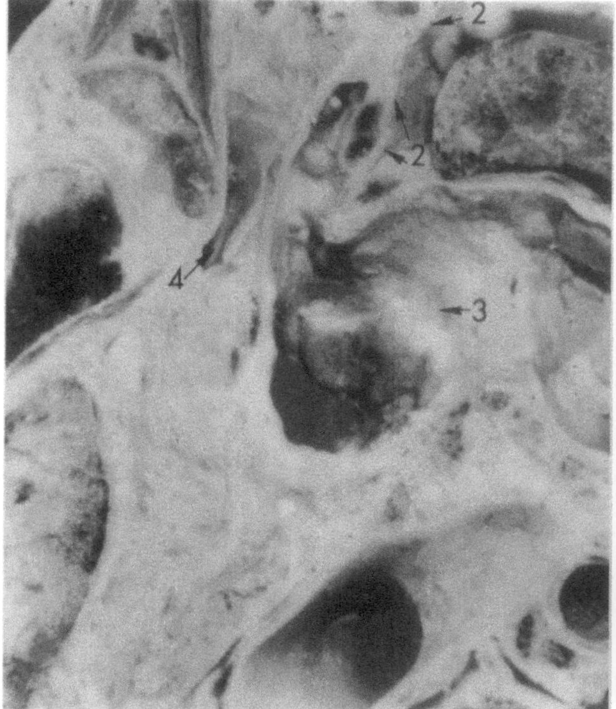

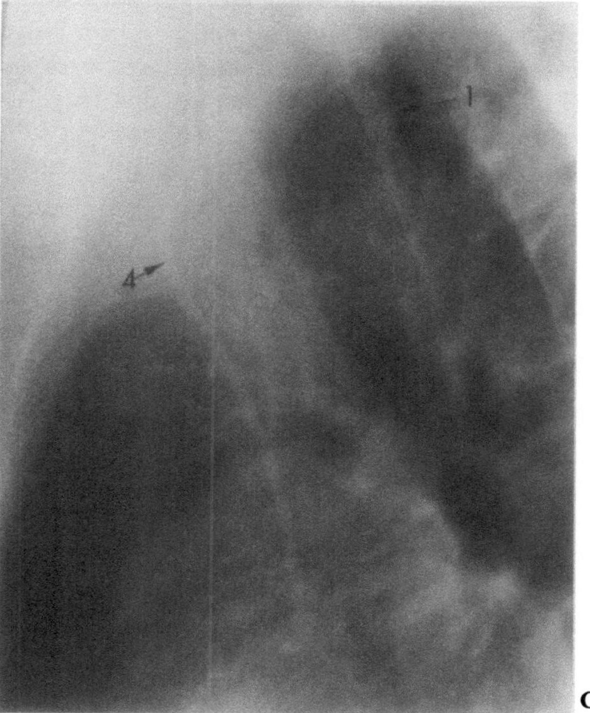

6.2.1.4 The Aberrant Right Subclavian Artery

An aberrant right subclavian artery (Figs. 6.15, 6.16, 6.17) may also be identified in the supra-aortic area on plain radiographs in some individuals. On PA radiographs of seven of 12 patients with this condition, Branscom and Austin noted a linear shadow extending upward and to the right from the aortic knob [7] (Figs. 6.16 and 6.17). They assumed this line to represent the contact of left lung with the anomalous vessel. A similar, although shorter line, was found in 20% of normal control patients. A study of the radiographs from this article suggests that this line in normal subjects may be produced by the left superior intercostal vein grooving the lung (see Fig. 6.22). In two of 12 patients with aberrant right subclavian arteries, the authors noted a prominent superior and posterior bulge from the aortic arch on lateral radiographs (Fig. 6.16). Aortography showed this bulge to represent the origin of the anomalous right subclavian artery. In a recent study of 101 patients

with anomalous right subclavian artery, Proto et al. [48] identified the linear shadow extending upward and to the right from the aortic knob in 60% of cases. They were also able to see the vessel through the tracheal air column in 43% of patients and observed it to produce a "mass" effect behind the medial aspect of the right clavicle in 32% (Fig. 6.16). On lateral radiographs, the vessel caused a retrotracheal opacity in 79%, obscured the aortic arch in 62%, and produced an imprint on the posterior tracheal wall in 49% of patients (Fig. 6.16). The diagnosis of anomalous right subclavian artery is readily made at computed tomography [37, 54] (Fig. 6.17), and, in fact, the anomalous vessel is not infrequently encountered as an incidental

Fig. 6.15A–C. Anomalous right subclavian artery. Drawing from anterior aspect (**A**) and from superior aspect (**B**). **C** AP arteriogram. Anomalous right subclavian artery (*2*) arises from medial aspect of aortic knob (*1*) and extends in an oblique retroesophageal course (**B**) through mediastinum on its way to right arm. (Courtesy G. Weinberger, Syracuse, NY)

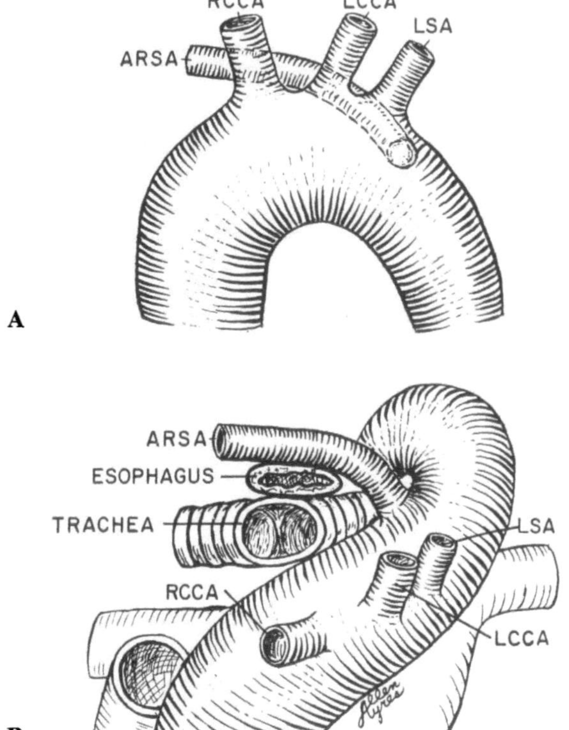

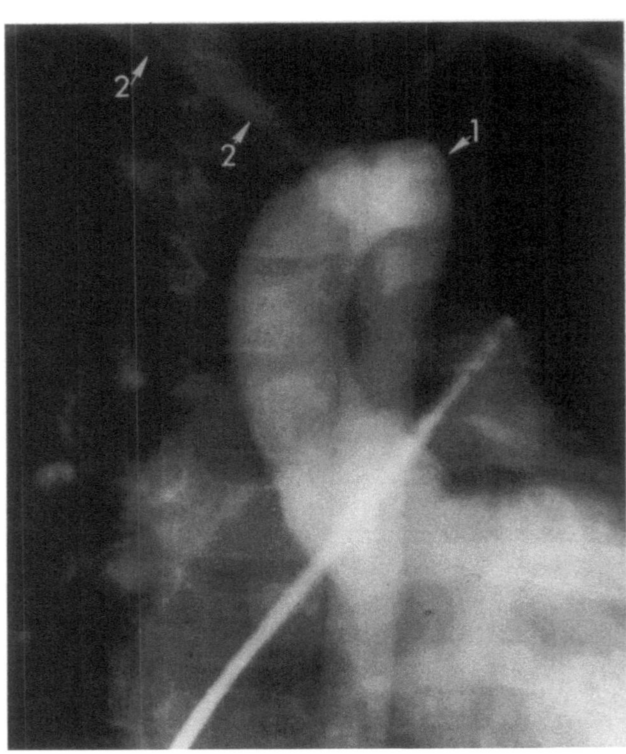

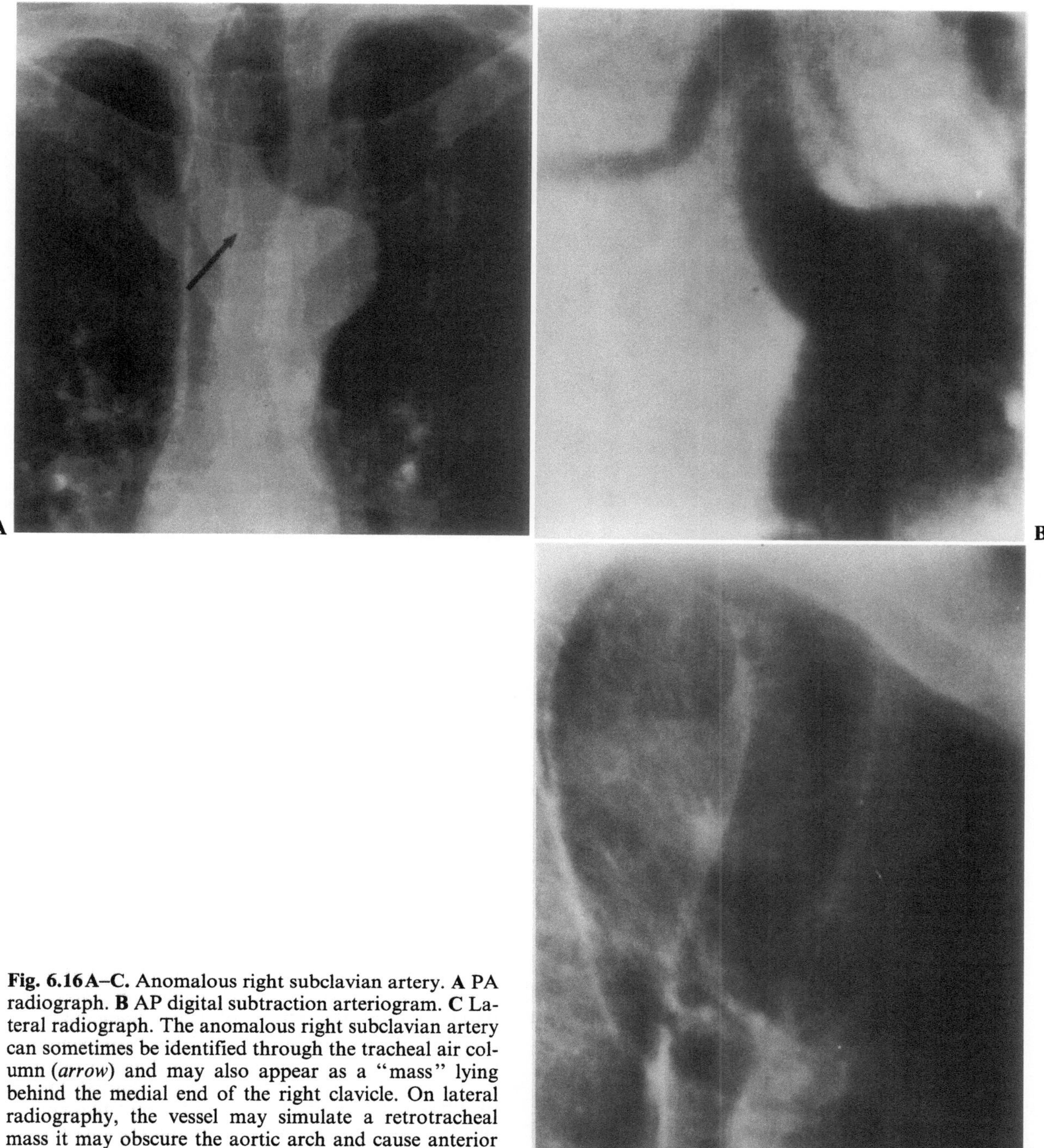

Fig. 6.16A–C. Anomalous right subclavian artery. **A** PA radiograph. **B** AP digital subtraction arteriogram. **C** Lateral radiograph. The anomalous right subclavian artery can sometimes be identified through the tracheal air column (*arrow*) and may also appear as a "mass" lying behind the medial end of the right clavicle. On lateral radiography, the vessel may simulate a retrotracheal mass it may obscure the aortic arch and cause anterior tracheal displacement

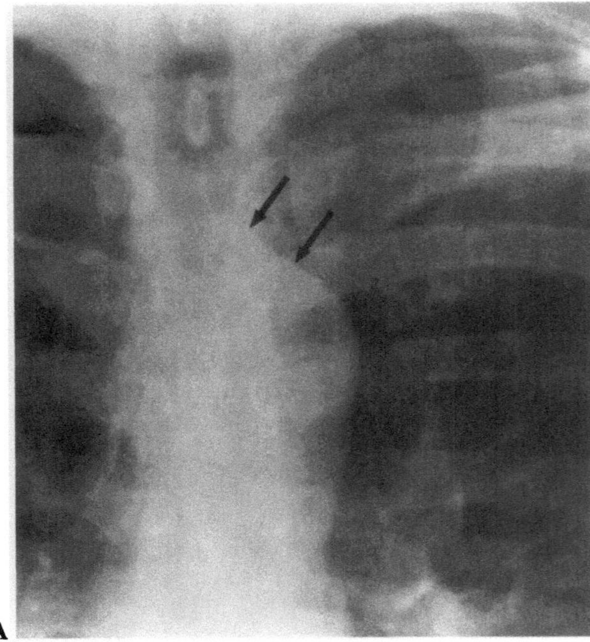

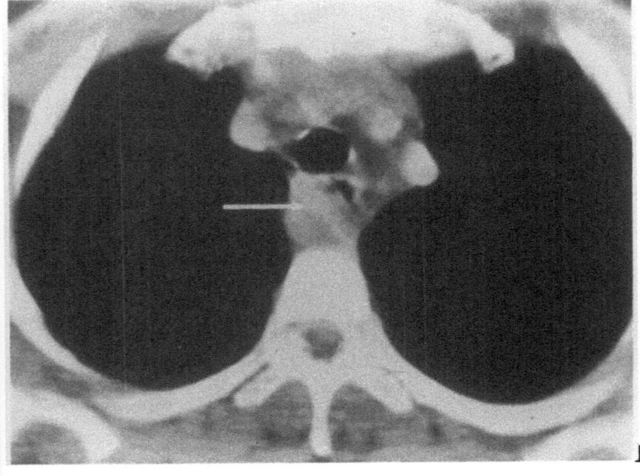

Fig. 6.17A, B. Anomalous right subclavian artery. **A** PA radiograph. **B** Computed tomogram. Not infrequently the PA radiograph provides a clue to the diagnosis of anomalous right subclavian artery. This clue is the presence of an interface extending upward and to the right from the aortic knob (*arrow*). The shadow represents the superior surface of the proximal portion of the anomalous vessel. Computed tomography is an ideal, noninvasive technique to establish the diagnosis of this common anomaly. The following findings are diagnostic: (a) a retroesophageal density continuous with the aortic arch which opacifies following contrast injection (*arrow*); (b) a course continous from the density to the usual position of the second and third portions of the vessel; (c) absence of the vessel in its usual position between the right innominate vein and the trachea; and (d) a small innominate artery

finding. This fact is not surprising since anomalous right subclavian artery is a common developmental abnormality [31].

Findings at computed tomography are diagnostic: (a) a retroesophageal density continuous with the aortic arch which opacifies following contrast injection; (b) a course continuous from the density to the usual position of the second and third portions of the vessel; (c) absence of the first portion of the vessel between the right innominate vein and the trachea; and (d) a small innominate artery (Fig. 6.17).

Occasionally, there is an outpouching at the origin of the anomalous right subclavian artery from the normal left-sided aorta; this aneurysm sometimes referred to as an "aortic diverticulum" or "aneurysm of Kommerell" [49] is another cause for a supra-aortic mass.

From the anatomic point of view, it should be possible at times to identify the left common carotid artery on frontal radiographs as it ascends from the aorta. In practice, such an interface is rarely seen (A.V. Proto, unpublished), in part because the lung-vessel interface is not tangential to the X-ray beam in frontal projections and because the left subclavian artery, situated behind the left common carotid artery, usually indents the lung more deeply, preventing contact of lung with the carotid (A.V. Proto, unpublished) (see Fig. 6.6C and D). Buckling of the left innominate artery simulating a supra-aortic mass has been reported by Sandler et al. [50]. A very prominent vertically oriented shadow in the supra-aortic area may be seen in the rarely encountered case of left innominate artery [45].

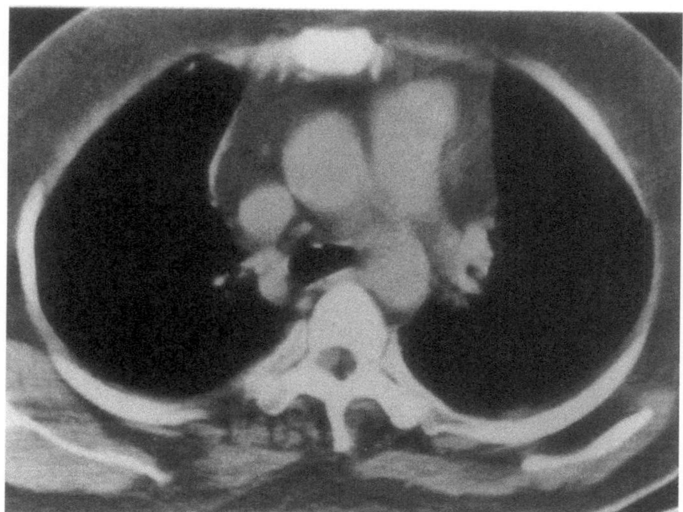

Fig. 6.18. The high left and main pulmonary arteries. Computed tomograms through the level of the aortic arch usually show the left lateral margin of the arch in contact with lung. When the main and left pulmonary arteries lie in a high (cephalad) position they can be imaged lateral to the arch as shown in this patient. In the case shown here, no diagnostic problems are presented, but in less striking examples a lateral aortic node or mass may be simulated (see chapter 7)

6.2.1.5 The High Left and Main Pulmonary Arteries

In normal subjects the left lateral aspect of the aortic arch is contacted by lung without interposition of any major vascular structure. In some individuals, however, high position of the main and left pulmonary arteries, sometimes accentuated by lack of deep inspiration during computed tomographic scanning, causes these vessels to be imaged lateral to the arch [38, 47] (Fig. 6.18). When this variant occurs, the imaged vessels may simulate a mass and represent a potential for misdiagnosis. A similar appearance may be seen when the left pulmonary artery is elevated secondary to left upper lobe collapse. This pitfall can be avoided by careful study of contiguous computed tomographic sections above, through, and below the aortic arch; if the shadow in question is shown to merge with the left pulmonary artery cephalad and the main pulmonary artery caudad, it can be confirmed as representing normal vasculature. Enhancement of the shadow following contrast administration is, of course, confirmatory.

6.2.1.6 The Left Paratracheal Reflection

The left lung infrequently contacts the left lateral wall of the trachea due to the interposition of the aortic arch below and the left common carotid and left subclavian arteries above (see Fig. 6.6). Nevertheless, such a line was found in 3.5% of the series of Bachman and Teixidor [2]. In his study of the left paratracheal reflection, Proto (unpublished) identified such an interface in 31% of normal PA radiographs. The interface projected medial to the left subclavian artery, presented a positive Mach band and, on correlated conventional and computed tomograms, was found anterior to the left subclavian artery in the same coronal plane as the trachea. Lung in this location abutted mediastinal fat surrounding the left common carotid artery in 94%, the left common carotid artery itself in 5%, and the left lateral tracheal wall in 1% of cases. Application of the anatomy of the left paratracheal reflection to radiologic interpretation is subject to the same constraints that apply to the right paratracheal line as discussed in chapter 8.

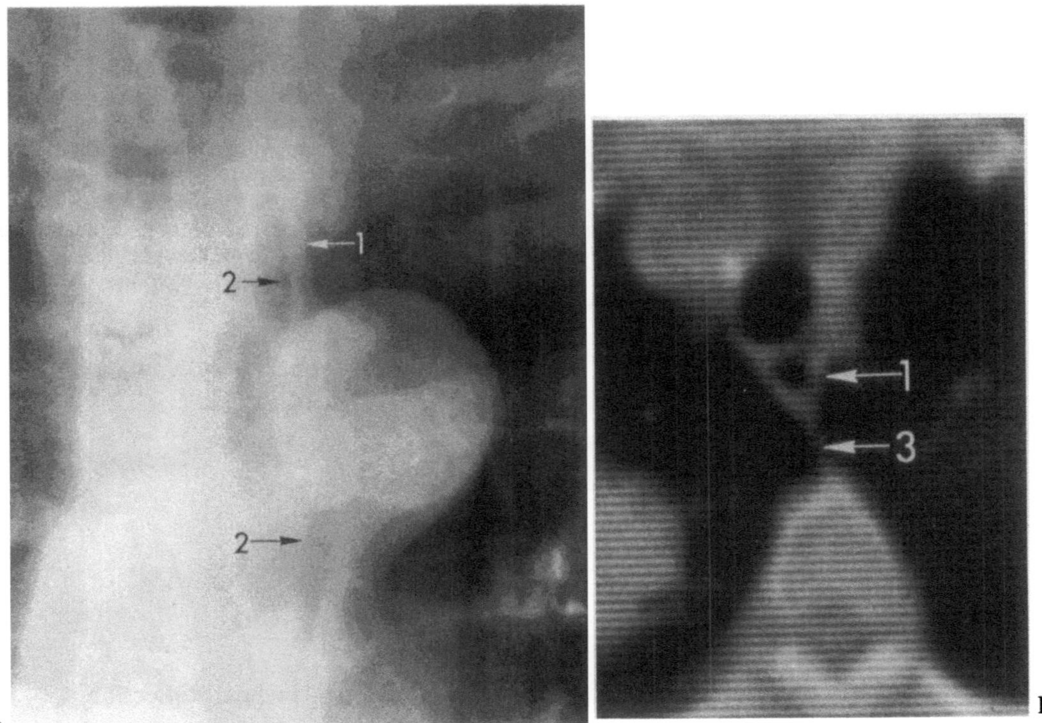

Fig. 6.19A, B. Left paraesophageal stripe. **A** PA radiograph. **B** Computed tomogram through plane slightly above carina. Left lung in supra-aortic area may contact left lateral wall of esophagus (*1*). This relationship, however, is far less constant than is contact of right lung in supra-azygos area with right lateral wall of esophagus. In **A**, note large amount of esophageal air (*2*), causing left esophageal wall to appear as line between luminal air and left lung. In patient shown in **B**, right and left lungs are in contact behind esophagus to produce posterior junction line (*3*)

6.2.1.7 The Left Paraesophageal Stripe

The paraesophageal stripe is less commonly seen on the left above the aortic arch than it is on the right above the azygos arch (Fig. 6.19). It was identified in six of 20 individuals in Gladnikoff's study [21]. Its application to radiologic interpretation is analogous to the way in which the concept of the right paraesophageal stripe is used. This is covered more fully in the chapter on the infra-azygos area (chapter 9).

6.2.1.8 The Posterior Junction Line

The posterior junction line above the level of the azygos and aortic arches will be discussed in the section on the supra-azygos area (chapter 8) and will not be elaborated upon here.

6.2.1.9 The Paraspinal Line

The left paraspinal line can be visualized above the level of the aortic arch. Its configuration is related to the anatomy of both the aorta and the left superior intercostal vein. Above the left superior intercostal vein, the paraspinal line lies closer to the vertebral bodies than it does below it. Woodring and Rhodes [60] have reported lobulated widening of the supra-aortic paraspinal line in 35% of patients with coarctation of the aorta. The change is attributed by them to dilated anastomoses of the posterior first and second intercostal arteries and branches of the inferior thyroid artery with the third and fourth intercostal arteries. The paraspinal line is reviewed more completely in chapter 7.

6.2.2 The Left Superior Intercostal Vein

The right and left superior intercostal veins drain the second, third, and fourth intercostal spaces (Fig. 6.20). The supreme intercostal veins carry blood from the first intercostal space on each side and empty into the right and left innominate (brachiocephalic) veins [57]. The right

Fig. 6.20. Left superior intercostal vein. Supra-aortic ▷ and supra-azygos areas (posterior aspect). Second, third, and fourth intercostal veins (*2, 3,* and *4*) sweep anteriorly off posterior chest wall to form left and right superior intercostal veins (*L.S.I.V., R.S.I.V.*). Note left superior intercostal vein swings laterally around aortic arch to its eventual termination in left innominate vein. *P.J.L.,* posterior junction line; *P.L.,* paraspinal line; *A.H.V.,* accessory hemiazygos vein; *A.V.,* azygos vein; *H.V.,* hemiazygos vein. (From [32])

Fig. 6.21 A, B. Anatomy of superior intercostal veins. **A** Coronal body section. **B** Radiograph of same coronal body section. **A** Shows wires (*1*) inserted into superior intercostal veins on each side. The prominence of right superior intercostal vein as it passes around spine is quite apparent; it is easy to visualize how this structure could groove posterior aspect of right lung. In similar manner, left superior intercostal vein may groove posterior aspect of left lung, particularly if vessel is not blanketed by mediastinal fat

▽

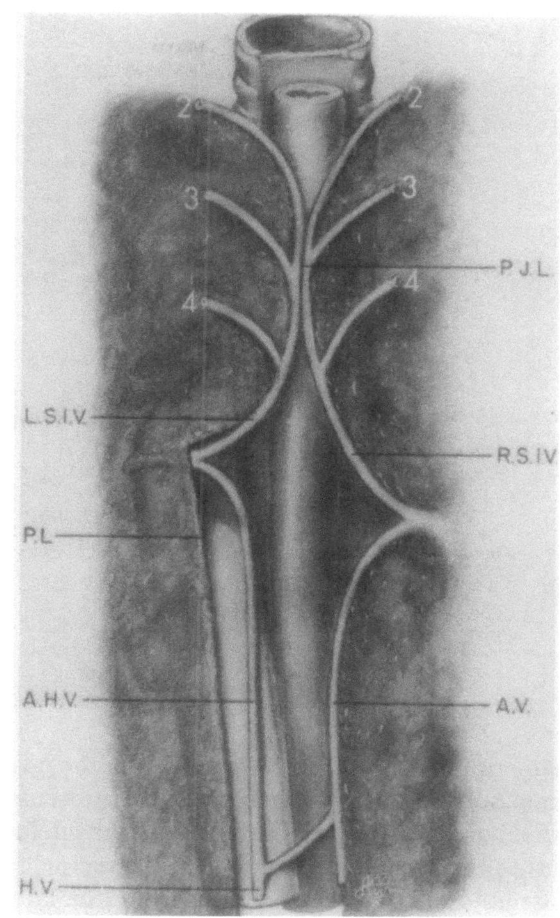

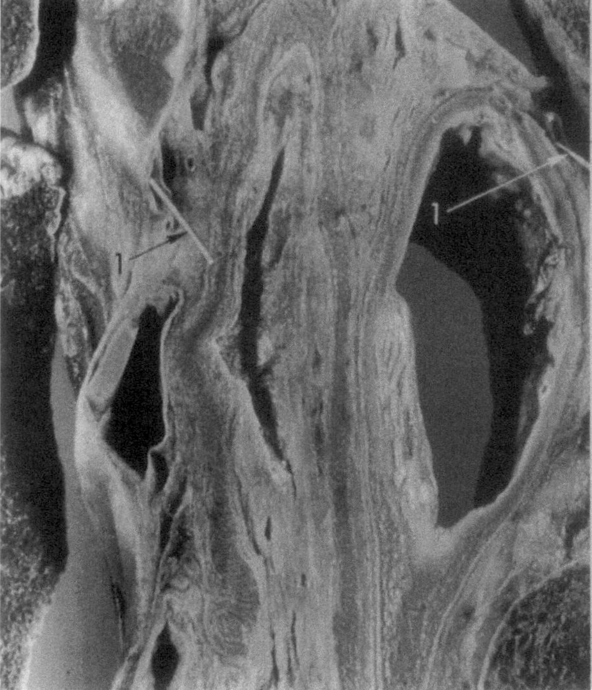

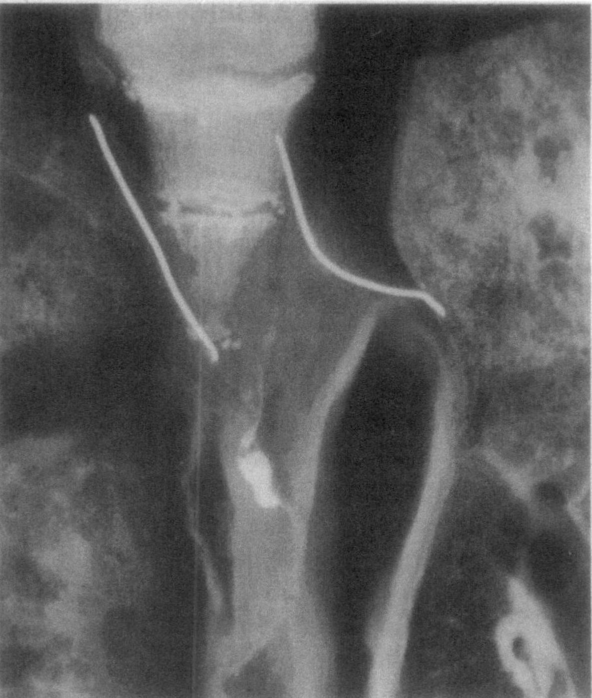

A   B

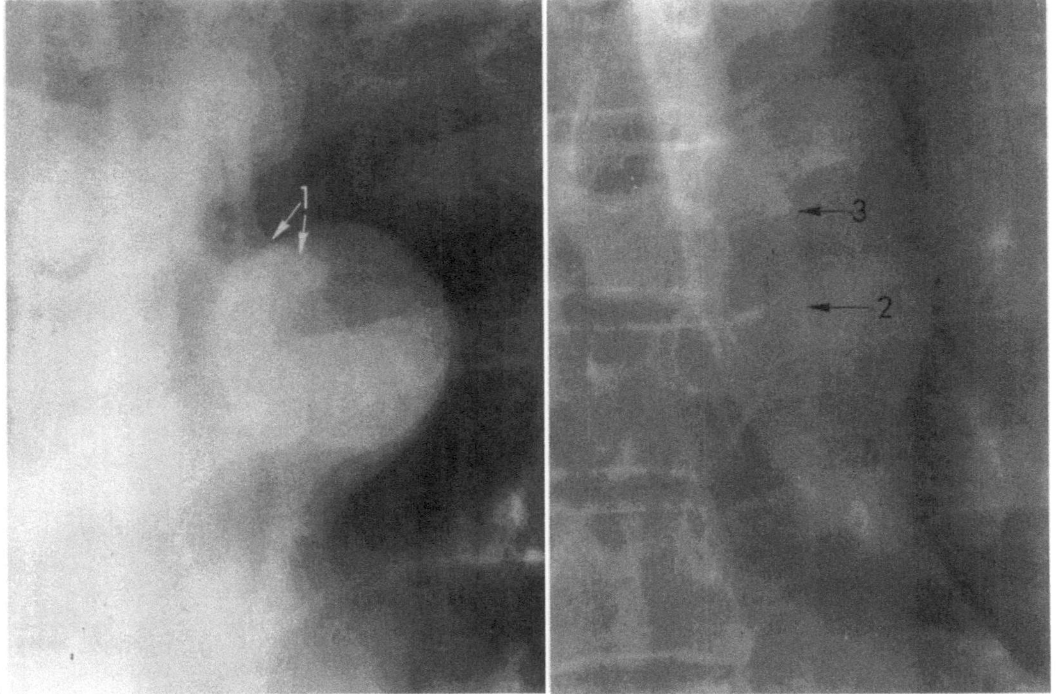

A   B

superior intercostal vein terminates in the posterior portion of the azygos arch and is discussed in detail in chapter 8. The left superior intercostal vein runs anteriorly from the paraspinal soft tissues and continues forward along the lateral aspect of the aortic arch (Fig. 6.21). It then swings upward in front of the left subclavian and common carotid arteries to terminate in the left innominate vein. In 75% of individuals there is a communication with the accessory hemiazygos vein behind the aortic knob [42].

As the left superior intercostal vein passes forward from its paraspinal to its para-aortic position, it frequently indents the medial portion of the left lung rather deeply. This groove in the lung is believed to be responsible for the abrupt medial angulation of the upper portion of the left paraspinal line so often seen on plain frontal radiographs and frontal tomograms [32] (Fig. 6.22). If the vein is blanketed by paraspinal fat, the configuration of the upper portion of the paraspinal line is more rounded. In front of the spine, the lungs frequently extend deeply into the mediastinum above the azygos and aortic arches to produce the posterior junction line; the lower portion of this line is intimately related to the paired superior intercostal veins.

Fig. 6.22 A, B. The impression of left superior intercostal vein on left lung. **A** PA radiograph. **B** AP tomogram. Contact of left lung with left superior intercostal vein can be seen through aortic knob in **A** (*1*). Configuration shown in **B** is more frequently encountered: left paraspinal line (*2*) can be followed cephalad to level of aortic knob, where it deviates sharply in medial direction (*3*). The sharp angulation in this portion of the paraspinal line is thought to represent the impression made by the left superior intercostal vein on the medial aspect of the left lung. The more medial extension of left lung above knob is apparently related to absence of descending aorta at this level. (**B** From [32])

At the lower end of the posterior junction line, the two lungs are draped over these veins which are thus responsible for the divergence of the caudal end of the posterior junction line to the right over the azygos arch and to the left over the aortic arch. On the left this interface of the left superior intercostal vein and lung may be simulated by the contact of an anomalous right subclavian artery with lung just above the aortic knob [7] (Figs. 6.17, 6.22).

In its position at the left side of the aortic arch, the left superior intercostal vein can be seen on 1.4%–9.5% of PA radiographs as a small protuberance from the aortic knob [3,

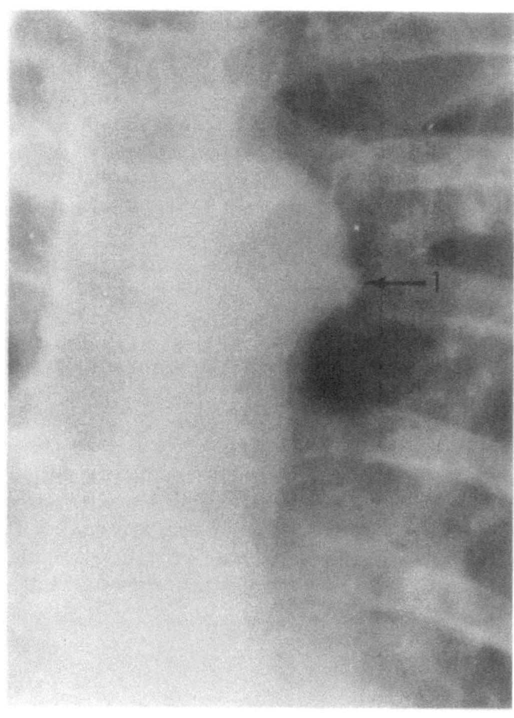

△

Fig. 6.23. Aortic nipple (PA radiograph). Shadow of normal left superior intercostal vein is seen in small percentage of individuals as it passes laterally around aortic knob (*1*). It has been given term "aortic nipple." Its position with respect to aortic knob is somewhat variable; in some patients it is seen adjacent to superolateral margin of knob (see Fig. 6.24), whereas in other patients it is seen in relation to inferolateral aspect of knob (*1*). It should not be mistaken for an enlarged lymph node

20, 35]. This projection has been termed "the aortic nipple" [35] (Figs. 6.23, 6.24). Its position with respect to the aortic knob is quite variable: in some patients it is seen superolaterally, in others, inferolaterally. Ball and Proto [3] point out that occasionally the shadow of the left superior intercostal vein may be seen through the aortic knob in a retroaortic position (Fig. 6.22). Although Friedman et al. [20] state that the upper limit of normal size for the aortic nipple is 4.5 mm; Pagniez et al. [42] report that the nipple can be as large as 10 mm in normal subjects. Like the azygos vein, the left superior intercostal vein becomes smaller during Valsalva's maneuver and enlarges in recumbency (Fig. 6.24).

The left superior intercostal vein can often be identified at computed tomographic examinations in both normal and abnormal states [3, 34] (see Figs. 6.26, 6.31). It has been stated that the left superior intercostal vein in

Fig. 6.24 A, B. Aortic nipple. **A** Erect PA radiograph. **B** Supine AP radiograph. Like azygos vein, configuration of aortic nipple may change from erect to recumbent position. In this patient, nipple is not evident on erect film but can be identified on supine study (*1*). Note in this patient, nipple is related to superolateral aspect of aortic knob

▽

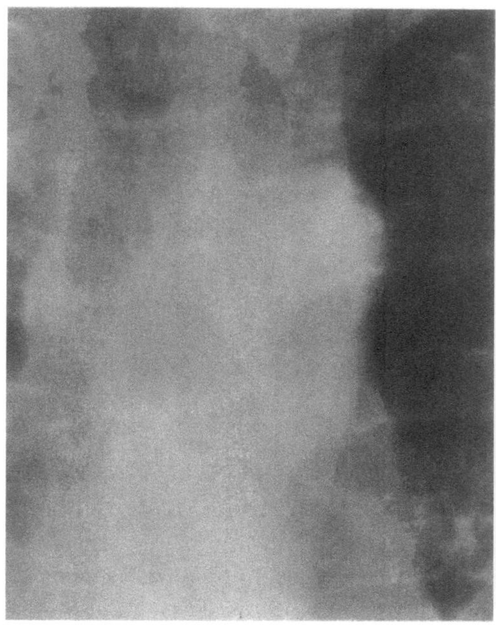

A

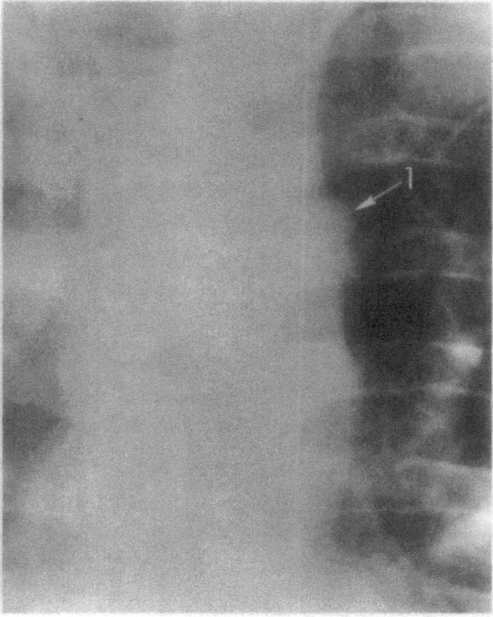

B

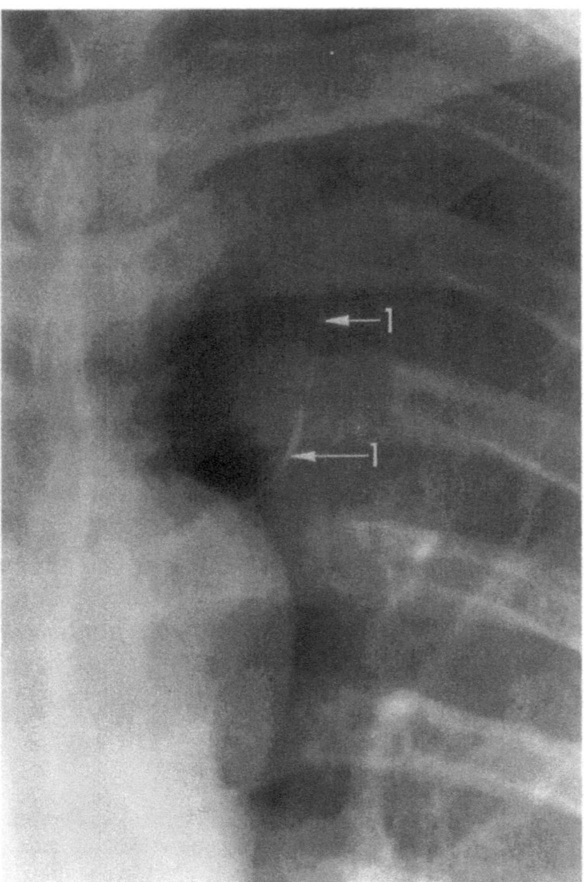

Fig. 6.25. Left azygos lobe (PA radiograph). Left azygos lobe is a much rarer anomaly than is right azygos lobe. Like azygos lobe it is demarcated from rest of upper lobe by anomalous fissure (*1*). On right side, azygos vein resides in inferior aspect of fissure; on left side left superior intercostal vein lies in inferior aspect of fissure. (From [32])

its location lateral to the aortic arch may be surrounded by air in cases of pneumomediastinum and may thus be better seen on both frontal and lateral radiographs in this condition [42]. Such a finding can be a potentially helpful one for the distinction of pneumomediastinum from paramediastinal pneumothorax [3].

Just as the azygos vein lies at the lower end of the azygos fissure in cases of azygos lobe, so the left superior intercostal vein lies at the lower end of the left azygos fissure in those rarely encountered examples of left azygos lobe (Fig. 6.25). Like the azygos vein, the left superior intercostal vein may become enlarged in left heart failure and in conditions producing in-

Fig. 6.26A–E. Hemiazygos continuation. **A** PA radio- ▷ graph. **B** AP tomogram. **C** and **D** AP films from thoracic angiogram performed following injection of contrast into inferior vena cava. **E** Computed tomogram. In this patient, inferior vena cava was continuous with hemiazygos vein and accessory hemiazygos vein (*1*). Accessory hemiazygos vein is shown to be directly continuous with anterior aspect of left superior intercostal vein (*2*), which is huge do to large volume of blood flow through it. Contrast material is seen to enter left innominate vein (*3*), which empties normally into a dilated superior vena cava (*4*). Also shown is reflux into posterior aspect of left superior intercostal vein (*5*), which is of normal size since it is not carrying an increased flow of blood. A very prominent aortic nipple is evident on PA radiograph and AP tomogram (*6*). Note negative Mach band about very large hemiazygos and accessory hemiazygos veins (*7*). Linear shadow medial to margin of dilated veins (*8*) is marginated by positive Mach band and hence must represent paraspinal line (see chapter 3). Shadow of descending aorta is therefore not visible and must lie medial to outlines of dilated veins and paraspinal line. (From [26])

creased pressure in the right heart. More frequently its enlargement is the result of an increase in blood flow through it. The vein may act as an accessory collateral pathway for venous return to the heart in cases of azygos continuation of the vena cava. In the very unusual example of hemiazygos continuation reported by Haswell and Berrigan [26], it is apparent that the vessel acted as the conduit through which the hemiazygos system drained into the left innominate (brachiocephalic) vein (Fig. 6.26). In this case the aortic nipple was very large.

Most often the enlarged left superior intercostal vein is associated with obstruction of the superior vena cava [53], the inferior vena cava, or the left innominate vein upstream from the point of entry of the left superior intercostal vein [42] (Figs. 6.27 and 6.28). Recently, Carter et al. [11] have reported demonstration of the aortic nipple several weeks before the superior vena caval syndrome became clinically manifest. In superior vena caval syndrome, the vessel is a dominant collateral pathway and is commonly enlarged [5, 32, 42]. Blood flows downward through the left superior intercostal vein into the hemiazygos and azygos veins and thence to the heart. Under these circumstances "downhill varices" of the esophagus may be encountered

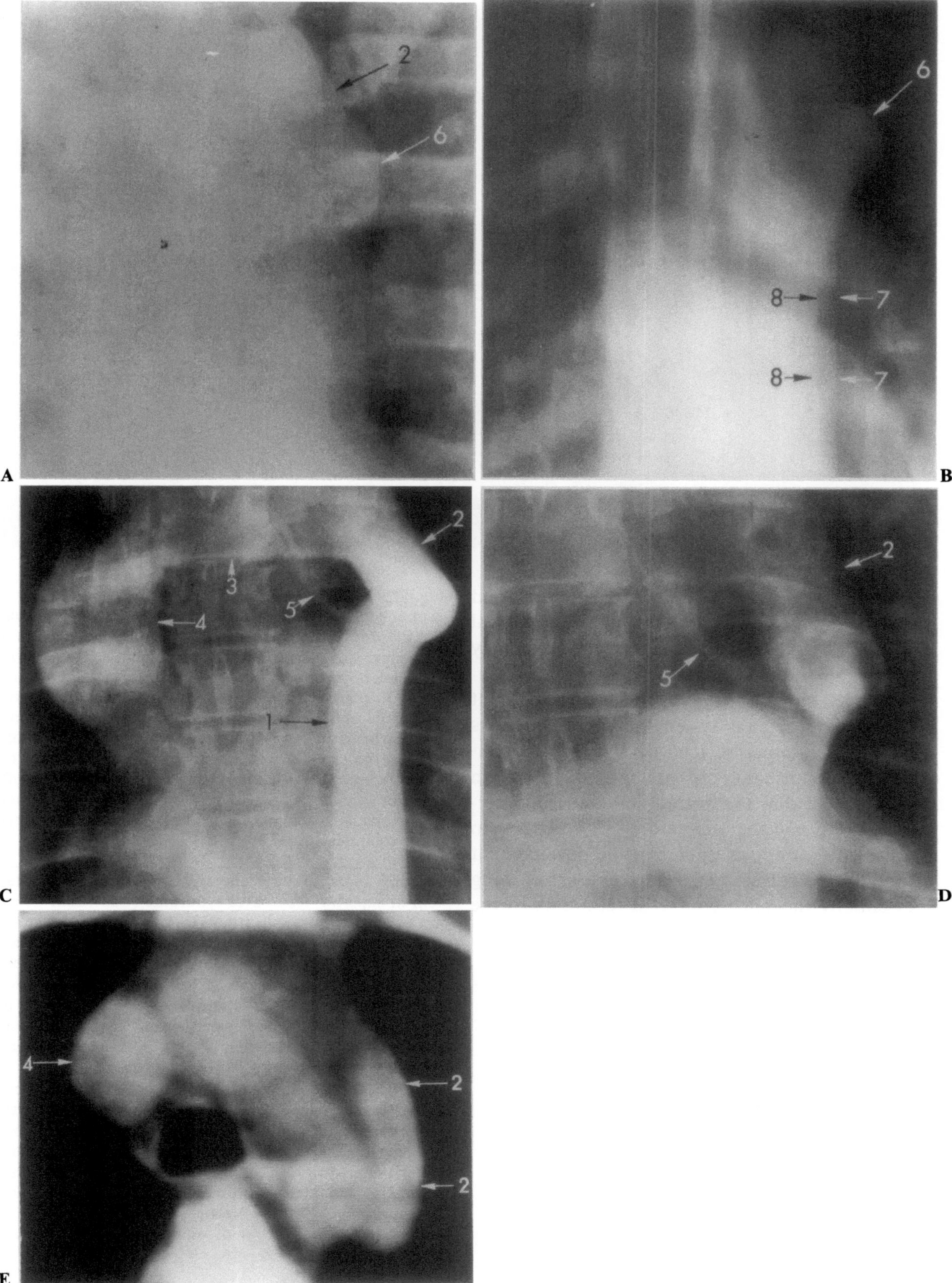

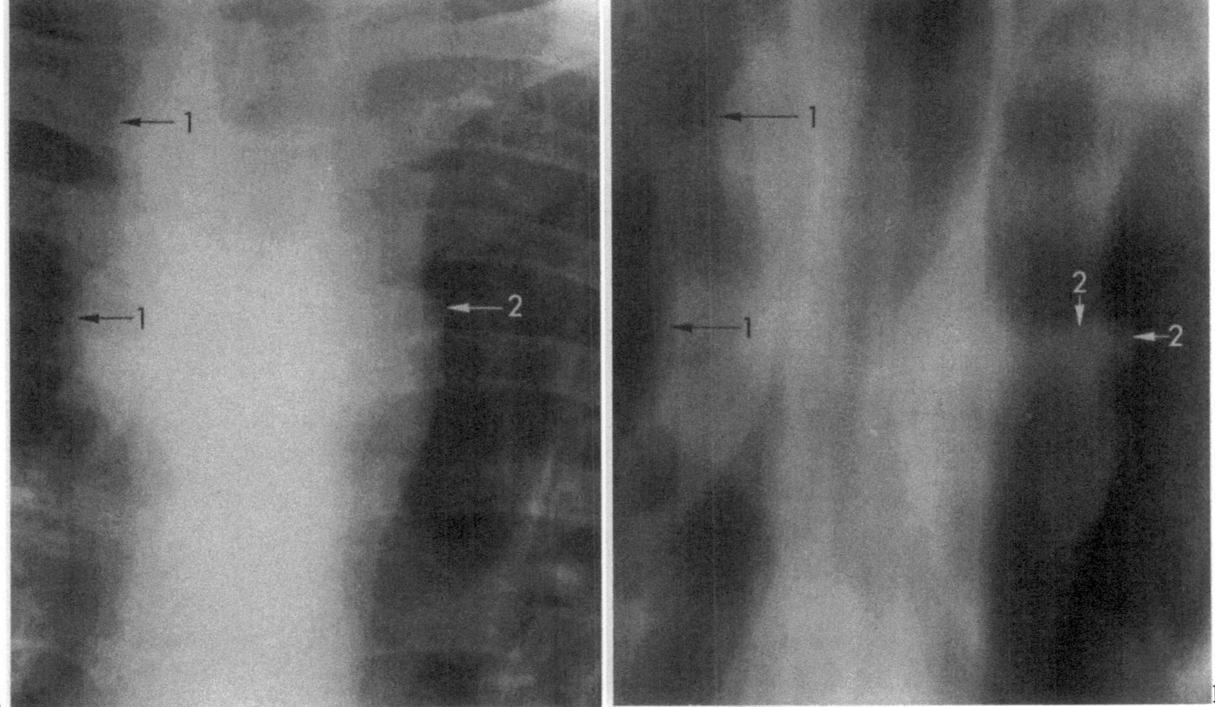

△

Fig. 6.27 A, B. Enlargement of left superior intercostal vein in superior vena caval syndrome. **A** PA radiograph. **B** AP tomogram. In this patient, superior vena caval syndrome was caused by very prominent right paratracheal adenopathy (*1*). In superior vena caval syndrome, superior intercostal veins may act as collateral pathway by means of which blood from upper portion of body reaches heart by way of azygos system. Prominent left superior intercostal vein (*2*) is clearly seen. Flow of blood from upper portion of thorax passes through left superior intercostal vein and then caudally through accessory hemiazygos and hemiazygos veins to enter azygos system. (From [32])

▷

Fig. 6.28 A–D. Enlargement of left superior intercostal vein in superior vena caval syndrome ("downhill" varices). **A** PA radiograph. **B** and **C** AP and lateral venous angiograms (not done simultaneously) following injection of both arms. **D** AP esophagram. Prominent left superior intercostal vein is seen at inferolateral aspect of aortic arch (*1*). Obstruction of superior vena cava is clearly shown (*2*). On left side, contrast can be seen in left superior intercostal vein (*3*) flowing caudad through accessory hemiazygos vein (*4*) into hemiazygos vein. On right side, some collateral flow is provided through internal mammary veins (*5*), which in turn communicate with vessels in anterior abdominal wall. Enlargement of veins in upper mediastinum may also involve vessels in wall of esophagus to produce varices (*6*). Since flow in these vessels is caudal, these prominent veins are sometimes referred to as "downhill" varices. Note that varices are present in upper portion of esophagus but not in its lower part

(Fig. 6.28). In this condition, collateral blood flow passing downward through esophageal veins to the azygos and hemiazygos veins may be demonstrated by barium swallow [19].

The left superior intercostal vein is a remnant of the left cardinal system of veins. It drains into the left superior vena cava when this congenital abnormality is present. It has been pointed out that the normal left superior intercostal vein and the anomalous left vertical vein represent variations in embryonic development of the cardinal system, both vessels following essentially the same course to terminate to the left innominate vein [42].

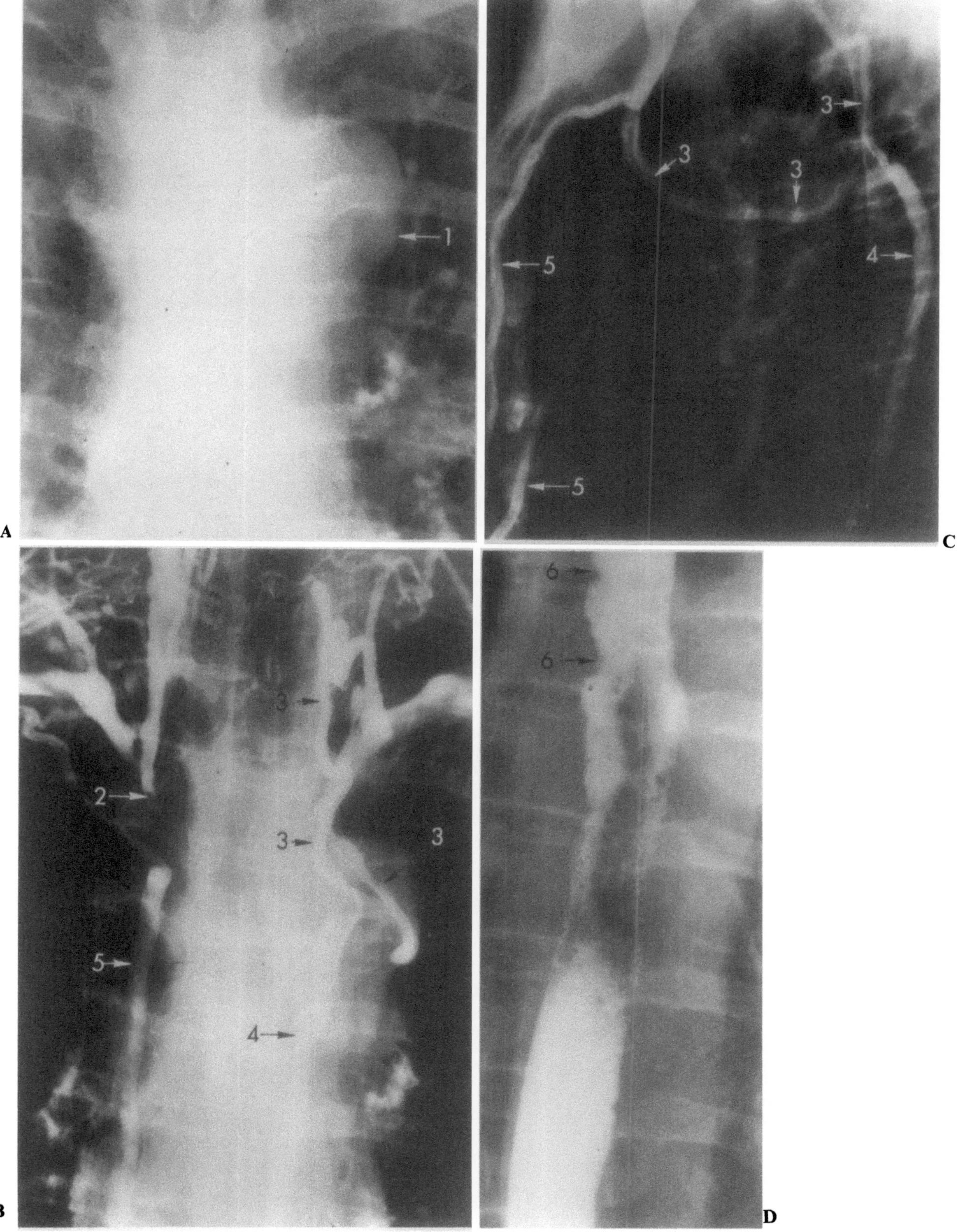
A
B
C
D
1
2
3
3
3
3
3
3
4
4
5
5
5
5
6
6

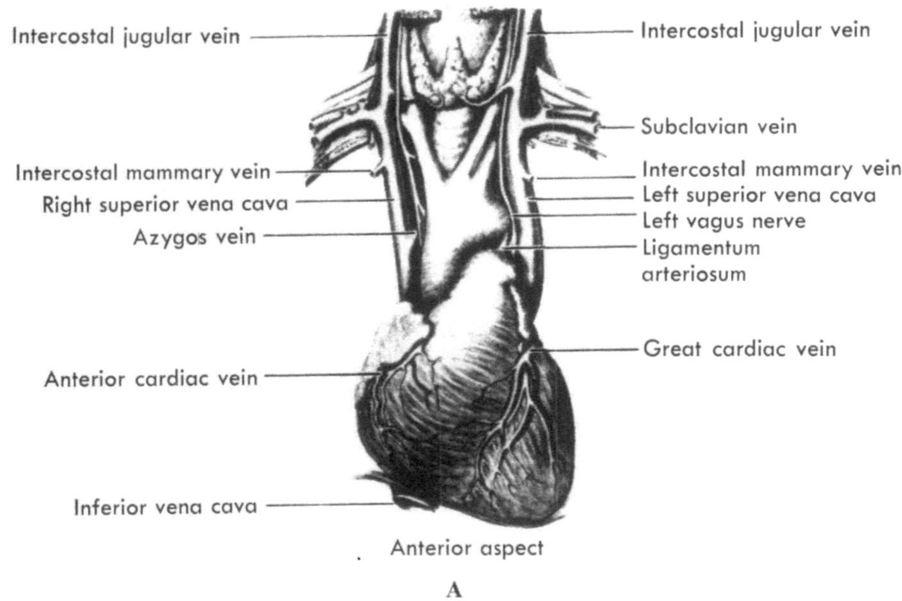

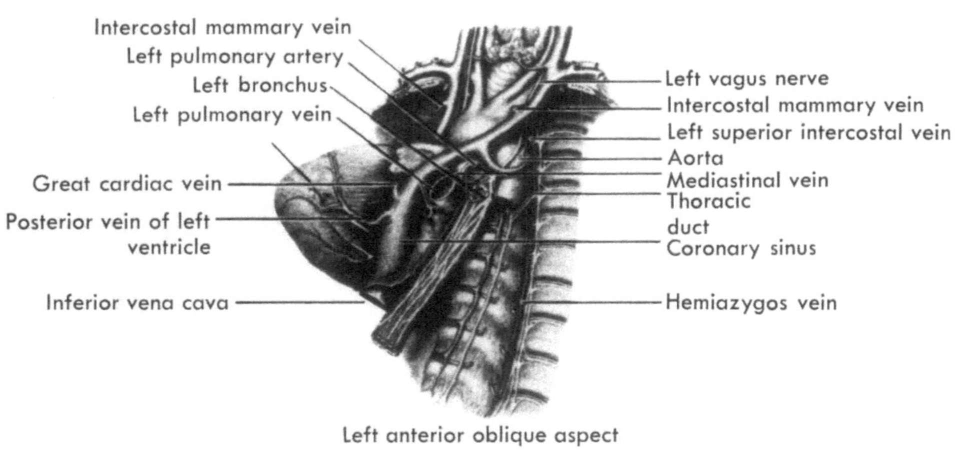

Fig. 6.29 A–D. Left superior vena cava. **A** Anterior aspect. **B** AP angiogram. **C** Left anterior oblique aspect. **D** Right posterior oblique angiogram. Anatomic features of left superior vena cava are clearly shown in **A** and **C**. Left superior vena cava is border forming in supra-aortic area. Note that it passes anterior to left lung root to enter coronary sinus. Angiograms (**B** and **D**) clearly depict course of left superior vena cava and its entry into coronary sinus. (From [59])

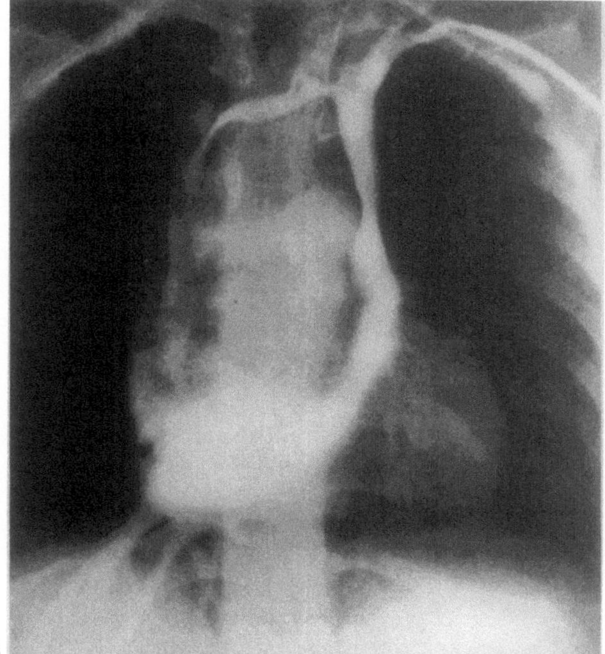

B

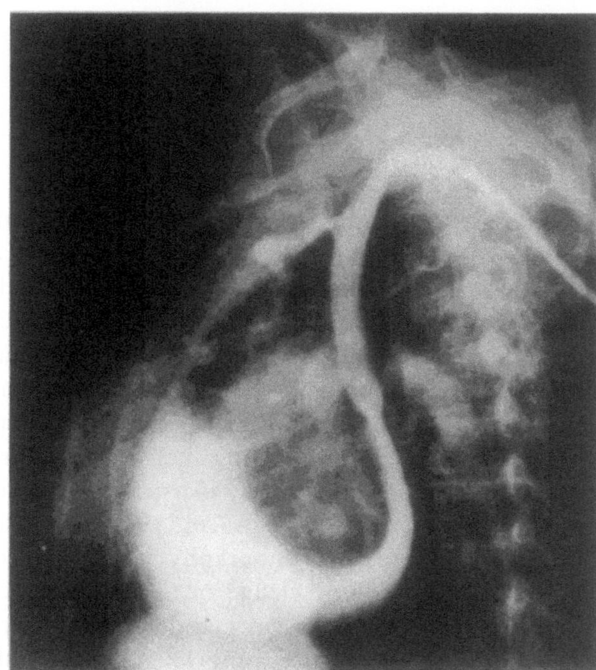

D

Fig. 6.29

6.2.3 Persistent Left Superior Vena Cava and Left Vertical Vein

Congenital anomalies in the development of the mediastinal veins may produce shadows simulating the aortic-pulmonary line or the pleural reflections over the subclavian artery. More often, they mimic the appearance of the mediastinum when it is involved by neoplastic or inflammatory disease. The left superior vena cava persists if the left common cardinal vein fails to be obliterated during fetal life [17, 18, 55]. In most cases, a right superior vena cava is present as well [59]. In about 40% of cases the left innominate vein connecting the two cavae is absent [59] strengthening the diagnosis of left superior vena cava at computed tomography [28].

The anomalous left superior vena cava descends vertically in front of the aortic arch close to and slightly lateral to the left vagus nerve (Fig. 6.29). It courses anterior to the left hilar structures and in front of the left superior pulmonary vein to enter the right atrium by way of the coronary sinus (Figs. 6.29, 6.30B). Rarely, it terminates in the left atrium [55]. In most reported cases the hemiazygos vein terminates in the lower end of the left superior vena cava [55].

In Winter's [59] series of 30 patients the presence of a persistent left superior vena cava was suspected on plain radiographs in only one case. Five patients had complete plain film study, including radiographs made during Müller's and Valsalva's maneuvers; the anomalous vessel was visible in only one of these cases, the questionable in two, and was not seen in two other patients. Winter concluded that "a shadow of the left superior vena cava can be identified on conventional chest films, but that the mediastinal contours as seen in the films of most patients with this anomaly are not sufficiently different from those of control subjects to establish with reliable accuracy the existence of this anomaly" [59]. Despite this pessimistic point of view, efforts should be made to recognize this condition because of its clinical significance and the fact that it is really not rare. The anomaly occurs in 0.3% of otherwise normal persons and in 3%–4% of patients with congenital heart disease [9, 12].

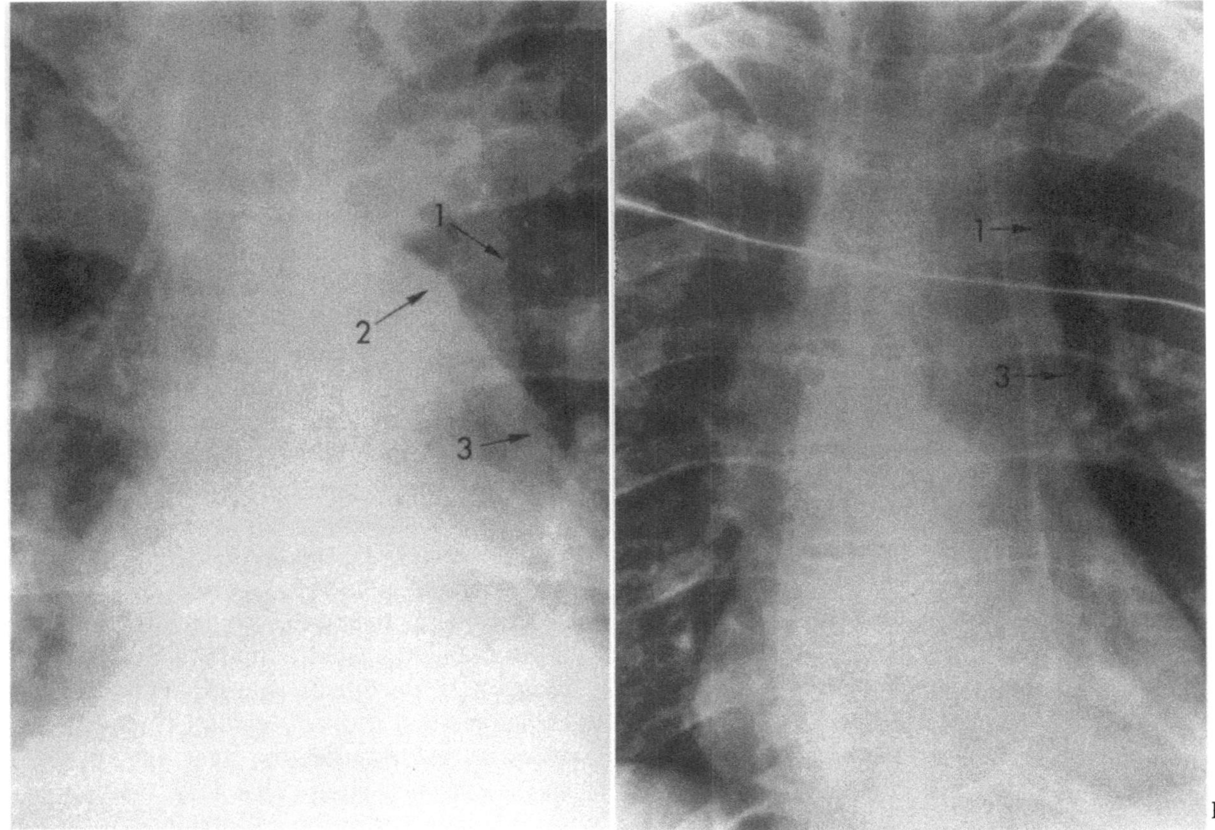

Fig. 6.30A, B. Left superior vena cava. **A** PA radiograph. **B** AP radiograph. These films demonstrate appearance of left superior vena cava in two different patients. Supra-aortic widening is noted in both (*1*). Note that shadows can be said to be anteriorly situated by application of cervicothoracic sign (see chapter 4). In patient shown in **A**, lateral margin of shadow passes well lateral of aortic knob (*2*) so that it cannot be first portion of left subclavian artery. Note also that inferior aspect of lateral margin of shadow crosses left hilum (*3*) unrelated to main pulmonary artery. In **B** transvenous catheter is seen passing through left innominate vein and pursuing a course along left superior mediastinum. Catheter has been passed through left superior vena cava and has entered right atrium by way of coronary sinus (see Fig. 6.29)

A better understanding of the normal contours of the supra-aortic area and their variants should cause the abnormal mediastinum to be recognized more easily; with persistent left superior vena cava the mediastinum above the aortic arch is widened to the left (Figs. 6.30, 6.31). The interface between the vessel and the left lung is vertical or slightly convex laterally and may

be seen to cross the shadow of the aortic knob and the left hilum (Figs. 6.30, 6.31). Such a shadow should raise suspicion of persistent left superior vena cava, particularly in the presence of a congenital heart disease or situs anomaly [9]. Recognition on PA radiographs that the supra-aortic area is abnormal is the key to correct diagnosis since following such a determination, computed tomography is usually a simple, noninvasive way to confirm the diagnosis [28, 58] (Fig. 6.31). Venography is, of course, also diagnostic. Knowledge of the anatomy of the left superior vena cava and, of course, of mediastinal venous anatomy is mandatory to an understanding of the unusual courses not infrequently taken by central venous catheters and pacemakers [23].

The left vertical vein should be distinguished pathologically from the persistent left superior vena cava [1, 12, 18]. The left vertical vein represents a persistence of a portion of the left common cardinal system when the left horn of the sinus venosus atrophies proximal to the entry

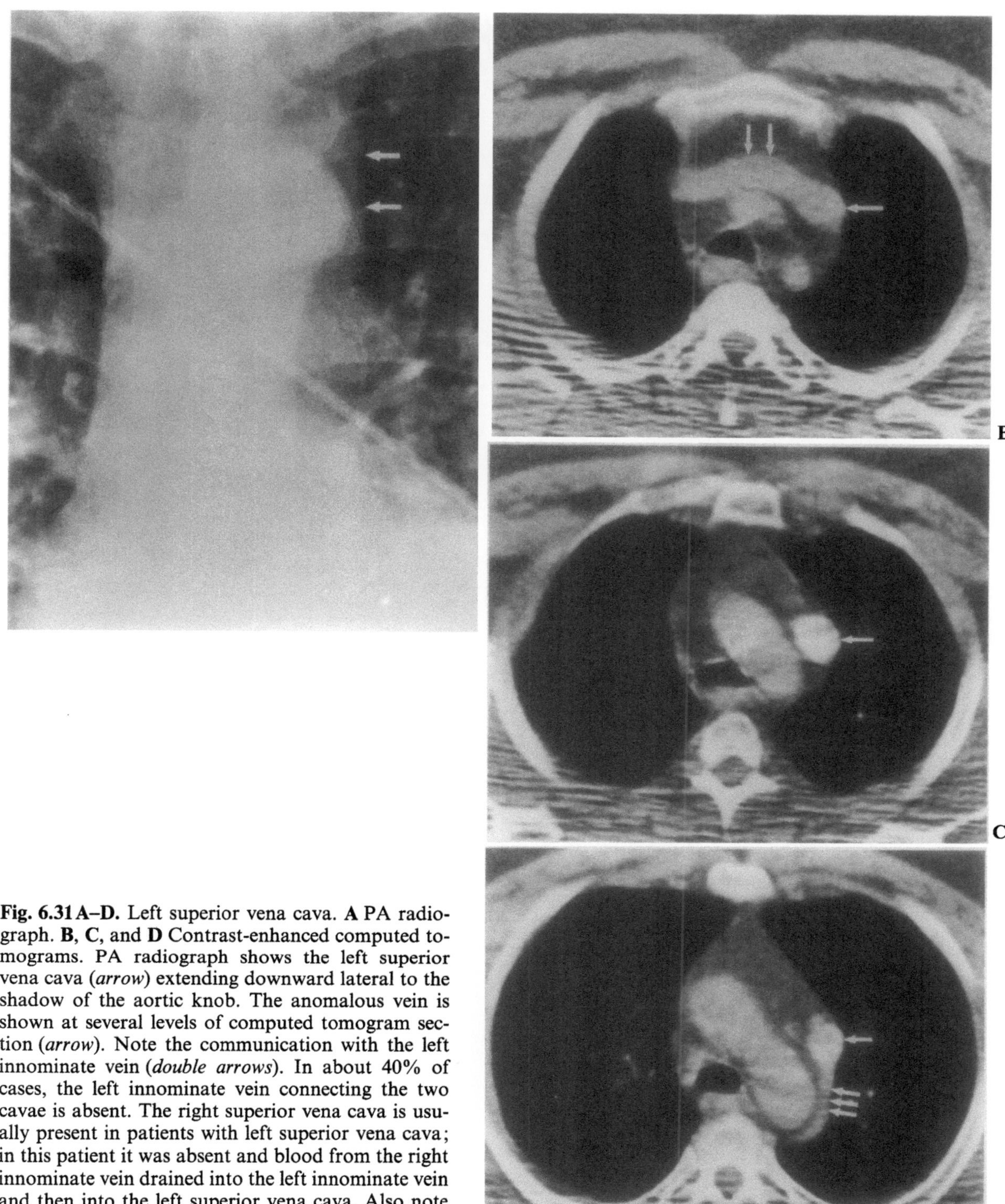

Fig. 6.31 A–D. Left superior vena cava. **A** PA radiograph. **B, C,** and **D** Contrast-enhanced computed tomograms. PA radiograph shows the left superior vena cava (*arrow*) extending downward lateral to the shadow of the aortic knob. The anomalous vein is shown at several levels of computed tomogram section (*arrow*). Note the communication with the left innominate vein (*double arrows*). In about 40% of cases, the left innominate vein connecting the two cavae is absent. The right superior vena cava is usually present in patients with left superior vena cava; in this patient it was absent and blood from the right innominate vein drained into the left innominate vein and then into the left superior vena cava. Also note the left superior intercostal vein (*triple arrows*) draining into the left cava

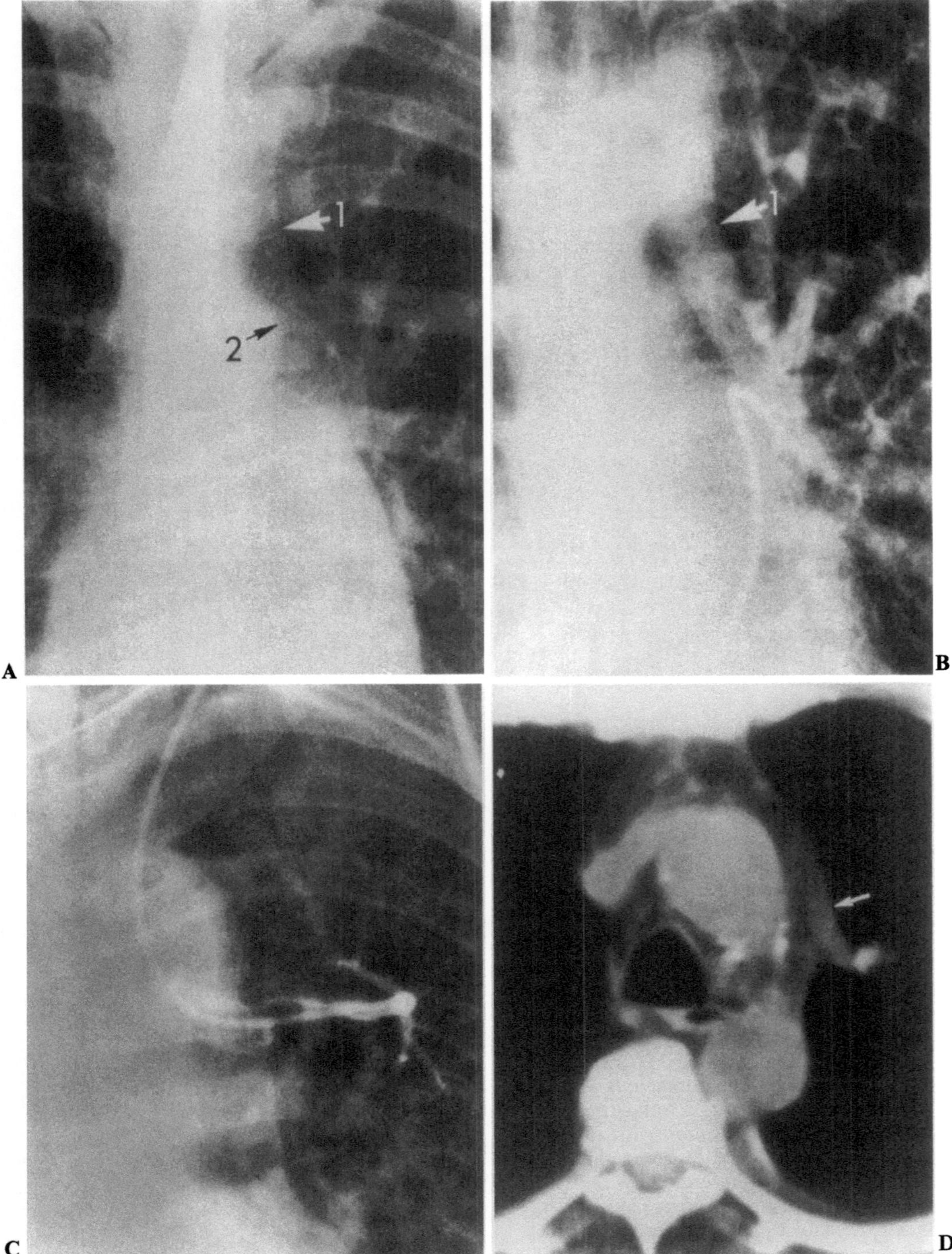

Fig. 6.32 A–D. Left vertical vein. **A** PA radiograph. **B** AP angiogram. **C** AP angiogram from another patient. **D** Computed tomogram of patient shown in **C**. Left vertical vein may simulate appearance of persistent left superior vena cava (*1*). Note lateral edge of vertical vein is projected to left of aortic knob (*2*). It may be small or large depending on quantity of blood flow through it, a condition dependent on amount of left lung drained by vessel. Flow in vessel is cephalad to left innominate vein. A smaller left vertical vein is demonstrated in **C**. At times, as shown in **D**, the anomalous vessel (*arrow*) can be demonstrated at computed tomography. (**A** and **B** From [1]; **C** and **D** from [23])

of the pulmonary veins [39]. In this condition, some or all of the left pulmonary veins drain into this structure which then carries the blood cephalad into the left innominate (brachiocephalic) vein. The vessel may be large when carrying a large volume of blood as in total anomalous pulmonary venous drainage; the typical "figure of eight" or "snowman" configuration of the heart and mediastinum results [8, 52]. With partial anomalous pulmonary venous return the left vertical vein is smaller and produces subtle supra-aortic abnormalities that may be impossible to distinguish on plain films from persistent left superior vena cava or from mediastinal disease (Fig. 6.32). Partial anomalous return to a left vertical vein shown can be demonstrated by computed tomography [23].

6.2.4 The Aortic Bodies and Paraganglioma

The aortic bodies are derived from the neural crest and are hence of ectodermal origin. They are classed with the paraganglia, small groups of chromaffin cells connected with the ganglia of the sympathetic trunk, and the ganglia of the celiac, renal, suprarenal, aortic, and hypogastric plexuses [56]. They can be the site of origin of a neoplasm that is analogous in many ways to the carotid body tumor [29]. These lesions are known by several synonyms – "chemodectoma," "glomus tumor," "aortic body tumor," and "paraganglioma." Totten [56] has reviewed the terminology used to describe these chromaffin tumors and has suggested "paraganglioma" as the preferred term.

Glenner and Grimley [22] have proposed a classification of paragangliomas in which those in the anterior mediastinum contiguous to the aortic arch (Fig. 6.33), or main pulmonary artery are termed "aorticopulmonary paragangliomas" and those lying posteriorly and arising from the sympathetic trunk are called "aorticosympathetic paragangliomas." Interestingly, most of the recorded examples of aorticopulmonary paraganglioma have not arisen from the aortic bodies but from nerve tissue located primarily along the vagus nerves or in the aortic adventitia. The tumor is often multicentric [33] and mediastinal paraganglioma associated with retroperitoneal paraganglioma may occur [25].

Paragangliomas of the mediastinum are rare. The first case involving the mediastinum was reported by Lattes [33] in 1950. In 1978, Olson and Salyer [41] stated that 47 mediastinal paragangliomas had been reported in the literature; 35 were aorticopulmonary and 12 were aorticosympathetic.

In 1982, Ogawa et al. [40] were able to find 25 cases of the aorticosympathetic type. Eight of the 25 were symptomatic tumors resulting in episodes of hypertension or sweating. Aorticopulmonary paragangliomas are rarely functional. They have a poor prognosis because of their tendency to invade adjacent tissues.

Carney [10] has recently reported a syndrome in young patients in which extra-adrenal paraganglioma, gastric leiomyosarcoma, and pulmonary chondroma are associated. The condition has come to be known as "Carney's triad" [10, 15]. In this syndrome, the paraganglioma is often in the thorax and in the case reported by Dajee et al. [15], the lesion was found in the mediastinum after careful surgical exploration which was initiated only because the patient presented with the other features of the triad. Occasionally patients show only two of the three tumors found in classical cases.

Thoracic paragangliomas present no distinguishing radiographic features. Paragangliomas are usually asymptomatic and are discovered incidentally (Fig. 6.33). They commonly show marked vascularity at angiography [16, 36, 44]. Sheps and Brown [51] have reported a case of mediastinal paraganglioma localized by ^{131}I-metaiodobenzylguanidine. The patient had Carney's triad.

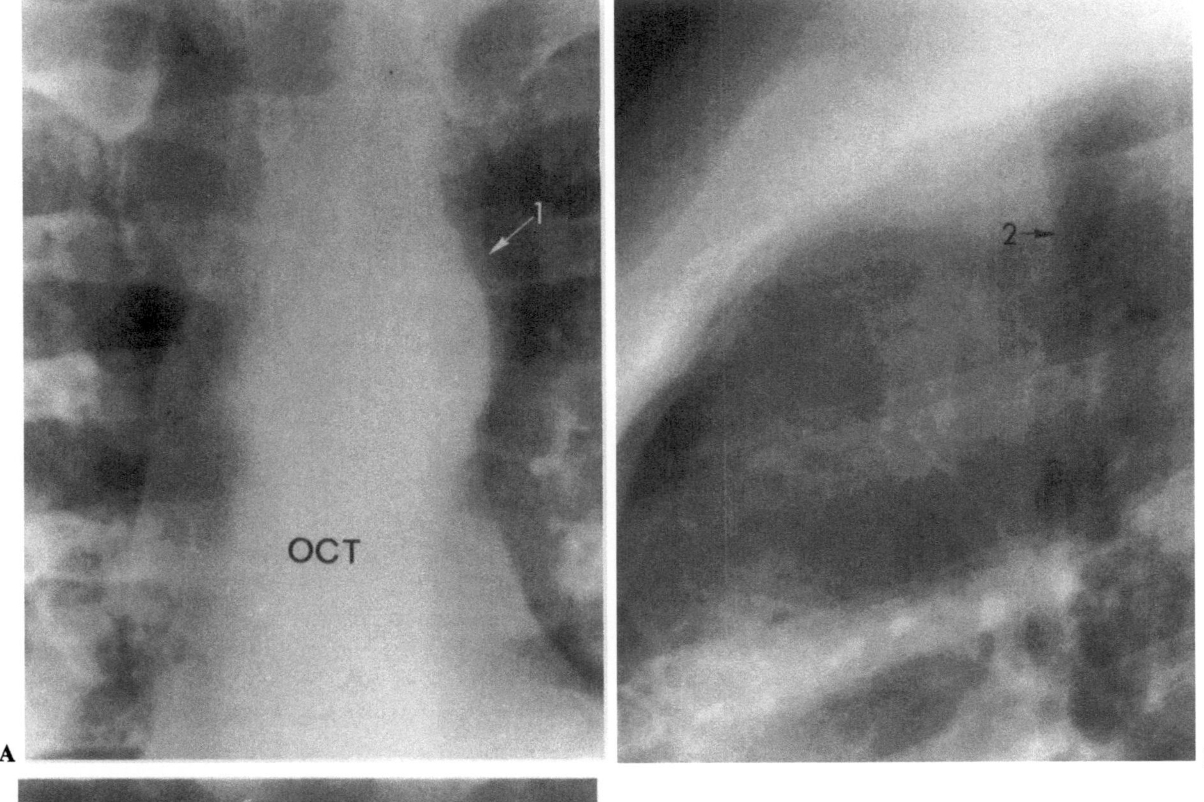

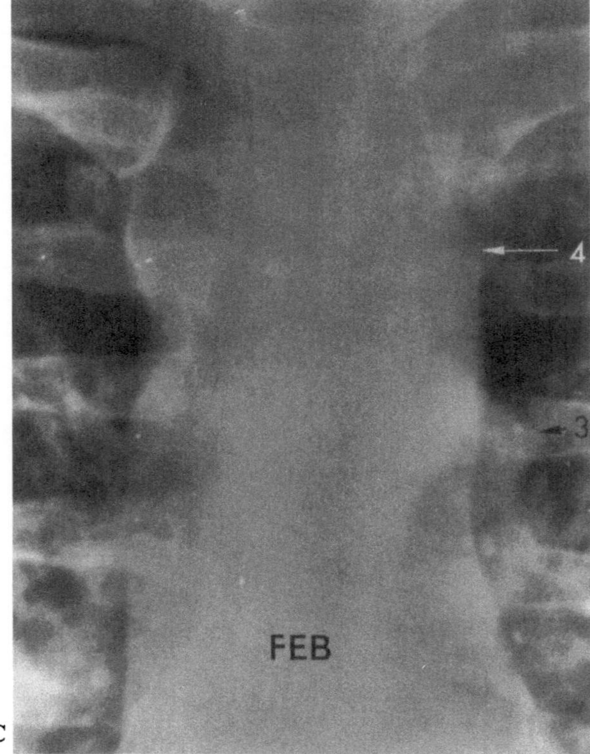

Fig. 6.33A–C. Paraganglioma. **A** and **B** PA and lateral radiographs. **C** PA radiograph made 4 months later. This patient was seen for recurrent bouts of severe substernal chest pain. Following such episodes, a distinct supra-aortic mass could be identified (*1*). As patient was observed, mass would gradually diminish in size only to recur after next episode of chest pain (**C**, *3*). At surgical exploration, mass was found related to aortic arch and contiguous structures; this proved to be paraganglioma, presumably arising from aortic body. Episodes of chest pain were thought to be related to bleeding within the tumor and, in turn, these bleeding episodes were thought to account for sudden increase in size of mass. Note impingement upon anterior wall of trachea (*2*) and progressive widening of supra-aortic area (*4*)

References

1. Adler SC, Silverman JF (1973) Anomalous venous drainage of the left upper lobe. Radiology 108:563–565
2. Bachman AL, Teixidor HS (1975) The posterior tracheal band: a reflector of local superior mediastinal abnormality. Br J Radiol 48:352–359
3. Ball JB Jr, Proto AV (1982) Variable appearance of the left superior intercostal vein. Radiology 144:445–452
4. Barrie JD (1961) Intrathoracic tumors of the carotid body type (chemodectoma). Thorax 16:78–86
5. Berk RN (1964) Dilation of the left superior intercostal vein. Radiology 83:419–423
6. Blank N, Castellino RA (1972) Patterns of pleural reflections of the left superior mediastinum – normal anatomy and distortions produced by adenopathy. Radiology 102:585–589
7. Branscom JJ, Austin JHM (1973) Aberrant right subclavian artery – findings seen on plain chest roentgenogram. Am J Roentgenol Radium Ther Nucl Med 119:539–542
8. Bruwer A (1956) Roentgenologic findings in total anomalous pulmonary venous connection. Mayo Clin Proc 31:171–176
9. Campbell M, Deuchar DC (1954) The left sided superior vena cava. Br Heart J 16:423–439
10. Carney JA (1979) The triad of gastric epithelioid leiomyosarcoma, functional extra-adrenal paraganglioma and pulmonary chondroma. Cancer 43:374–382
11. Carter MM, Tarr RW, Mazer MJ, Carroll FE (1985) "Aortic nipple" as a sign of impending superior vena cavae syndrome. Chest 87:775–777
12. Cha EM, Khoury GH (1972) Persistent left superior vena cava. Radiology 103:375–381
13. Cheng TO (1970) Pseudocoarctation of the aorta – an important consideration in the differential diagnosis of superior mediastinal mass. Am J Med 49:551–555
14. Cimmino CV (1975) Contacts of the left lung with the mediastinum – sources of diagnostic error. Am J Roentgenol Radium Ther Nucl Med 124:412–416
15. Dajee A, Dajee H, Hinrichs S, Lillington G (1982) Pulmonary chondroma, extra-adrenal paraganglioma and gastric leiomyosarcoma. Carney's triad. J Thorac Cardiovasc Surg 84:377–381
16. Drucker EA, McLoud TC, Dedrick CG, Hilgenberg AD, Geller SC, Shepard JO (1987) Mediastinal paraganglioma: radiologic evaluation of an unusual vascular tumor. AJR 148:521–522
17. Edwards JE (1953) Pathological and developmental considerations in anomalous pulmonary venous connection. Mayo Clin Proc 28:441–452
18. Edwards JE, Helmholz HF Jr (1953) A classification of total anomalous pulmonary venous connection based on developmental considerations. Mayo Clin Proc 28:441–452
19. Felson B, Lessure AP (1964) "Downhill" varices of the esophagus. Dis Chest 46:740–746
20. Friedman AC, Chambers E, Sprayregen S (1978) Normal and abnormal superior intercostal vein. AJR 131:599–602
21. Gladnikoff H (1948) A radiographic study of the mediastinum in health and pulmonary carcinoma. Acta Radiol [Suppl] 73:1–87
22. Glenner GG, Grimley PM (1974) Tumor of the extra-adrenal paraganglion system (including chemoreceptors). Armed Forces Institute of Pathology, 2nd series, fascicle 9, Washington DC
23. Godwin JD, Chen JTT (1986) Thoracic venous anatomy. AJR 147:674–684
24. Gondos B (1961) Roentgen image of the subclavian artery in the pulmonary apex. Am J Roentgenol Radium Ther Nucl Med 86:1058–1060
25. Haber S (1964) Retroperitoneal and mediastinal chemodectoma – report of a case and review of the literature. Am J Roentgenol Radium Ther Nucl Med 92:1029–1041
26. Haswell DM, Berrigan TJ Jr (1976) Anomalous inferior vena cava with accessory hemiazygous continuation. Radiology 119:51–54
27. Hewitt RL, Ichinose H, Weichert RF III, Drapanas T (1972) Chemodectomas. Surgery 71:275–282
28. Huggins TJ, Lesar MSL, Friedman AC, Pyatt RS (1982) CT appearance of left superior vena cava. J Comput Assist Tomogr 6:294–297
29. Karnauchow PN (1965) The carotid body: a pathologist's view. Can Med Assoc J 92:1298–1302
30. Keats TE (1972) The aortic-pulmonary mediastinal stripe. Am J Roentgenol Radium Ther Nucl Med 116:107–109
31. Klinkhamer AC (1966) Aberrant right subclavian artery clinical and roentgenologic aspects. Am J Roentgenol 97:438–446
32. Lane EJ, Heitzman ER, Dinn WM (1976) The radiology of the superior intercostal veins. Radiology 120:263–268
33. Lattes R (1950) Non-chromaffin paraganglioma of ganglion nodosum, carotid body and aortic arch bodies. Cancer 3:667–694
34. Lund G (1982) CT appearance of the superior intercostal veins. Eur J Radiol 2:122–124
35. MacDonald CJ, Castellino RA, Blank N (1970) The aortic "nipple" – the left superior intercostal vein. Radiology 96:533–536
36. Mapp EM, Krause TB, Fox EF, Foci G (1969) Chemodectoma of the anterior mediastinum – report of a case of probable aortic body origin with arteriographic findings. Radiology 92:547–548
37. McLoughlin MJ, Weisbrod G, Wise DJ, Yeung HPH (1981) Computed tomography in congenital anomalies of the aortic arch and great vessels. Radiology 138:399–403
38. Mencini RA, Proto AV (1982) The high left and main pulmonary arteries: a CT pitfall. J Comput Assist Tomogr 6:452–459
39. Neill CA (1956) Development of pulmonary veins – with reference to the embryology of anomalies of pulmonary venous return. Pediatrics 18:880–887

40. Ogawa J, Inove H, Koide S, Kawada S, Shohtsu A, Hata J (1982) Functioning paraganglioma in the posterior mediastinum. Ann Thor Surg 33:507–510

41. Olson JL, Salyer MW (1978) Mediastinal paragangliomas (aortic body tumor): a report of four cases and a review of the literature. Cancer 41:2405–2412

42. Pagniez B, Benies JL, DuPuis C, Remy J (1975) The left superior intercostal vein. J Radiol Electrol Med Nucl 56:285–298

43. Parkinson J, Bedford DE (1936) The aortic triangle – a radiological landmark in the left oblique projection. Lancet 2:909–911

44. Phillips LA (1963) Mediastinal chemodectoma and thoracic aortography – a case report. Clin Radiol 14:129–132

45. Poker N, Finby N, Steinberg I (1958) Subclavian arteries: study in health and disease. Am J Roentgenol Radium Ther Nucl Med 80:193–216

46. Proto AV, Chaliff MI (1986) Apical opacity: a normal finding on posteroanterior chest radiographs. Radiology 161:429–432

47. Proto AV, Rost RC Jr (1985) CT of the thorax: pitfalls in interpretation. Radiographics 5:693–698

48. Proto AV, Cuthbert NW, Raider L (1987) Aberrant right subclavian artery: further observations. AJR 148:253–257

49. Salomonowitz E, Edwards JE, Hunter DW, Casteneda-Zuniga WR, Lund G, Cragg AH, Amplatz K (1984) The three types of aortic diverticulae. AJR 142:673–679

50. Sandler CM, Toombs BD, Lester RG (1979) Buckling of the left common carotid artery simulating mediastinal neoplasm. AJR 133:312–313

51. Sheps SG, Brown ML (1985) Localization of mediastinal paragangliomas (pheochromocytoma). Chest 87:807–809

52. Snellen HA, Albers FH (1952) The clinical diagnosis of anomalous pulmonary venous drainage. Circulation 6:801–816

53. Steinberg I (1962) Dilatation of the hemiazygous veins in superior vena caval occlusion simulating mediastinal tumor. Am J Roentgenol Radium Ther Nucl Med 87:248–257

54. Taber P, Chang LWM, Campion GM (1979) Diagnosis of retroesophageal right aortic arch by computed tomography. J Comput Assist Tomogr 3:684–685

55. Taybi H, Kurlander CJ, Lurie PR, Campbell JA (1965) Anomalous systemic venous connection to the left atrium or to a pulmonary vein. Am J Roentgenol Radium Ther Nucl Med 94:62–77

56. Totten RS (1973) Terminology of carotid body tumors: confusion at the crossroads (bifurcation). Hum Pathol 4:453–454

57. Warwick R, Williams PR (1973) Gray's anatomy, 35th edn. Saunders, Philadelphia

58. Webb WR, Gamsu G, Speckman JM, Kaiser JA, Federle MP, Lipton MJ (1982) Computed tomographic demonstration of mediastinal venous anomalies. AJR 139:157–161

59. Winter FS (1954) Persistent left superior vena cava – a survey of the world literature. Angiology 5:90–132

60. Woodring JH, Rhodes RA (1985) Posterosuperior mediastinal widening in aortic coarctation. AJR 144:23–25

7 The Infra-aortic Area

7.1 General Anatomic Considerations

The portion of the mediastinum to be considered in this chapter lies below the aortic arch and behind the left side of the anterior mediastinum. The anatomy of the thoracic aorta has been discussed in detail in chapter 6. The proximal portion of the main pulmonary artery is situated anterior to the root of the aorta (see Fig. 6.2). As the pulmonary artery ascends, it comes to lie to the left of the ascending aorta; at this point the two great vessels are in the same coronal plane (see Fig. 6.3). This plane marks the anterior boundary of the infra-aortic area; the posterior margin of the anterior mediastinum is the pericardium covering the great vessels and the heart [27, 154].

Along the anterior aspect of the infra-aortic area, lung contacts heart in front of the left inferior pulmonary ligament. The configurations produced by the contact of lung with the left atrium and left ventricle are well known, having been considered in detail in many articles and texts. They will not be reviewed here, although the appearances of the left pulmonary veins as they enter the atrium will be discussed. This chapter will be concerned, therefore, with a review of the anatomy of the mediastinal structures situated below the aortic arch; the aortic pulmonic window, the preaortic area behind the heart, and the left paraspinal area will be considered.

7.2 Radiologic Correlations with Anatomy and Pathology

7.2.1 The Aortic-Pulmonic Window

The portion of the infra-aortic area of the mediastinum encompassed by the arch of the aorta above and by the left pulmonary artery below is sometimes known as the "aortic-pulmonic window." The origin of this term is obscure, although Parkinson and Bedford state that it was in common usage in Vienna many years ago [112]. These authors view the aortic-pulmonic window as being circumscribed by the aortic arch above and the left atrium below with the left pulmonary artery dividing the window. Since the view of the mediastinum provided by the window is entirely above the left pulmonary artery, we have preferred to use the aortic arch and the left pulmonary artery as boundaries of the window [68]. This region of the mediastinum has considerable radiologic importance since it can usually be identified on PA, lateral, and oblique chest radiographs and because it contains many vital anatomic structures or is bordered by them. Neoplastic disease frequently involves the aortic-pulmonic window; metastatic disease and lymphoma commonly involve the lymph nodes that lie within its confines.

Mediastinoscopy, commonly used to assess mediastinal nodal disease [47, 55, 76, 134], is much less accurate for the evaluation of the left side of the mediastinum than it is for the right side [79, 115]. Only the nodes at the medial aspect of the aortic-pulmonic window can be visualized with this technique; those lying at the infero-lateral margin of the aortic arch cannot be seen [115]. For this reason, assessment of

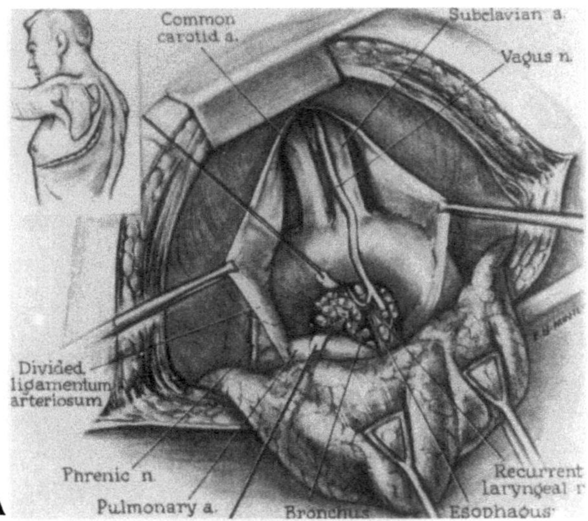

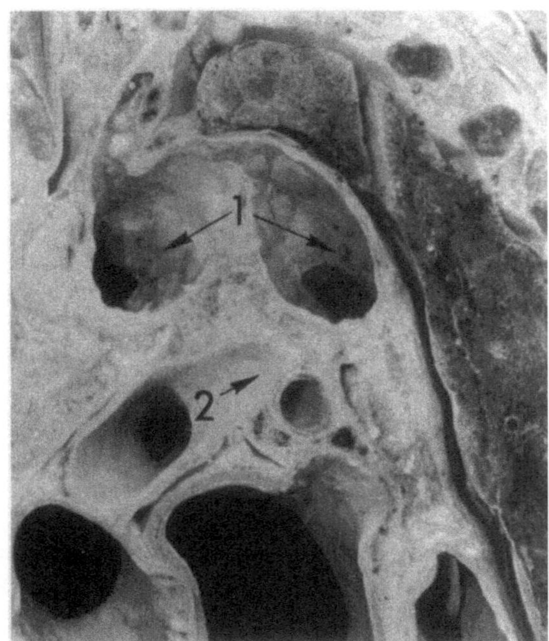

Fig. 7.1A, B. Aortic-pulmonic window. **A** Aortic-pulmonic window viewed from left side at surgery. **B** Sagittal body section through the aortic-pulmonic window. Aortic-pulmonic window is that portion of left side of mediastinum between aortic arch (*1*) and left pulmonary artery (*2*). (**A** From [38])

disease in this area must rely heavily upon radiologic investigation.

From its point of origin the left pulmonary artery courses posteriorly and laterally from a point immediately behind the posterior wall of the ascending aorta (Fig. 7.1). The aortic arch passes cephalad, posteriorly, and to the left. The area thus circumscribed, the aortic-pulmonic window, is filled with areolar tissue and fat (Fig. 7.2) and contains the so-called ductus lymph nodes, usually one or two in number, and some of the inferior nodes in the left tracheobronchial lymph node chain (Fig. 7.2), the left bronchial arteries, and the left recurrent laryngeal nerve (Figs. 7.1 and 7.2). Webb [157] has reported an unusual case in which the left brachiocephalic vein crossed the window and passed anterior to the trachea to join the right brachiocephalic vein.

Laterally, the aortic-pulmonic window is bordered or "closed" by the mediastinal pleura subtending inferiorly from the aortic arch (Fig. 7.2). The window extends posteriorly to a point where the descending aorta and left pulmonary artery are intimately related (see Fig. 7.13). Below this region lung may extend into the back of the window to contact the back of the left main and/or lower lobe bronchi [157] (see Fig. 7.22). In many normal patients, the presence of a large quantity of fat in the aortic-pulmonic window allows one to visualize the window rather clearly. The normal appearance on frontal radiographs is that of a "bow tie" (Fig. 7.3). Occasionally, the ligamentum arteriosum is outlined by fat within the window. It also may be identified when calcified (Fig. 7.4). Currarino and Jackson [29] state that calcification in the ductus is a common finding in children, developing a few months to several years after the normal closure of the ductus. Apparently, in many cases calcification disappears as children grow older.

The left recurrent laryngeal nerve has a long intrathoracic course and is more vulnerable to disease than the right recurrent laryngeal nerve. It arises from the vagus nerve lateral to the aortic arch (Figs. 7.1 and 7.2), sweeping through the aortic-pulmonic window behind the ligamentum arteriosum to ascend beside the trachea

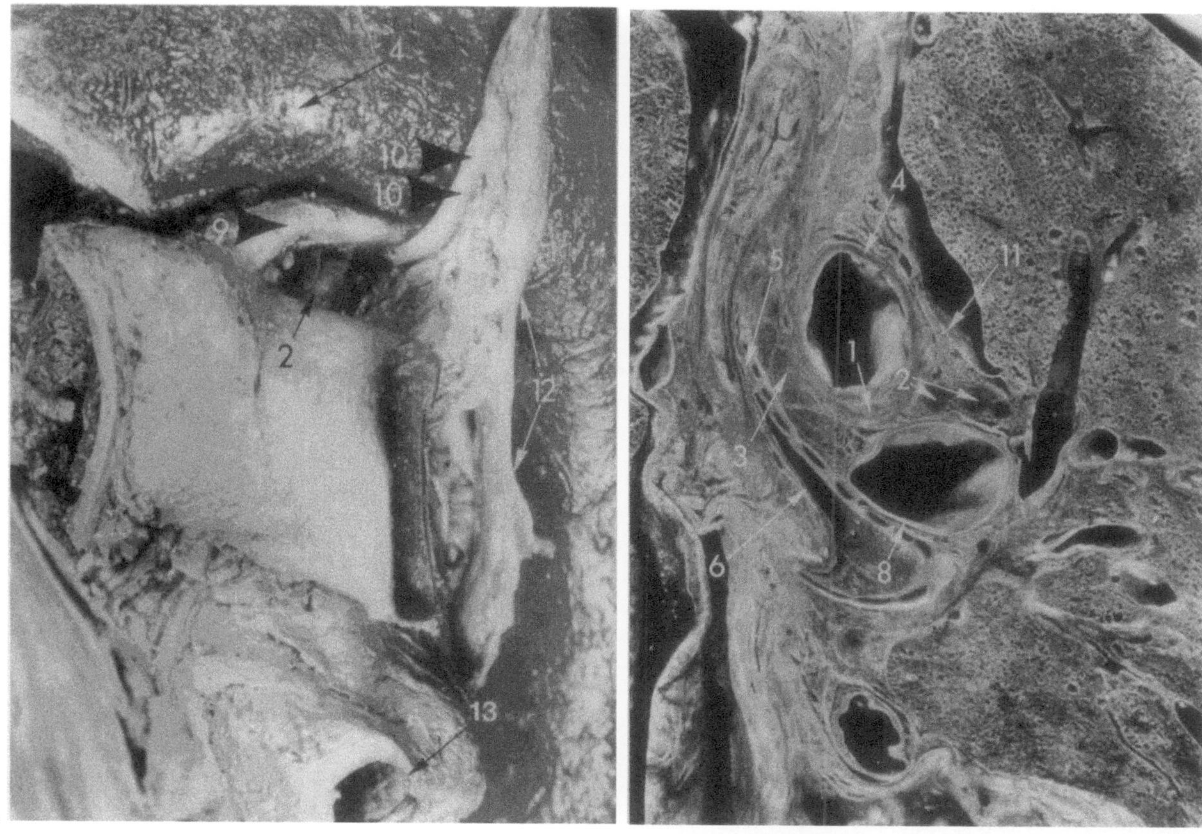

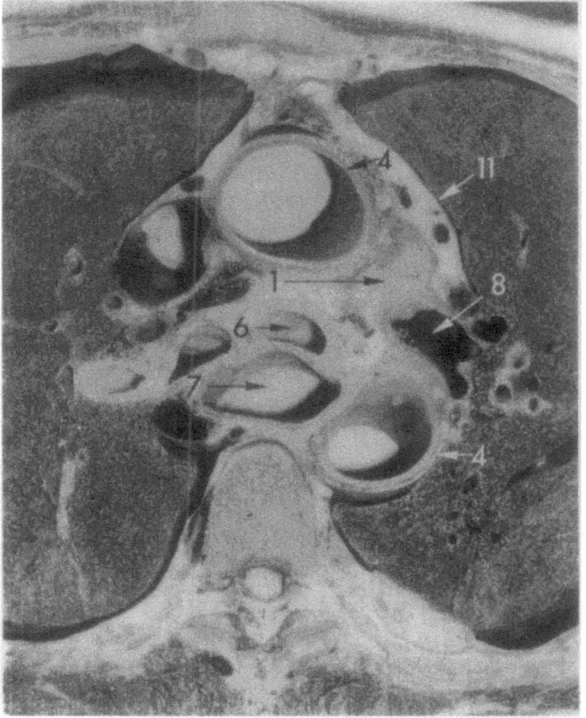

Fig. 7.2 A–C. Aortic-pulmonic window viewed from left side with mediastinal pleura removed (**A**) and coronal and transverse body sections through aortic-pulmonic window (**B** and **C**). Aortic-pulmonic window is filled with areolar tissue and fat (*1*). It contains several vital structures. At its lateral margin lie ductus nodes (*2*); at its medial edge, inferior nodes of left tracheobronchial chain (*3*) separate aortic arch (*4*) from trachea (*5*) and left main bronchus (*6*) in front and esophagus behind (*7*). Left pulmonary artery (*8*) lies below. Window is transversed by ligamentum arteriosum (*9*) and left recurrent laryngeal nerve (*10*). Mediastinal pleura can be seen "closing" window laterally (*11*). Incidentally shown is vagus nerve (*12*) and left upper lobe bronchus (*13*). (From [68])

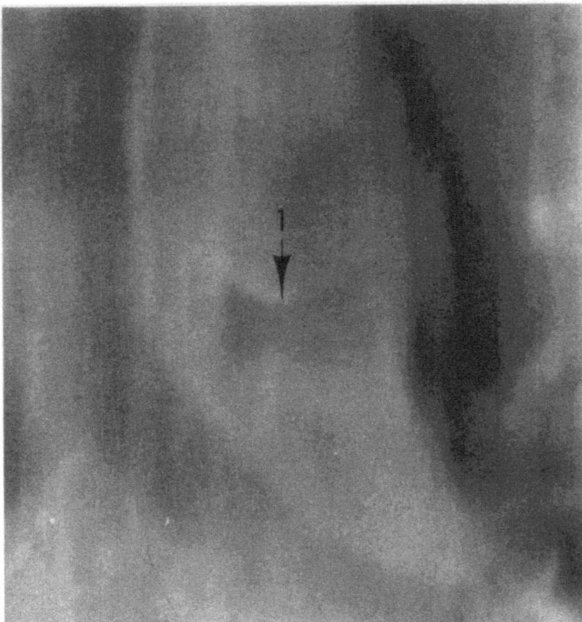

Fig. 7.3. Fat in the aortic-pulmonic window (AP tomogram). The considerable quantity of fat normally present in aortic-pulmonic window may be visualized in a small percentage of patients. Appearance of fat typically presents a "bow tie" appearance (*1*) due to intrusion of convex lower margin of aortic arch from above and convex upper margin of left pulmonary artery from below. (From [68])

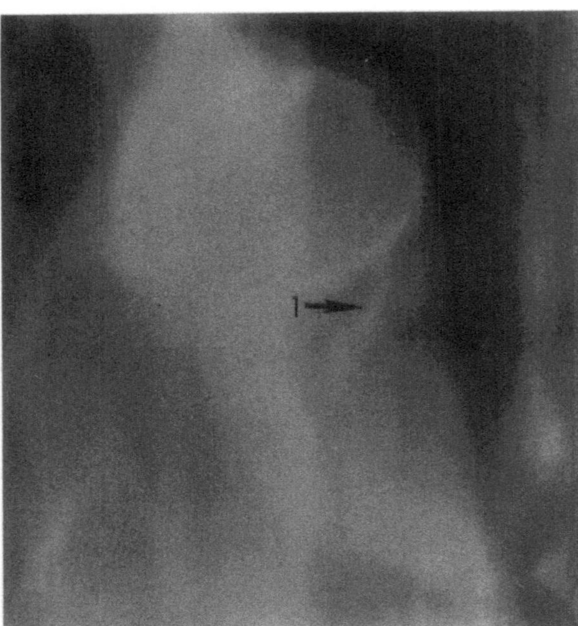

Fig. 7.4. Demonstration of ligamentum arteriosum in aortic-pulmonic window (AP tomogram). Infrequently, ligamentum arteriosum may be seen outlined by fat in aortic-pulmonic window. Somewhat more commonly it is visualized because it is calcified (*1*). (From [68])

just anterior to the esophagus. As the recurrent nerve passes medially through the upper portion of the aortic-pulmonic window, it is in contiguity with inferior lymph nodes in the left tracheobronchial chain (Fig. 7.2). It is at this point that mediastinal nodal metastases frequently involve the recurrent nerve, causing left vocal cord paresis. Of course, if ductus nodes lying laterally in the inferior portion of the window enlarge to sufficient size, they too may compromise the recurrent nerve. In every patient with an unexplained complaint of hoarseness, a careful study of the mediastinum must be undertaken to exclude a lesion that could compromise either recurrent laryngeal nerve. The right recurrent laryngeal nerve arises from the vagus nerve in front of the right subclavian artery, looping under that vessel to ascend beside the trachea and behind the common carotid artery. It is less frequently involved by mediastinal disease than is the left recurrent laryngeal nerve.

7.2.1.1 Lateral "Closure" of the Aortic-Pulmonic Window

At the anterior margin of the aortic-pulmonic window, the mediastinal pleura extending inferiorly from the aortic arch reflects over the main pulmonary artery onto the left superior pulmonary vein as this vein passes anterior to the left main bronchus to enter the left atrium. The interface of lung and pleura in this area produces a characteristic tongue-like appearance with a rounded extremity extending inferiorly and medially (Fig. 7.5). Radiographic demonstration of this reflection is, however, relatively infrequent.

Fig. 7.5A–E. Lateral "closure" of aortic-pulmonic window (anterior). **A** PA radiograph. **B** AP tomogram. **C** Coronal body section. **D** Radiograph of same section. **E** Left side of mediastinum with pleura removed. At anterior margin of aortic-pulmonic window, mediastinal pleura extending inferiorly from aortic arch reflects over main pulmonary artery (*1*) onto left superior pulmonary vein (*2*) as this vessel passes anterior to left main bronchus. This interface of lung and mediastinum has characteristic tongue-like appearance with rounded extremity extending inferiorly and medially (*3*). Left phrenic nerve passing anterior to left hilum is in intimate association with this region of contact between lung and mediastinum (*4*). (**B, C,** and **D** From [68]; **E** from [117])

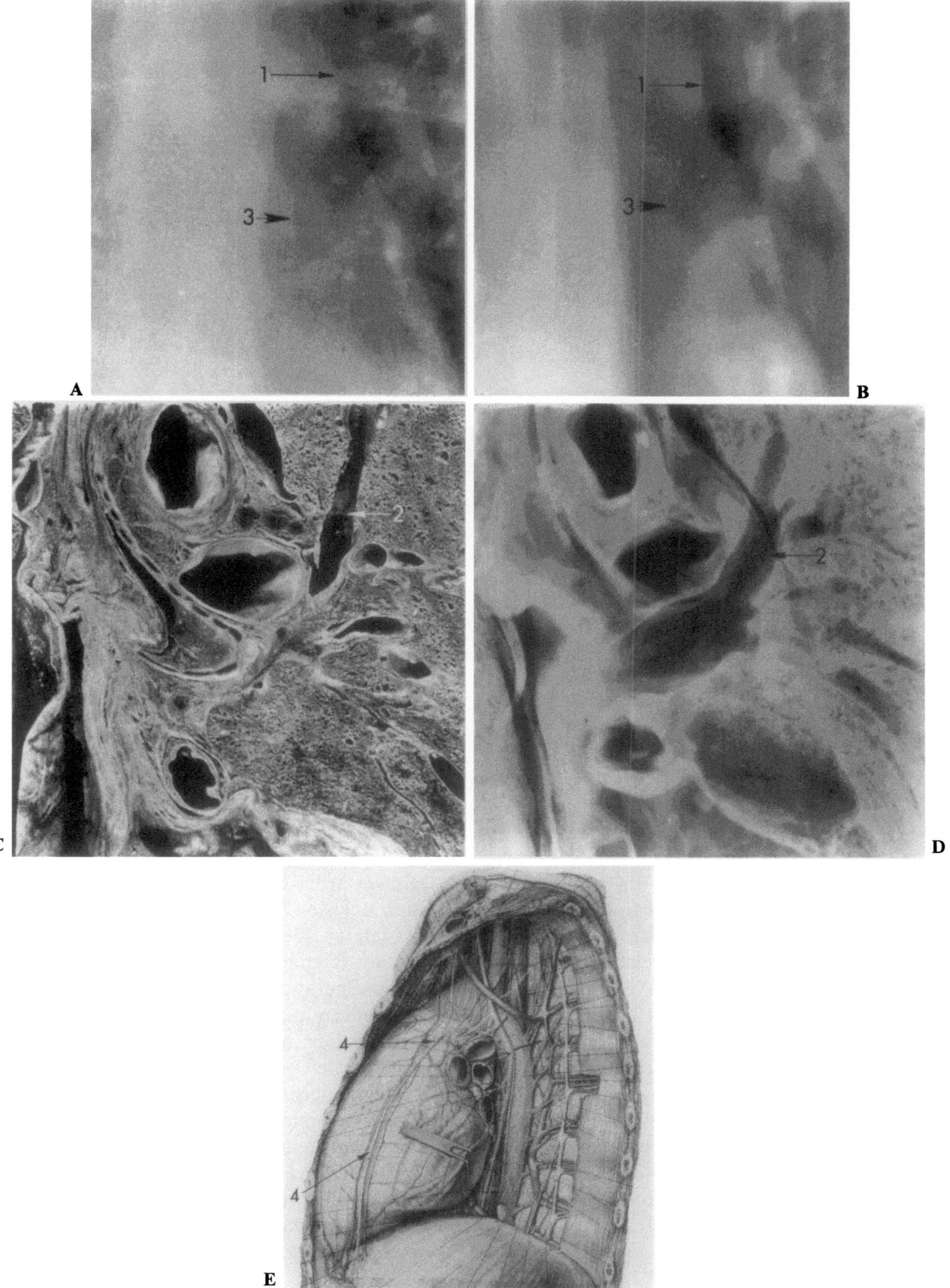

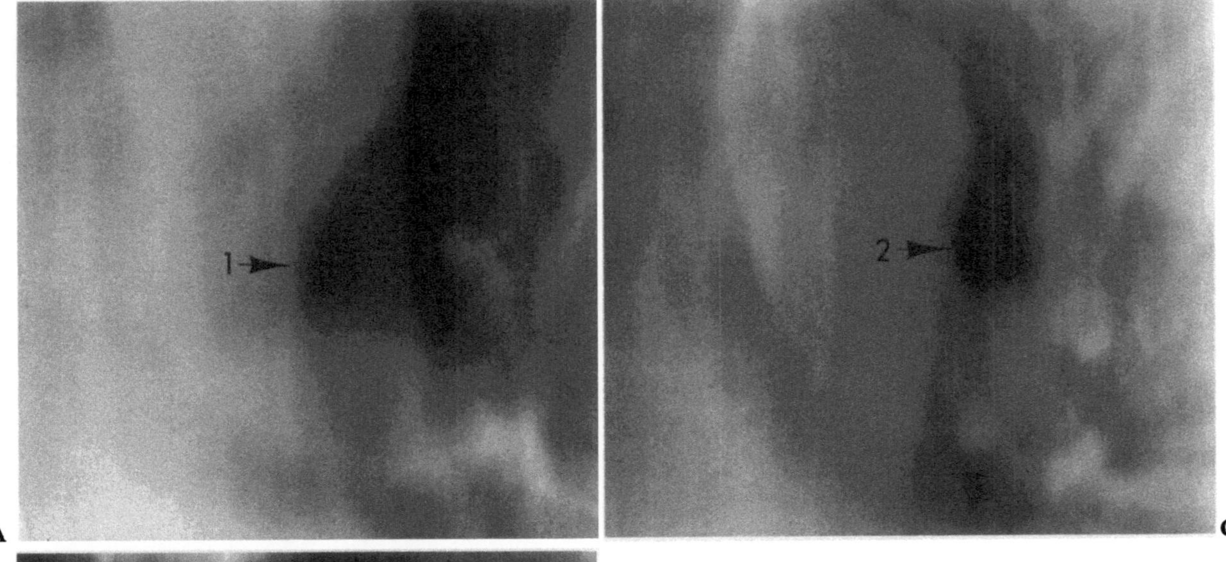

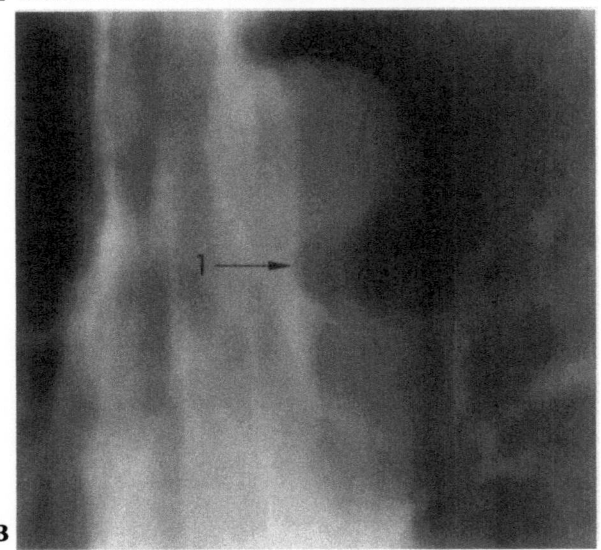

Fig. 7.6 A–C. Lateral "closure" of aortic-pulmonic window. (Midpoint) AP tomograms. Reflections of mediastinal pleura from the aortic arch onto left pulmonary artery "close" lateral aspect of the aortic pulmonary window midway from front to back. Appearance of this reflection is quite variable. As shown in **A** and **B**, deep intrusions of lung into window may be seen (*1*). This finding is seen in individuals with ectasia of the aorta and/or prominent pulmonary arteries and in most patients with emphysema. Such an appearance virtually excludes enlargement of ductus nodes. More often, configuration of this pleural reflection is straight, as shown in **C** (*2*). (**A** and **C** From [68])

After descending through the upper thorax lateral to the left common carotid artery and in front of the left subclavian artery, the left phrenic nerve passes to the left of the aortic arch anterior to the vagus nerve. It then courses over the surface of the left atrial appendage anterior to the entry of the left superior pulmonary vein. At this point it is situated just in front of the aortic-pulmonic window and can be compromised by disease processes extending anteriorly from the window, resulting in diaphragmatic paralysis. Below this level the phrenic nerve passes along the anterolateral aspect of the pericardium over the left ventricle to the diaphragm (Fig. 7.5).

Midway from front to back, the pleural reflection "closing" the aortic-pulmonic window on its lateral side passes from the midportion of the aortic arch onto the left pulmonary artery. Configurations produced by this area of pleural reflection are quite varied, ranging from deep incursions of lung into the mediastinum above the left pulmonary artery (Figs. 7.6 and 7.7) to appearances in which the pleural reflection is essentially vertical (Fig. 7.6) or demonstrates only a mild concavity directed laterally. Deeper extensions into the mediastinum are commonly observed in patients with chronic obstructive pulmonary disease and in those individuals with ectatic aortas and large left pulmo-

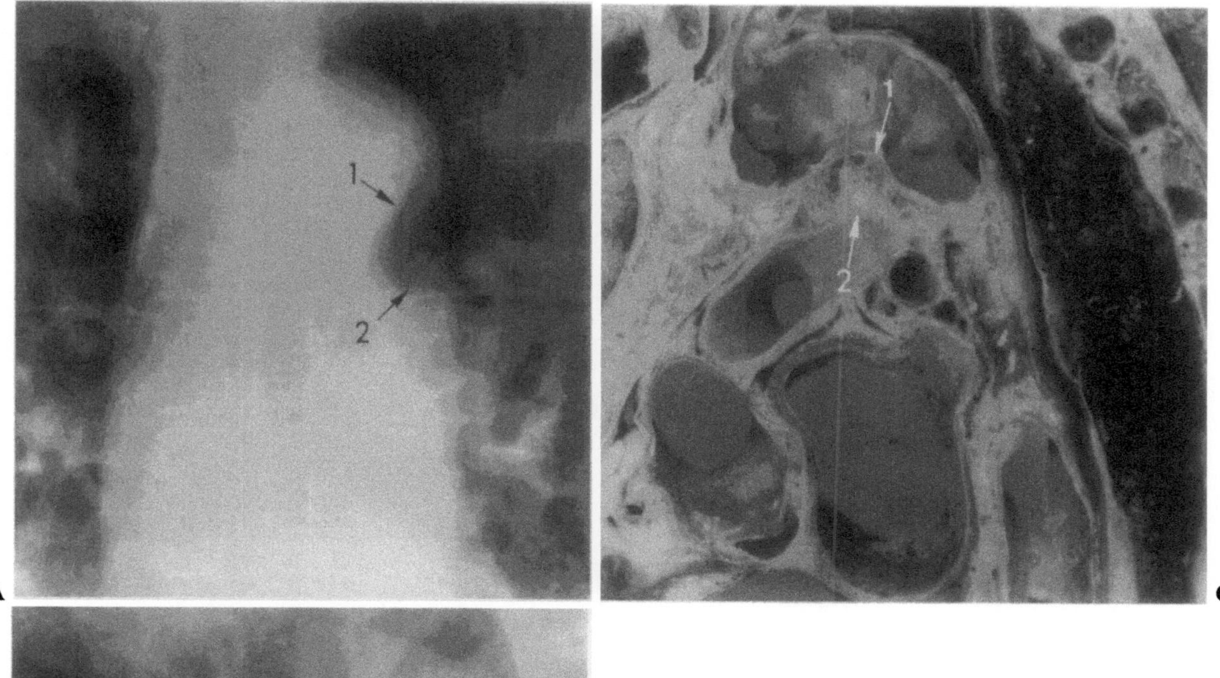

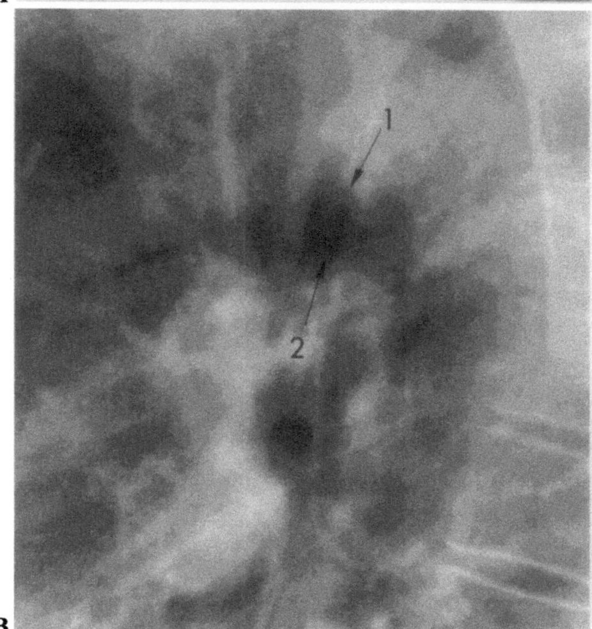

Fig. 7.7A–C. Lateral "closure" of aortic-pulmonic window (midpoint). **A** and **B** PA and lateral radiographs. **C** Sagittal body section. Deep intrusion of lung into aortic-pulmonic window can frequently identified on lateral radiographs; lung in window outlines inferior aspect of aortic arch (*1*) and superior aspect of pulmonary artery (*2*). Presence of such an appearance on lateral radiographs again confirms there is no gross nodal enlargement or other mass at lateral aspect of window

nary arteries (Fig. 7.6). An unusual condition in which the aortic-pulmonic window is filled with lung is congenital absence of the left pericardium. In this abnormality the left parietal pleura is deficient, permitting lung to make intimate contact with the aortic arch and pulmonary artery, since in effect the window is not closed laterally [40, 104, 108]. The defect apparently represents a disturbance in the development of the left pleuropericardial membrane [40]. When the left pericardium is absent

only in part, soft tissue herniation may occur through the defect [35, 40, 104]. The herniated tissue may be the left atrial appendage [35, 40, 104]. The relationship of such a hernia to the aortic-pulmonic window is apparently variable, but it may be seen as a mass in the left hilum [40].

Although the radiographic appearances do vary, a configuration of the lateral closure of the aortic-pulmonic window demonstrating a convexity directed laterally should raise the con-

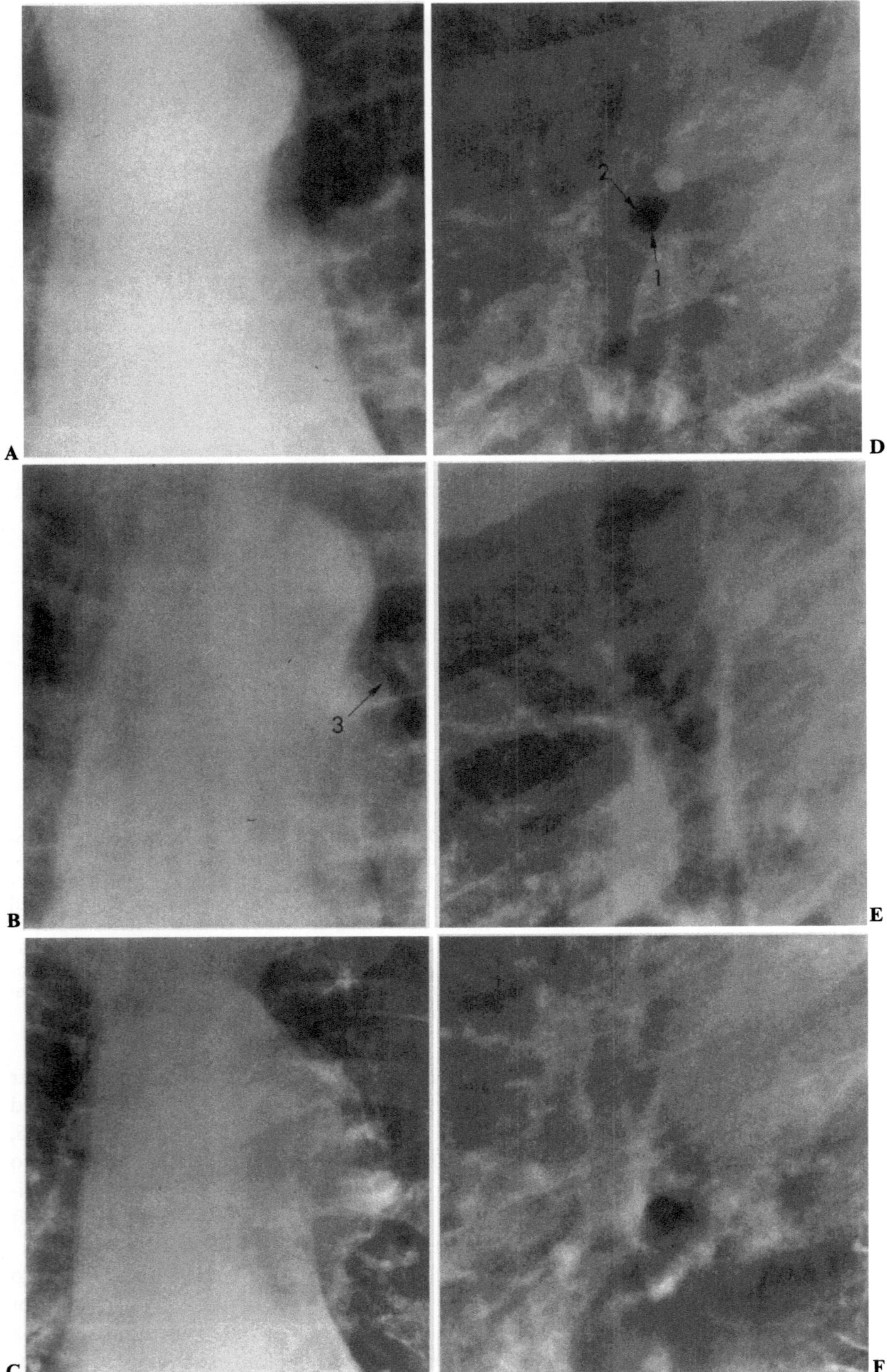

◁ **Fig. 7.8 A–F.** Development of mass in aortic-pulmonic window. **A–C** PA radiographs. **D–F** Lateral radiographs. In **A** and **D** note intrusion of lung into aortic-pulmonic window. On lateral view (**D**), top of left pulmonary artery can be seen (*1*) superimposed on shadow of right upper lobe bronchus (*2*). Subsequent PA films (**B**) show that lateral closure of aortic-pulmonic window has developed distinct lateral convexity (*3*). Such a convex configuration should always be considered abnormal until proven otherwise. Note that in **E** the superior surface of left pulmonary artery is less well demonstrated. One year later, PA and lateral radiographs (**C** and **F**) demonstrate huge mass filling aortic-pulmonic window. Disease was bronchogenic carcinoma with nodal metastases

Fig. 7.9 A, B. Lateral "closure" of aortic-pulmonic window. Mediastinal pleura "closing" posterior aspect of aortic-pulmonic window (AP tomograms). Mediastinal pleura closing posterior aspect of aortic-pulmonic window sweeps off posterior aspect of aortic arch and extends caudally behind left pulmonary artery and left main bronchus in front of descending aorta. This interface of preaortic lung and mediastinum is sometimes called "preaortic" line (*1*). In contrast to normal appearance of line in **A**, the presence of masses or enlarged lymph nodes in posterior aspect of window as shown in **B** or complete filling of window by very large masses will cause upper portion of preaortic line to be displaced laterally (*2*), frequently extending further to left than aortic knob (*3*). (From [68])
▽

sideration of a mass in this area (Figs. 7.8, 7.9, and 7.18). Statistically, this will most often turn out to by lymph node enlargement. Subtle changes can be very difficult to detect, and comparison of serial examinations is often vital to correct diagnosis, as pointed out by Blank and Castellino [10] (Figs. 7.8 and 7.18). These authors have provided a statistical study of the variations in the radiographic appearance of the pleural reflection from the aortic arch to the left pulmonary artery, an interface that they have termed reflection "B."

Lateral radiographs are often helpful to confirm disease in the aortic-pulmonic window; if lung extends deeply into the window, the inferior surface of the aortic arch and the superior surface of the left pulmonary artery are usually easily identified (Fig. 7.7). These contours cannot be visualized on the lateral roentgenogram when masses or lymphadenopathy exclude lung from the window (Fig. 7.8).

In addition to producing a prominent convex bulge in the lateral closure of the aortic-pulmonic window, large masses in this area, their growth restricted by the aortic arch above, may

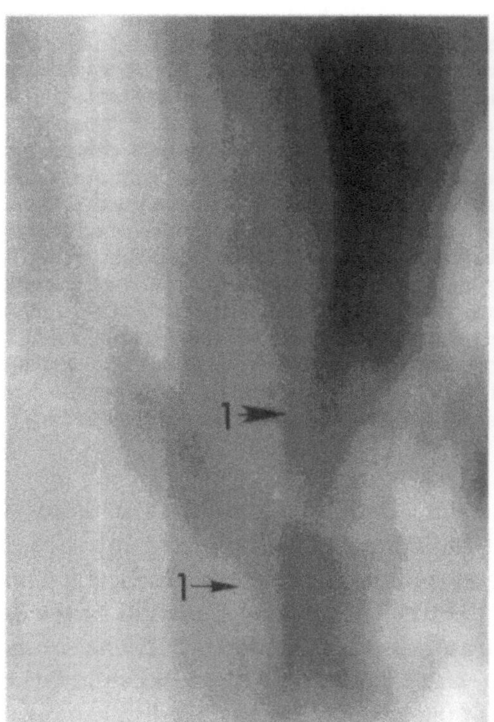

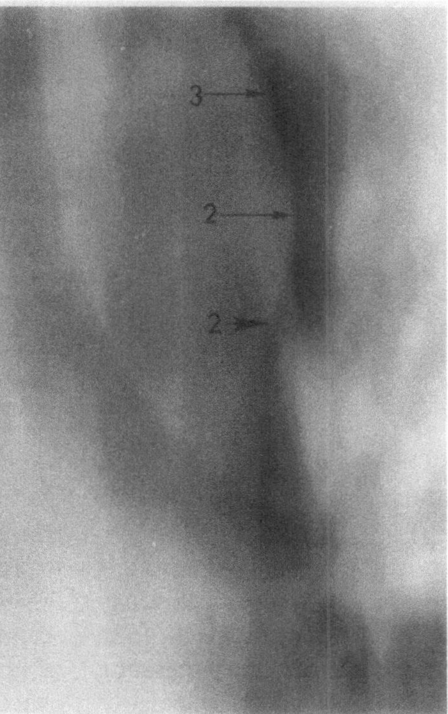

A   **B**

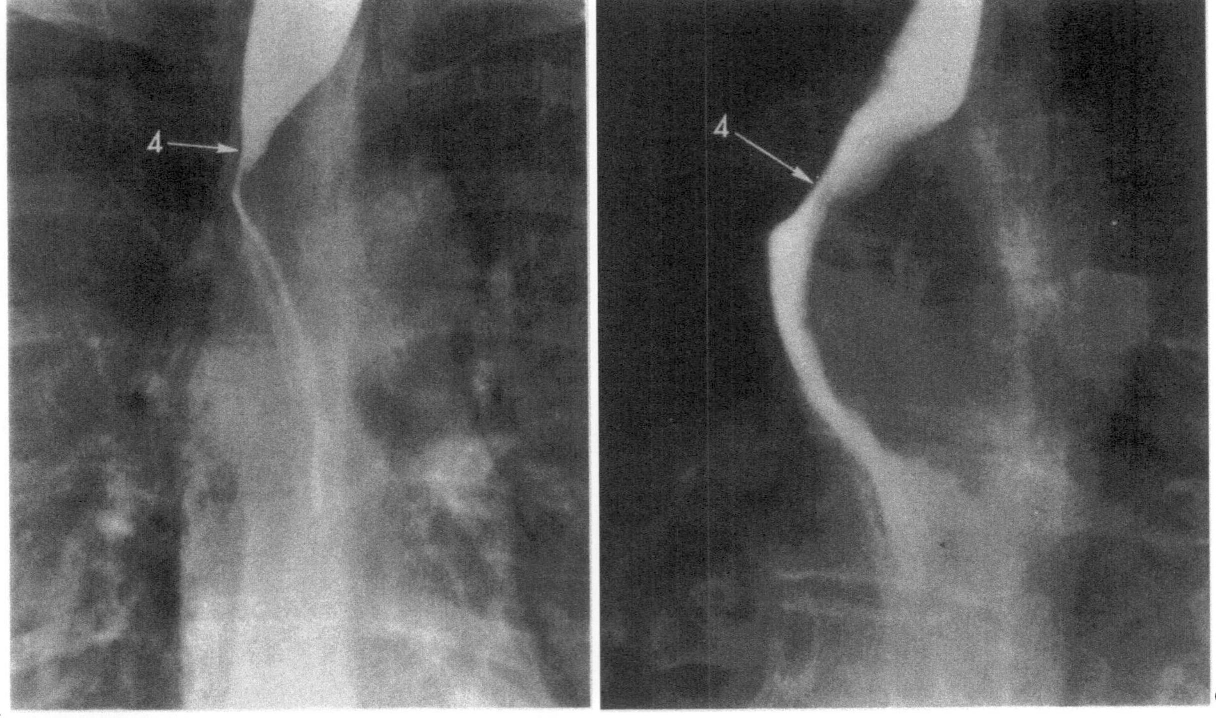

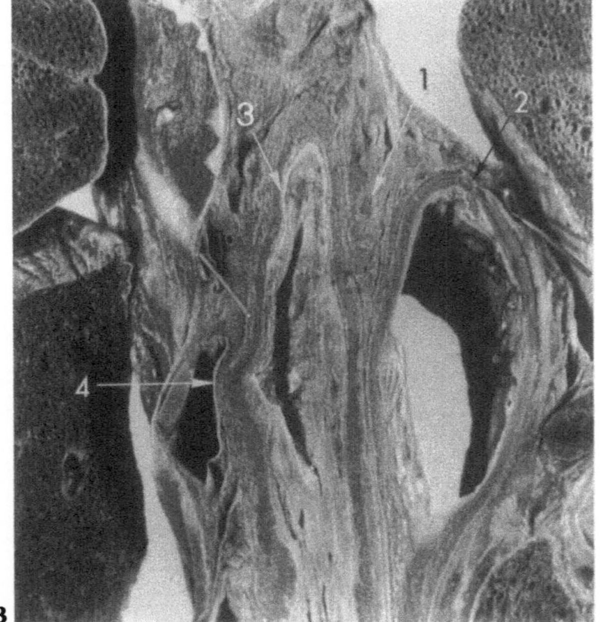

Fig. 7.10A–C. Medial "closure" of aortic-pulmonic window. Separation of esophagus from aortic arch. A PA radiograph with barium in esophagus. B Coronal body section through level of aortic arch. C AP radiograph with barium in esophagus. Behind trachea and left main bronchus, esophagus lies at posteromedial aspect of aortic-pulmonic window. Immediately above this point, its left lateral aspect is in intimate contact with aortic arch. Separation of esophagus from aortic arch should suggest presence of mass between the two. Nodes in inferior portion of left tracheobronchial chain (*1*) are found between aortic arch (*2*) and esophagus (*3*) (see also Fig. 7.2B). In A these nodes were enlarged by metastatic carcinoma. In this example, esophagus is displaced for short distance above aortic arch. Exceptionally, a lesion of esophagus (in C a leiomyoma) may produce same effect. Note that in A and C esophagus has been driven against restraining influence of azygos arch (*4*)

drive the left pulmonary artery downward as they increase in size (Fig. 7.12).

Posteriorly, the aortic-pulmonic window is "closed" on its lateral side by the pleural reflection subtending from the posterior aspect of the arch and the upper portion of the descending aorta. The resulting lung-pleura interface produces a line that is commonly visualized on frontal radiographs; it is directed medially as it progresses caudally from the aortic arch and lies to the right of the lateral margin of the descending aorta (Figs. 7.9 and 7.22). The contact of lung with the pleura, which closes the lateral aspect of the aortic-pulmonic window posterior-

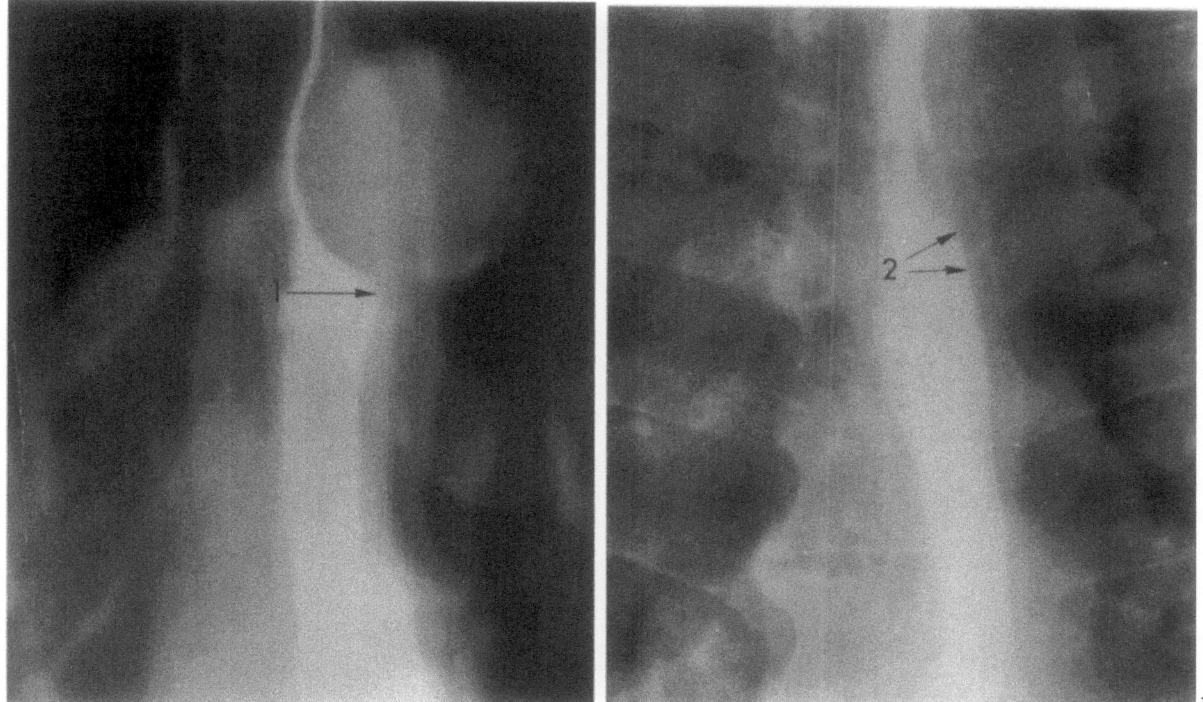

A   B

Fig. 7.11 A, B. Medial "closure" of aortic-pulmonic window. Effacement of subaortic outpouching of esophagus. A AP tomogram with barium in esophagus. B PA radiograph with barium in esophagus. Normally, esophagus intrudes under aortic arch, causing beak-like encroachement upon aortic-pulmonic window medially and posteriorly (1). Outpouching is more severe when aortic arch is dilated (A). In B this normal outpouching is not seen, and barium-filled esophagus appears flattened in this area (2). This finding on an esophagram virtually assures the diagnosis of metastatic disease in the aortic-pulmonic window

ly and its extension caudally from this point, is referred to as the "preaortic line" [68]. This line has been thought by some observers to be a shadow produced by the contact of lung with the left lateral margin of the ascending aorta. In our experience the normal ascending aorta infrequently makes an interface with left lung (see Fig. 7.35). Enlarged nodes in the aortic-pulmonic window, especially more posteriorly situated ones, commonly displace the preaortic line laterally (Fig. 7.9). The line will be discussed in greater detail later in this chapter.

7.2.1.2 Medial "Closure" of the Aortic-Pulmonic Window

At the medial margin of the aortic-pulmonic window, the trachea and left main bronchus course anterior to the esophagus (Fig. 7.2). The inferior nodes of the left tracheobronchial chain lie lateral to these structures and between them and the aortic arch (Fig. 7.2). When these nodes

are enlarged, they may be detected radiographically since they sometimes displace the trachea and the esophagus away from the shadow of the aortic arch (Fig. 7.10). Below the impression produced by the aortic arch, the esophagus is commonly seen to bulge laterally into the medial side of the aortic-pulmonic window [7] (Fig. 7.11). When this outpouching is effaced or the esophagus displaced medially at this level, a mass or lymphadenopathy in the window should be suspected (Figs. 7.11, 7.12) [68]. Care

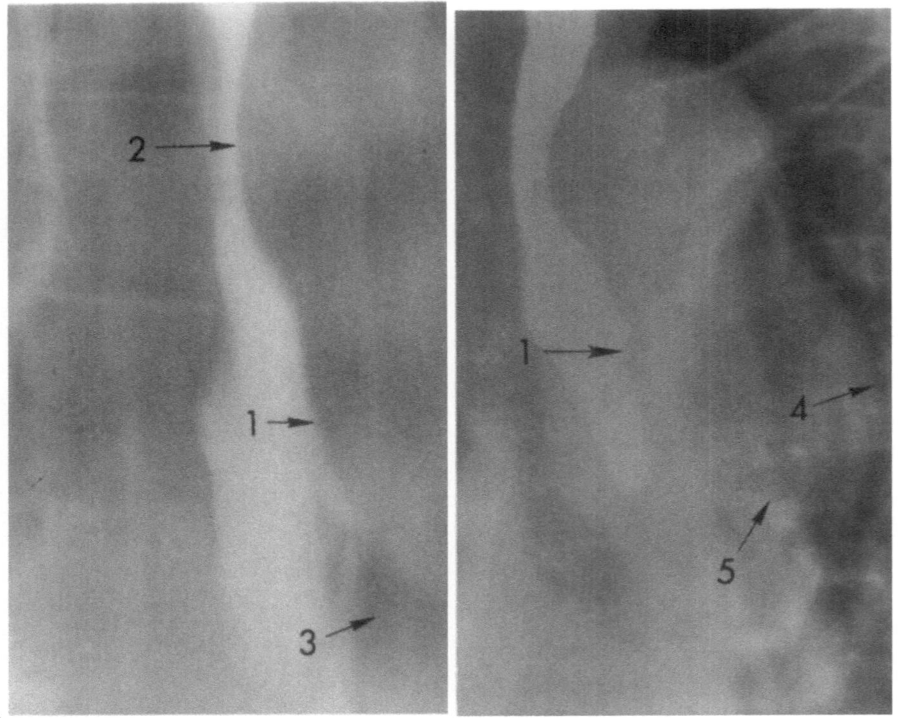

Fig. 7.12A, B. Medial "closure" of aortic-pulmonic window. Effacement of subaortic outpouching of esophagus. **A** AP tomogram with barium in the esophagus. **B** PA radiograph with barium in the esophagus. In these two patients large masses in aortic-pulmonic window efface normal subaortic outpouching of esophagus (*1*). In **A** an impression is made on left wall of esophagus below impression of aortic knob (*2*) and above impression of left main bronchus (*3*). In **B** there is marked convex bulging of lateral closure of aortic-pulmonic window (*4*); left pulmonary artery (*5*) is depressed. (**B** From [68])

should be taken not to mistake such an imprint for that produced by the impression of the left main bronchus on the esophagus [52, 128, 129].

7.2.1.3 Posterior "Closure" of the Aortic-Pulmonic Window

At its extreme posterior aspect, the aortic-pulmonic window is "closed" by the descending aorta above and the left pulmonary artery bronchus below (Fig. 7.13). The left pulmonary artery lies anterolateral to the descending aorta

at the point where it "closes" the window posteriorly (Fig. 7.13). Lung commonly intrudes between the aorta and the left pulmonary artery producing a pointed or "beak-like" configuration directed centrally on computed tomograms (Fig. 7.13). A lymph node commonly lies at the apex of the point (Fig. 7.13). Enlargement of this node or other mass in the back of the window will efface the pointed configuration. A convex bulge lateral to the descending aorta and medial to the left pulmonary artery strongly suggests mass, just as a convex bulge in the lateral closure of the window does (Fig. 7.14).

Below the approximation of the descending aorta and the left pulmonary artery lung may extend centrally to contact the posterior wall of the left main or lower lobe bronchus [156] (see Fig. 7.22). Webb [156] noted the contact of lung with the posterior wall of the left main and lower lobe bronchi on 86% of computed tomograms on normal patients. This retrobronchial stripe was seen by Proto [122] in 43% of plain chest radiographs; thickening of this stripe to more than 2 mm is abnormal, often reflecting the presence of peribronchial tumor.

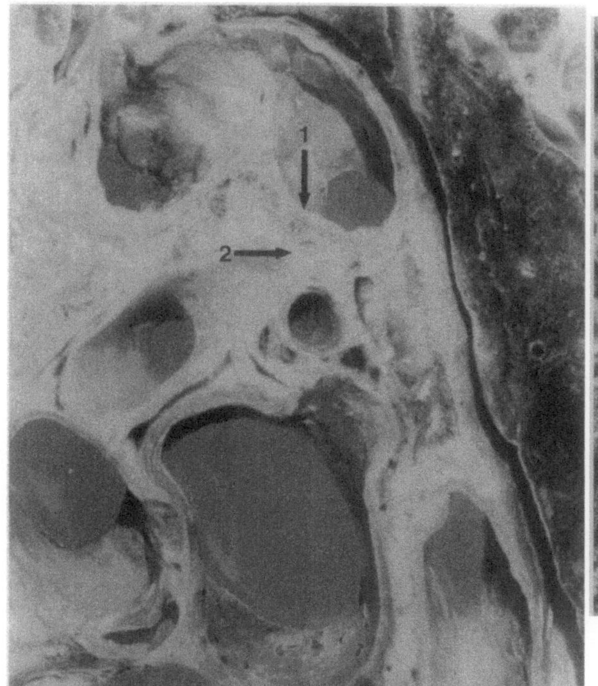

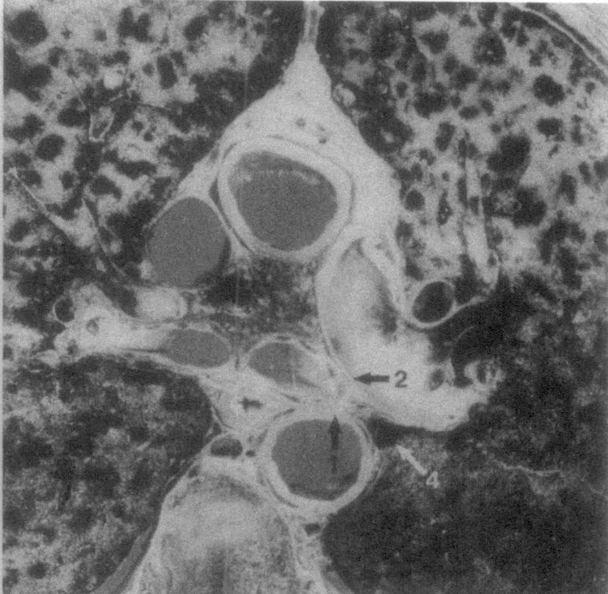

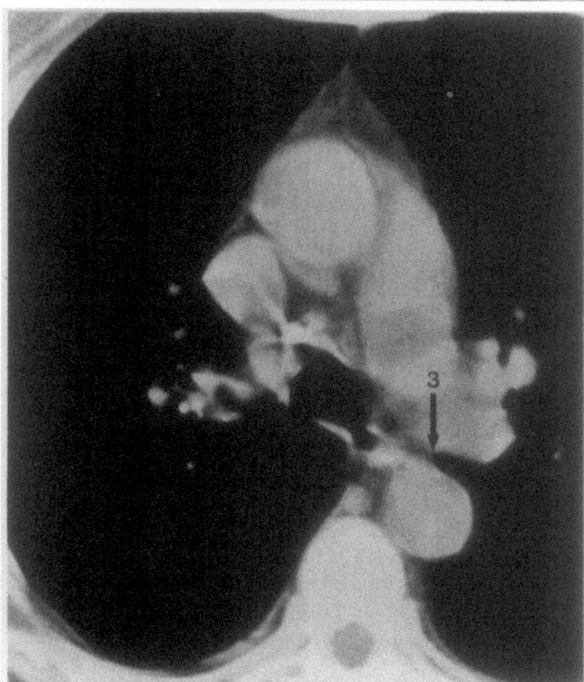

Fig. 7.13A–C. Posterior "closure" of the aortic-pulmonic window. A Sagittal body section through the aorta. B Transverse body section at the level of the left pulmonary artery. C Computed tomogram at the same level. The aortic-pulmonic window is "closed" posteriorly by contact of the aorta (1) above with the left pulmonary artery (2) below. The left pulmonary artery lies anterolateral to the descending aorta, and between the two there is a normal, beak-like intrusion of lung (3). This lung is preaortic in position. At the apex of the "beak" a lymph node is constantly formed (4). Effacement of the beak-like intrusion suggests a mass

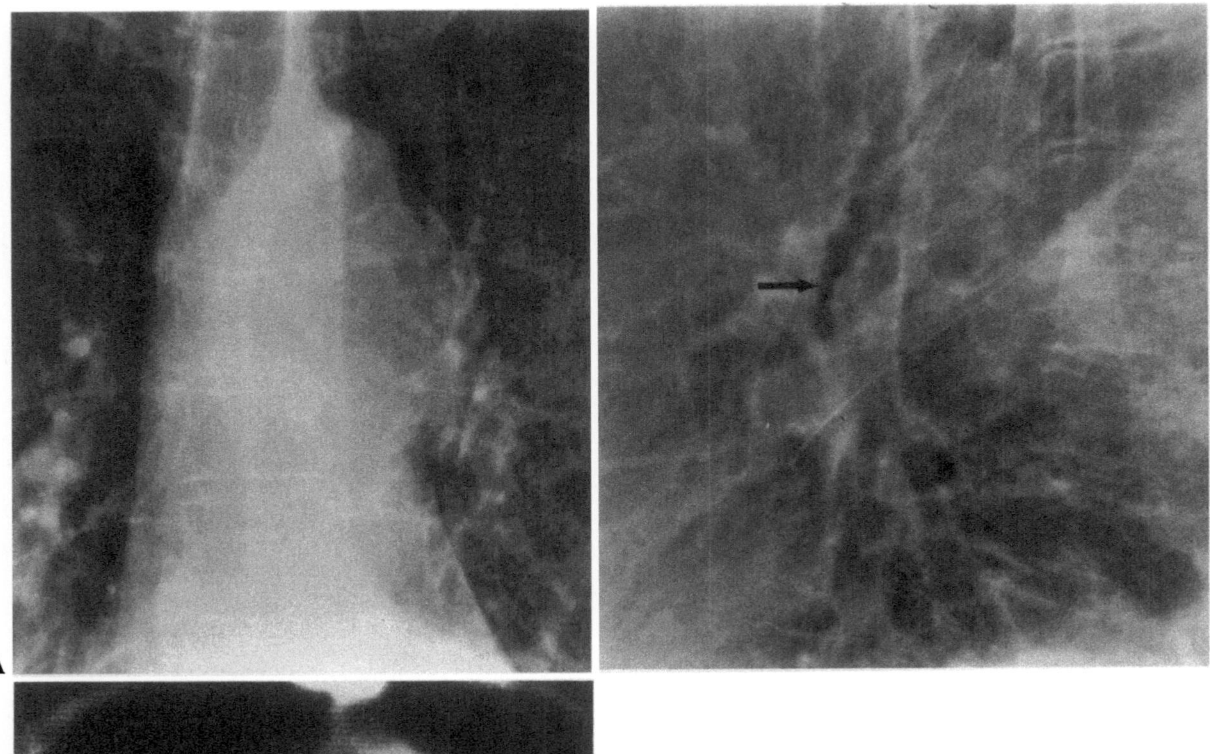

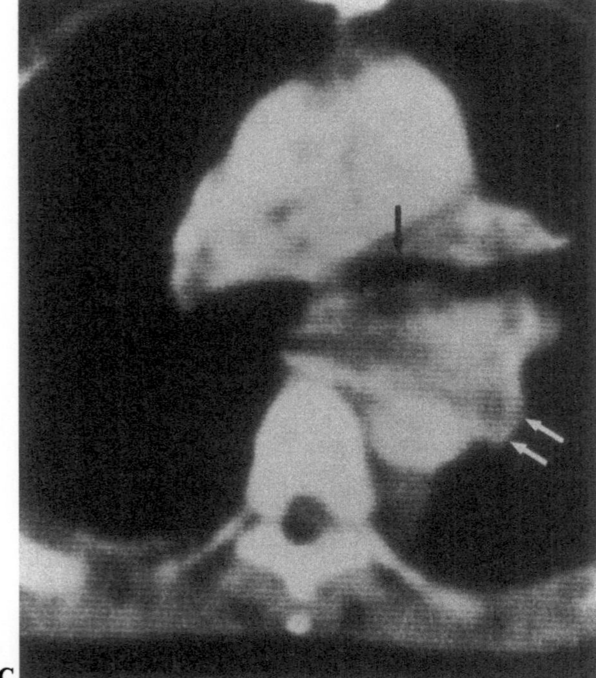

Fig. 7.14A–C. Development of a mass in the aortic-pulmonic window. **A** PA radiograph. **B** Lateral radiograph. **C** Computed tomogram. In this patient with the sudden onset of posterior chest pain, dissecting aneurysm was considered a probable diagnosis. Chest radiographs showed a mass in the region of the aortic-pulmonic window posteriorly. On the lateral radiograph, the left main bronchus is displaced anteriorly (*single arrow*). The computed tomogram also shows the anterior displacement of the left main and upper lobe bronchi (*single arrow*). The descending aorta is normal. A convex bulge (*double arrows*) at the posterior aspect of the window replaces the normal beak-like configuration and was found at surgery to be nodal enlargement secondary to bronchogenic carcinoma

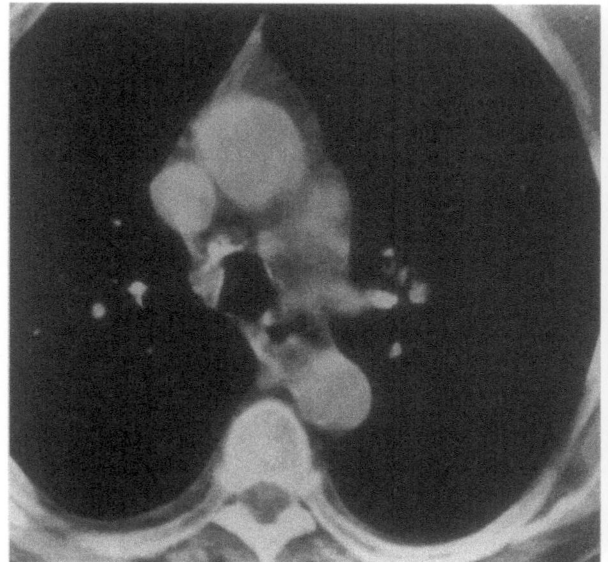
A

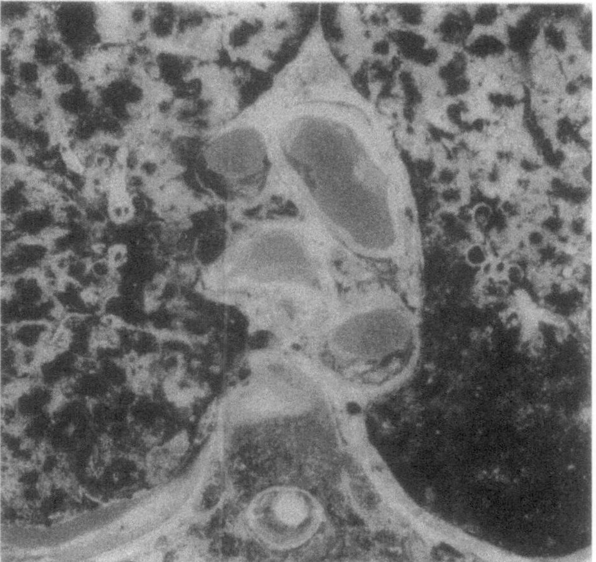
B

7.2.1.4 The Aortic-Pulmonic Window on Computed Tomograms

The aortic-pulmonic window is often difficult to evaluate on computed tomograms. The cephalo-caudad dimension of the window is not great and standard examinations made with axial images 1 cm in thickness commonly demonstrate the window on only one section (Fig. 7.15). Furthermore, partial volume effect may cause the lower portion of the aortic arch or the top of the pulmonary artery (Fig. 7.15) to appear as ill-defined opacity in the window area. When necessary, thin sections can be obtained to obviate these problems. Despite these difficulties, computed tomography is a very valuable adjunct to plain films in the evaluation of the window; nodes can be demonstrated in the window and the effect of nodal enlargement or mass on window "closure" is often well demonstrated [78] (Figs. 7.14, 7.17, and 7.18).

It should be emphasized that the aortic arch is "ringed" by lymph nodes (Fig. 7.16). When nodes in the window are enlarged, nodes lateral to the aortic arch, the lateral aortic nodes, are commonly enlarged; nodes lateral to the aortic arch, the lateral aortic nodes, are commonly enlarged as well (Fig. 7.18). Nodes in this location are difficult to see on PA or lateral chest radiographs because their contact with lung is not

Fig. 7.15A, B. The aortic-pulmonic window on computed tomograms. **A** Computed tomogram. **B** Transverse body section. The aortic-pulmonic window has a short cephalocaudad dimension and is often seen on only one image if the examination is performed using contiguous sections 1 cm in thickness. The inferior aspect of the aortic arch or the top of the left pulmonary artery (see Fig. 7.13B) may be partially volumed in the section

parallel to the X-ray beam in either plane (Figs. 7.17 and 7.18). Sometimes these nodes can be appreciated on frontal radiographs if they are sufficiently bulky to add to the density of the aortic knob over which they are superimposed (Fig. 7.17).

Lateral aortic (para-aortic) nodes are readily shown on computed tomograms (Figs. 7.17 and 7.18). Care should be taken to avoid mistaking confluent lateral aortic nodal involvement for a partially volumed main or left pulmonary artery (Fig. 7.19). These vascular structures may be seen in part, lateral to the aortic arch, when they are high in position (see chapter 6). Contrast enhancement resolves this dilemma. Another pitfall in the diagnosis of nodal enlargement as the lateral aspect of the aortic-pulmonic window is to mistake the left superior pulmonary vein for a node (see chapter 10). Again, repeat scanning following contrast injection clarifies the problem when comparison of

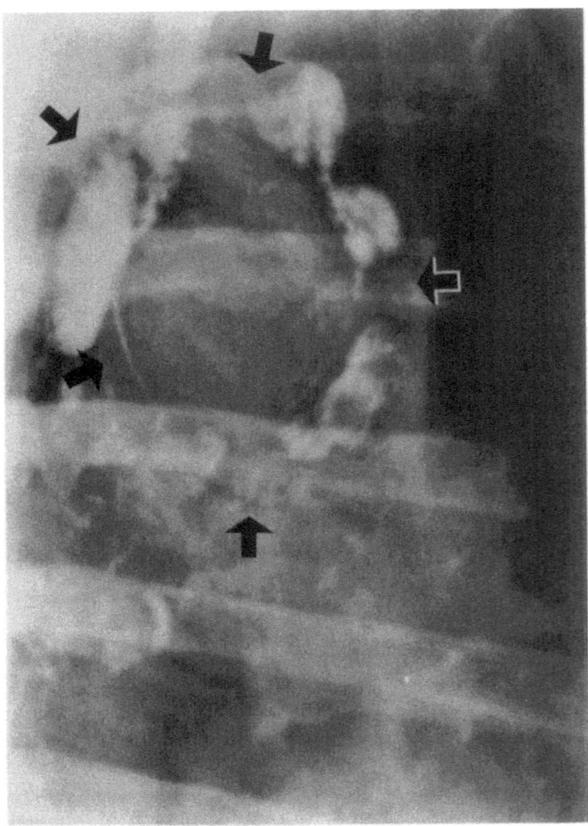

Fig. 7.16. Location of lymph nodes around the aortic arch. Left posterior oblique chest radiograph made after pedal lymphangiography (*arrows*). Lymph nodes ring the aortic arch. It is common for disease involving lymph nodes in the aortic-pulmonic window to involve also lateral aortic (para-aortic) nodes and left lower paratracheal nodes. Filling of normal mediastinal lymph nodes with contrast following lymphangiography is not uncommon. (Courtesy G. Tricomi, Rome, Italy)

Fig. 7.17A, B. Enlargement of lateral aortic (para-aortic) lymph nodes. **A** PA radiograph. **B** Computed tomogram. The PA radiograph shows no definite evidence of mass although the shadow of the aortic knob is questionably more dense than normal. The computed tomogram clearly demonstrates a large lateral aortic (para-aortic) nodal mass (*arrows*). Note that the position of the mass is such that it will not be seen in profile on either PA or lateral examinations. (A right anterior oblique radiograph would show it.) The added soft tissue anterior to the aortic knob results in the knob appearing to be more dense on the PA film

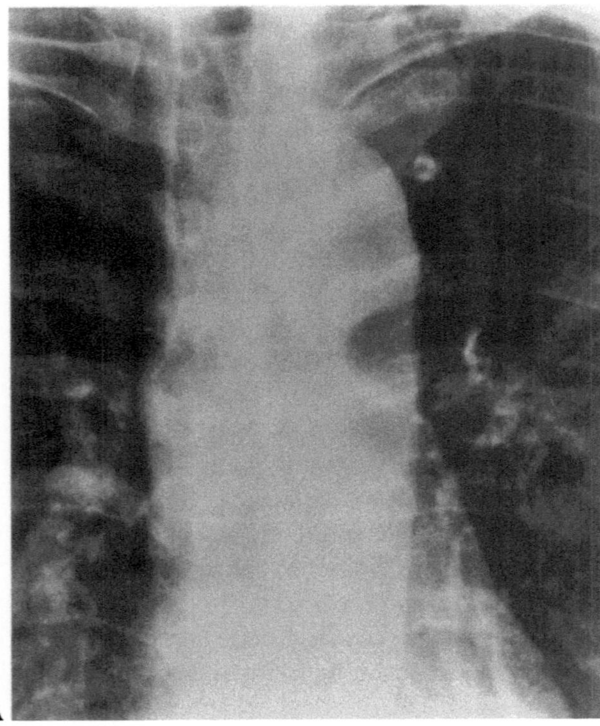

A

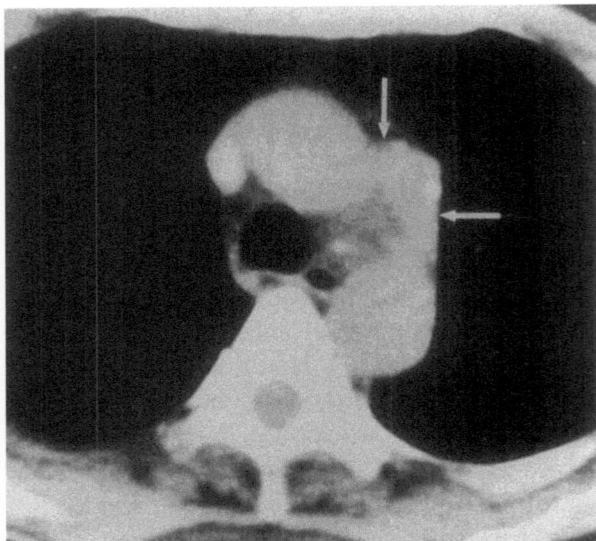

B

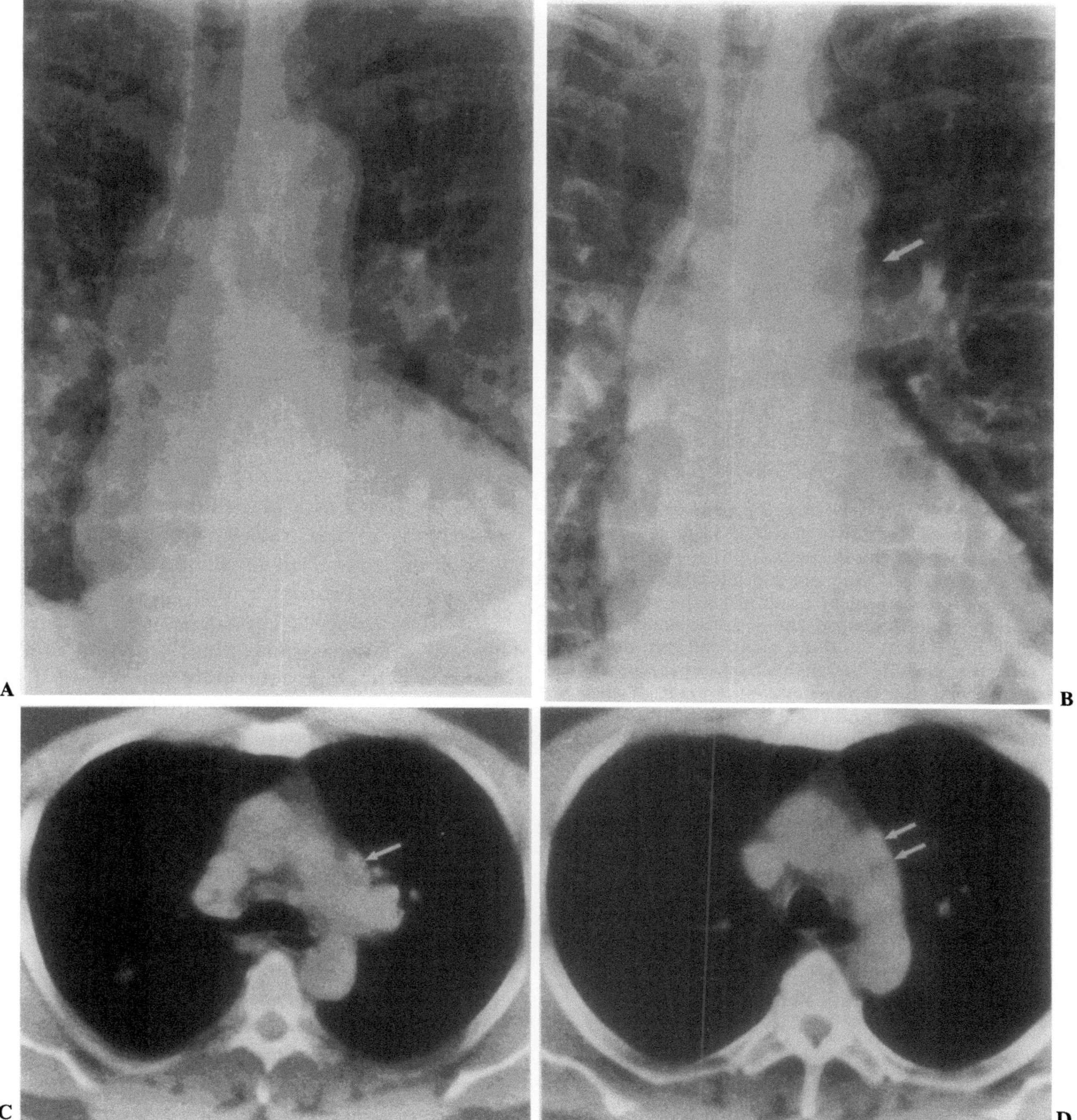

Fig. 7.18A–D. Enlargement of lateral aortic (para-aortic) lymph nodes. **A** and **B** PA radiographs. **C** and **D** Computed tomograms. The PA radiographs made approximately 1 year apart show development of a mass in the aortic pulmonic window. Note the new convex bulge above the left pulmonary artery (*arrow*) in **B**. The nodal enlargement responsible for this shadow is demonstrated in **C** (*arrow*). Lateral aortic (para-aortic) nodes are also seen to be enlarged in **D** (*arrows*). Enlargement of lateral aortic nodes is a common accompanyment of enlarged window nodes. Note that the enlarged lateral aortic nodes cannot be appreciated in **B**

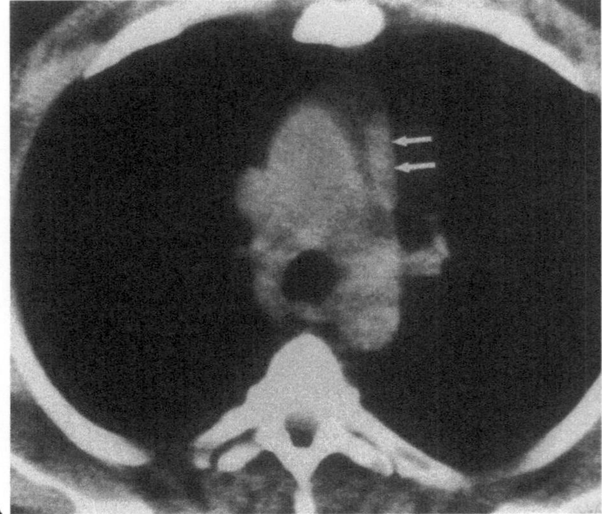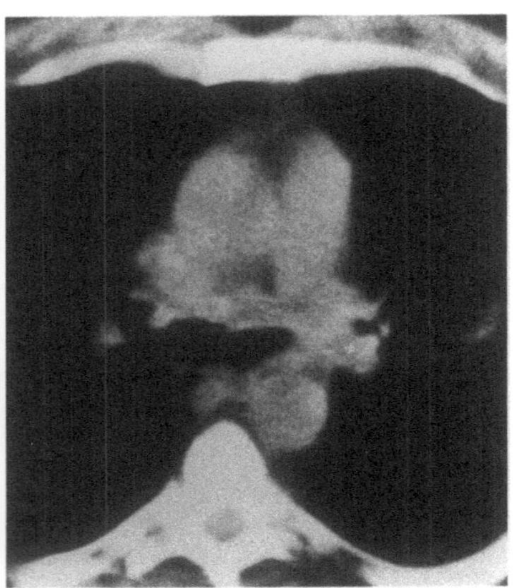

A   B

Fig. 7.19A, B. Partially volumed main and left pulmonary arteries. A simulant of enlarged lateral aortic (para-aortic) nodes. **A** and **B** Computed tomograms. Note that in **A** a portion of the main and left pulmonary arteries is shown (*arrows*) as the result of partial volume effect. It can simulate enlarged lateral aortic nodes (compare with Fig. 7.18D). In **B** the main and left pulmonary arteries are readily identifiable. Sometimes repeat examination with thin sections and/or contrast enhancement is necessary to confirm that a questionable density in this area is due to partial volume effect involving the main and/or left pulmonary arteries

serial sections does not definitely confirm the shadow as being a vessel. At times, left superior vena cava and the left superior intercostal vein may also cause confusion (see chapter 6).

7.2.2 The Left Main Bronchus

The position of the left main bronchus is an important landmark that can be critical to the proper localization of mediastinal and sometimes pulmonary processes. The left atrium is situated at the anterior and inferior boundary of the aortic-pulmonic window and lies immediately in front of the lower portion of the left main bronchus and the origin of the left lower lobe bronchus. Lane and Whalen [85] have pointed out that left atrial enlargement will cause posterior displacement of the left main bronchus. The left upper lobe bronchus is displaced posteriorly as well and may be identified

on lateral films as a black dot behind the coronal plane of the trachea. On frontal radiographs the carinal angle (the angle formed by the two main bronchi at their origin from the trachea) is reduced. The rotation of the main bronchi off the coronal plane tends to make the carinal angle appear more acute than it is normally. The normal carinal angle should measure 60° in men and 70° in women. The angle is variable in children [102]. Similarly, aneurysmal dilatation of the main pulmonary artery, located in front of the proximal portion of the left main bronchus, will displace the bronchus posteriorly.

Anterior displacement of the left main bronchus suggests a lesion at the posterior aspect of the aortic-pulmonic window (Fig. 7.14). Traumatic rupture of the aorta is such a process. 95% of traumatic aneurysms occur at the aortic isthmus – that portion of the aortic arch between the left subclavian artery and the ligamentum arteriosum [133]. Anterior and inferior displacement of the left main bronchus was a helpful diagnostic finding in the series reported by Sanborn et al. [133] (see Fig. 7.39) and heightened the suspicion of rupture when mediastinal contours were equivocal. Other observers, however, have considered this finding to be of less value [103]. At times, if the injury has occurred in the distal portion of the aortic isthmus, anterior bronchial displacement without inferior displacement is encountered. Again, the rotation

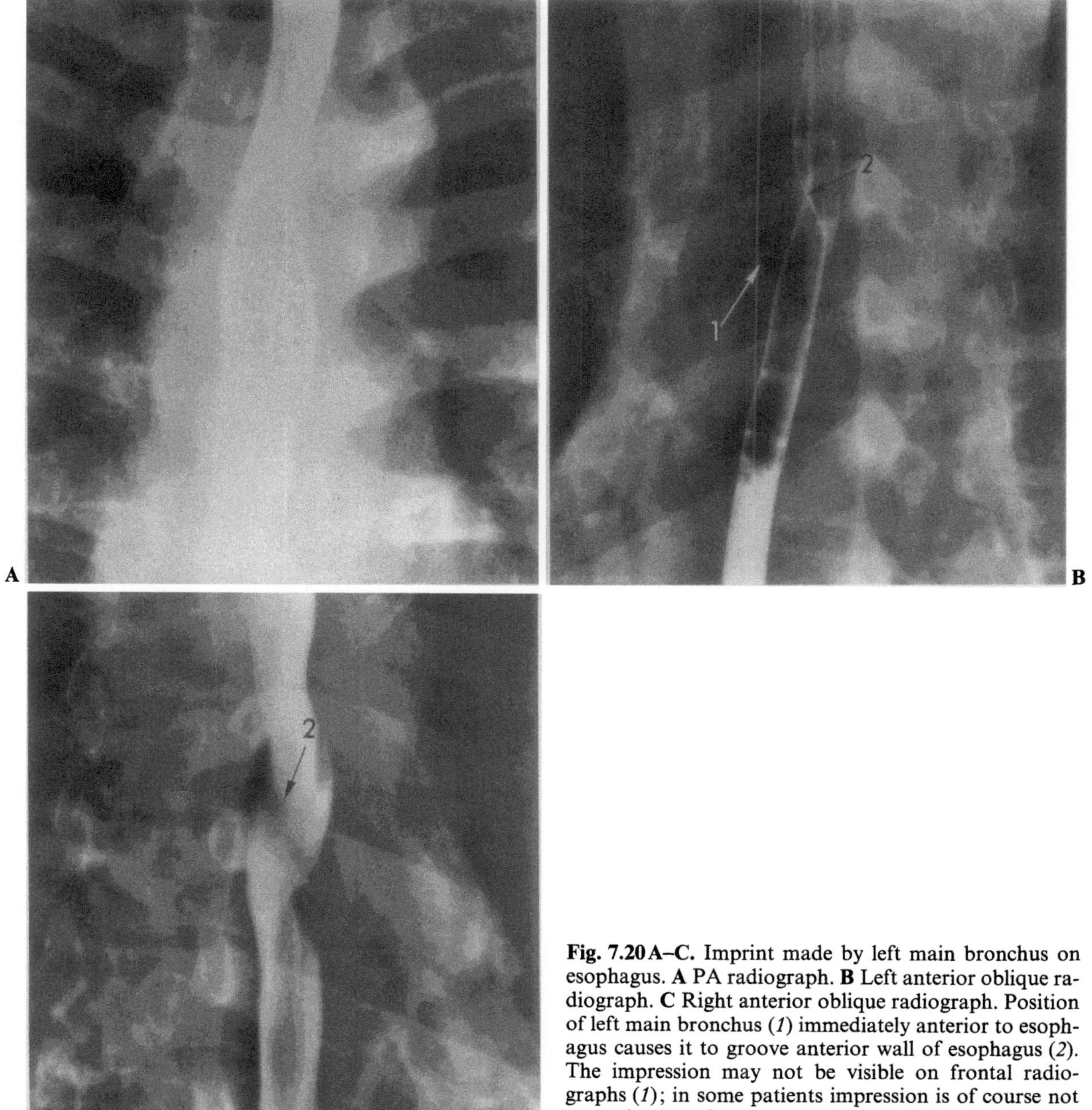

Fig. 7.20A–C. Imprint made by left main bronchus on esophagus. **A** PA radiograph. **B** Left anterior oblique radiograph. **C** Right anterior oblique radiograph. Position of left main bronchus (*1*) immediately anterior to esophagus causes it to groove anterior wall of esophagus (*2*). The impression may not be visible on frontal radiographs (*1*); in some patients impression is of course not seen when esophagus descends immediately behind carina; to be impressed upon by left main bronchus, esophagus must descend at least slightly to left of midline (**A**)

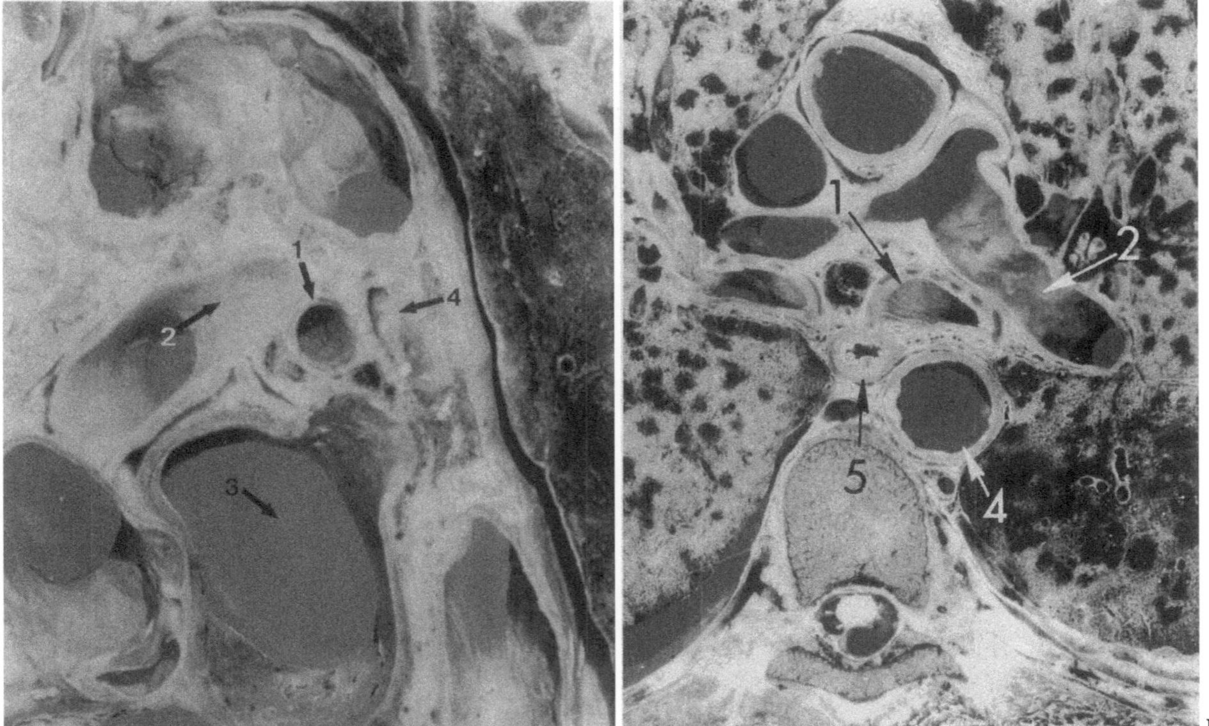

Fig. 7.21 A, B. The anatomic relationships of left main bronchus. **A** Sagittal body section. **B** Transverse body section. Left main bronchus (*1*), extending inferiorly along posteromedial aspect of aortic-pulmonic window, swings under the left pulmonary artery (*2*) and above the left atrium (*3*). Its posterior aspect is in intimate relationship to descending aorta (*4*). Esophagus (*5*) also lies posterior to bronchus and is often somewhat medially situated with respect to bronchus. Buckling of descending aorta carries esophagus laterally, placing it more directly behind bronchus

of the main bronchi will cause apparent narrowing of the carinal angle on frontal films, a finding that often creates the illusion of inferior bronchial displacement.

Gross increase in size of the left pulmonary artery passing over the bronchus will depress it. Left lower lobe atelectasis will also cause inferior and sometimes posterior bronchial displacement [158]. Marked left atrial enlargement often causes this chamber to extend beneath the bronchus elevating it (see Fig. 9.25). Left upper lobe atelectasis raises the bronchus toward the under aspect of the aortic arch, foreshortening

the aortic-pulmonic window in its cephalocaudad dimension.

The left main bronchus frequently impinges against the esophagus to produce an indentation that should not be misinterpreted as evidence of a node or a mass. This contact of the left main bronchus is evident on esophagrams as a groove in the anterior esophageal wall running obliquely downward and to the left (Fig. 7.20). According to Gladnikoff [52], the impression produced by the left main bronchus on the esophagus is due to displacement of the esophagus against the bronchus by the descending aorta (Fig. 7.21). It is less evident when tortuosity of the aorta causes that vessel and the esophagus to buckle away from the bronchus. Gladnikoff was able to identify the impression in 61 of 75 patients; in 13 of the 14 cases not showing the impression of the esophagus passed downward directly behind the trachea rather than behind the left main bronchus. In common with other normal esophageal impressions, this one should be recognized as a normal anatomic finding and should not be misinterpreted as a pressure defect caused by a node or a mass.

Below the left bronchial imprint the esophagus often demonstrates a minimal protrusion forward and to the left called by Gladnikoff the "bifurcation bulge." It is more commonly seen when the aorta is not ectatic and the esophagus lies more nearly in the midline. When visualized, this finding militates against the presence of subcarinal nodes. Further discussion of the radiographic appearance of the left main bronchus appears in chapter 10.

7.2.3 The Preaortic Area

7.2.3.1 The Preaortic Line

In some individuals the left lower lobe extends to the right in front of the descending aorta to produce an interface with the soft tissues of the mediastinum (Fig. 7.22). This contact of lung with mediastinum can be visualized on frontal radiographs and is called the "preaortic line" (Figs. 7.22 and 7.23). In many ways the medial extension of the left lower lobe anterior to the aorta is analogous to the extension of the right lower lobe in front of the azygos vein into the azygoesophageal recess.

At its upper extent this line is the pleural interface that "closes" the lateral aspect of the aortic-pulmonic window posteriorly. This upper end of the preaortic line usually deviates laterally as it becomes continuous with the pleura over the aortic arch (Fig. 7.22). It has been mentioned previously that some observers have felt that the line represents the interface of the left side of the ascending aorta silhouetted against left lung. Our studies of frontal thoracic aortograms and computed axial tomograms in normal individuals indicate this anatomic situation is unusual (see Fig. 7.35). Sometimes, the preaortic line is visualized as a straight vertical line meeting the undersurface of the aortic knob at the six o'clock position (Fig. 7.23) rather than deflecting to become continuous with the lateral margin of the aortic arch. The line can be followed inferiorly, paralleling the descending aorta, to about the T-10 level, where, like the medial margin of the azygoesophageal recess, it is diminished or lost as the aorta swings from

its course lateral to the spine to occupy a more prespinal position. It does not extend very far toward the right side, rarely reaching the midline. The left lung adopts a more preaortic position in patients with emphysema and with kyphosis than it does normally; this situation is also found with aortic ectasia.

The preaortic line is visualized far less often than is the medial margin of the azygoesophageal recess. Gladnikoff [52] identified the line in only three of 200 patients. In our material, portions of the line have been seen much more often than in Gladnikoff's study. We have accumulated no statistics as to its incidence on plain films or conventional tomograms, but it was identified on 55% of 80 computed tomograms that we reviewed (Figs. 7.13 and 7.22).

The veins draining the left upper lobe and the left lower lobe not infrequently join before entering the left atrium [27, 154]. On radiographs, this confluence is visualized behind the heart as a rounded density outlined against lung in a preaortic location (Fig. 7.24). In addition the left confluence may produce an impression on the left anterolateral wall of the esophagus (see Fig. 3.1). Although the shadow produced by confluence of the right pulmonary veins is usually readily recognized, the confluence of the left pulmonary veins seems to be less well known and is sometimes mistaken for a retrocardiac mass. Conventional or computed tomograms that demonstrate the pulmonary veins entering the structure in question are usually sufficient to prove the shadow to be the left confluence (Fig. 7.24). Rarely, a pulmonary angiogram may be required.

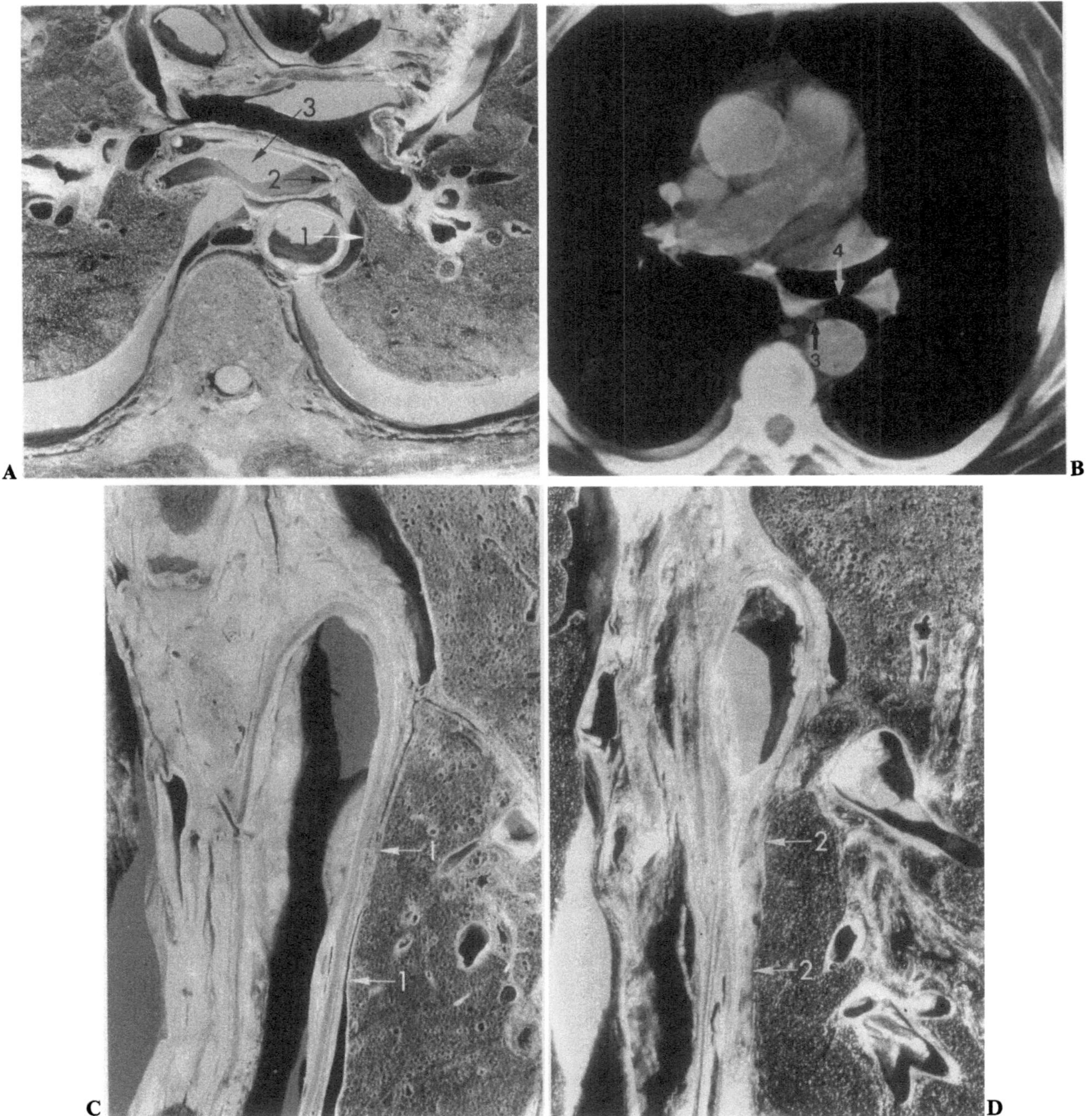

Fig. 7.22 A–D

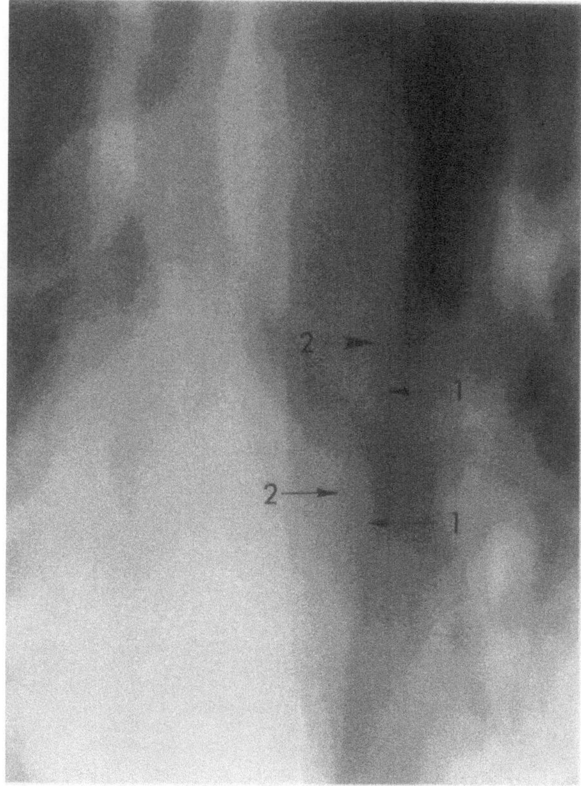

Fig. 7.22 E

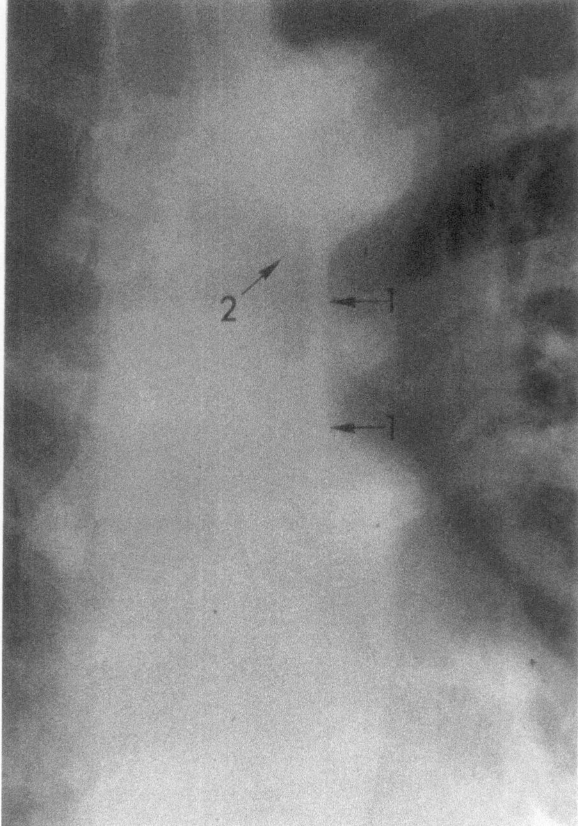

Fig. 7.22 A–E. Anatomy of preaortic line. **A** Transverse body section. **B** Computed tomogram. **C** and **D** Coronal body sections. **E** AP tomogram. Contact of left lower lobe with left wall of descending aorta (*1*) is demonstrated in **A–C.** In a coronal plane slightly more forward (**A, B,** and **D**), lung can be seen to extend medially in front of descending aorta, meeting left lateral wall of esophagus (*3*). This contact of lung with mediastinum anterior to descending aorta is called "preaortic line" (*2*) and can be considered analogous to contact of right lung in the azygoesophageal recess with the mediastinum. In **B** note the contact of preaortic lung with the posterior wall of the left lower lobe bronchus (*4*). (**D** From [68])

Fig. 7.23. Preaortic line (PA radiograph). Preaortic line sometimes ascends in direct vertical fashion to contact undersurface of aortic arch in posterior aspect of aortic-pulmonic window (*1*). In this example, right side of line is outlined by esophageal air (*2*). (Courtesy J. Wiot, Cincinnati, Ohio)

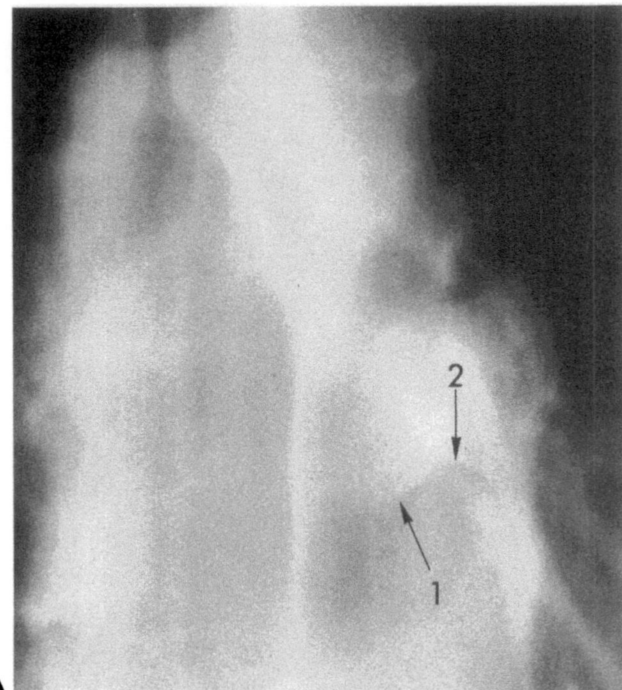

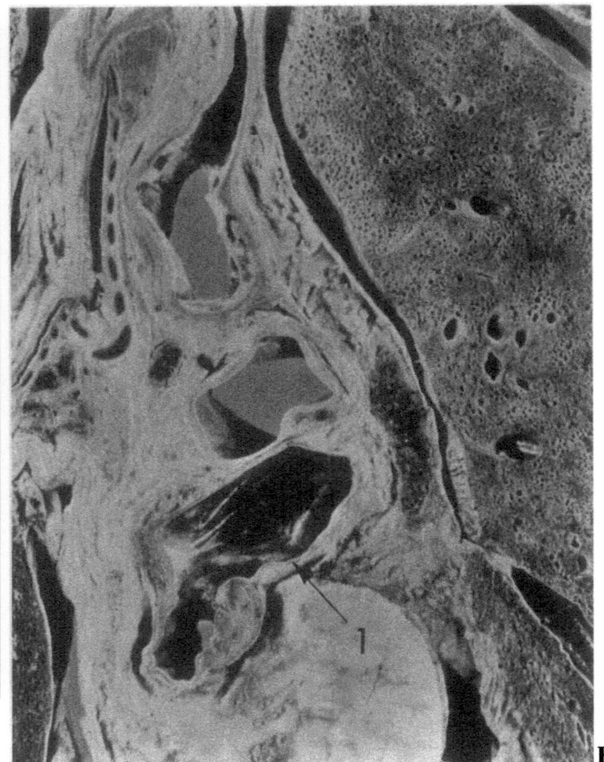

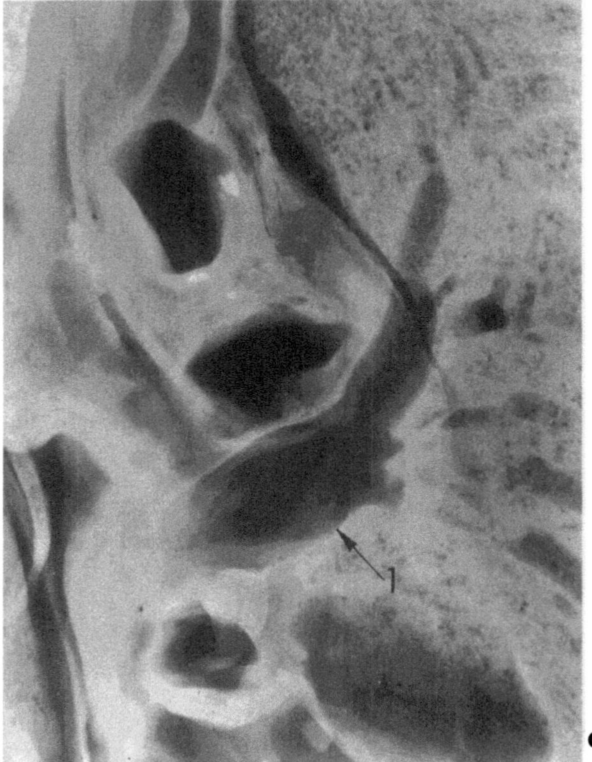

Fig. 7.24A–C. Confluence of left pulmonary veins. **A** AP tomogram. **B** Coronal body section. Confluence of right pulmonary veins commonly produces shadow behind right atrium. This appearance is well known and not often mistaken for pathologic process. The confluence of left pulmonary veins (*1*), however, is less commonly appreciated and seems more frequently to be misconstrued as a mass. Demonstration of veins entering structure (*2*) proves vascular nature of mass shadow. (**A** From [67])

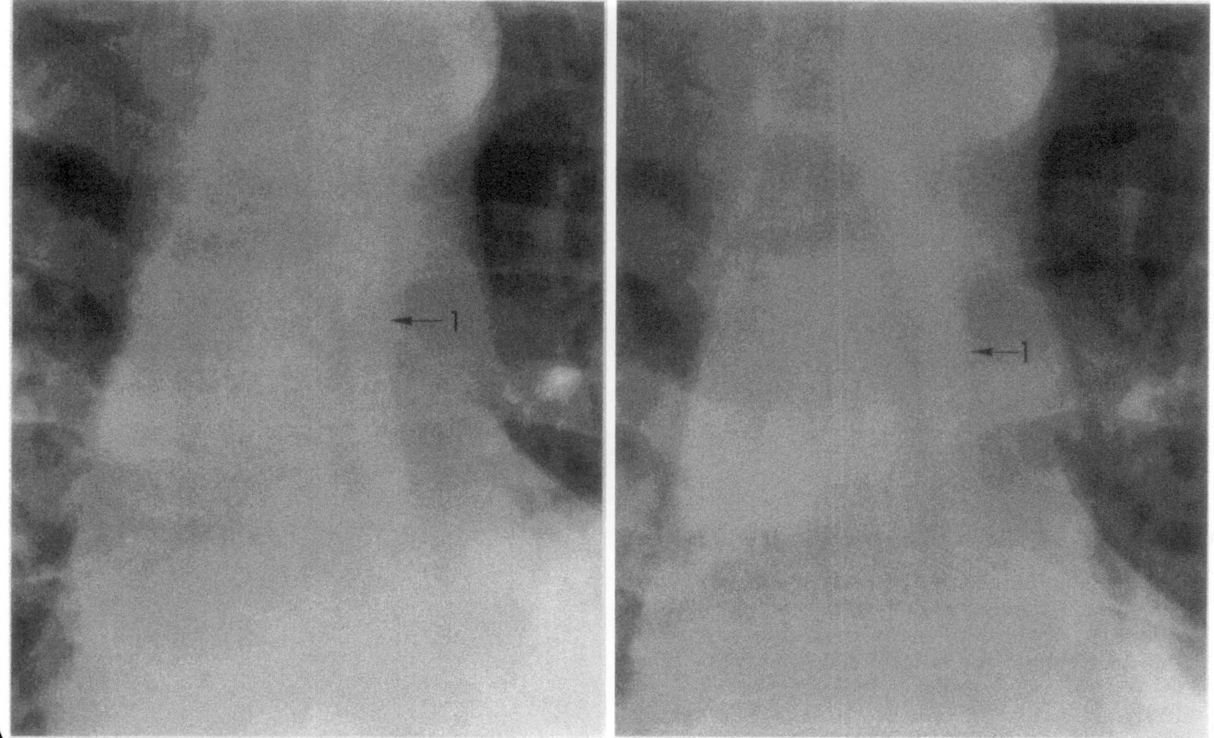

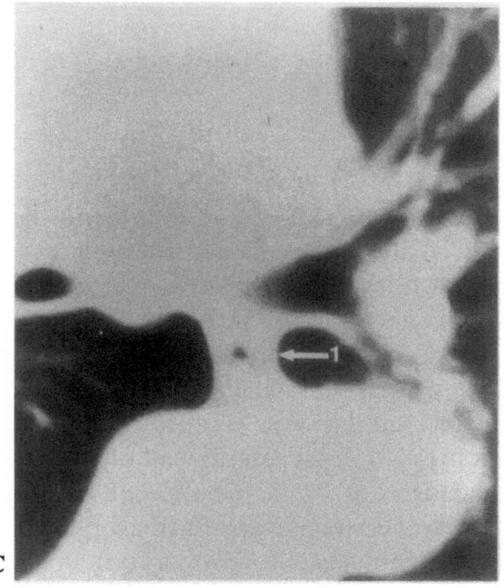

Fig. 7.25 A–C. Left pleuroesophageal stripe. A PA radiograph. B PA radiograph with barium in esophagus. C Computed tomogram. Lung in preaortic position contacts mediastinum to produce preaortic line. In some patients, this point of contact is against left lateral wall of esophagus to produce left pleuroesophageal stripe (*1*). Like relationship of lung in azygoesophageal recess to right esophageal wall, relationship of preaortic lung to left esophageal wall is variable. In C note the contact of preaortic lung with the posterior wall of the left lower lobe bronchus. (Courtesy J. Wiot, Cincinnati, Ohio)

7.2.3.2 The Left Pleuroesophageal Stripe

Just as the right lung in the azygoesophageal recess can contact the right lateral or posterior esophageal wall [22, 24], so can the left lung in a preaortic position meet the left lateral or posterior esophageal wall to produce a left pleuroesophageal stripe (Figs. 7.25 and 7.27). Since the left lung only occasionally extends in front of the aorta, it does not often contact the esophagus, and hence a left pleuroesophageal stripe is not often encountered. As on the right side, one should not use the position of the preaortic line to predict the position of the esophagus. Left lung in front of the aorta may contact the esophagus, but very often it does not extend

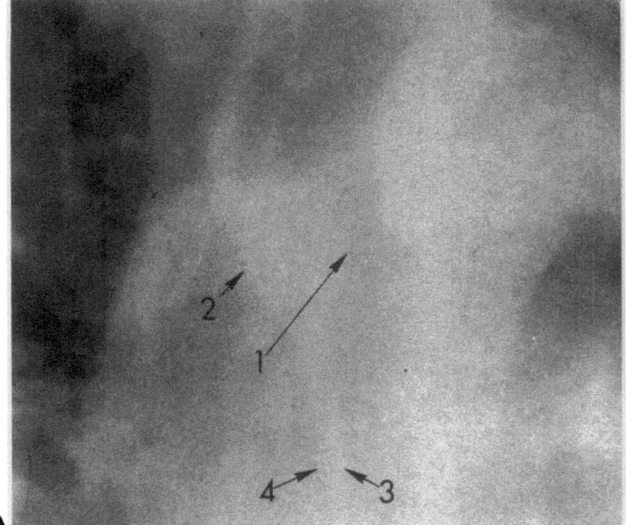

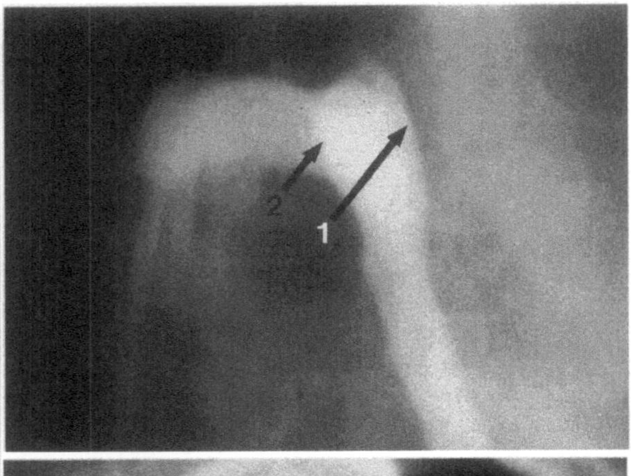

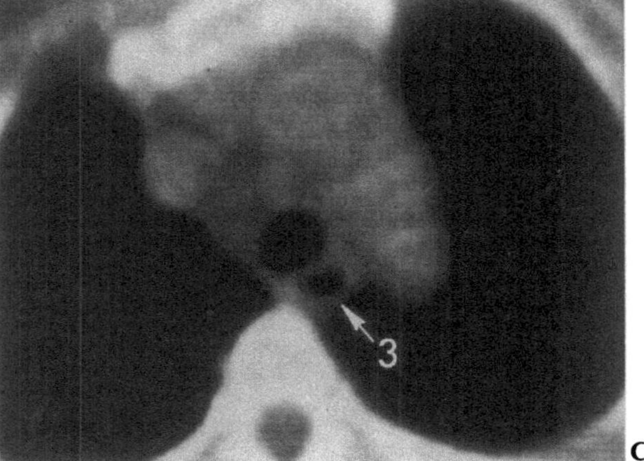

Fig. 7.26 A–C. Air in esophagus. **A** PA radiograph. **B** AP azygogram. **C** Computed tomogram through level of aortic arch. Presence of air in esophagus is common radiologic finding. Air is most commonly seen below level of aortic arch and slightly less often above it. Infrequently, as in **A** and **C**, air can be seen in esophagus medial to aortic arch. In **A** elliptical configuration of posterior turn of azygos arch, the azygos "knob" (see chapter 8), can be seen outlined on its left side by air in the esophagus (*1*) and on its right side by contact with the right lung (*2*). Subtending inferiorly from it can be seen right lateral esophageal wall outlined between gas in esophagus (*3*) and lung in azygoesophageal recess (*4*)

that far medially. Cimmino [25] has correlated the plain film appearances of the pleuroesophageal stripe with computed tomograms.

The esophagus often contains considerable quantities of air, even in normal subjects, and frequently this can be demonstrated on radiographs [23, 121]. Proto and Lane [121] found air to be present in the esophagus in 36% of 200 normal subjects studied by them. Air was present slightly more often below the aortic arch than above it; occasionally it was encountered medial to the aortic knob (Fig. 7.26). When the esophagus is particularly well filled with air, it is sometimes possible to identify its right lateral wall outlined between air in the lumen and air in the azygoesophageal recess or its left lateral wall outlined between air in the lumen and air in the preaortic lung. Exceptionally, both walls are visible on frontal radiographs (Fig. 7.27).

If the esophagus just medial and inferior to the aortic arch is filled, the left pleuroesophageal stripe may be followed cephalad to the undersurface of the aortic arch where the subaortic bulge of the esophagus can be identified. The air-filled esophagus in this location adopts a diamond-like configuration frequently crossed by a line representing the lateral wall of the left main bronchus (Fig. 7.27). Knowledge of the normal appearances of the gas-filled esophagus is of major significance to proper radiologic analysis of the mediastinum [23, 121]. Obviously the contours of the gas-filled esophagus are identical to those encountered in the barium-filled esophagus (Fig. 7.27). At times, however, esophageal air can be mistaken for air in lung or even air free in the mediastinum. On other occasions, mediastinal abnormalities may be misinterpreted if the appearance of these esophageal gas shadows and their variations are not appreciated (Figs. 7.28–7.30).

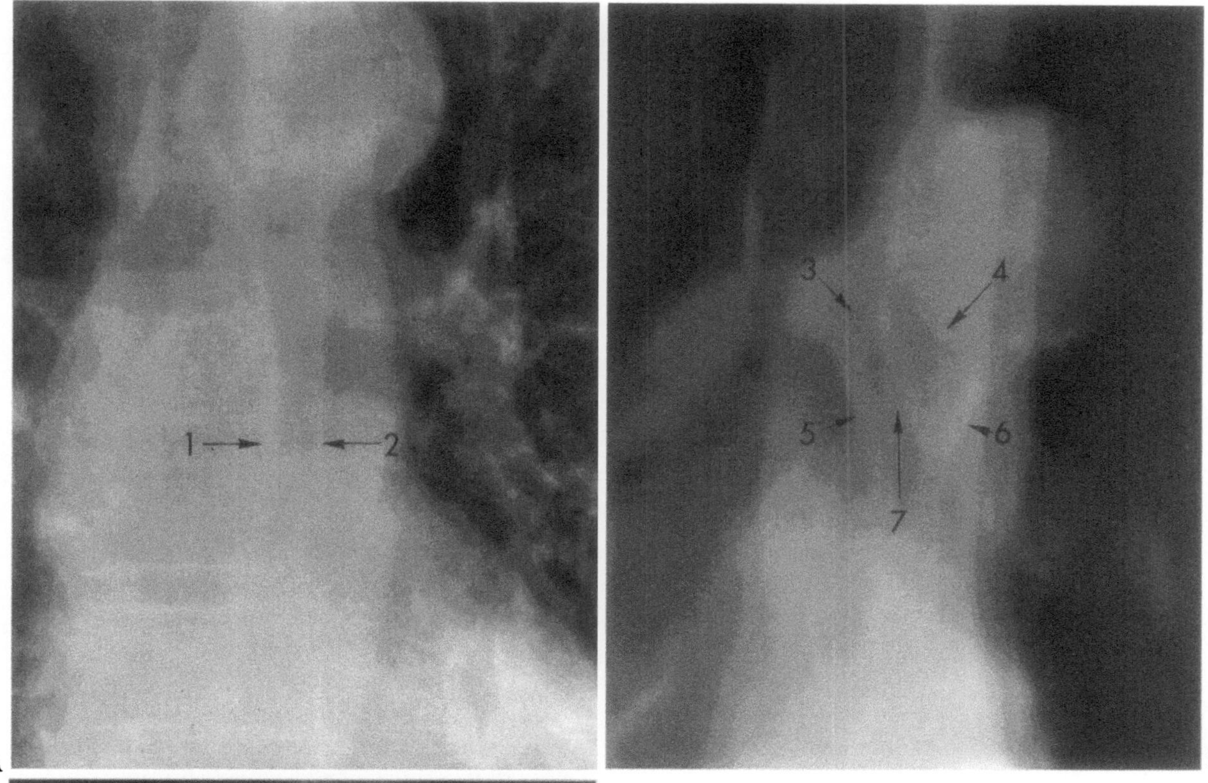

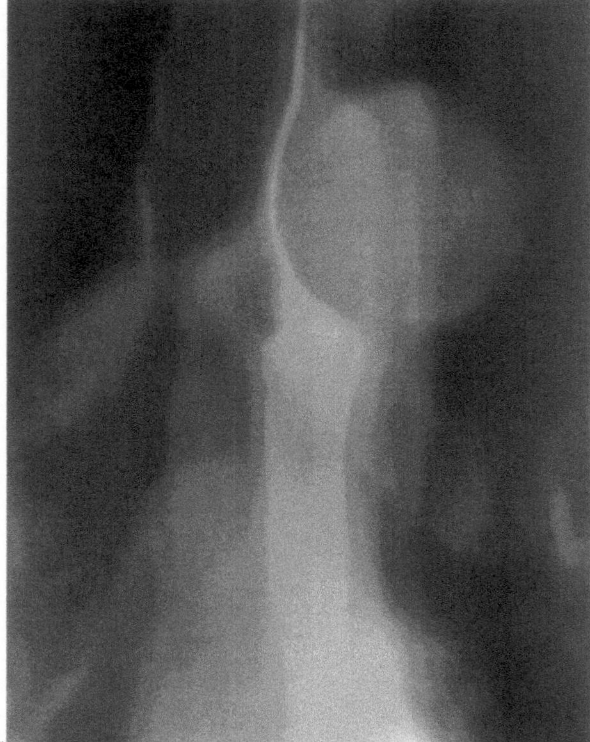

Fig. 7.27 A–C. Air in esophagus. **A** PA radiograph. **B** AP tomogram. **C** AP tomogram of patient shown in **B** with barium in esophagus. Occasionally, both right and left lateral walls of esophagus will be visualized on plain films or tomograms. Lung in azygoesophageal recess and air in esophageal lumen outlines right lateral esophageal wall (*1*), whereas air in preaortic left lung and air in esophageal lumen outlines left lateral esophageal wall (*2*). Air in esophageal lumen immediately below aortic arch may adopt diamond-shaped configuration produced by impressions of azygos knob (*3*) and aortic knob (*4*) above and lung in azygoesophageal recess (*5*) and preaortic left lung (*6*) below. The resulting diamond-shaped air shadow is crossed by superior wall of left main bronchus (*7*). (**A** Courtesy R. Fraser, Birmingham, Alabama)

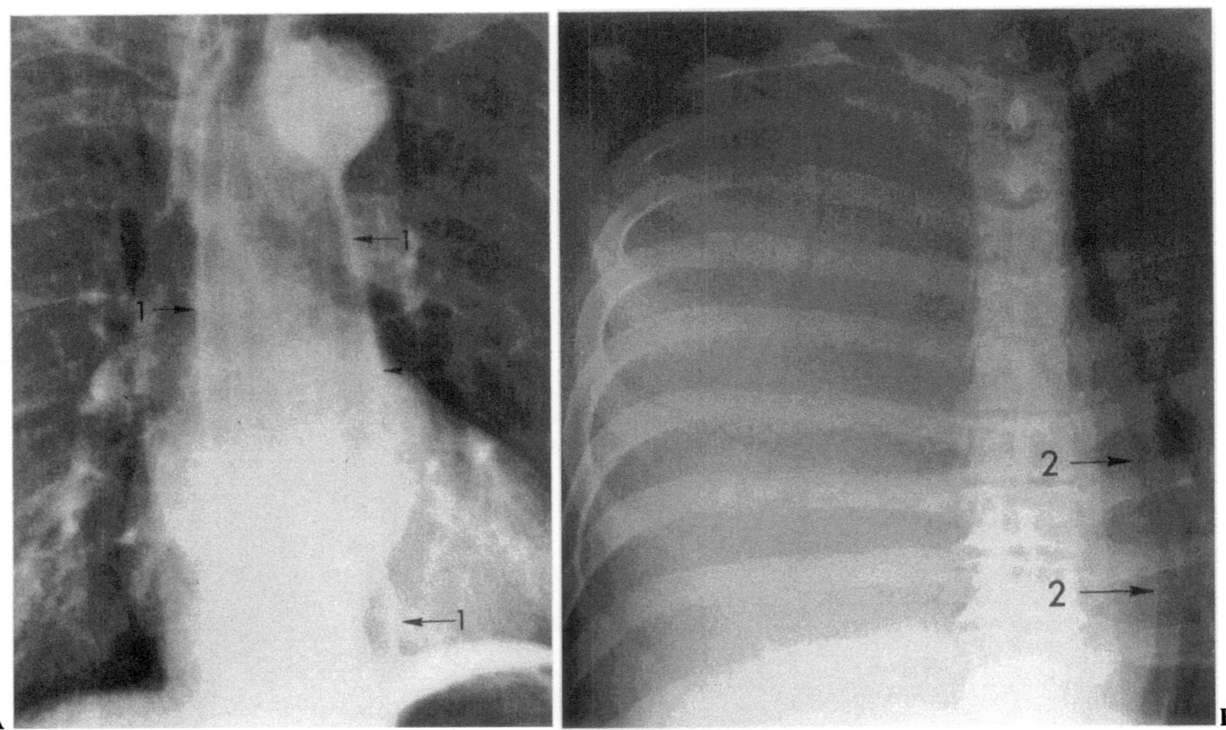

Fig. 7.28A, B. Variation in appearance of esophageal air. **A** PA radiograph. **B** AP radiograph. Extensive filling of esophagus with air suggests diagnosis of achalasia or of scleroderma. However, in **A**, marked distention of esophagus (*1*) could not be related to any known cause. In **B**, gas-filled esophagus (*2*) is displaced far to left side by massive right-sided pleural effusion secondary to Hodgkin's disease

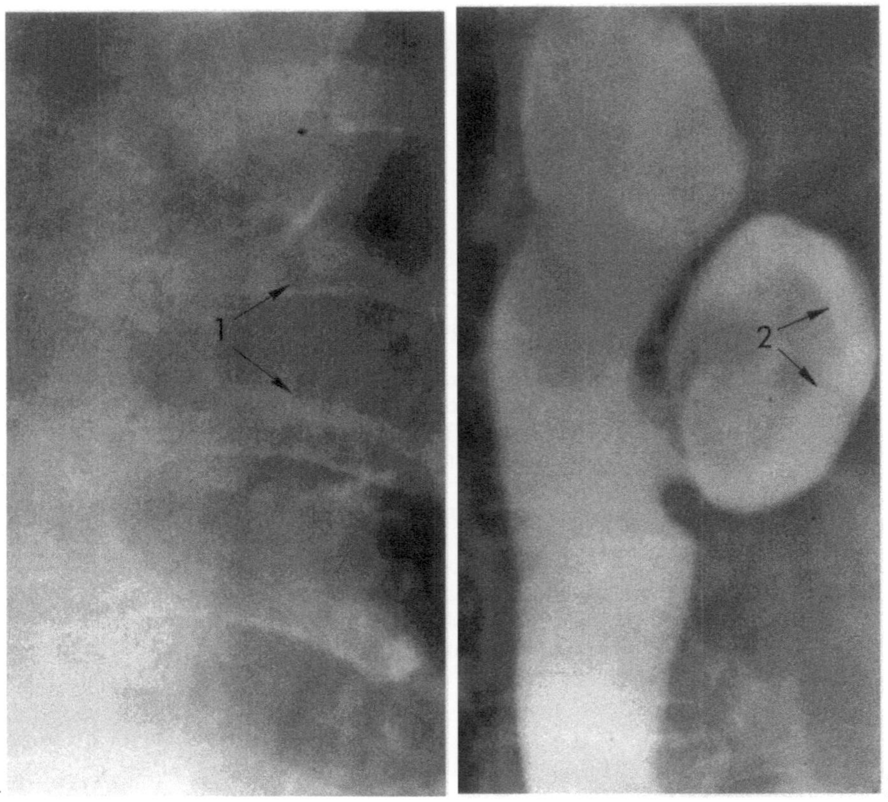

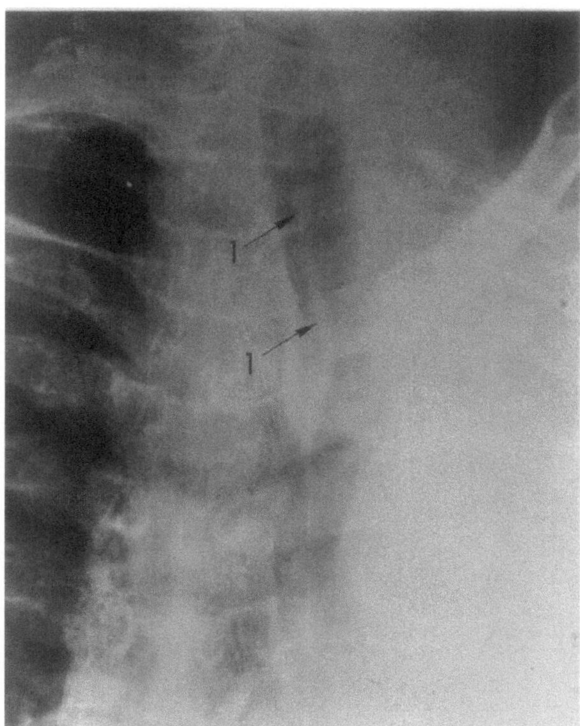

Fig. 7.30. Variation in appearance of esophageal air (PA radiograph). In this patient linear shadow of increased density visualized through trachea simulates posterior junction line (*1*). However, left pneumonectomy had been performed. The linear shadow represents right esophageal wall outlined between air in right lung and air in esophageal lumen. (Courtesy L. Santini, Danville, PA)

◁───────────────────────────────────

Fig. 7.29 A, B. Variation in appearance of esophageal air. **A** PA radiograph. **B** AP radiograph with barium in esophagus. In this patient arcuate radiolucent shadow (*1*) seen in region of aortic-pulmonic window posed diagnostic dilemma. Barium swallow clearly demonstrates that arcuate radiolucency was crescent of air surrounding bolus of foreign material (*2*) in an esophageal diverticulum. In evaluation of unusual gas shadows in mediastinum, esophagram is required

7.2.3.3 The Posterior Junction Line

The posterior junction line will be discussed in detail in chapter 9. It is mentioned here for the sake of completeness and to point out that the visceral and parietal pleurae over the left lung in a preaortic location form the left half of the posterior junction line [26] (see Fig. 9.18).

7.2.4 The Thoracic Duct

The thoracic duct ascends through the lower mediastinum between the azygos vein and the aorta. The duct has an intimate relationship to the aorta and often lies to the left of the midline, hence its inclusion here in the infra-aortic area. The thoracic duct extends cephalad from the cisterna chyli, entering the thorax through the aortic hiatus in the diaphragm (see Fig. 7.49). As it ascends in front of the spine on the left side of the azygos vein, it lies to the right of the descending aorta and is rather closely bound to it (Fig. 7.31). When an ectatic aorta buckles into the left chest, lymphangiograms have shown that the thoracic duct follows the aorta [131]. At the level of the aortic arch the thoracic duct turns forward from behind the aortic knob to pass behind the proximal portion of the left subclavian artery. Van Pernis [152], in a study of 1081 ducts, found that the forward turn occurred at the T-5 level in 480 cases and at the T-6 level in 601. In its upper thoracic course the duct is closely applied to the left lateral wall of the esophagus. It passes into the root of the neck to terminate at the point of junction of the left subclavian and left internal jugular veins.

Congenital variations in the thoracic duct are extremely common [152]. Rosenberger and Abrams [131] found the maximum diameter of the normal duct to be 7 mm. The radiologic significance of the thoracic duct is rather minimal and is limited almost entirely to problems of duct obstruction, duct displacement, and duct laceration [131].

Primary tumors are not known to involve the duct, but obstruction of the duct secondary to mediastinal neoplasm is apparently not rare [94]. A sharp cut-off of the duct and de-

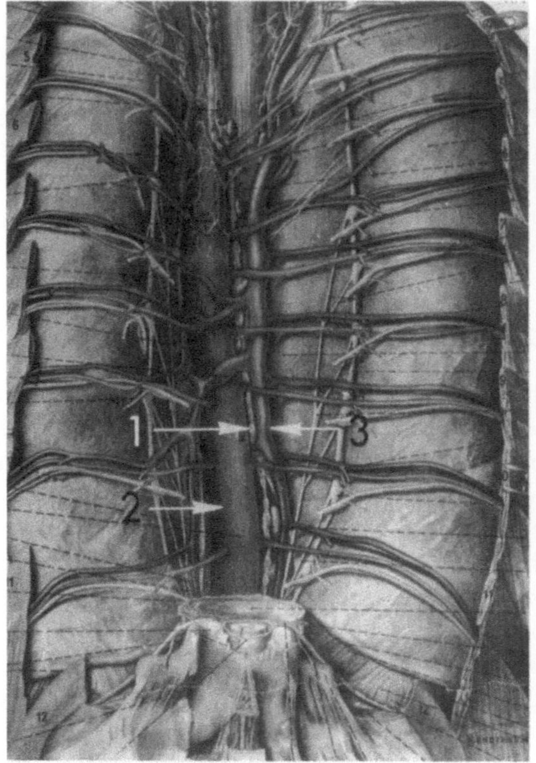 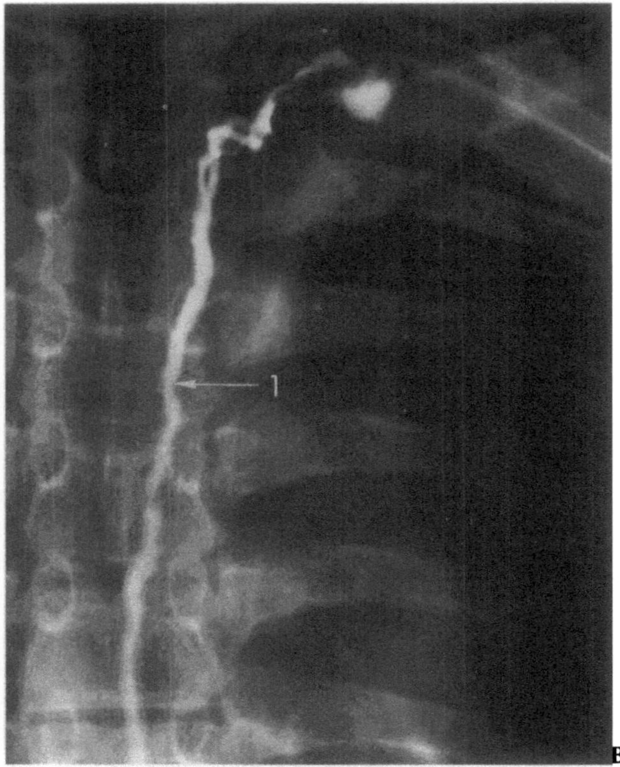

A   B

Fig. 7.31 A, B. Thoracic duct. **A** Relationships of descending aorta, thoracic duct, and azygos and hemiazygos veins viewed from posterior aspect. **B** AP radiograph with contrast material in thoracic duct. Thoracic duct (*1*) ascends in prespinal location lying between aorta (*2*) and azygos vein (*3*). At level of aortic arch, thoracic duct turns forward from behind aortic knob to pass behind proximal portion of left subclavian artery. (**A** From [117])

layed duct emptying are considered the best indicators of obstruction at lymphangiography [131]. Opacification of mediastinal lymph nodes is seen with duct obstruction but sometimes occurs without it [3], especially when duct anomalies are present.

Displacement of the duct by mediastinal masses may be demonstrated. Rosenberger and Abrams [131] have stated that if the thoracic duct is separated from the trachea by more than 10 mm, mediastinal abnormality should be suspected. It is felt that this criterion should be used with caution; in the upper thorax the duct is closely applied to the left lateral wall of the esophagus, and it is well known that the anatomic relationship of the trachea and the esophagus is quite variable.

Traumatic disruption of the thoracic duct is uncommon but not rare [9, 94, 116]. Initially, following laceration, chyle accumulates in the mediastinum, most often diffusely widening it [71] but sometimes causing a localized mass [15] (see Fig. 7.56). Commonly, there is a latent period of 1–6 weeks before chylothorax develops. In at least one reported case, however, there was a latent period of several months [15]. Damage to the lower portion of the duct is usually indirect, occurring as a result of blunt trauma, and tends to produce right chylothorax. It has been conjectured that hyperextension injuries cause the duct to be sheared by the diaphragmatic crura marginating the aortic hiatus [15] (see Fig. 7.56). Laceration of the cephalad portion of the thoracic duct is more commonly produced by direct injury; because the upper duct is in contact with the left mediastinal pleura, left chylothorax often results [90]. Laceration of the thoracic duct can be life threatening. Fluid loss can be great, since lymph flow through the thoracic duct has been estimated at 60–90 ml/h by Drinker and Yoffee [34] and at 14–110 ml/h by Shafiroff and Kan [137]. A flow of up to 2500 ml in 24 h has been reported from the cannulated duct [155]. Exact localization of the point of duct injury is difficult to determine clinically or at surgery but is important to proper management. Lymphangiography can be most helpful in locating the laceration [66]. Ligation of the thoracic duct is an effective form of treatment for duct laceration [57, 90]; following duct ligation, collateral channels develop quickly [119].

7.2.5 The Paraspinal Area

The paraspinal area on the left side is confined laterally by the parietal pleura over the paraspinal soft tissues; medially it lies against the lateral margin of the vertebral bodies (Fig. 7.32). Below the level of the fourth thoracic vertebra it is situated posterior to the descending aorta. The area contains many vital structures. The sympathetic trunks follow a cephalocaudad course along the anterolateral aspect of the vertebral bodies; behind the left sympathetic trunk

run the hemiazygos and accessory hemiazygos veins. The intercostal arteries course still more posteriorly from their points of origin from the posterior aspect of the descending aorta. They are accompanied by the intercostal veins and nerves. The intercostal lymph nodes are found in the posterior portion of the intercostal spaces in relationship to the intercostal vessels [27, 154]. All of these structures lie in a bed of areolar tissue and fat. Disease processes may involve any of these structures and may alter

Fig. 7.32 A, B. Paraspinal area. **A** Transverse body section. **B** Coronal body section. Paraspinal areas are confined medially by lateral margins of vertebral bodies (*1*) and laterally by parietal pleura covering mediastinal soft tissues (*2*). Note that paraspinal area is wider on left side than it is on right; this is commonly attributed to left-sided position of descending aorta. Interface of left lung with paraspinal soft tissues is usually oriented in plane parallel to frontal X-ray beam (*long arrow*), again apparently related to the left-sided position of descending aorta. Interface of right lung and right paraspinal musculature is not parallel to frontal X-ray beam (*long arrow*). Frequently it is better demonstrated in left anterior oblique or right posterior oblique projections. Note also there is considerable quantity of fat in left side of mediastinum behind aorta (*3*) and that there is considerably less fat on right side. Above T-4 the width of paraspinal fat on each side is the same

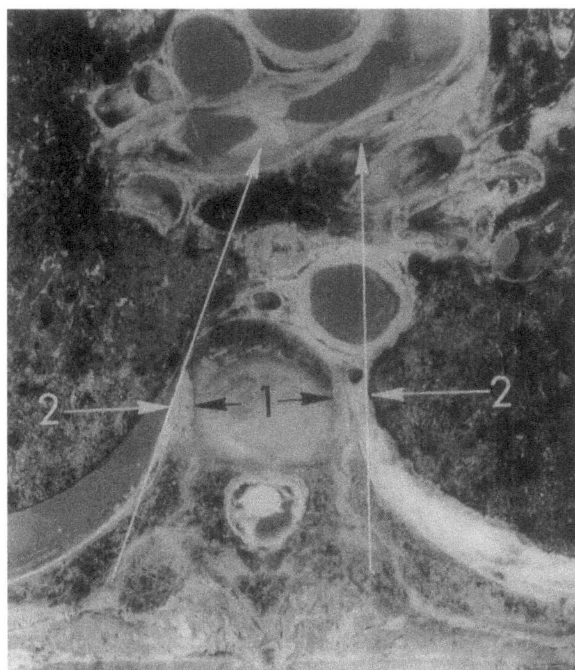

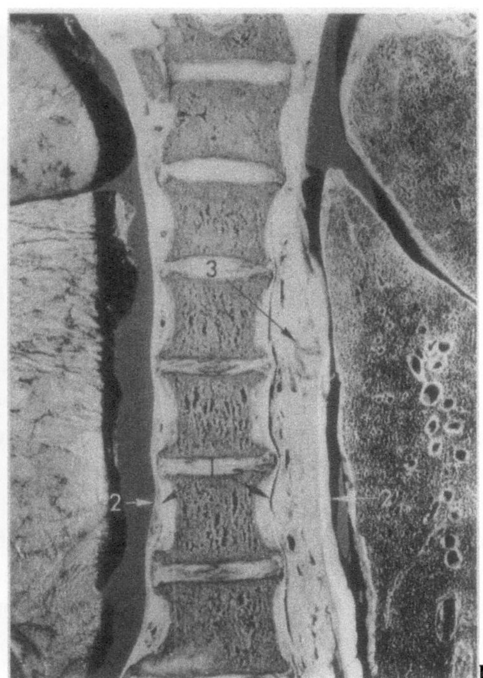

A   B

the paraspinal area and its major counterpart in radiologic anatomy – the paraspinal line. Kittredge [81] has provided a review of the anatomy of the area as demonstrated at computed tomography. The ensuing discussion will concern the paraspinal line and some pathologic processes that distort it.

7.2.5.1 The Paraspinal Line

The paraspinal line represents an interface of paraspinal soft tissues and contiguous lung. This seems a rather obvious statement in light of present day knowledge about correlated radiographic anatomy, but only four decades ago the nature of the line was the subject of considerable debate in the radiologic literature [49, 50]. In an editorial appearing in Radiology in 1942, Garland [49] suggested that the line might be related to the hemiazygos veins and asked for opinions concerning this possibility, at the same time soliciting other explanations. Several responses were received, including one from Brailsford [14] in which he produced evidence to show that the line represented the contact of lung with the paraspinal soft tissues. This opinion was soon supported by the studies of Billing [8].

The right paraspinal line is not seen as frequently as the left and is usually not as wide (Figs. 7.32 and 7.33). The hypothesis most frequently used to explain this difference is that the position of the descending aorta causes the interface of left lung against paraspinal soft tissues to be oriented in a true sagittal plane parallel to a frontal X-ray beam [14, 30] (Fig. 7.32). This contention is supported by the frequent visualization of a right paraspinal line when a right-sided descending aorta is present [30]. Normally, the contact of right lung with the paraspinal soft tissues is in an oblique plane and is better seen in left anterior or right posterior oblique projections. Doyle et al. [32] have made the interesting observation that the paraspinal line widens somewhat with advancing age and attributes this fact to the development of osteophytes along the thoracic spine and to dilatation of the descending aorta.

At the level of the aortic arch the upper end of the left paraspinal line deviates medially to lie much closer to the spine. Often the medial course of the paraspinal line at the level of the arch is sharply angulated rather than gently tapering (Fig. 7.33). The angulation is commonly identified through the shadow of the aortic knob. Should there be any doubt on a frontal radiograph concerning which of several vertical lines is the paraspinal line, the sharp medial angulation at the level of the aortic knob allows certain identification of the paraspinal line. It is felt that the angulation in the line at this point is caused by intrusion of the left lung into the supra-aortic area over the left superior intercostal vein [86] (see Figs. 6.21 and 6.22). The vein grooves the lung deeply at the point of angulation. When the upper end of the paraspinal line is rounded rather than sharply angulated, it is felt that the left superior intercostal vein is blanketed by fat. In those rare instances when a left azygos lobe is present, the hemiazygos fissure may be followed inferiorly and medially to the point of angulation, where it divides to encompass the left superior intercostal vein just as the azygos fissure encloses the azygos vein.

The lower aspect of the left paraspinal line can be followed inferiorly to the diaphragm in most instances. Commonly it is as wide or wider inferiorly than above, even though the descending aorta below T-10 adopts a more prespinal position than a paraspinal one (Figs. 7.33 and 7.34). This observation tends to cast some doubt on the thesis that the position of the left paraspinal line is predicated totally on the location of the aorta. In anatomic specimens, areolar tissue and fat fill the paraspinal area behind the descending aorta and do not diminish in thickness below the T-10 level (Figs. 7.32 and 7.33). This anatomic point also may be a significant factor accounting for the greater prominence of the left paraspinal line as compared to the right. Why there should be more fat and areolar tissue paraspinally on the left than on the right is not known.

In some individuals the left paraspinal line is seen as a line rather than as a lung-soft tissue interface. That is, the paraspinal line may appear as a white stripe between two areas of

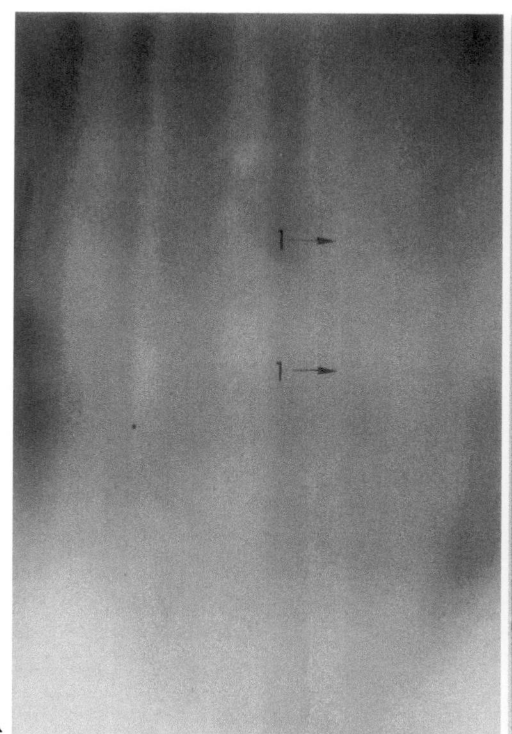

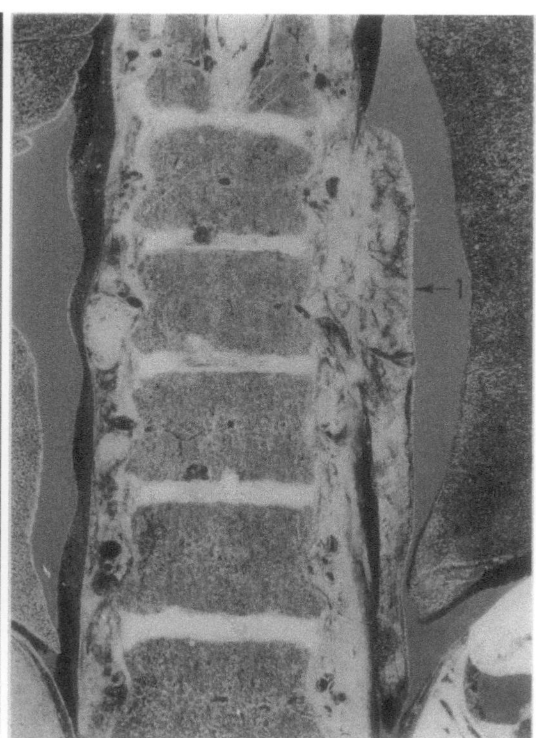

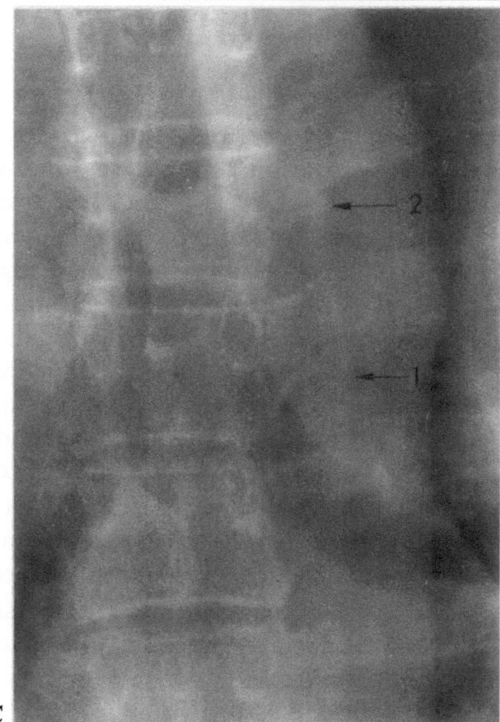

Fig. 7.33 A–C. Paraspinal line. **A** AP tomogram. **B** Coronary body section made from same patient. **C** AP radiograph. Presence of considerable amount of left paraspinal fat causes left paraspinal line to be seen further lateral than right paraspinal line. Paraspinal line often appears as white stripe representing opposed visceral and parietal pleurae between radiolucent left lower lobe and paraspinal fat (*1*). Note that paraspinal line is less wide superiorly (**C**); this is apparently due to fact that there is less paraspinal fat above level of aortic knob than there is below (**B**). Sharp angulation of line at level of aortic knob (*2*) is felt to be caused by left superior intercostal vein which grooves left lung as it courses forward about lateral aspect of aortic knob

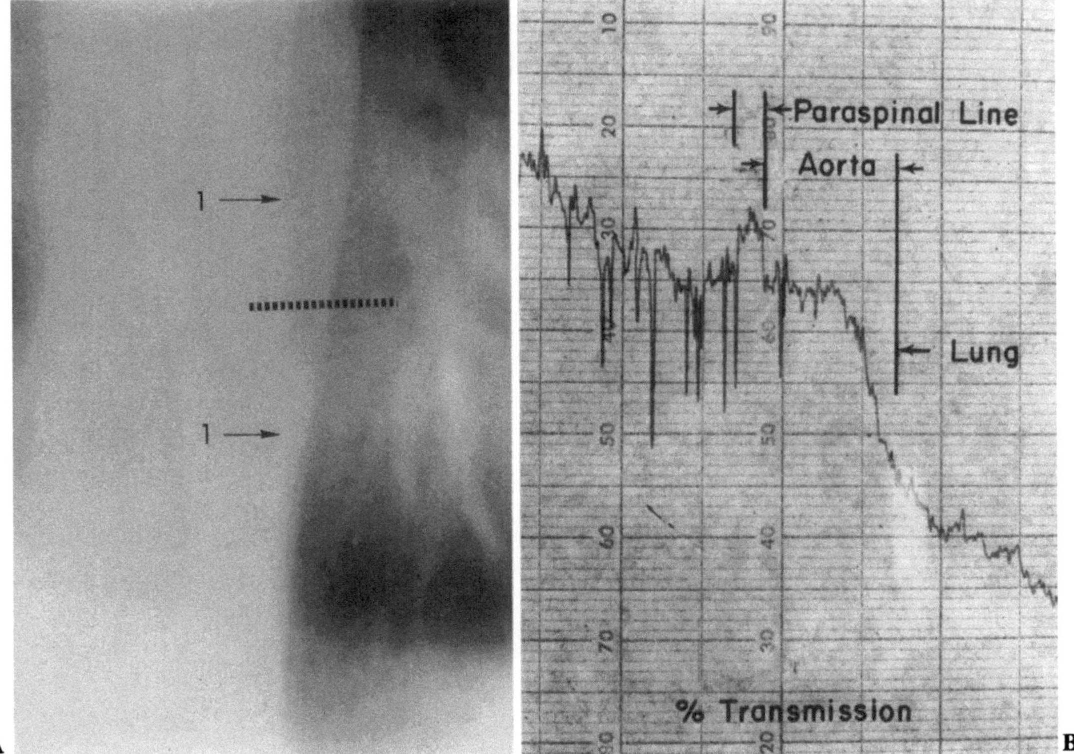

Fig. 7.34A, B. Paraspinal line. **A** PA radiograph. **B** Photodensitometric tracing. Although at times the white stripe of paraspinal line (*1*) may actually be due to increased pleural density between areas of lesser density, on other occasions appearance can be spurious and is due to Mach effect. Without photodensitometric determination it is often not possible to determine whether line is real or spurious. In this example, photodensitometric tracing across *dotted line* shown in **A** proves paraspinal line to be reflective of true change. At times it is possible to prove presence of Mach effect by masking margins of paraspinal line with dark paper. If line disappears, it is due to Mach effect. Factors producing the paraspinal line are still the subject of debate (see text)

greater radiolucency (Figs. 7.33, 7.34, and 7.47). Under these circumstances, photodensitometric studies often confirm that there is a greater density at the pleural interface than there is on either side of it (Fig. 7.34), but sometimes they do not. In the former case the explanation is a simple one: the visceral and mediastinal pleurae are being outlined between lung and paraspinal fat. In the latter situation, when photodensitometry clearly proves that the apparent visualization of a line between the two areas of radiolucency is spurious, the explanation for the illusion is the Mach effect [87] (see chapter 3). Under appropriate physical circumstances the Mach effect produces a type of edge enhancement that will cause anatomic structures or pathologic processes to be marginated by a rim of greater or lesser density, depending upon their contour. The paraspinal line appears to be edged by white, a positive Mach band, because a concave area of greater luminance, the paraspinal soft tissues, is in contact with a convex area of greater luminance, the lung (Fig. 7.33). The descending aorta appears edged by black, a negative Mach band, since the physical conditions producing the Mach effect are reversed. The difference in the Mach bands marginating the descending aorta and the paraspinal line permits them to be distinguished from one another when other radiographic findings are equivocal (Fig. 7.35, see also Fig. 6.26).

Genereux [51] has presented the argument that the paraspinal line appears as a line solely due to Mach effect. In eight cases studied by him, photodensitometry failed to show a density to be present on the film even though a line appeared to be present. He also feels that the paraspinal line is often wider than can be accounted for by the aggregate thickness of the visceral and parietal (mediastinal) pleurae. Another argument offered by Genereux is that if the paraspinal line can result from the pleurae outlined between fat medially and lung laterally, why then is a thin layer of paramediastinal fluid not seen as a thicker line? He claims that he has never seen such an example and we cannot say that we have either. Suffice it to say that the factors which cause the paraspinal line to be visualized are debatable. We continue to feel that the apposed pleurae can be seen as a line, independent of Mach effect, at least in some cases. Our photodensitometric studies support such a conclusion.

The appearance of the paraspinal line on radiographs as a line rather than an interface can be useful in radiologic interpretation, whether it is a real line or a spurious one. If along its course the line can no longer be seen as a line but only as an interface, paraspinal disease medial to this should be inferred (Fig. 7.36). If the line is a real one, it can be assumed that paraspinal fat is infiltrated, rendering it of soft tissue density. If the line is spurious, the same conclusion must be drawn, since the Mach effect should not occur at one point along the paraspinal line without occurring at another unless the physical conditions affecting its visualization were different at the two points.

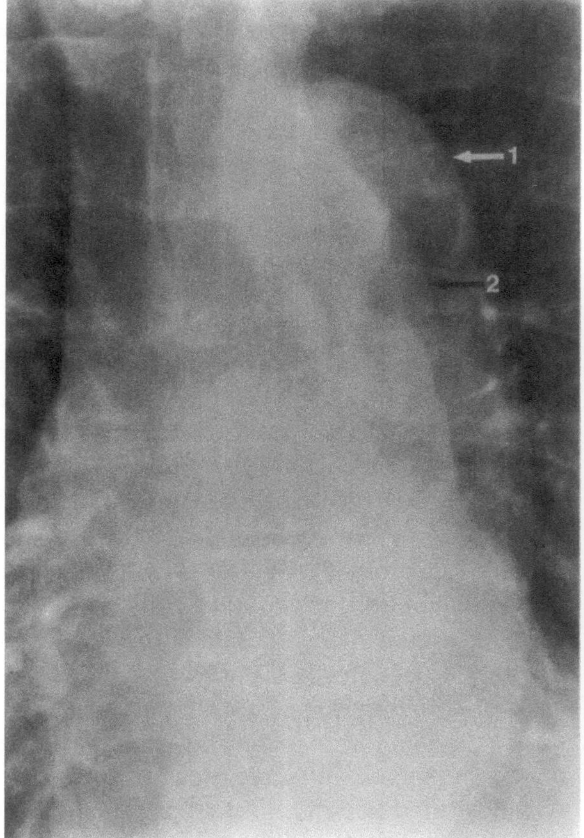

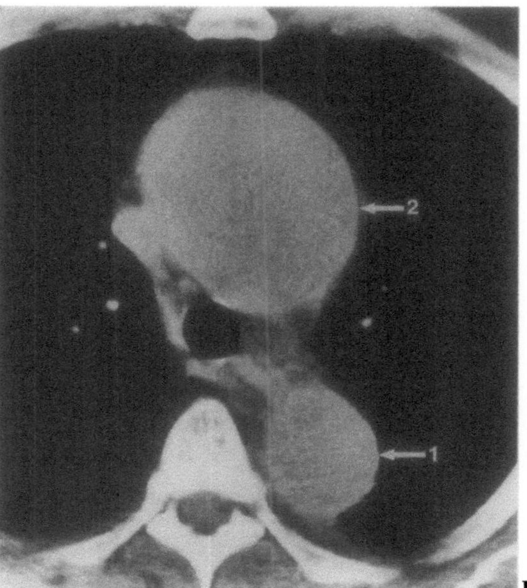

Fig. 7.35 A, B. Mach effect. Usefulness in radiographic analysis. A PA radiograph. B Computed tomogram. In the analysis of the PA radiograph, the lateral margin of the descending aorta (1) was readily identified, but the arcuate shadow (2) medial to it presented a diagnostic problem. At first glance it may be thought to represent the paraspinal line, but the shadow is edged in black, a negative Mach band, and therefore cannot represent the paraspinal line. Therefore, a mediastinal mass cannot be excluded. The computed tomogram shows that the shadow represents contact of the ascending aorta with the left lung. This is an unusual occurrence, but may occur when the ascending aorta is dilated

A   B

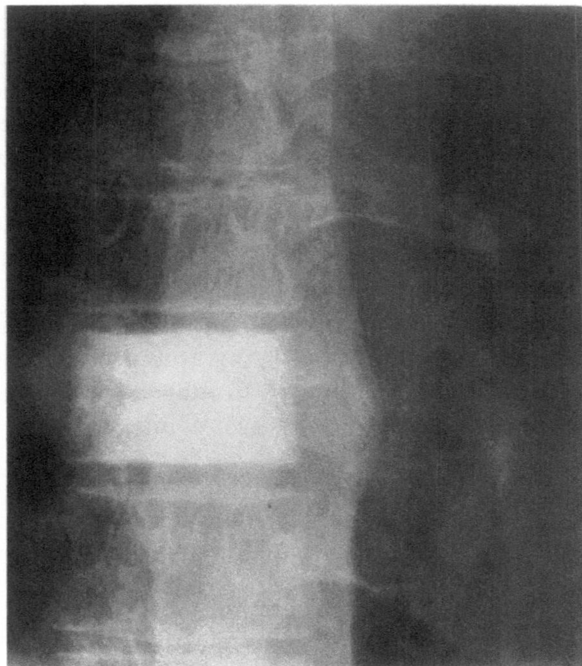

Fig. 7.36. Paraspinal line. Loss of paraspinal line as indication of paraspinal disease (AP radiograph). The paraspinal area is shown to protrude laterally into left lung adjacent to osteoblastic process involving body of T-9. Note that white stripe representing paraspinal line can be followed inferiorly to T-8, is lost adjacent to T-9, and resumes its appearance as white line at T-10 level. Loss of white line is reflective of paraspinal disease. If paraspinal line in this case is a real one, it can be assumed that paraspinal fat is infiltrated, rendering it of soft tissue density. If line is result of Mach effect, same conclusion must be drawn since this effect should not occur at one point along paraspinal line without occurring at another unless physical conditions affecting its visualization were different at the two points. This is an extreme example, but sometimes very subtle changes in appearance of paraspinal line can be analyzed in this manner to diagnose paraspinal disease

7.2.5.2 Disease Altering the Paraspinal Line

Hemorrhage: Traumatic Rupture of the Thoracic Aorta

Bleeding is a common cause for widening of the paraspinal line. Hemorrhage may result from injury to small vessels as is usually the case with fractures of the thoracic spine or from larger vessels. A prototype of the latter type of injury is traumatic rupture of the aorta.

Rupture of the aorta following chest trauma is becoming increasingly more frequent [6, 60, 93] with most cases occurring as the result of vehicular accidents. Several comprehensive reviews of the subject can be found in the literature [18, 44, 88, 103, 113, 114, 133]. Several mechanisms of injury have been postulated, the most common being rapid deceleration with "whipping" of the more mobile anterior portion of the aortic arch on the more fixed posterior arch and paraspinal aorta. Posterior displacement and rotation of the heart and proximal aorta up to the point of maximal fixation of the aorta have also been suggested as a possible cause [18]. Lundevall [93] emphasizes the role played by rapidly altered fluid dynamics within the aorta.

Approximately 95% of all aortic ruptures occur in the region of the aortic isthmus at the site of the ligamentum arteriosum (Fig. 7.37). The remaining 5% occur immediately above the aortic valve [133]. Since this portion of the aorta is intrapericardial, bleeding from a ruptured ascending aorta into the mediastinum or pleura is rare. Death frequently occurs from cardiac tamponade. Most injuries to the aortic isthmus are severe, and complete transection of the aorta is common; indeed, some series indicate that complete transection occurs in as many as 40% of all aortic ruptures [1]. Complete transection is not incompatible with survival; in some cases, blood is contained by the adventitia and surrounding tissues (Fig. 7.37) with eventual development of a false aneurysm. Traumatic aneurysms secondary to penetrating wounds of the thorax are uncommon since laceration through the adventitia and adjacent tissues generally results in immediate fatal hemorrhage [6].

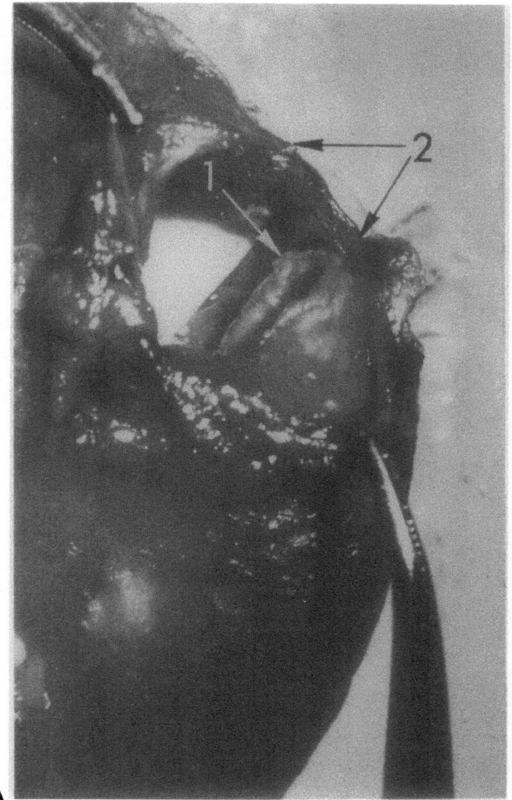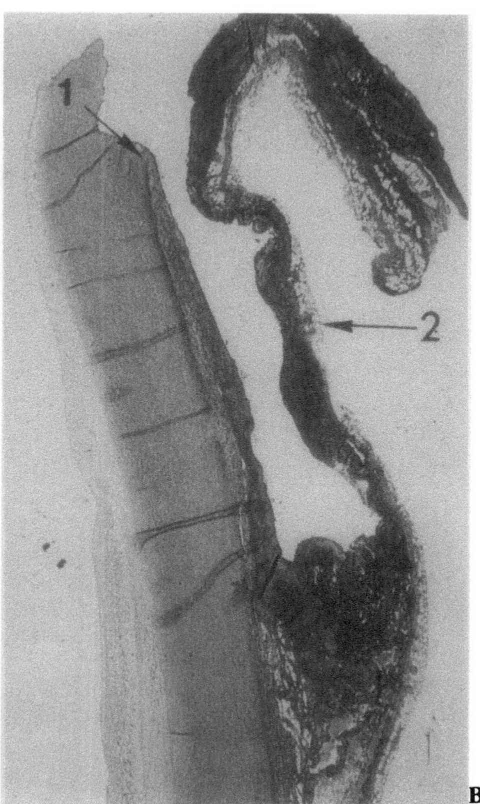

Fig. 7.37 A, B. Traumatic rupture of thoracic aorta. **A** Upper descending aorta viewed through incised adventitia. **B** Low-power photomicrograph. Complete disruption of intima and media of aorta (*1*) in usual location is demonstrated. Of traumatic fractures of the aorta, 95% occur just below aortic knob. Such injury to intima and media occurs commonly in aortic rupture, but exanguination may not result if blood remains contained by intact aortic adventitia (*2*). (From [133])

Immediate death is the usual result of aortic rupture, but 10%–20% of all patients with this injury will live for longer than 1 h. In our series of more than 60 patients, one in six survived to have adequate clinical and radiologic evaluation [133]. Fewer than 5% of all patients live long enough for a chronic traumatic aneurysm to develop [6]. Only three patients in our study had documented aneurysms of greater than 2 months' duration [133] (see Fig. 7.42).

Evidence of major thoracic injury with or without shock should alert the radiologist to the possibility of aortic rupture. Severe chest pain, often intrascapular, is a common symptom. Dysphagia may result from compression of the esophagus, and increasing respiratory distress may occur from airway compromise caused by a mediastinal hematoma. Changes in blood pressure or pulse in the neck or arms may occasionally be noted [84] (Fig. 7.38), and a systolic murmur may infrequently be audible in the left second parasternal interspace [99]. Hypertension in the arms following aortic rupture has been attributed to compromise of the aortic lumen by a surrounding hematoma [48]. Such compromise has not been encountered in any of our angiograms or pathologic specimens, and it is our assumption that hypertension is the result of functional obstruction caused by flow turbulence at the rupture site. In some instances the development of a hemothorax, particularly one that develops rapidly, is an important diagnostic clue, as is persistent active bleeding from a chest tube (Fig. 7.40).

Prompt recognition of thoracic injury is important since the local nature of the injury and the fact that the adjacent aorta is usually normal

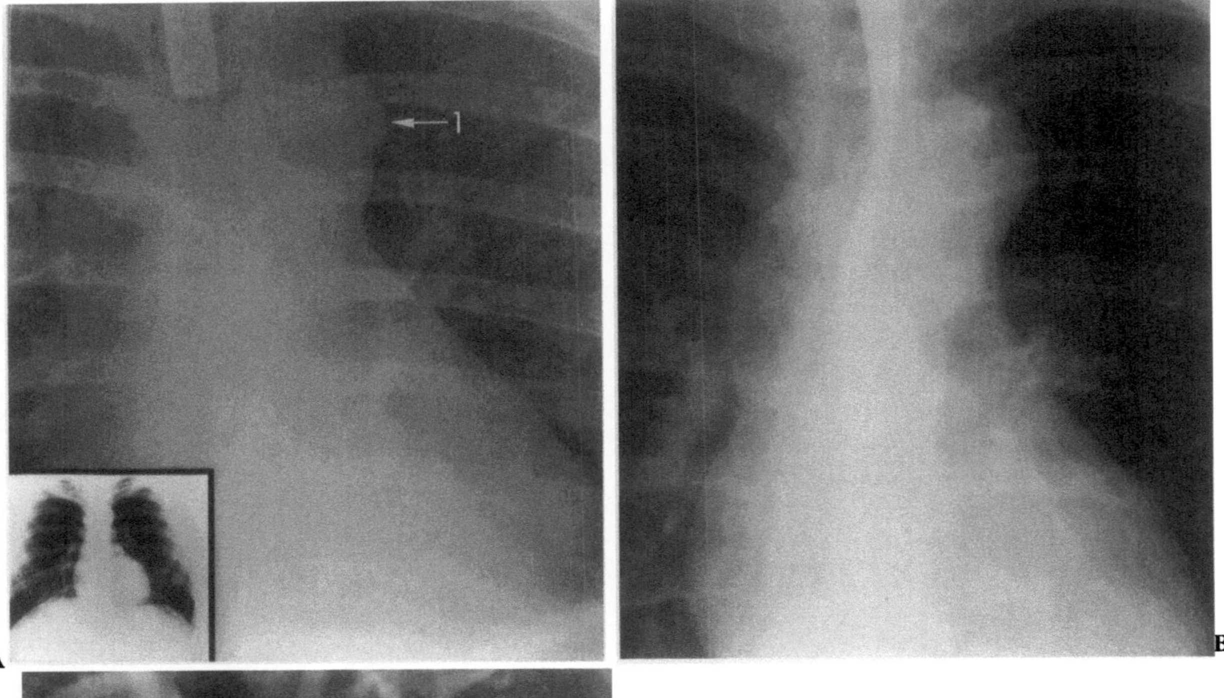

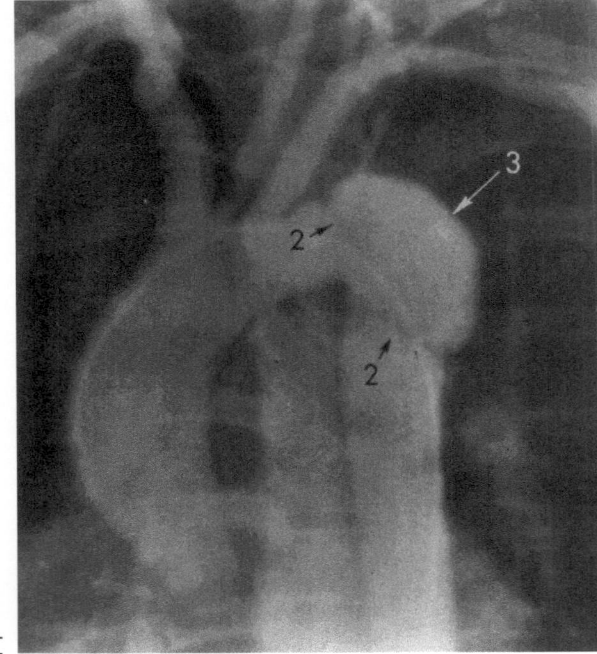

Fig. 7.38 A–C. Traumatic rupture of thoracic aorta. Localized mediastinal hemorrhage. **A** AP radiograph. **B** PA radiograph. **C** Right posterior oblique radiograph from thoracic aortogram. Abnormalities produced on plain radiographs by traumatic aortic rupture may be minimal. As in this case, changes may be slight, although complete transection of aorta has resulted. Minimal angulation at lateral aspect of aortic knob (*1*) was not thought significant in this patient who had sustained major trauma in automobile accident, even though configuration was somewhat different than it was on photofluorogram made a few months earlier (*insert*). Patient subsequently became hypertensive in arms. During evaluation of this problem 6 weeks after accident, PA chest radiograph revealed configuration of aortic knob to be markedly changed and very prominent. An aortogram demonstrated false aneurysm. At surgery, aorta was found to be totally transected and its end (*2*) was incorporated into false aneurysm (*3*). Successful repair was achieved

permit a favorable diagnosis if surgical repair can be performed in time [1, 75, 114]. However, the lesion may be clinically occult or go undetected because signs and symptoms of aortic injury are obscured by a multiplicity of other injuries. The diagnosis of aortic rupture can be suspected on plain chest radiographs and confirmed by aortography. The plain film diagnosis may be difficult, since films must usually be obtained with the patient in a supine position, with short tube-film distances, and often in a relatively expiratory phase of respiration.

As a result of these factors the mediastinum may be extremely difficult to evaluate. Fracture of the first and/or second ribs is not of predictive value for major vessel injury. In a study of 214 patients with chest trauma, Fisher et al. [43] divided them into two groups depending upon whether they did or did not have fractures of the first and/or second ribs. The frequency of major vascular injury was the same in both groups. The roentgen findings in acute aortic rupture may be grouped into three categories.

Localized Mediastinal Hemorrhage. In some experimentally produced aortic ruptures and in a large number of clinical cases the most minimal lesion has been a transverse intimal tear [133]. With more severe injury, tears of the intima and media occur, and subadventitial accumulations of blood develop (Fig. 7.37). Patients presenting with such localized hematomas may have few or no clinical signs, but still have a grave prognosis. Such cases are often unrecognized, and the patient may show only a prominent, poorly defined, or irregular aortic knob (Fig. 7.38). In a recent study, this finding was one of the two most frequent radiographic signs of aortic rupture, the other being mediastinal widening [135]. As a hematoma enlarges, the trachea may be displaced to the right (Fig. 7.40), and the left main bronchus may be deviated anteriorly, inferiorly, and to the right [97] (Fig. 7.39). This bronchial displacement is easily understood in light of the anatomic relationships in the aortic-pulmonic window. Displacement of a nasogastric tube to the right at the level of T-4 may be a helpful sign [97], but certainly this finding is often not present [153].

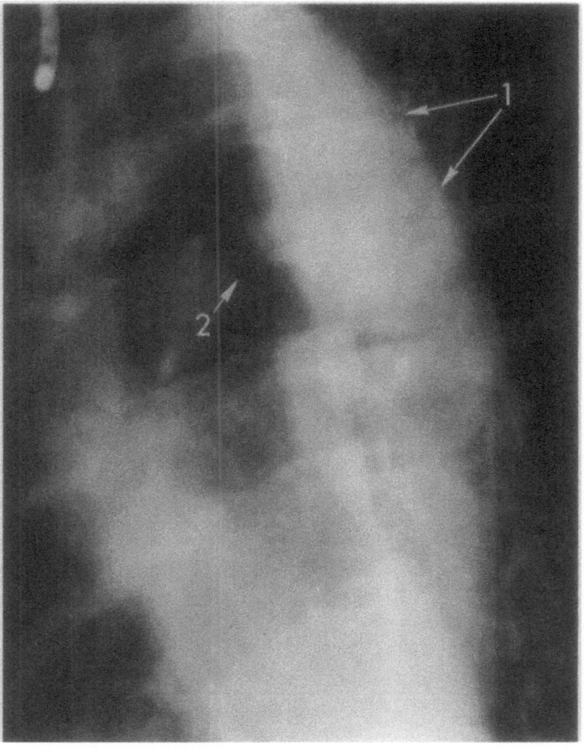

Fig. 7.39. Traumatic rupture of thoracic aorta. Localized mediastinal hemorrhage. Right posterior oblique radiograph from thoracic angiogram. Fusiform dilation of upper portion of descending aorta due to false aneurysm is identified (*1*). Note that left main bronchus (*2*) is displaced forward and downward. (From [133])

Generalized Mediastinal Hemorrhage. Generalized mediastinal bleeding resulting from acute aortic injury frequently produces widening of the mediastinum. In some cases it is difficult to determine whether the mediastinum is truly abnormal or whether technical factors have accentuated its normal outline. Some observers have emphasized the importance of the mediastinal width/chest width ratio [136], but others [98] have disputed its value. We have found it to be an unreliable criterion. Simeone et al. [144] have reported the presence of a left apical cap in traumatized patients to be a good indicator of generalized bleeding. This is a useful sign, especially if previous films do not show the cap or if it enlarges on serial examinations. In some patients, obliteration of the normal imprints made on the adjacent lung by the mediastinal contents indicates that disease is truly present (Fig. 7.40). Widening of the paraspinal line

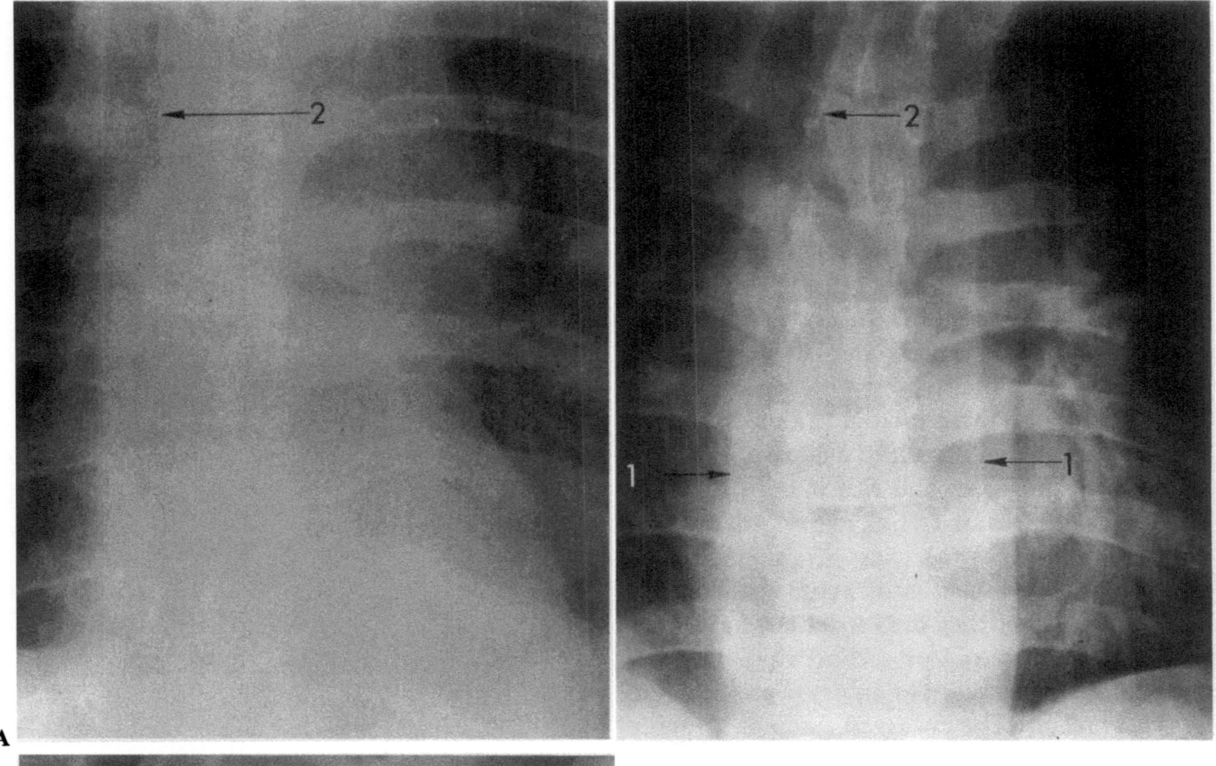

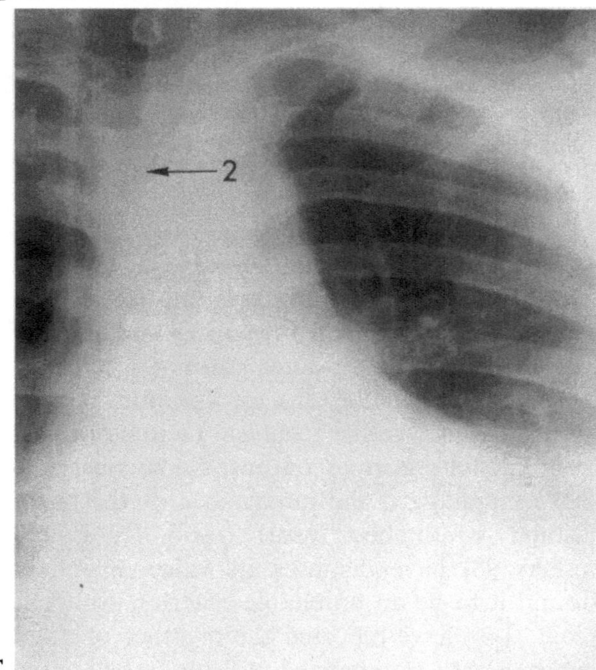

Fig. 7.40 A–C. Traumatic rupture of thoracic aorta. Generalized mediastinal hemorrhage. **A** and **C** PA radiographs. **B** AP radiograph. Traumatic rupture of aorta can produce generalized dissection of blood through connective tissue planes of mediastinum. In **A** loss of normal contours in supra-aortic and supra-azygos areas is apparent. In **B** there is generalized widening of paraspinal line on each side (*1*), whereas in **C** bleeding into pleural space has occurred. In last patient, traumatic rupture of aorta was not considered initially, even though there was brisk bleeding from chest tube. In all three patients, marked tracheal displacement is evident (*2*). (**B** and **C** From [133])

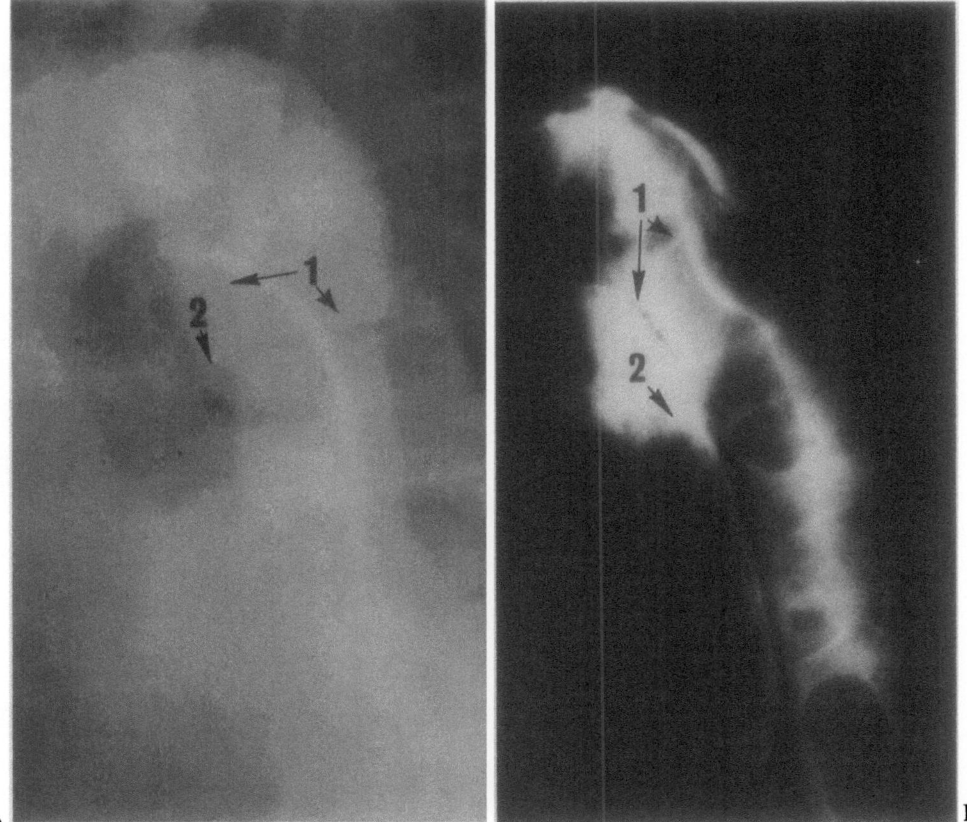

to the right or left or bilaterally is very helpful (Fig. 7.40).

To be sure, not all patients with mediastinal hematoma following trauma suffer aortic rupture; bleeding may occur from smaller arteries or veins. Displacement of the left main bronchus is characteristic and is helpful in distinguishing mediastinal widening due to a ruptured aorta from bleeding of other origin. Although the carinal angle was normal in six patients with mediastinal hemorrhage who were found by angiography to have an intact aorta, it averaged 10° less than normal in our cases of mediastinal hemorrhage due to aortic rupture [133].

Hemothorax. In many cases, bleeding is only partially confined to the mediastinum. Hemorrhage into the pleural space is common and may be erroneously thought to be the result of left-sided rib fracture. A rapidly accumulating hemothorax or persistent active bleeding from a chest tube should suggest the diagnosis (Fig. 7.40). In the final analysis, many patients with suspect injury to the aorta will require aor-

Fig. 7.42A–B. Traumatic rupture of thoracic aorta. Chronic traumatic aneurysm. **A** PA radiograph. **B** Photograph of opened surgical specimen. **C** Low power photomicrograph. In this patient with history of severe thoracic trauma in the past, the diagnosis of chronic traumatic aortic aneurysm was made. At surgery, well-established false aneurysm incorporated transected ends of aorta. Aortic intima and media (*1*) can be seen intruding into false aneurysmal sac (*2*)

tography to prove or disprove the diagnosis (Fig. 7.38). Considering the obvious importance of correct diagnosis of aortic rupture, aortograms should be done freely if any reasonable suspicion exists [4]. A relatively high percentage of normal studies is acceptable to avoid missing the injury. Although computed tomography has been reported to diagnose aortic rupture without false positive or false negative diagnoses in a small number of patients [65], we have preferred to use aortography as the "gold standard" to establish the diagnosis.

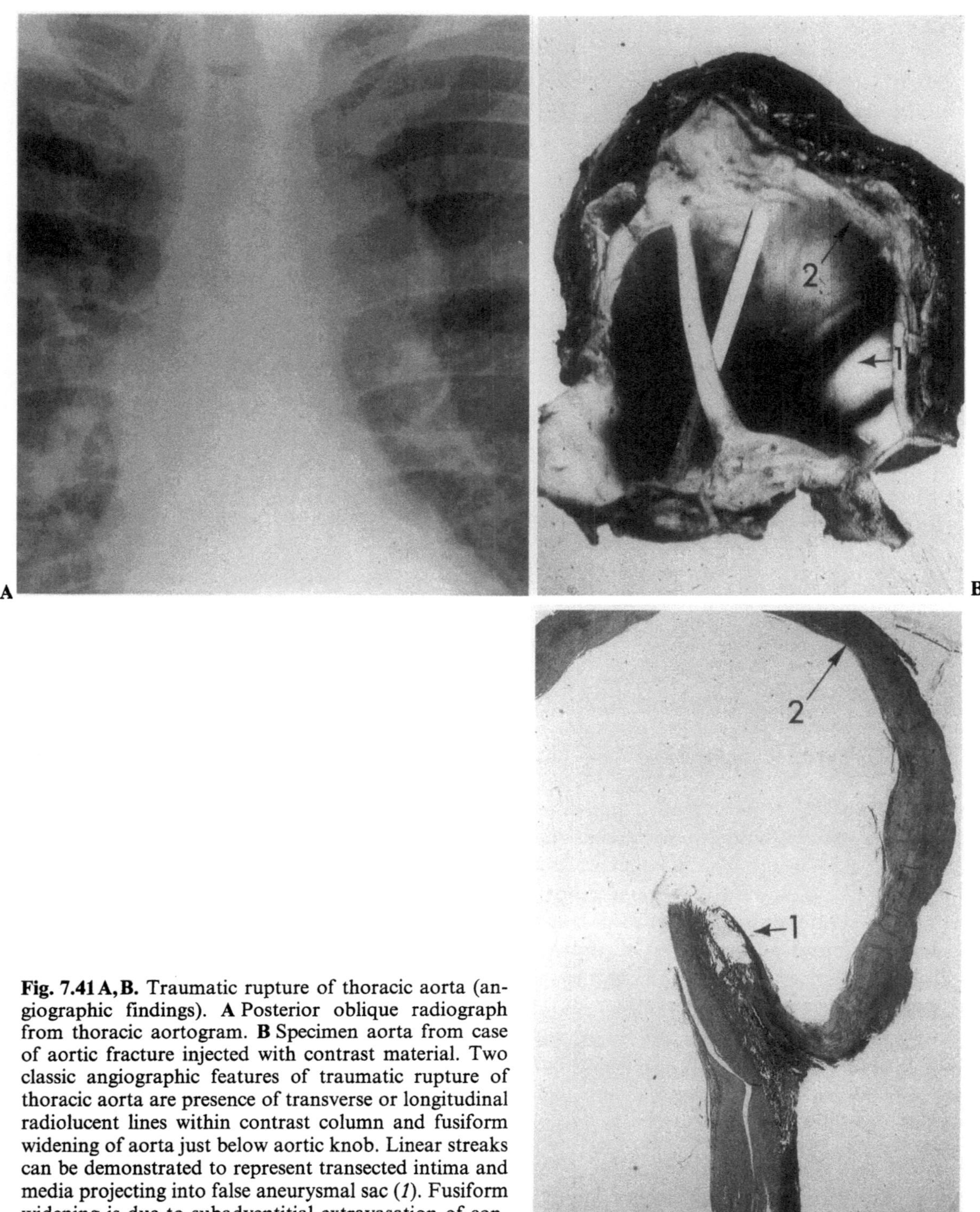

Fig. 7.41 A, B. Traumatic rupture of thoracic aorta (angiographic findings). **A** Posterior oblique radiograph from thoracic aortogram. **B** Specimen aorta from case of aortic fracture injected with contrast material. Two classic angiographic features of traumatic rupture of thoracic aorta are presence of transverse or longitudinal radiolucent lines within contrast column and fusiform widening of aorta just below aortic knob. Linear streaks can be demonstrated to represent transected intima and media projecting into false aneurysmal sac (*1*). Fusiform widening is due to subadventitial extravasation of contrast material (*2*). (From [133])

The angiographic appearance of a traumatic aortic aneurysm is variable, ranging from a slight irregularity in the contour of the aortic isthmus to an obvious false saccular aneurysm. A localized, slightly irregular fusiform widening of the aorta just distal to the arch is a frequent finding and can be shown to be the result of subadventitial extravasation of the contrast agent through the traumatic defect in the intima and media, producing a fusiform periaortic hematoma that becomes opacified during angiography (Fig. 7.41). A sharply defined linear defect may sometimes be seen in the dye column at the proximal or distal margin of the aneurysm. This defect is produced by protrusion of the transected portions of the aorta into the false aneurysm (Fig. 7.41). Chronic traumatic aneurysms cannot be distinguished from aneurysms of other etiology on plain films (Fig. 7.42). If they are suspected because of a past history of significant chest trauma, surgery is usually advised [70].

Abscess: Rupture of the Esophagus

The presence of infected material in the paraspinal area can also result in widening of the paraspinal line. Spontaneous rupture of the esophagus is a prototype of this phenomenon. Spontaneous rupture of the esophagus, also known as "Boerhaave's syndrome," is caused by a sudden increase in intraluminal pressure in the distal esophagus and is to be differentiated from laceration produced during esophagoscopy or by penetrating wounds. It is an unusual condition, but one which is of considerable importance in chest radiology because of the significant role played by the radiographic examination in the establishment of the diagnosis [11, 16, 21, 56, 101, 105, 110, 118, 130, 149]. Early diagnosis, often first suggested from chest roentgenograms, is vital if patients with this condition are to survive. Although many patients with Boerhaave's syndrome have diffuse mediastinal abnormalities on radiographs, the tendency of the esophagus to rupture along its left posterolateral aspect most often causes the earliest roentgenographic changes to occur in the left side of the mediastinum posteriorly

above the diaphragm [130]. The left paraspinal line is almost always widened or obliterated, hence the discussion of this entity with other conditions that distort the paraspinal line.

Boerhaave's syndrome is named after Hermann Boerhaave, a Dutch physician of the early eighteenth century [130]. It occurs when the fluid pressure within the lumen of the distal esophagus exceeds the tensile strength of the esophageal wall. In most instances, gastric distention precedes the episode that is initiated by elevation of intragastric pressure due to vomiting, or less likely, by forceful contraction of the abdominal musculature occurring in childbirth, coughing, convulsive seizures, weight lifting, or status asthmaticus [130]. Relaxation of the distal esophageal sphincter then allows the sudden imposition of elevated hydrostatic pressure against the wall of the lower end of the esophagus. Esophageal rupture is often due to instrumentation, especially balloon dilatation [83, 147] of the esophagus. In fact, Stewart et al. [147] have emphasized the desirability of contrast study of the esophagus following balloon dilatation.

Most ruptures occur along the left posterolateral aspect of the distal third of the esophagus, although occasionally, tears may occur along the right posterolateral wall or along the left anterior wall. Therefore, the abnormal radiographic findings are usually first encountered on the left side. Following a rupture of the left posterolateral esophageal wall, the extravasated fluid may dissect posteriorly through the perivisceral fascial space either medial or lateral to the descending aorta. In most cases, dissection in both directions undoubtedly occurs. Posterior spread that extends primarily medial to the descending aorta will reach the tough prespinal fascia and will be diverted into the left paraspinal space and sometimes into the right paraspinal space as well. Widening of the paraspinal line, often bilaterally, is the result seen on radiographs (Fig. 7.43). Such widening may be localized or diffuse, but commonly it is initially focal, with rather extensive broadening of the paraspinal line developing subsequently. Posterior dissection lateral to the aorta will alter the preaortic line, if it is present, and will later obliterate the shadow of the lateral margin of the de-

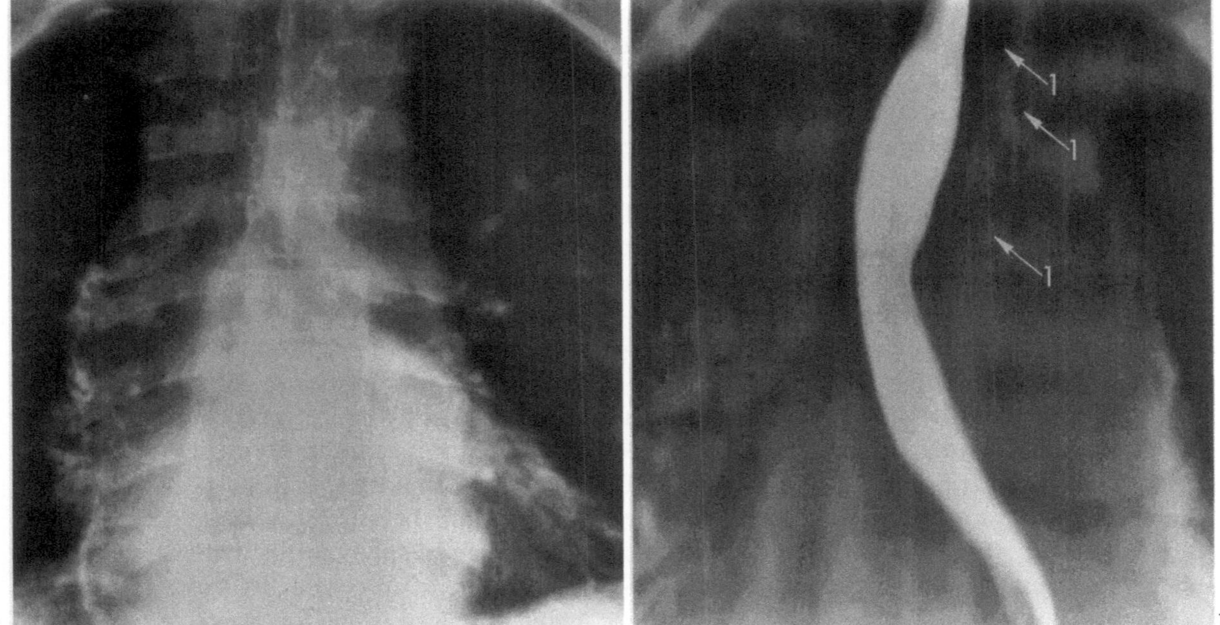

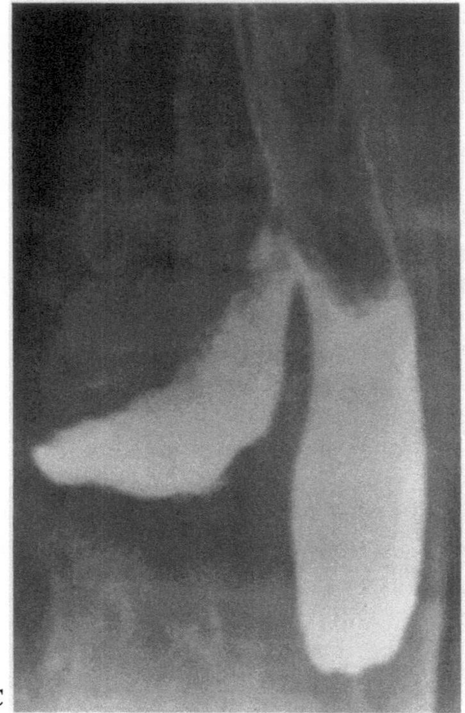

Fig. 7.43 A–C. Spontaneous rupture of esophagus (Boerhaave's syndrome). **A** AP radiograph. **B** AP tomogram with barium in esophagus. **C** AP radiograph with barium in esophagus made several days after **A** and **B**. Spontaneous rupture of esophagus is due to sudden development of markedly elevated intraluminal pressure within lower end of esophagus. In this patient, rupture occurred 48 h previously. Initial radiograph (**A**) showed diffuse bilateral mediastinal widening; normal mediastinal imprints are lost. Although no extravasation occurred at barium swallow (**B**), presence of air in mediastinum (*1*) coupled with history of vomiting made esophageal rupture a virtual certainty. Note significant air bronchogram in **B** due to lateral displacement of mediastinal pleurae about central bronchi. Although rupture is most commonly through left posterolateral wall of esophagus, an esophagram several days later (**C**) demonstrated perforation in this patient to be right sided

scending aorta. Continued posterior extension will widen the paraspinal line. Escape of fluid into the mediastinum and subsequent mediastinitis may ultimately cause diffuse mediastinal widening as demonstrated in Fig. 7.43. Initially, there may be localized collections of gas in the mediastinum (Fig. 7.43). At times gas dissects both paraspinally and beneath the parietal pleura of the left diaphragm to form a radiolucent angle resembling the letter V. This finding is referred to as the "V sign of Naclerio" [105] (see Fig. 3.19). As the process progresses, gas often dissects throughout the mediastinum and into the neck. Irritation of the pleura results in pleural effusion, which develops more commonly on the left side. Direct rupture of the process into the pleural space may occur. Perforation of the lower esophagus usually results in left pleural effusion while perforation of the midesophagus commonly results in right pleural effusion [63].

In most cases the diagnosis is readily confirmed by means of contrast examination of the esophagus. Iodinated contrast material is preferred if mediastinal or pleural perforation is suspected [46, 147]. Barium has been found to produce inflammatory foreign body reaction leading to fibrosis if it is introduced into the mediastinum in experimental animals [76]. Barium is safe, and preferred, if only a mucosal tear is suspected [31], and, according to some observers [46], should be used after a negative study with iodinated contrast material since the latter agent may fail to demonstrate a small percentage of tears.

In general, Boerhaave's syndrome carries an ominous prognosis, but the outcome is directly related to the promptness of diagnosis. The reported mortality associated with the delay of 12 h or less in the establishment of diagnosis and treatment is about 25%, but rises to 60% if the delay is over 12 h and up to 90% if the delay exceeds 48 h [130, 149]. Neff and Lawson [106] have reported a case successfully managed by balloon occlusion of the fistula.

Neurogenic Tumors

Tumors of neurogenic origin represent about 90% of all localized masses distorting the para-

spinal area and the paraspinal line [95]. With few exceptions, neurogenic tumors are posteriorly situated; they arise from structures within the spinal canal, the nerve roots, the intercostal nerves, and the sympathetic trunks. Tumors developing from the phrenic and vagus nerves are found further forward [124]. Histologically, neurogenic tumors may be neurofibromas, neurilemmomas, ganglioneuromas, ganglioneuroblastomas, or neuroblastomas. Mediastinal neuroblastoma is said to have a somewhat more favorable prognosis than neuroblastoma arising elsewhere [61].

Ganglioneuromas and ganglioneuroblastomas tend to arise more frequently from the sympathetic trunk, and although still posterior in position at the anterolateral margin of the spine, they tend to be located somewhat forward of the other neurogenic tumors. They are also more often fusiform in shape [95, 126]. Neurofibromas and neurilemmomas are found more posteriorly in the paraspinal area and adopt a round or oval shape [95, 126] (Figs. 7.44 and 3.11). They tend to produce rib separation or erosion of the ribs or spine. Absence of bony changes should not exclude a diagnosis of neurogenic tumor; large lesions of this type may be present without causing bony abnormality (see Fig. 3.11).

The various forms of foregut malformation may produce cystic lesions which are difficult or impossible to distinguish from neurogenic tumors [125]. Neurenteric cysts may also be difficult to differentiate. Vertebral body defects associated with spinal dysraphism are often a helpful clue to the diagnosis of neurenteric cyst [95, 107, 160]. Lymphoma and metastatic carcinoma should be considered in the differential diagnosis of neurogenic tumors since they, too, frequently produce paraspinal masses. Such masses are usually found in association with bone destruction. Many other much less common lesions, including abscess and hematoma, can affect the paraspinal area. Two of these rare processes, mediastinal varices and extramedullary hematopoesis, distort the paraspinal line in unique and often characteristic ways. They will be discussed briefly.

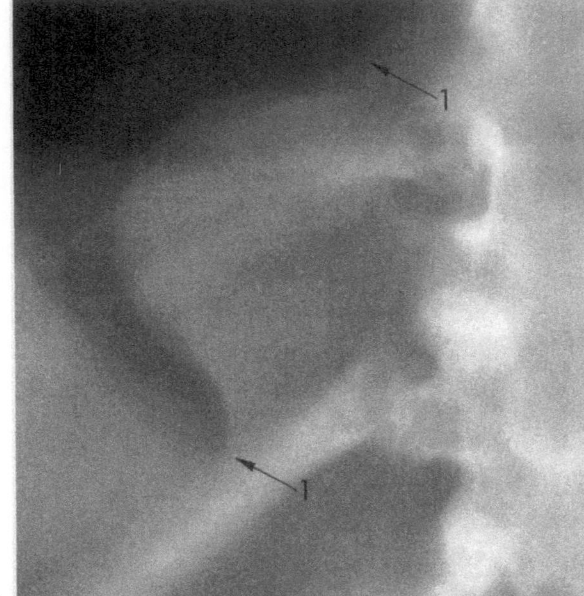

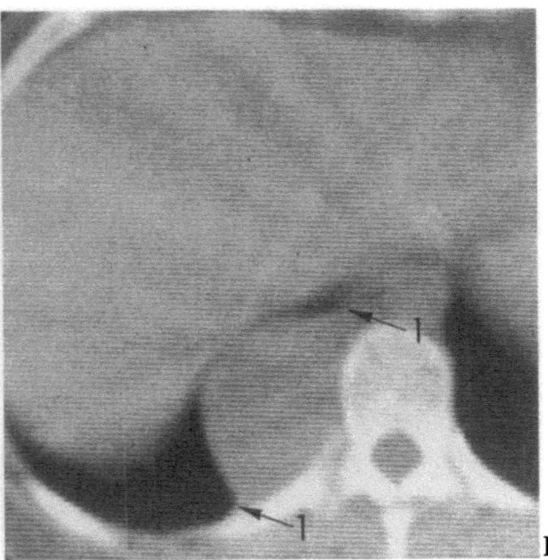

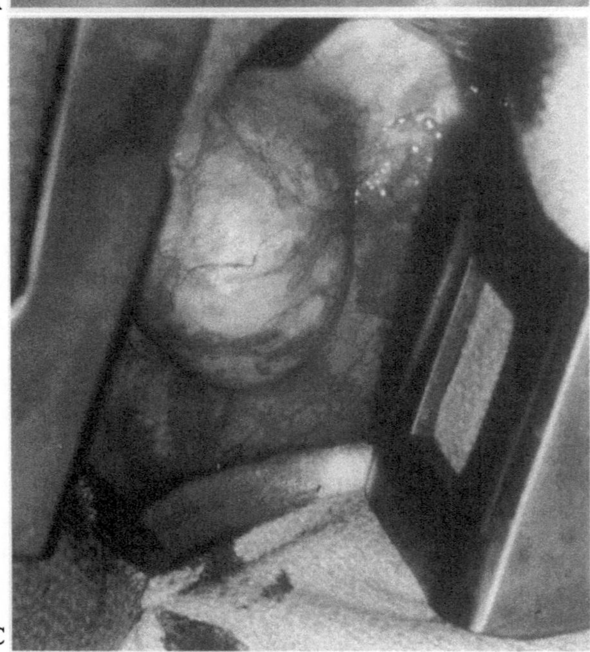

Fig. 7.44 A–C. Neurogenic tumor. **A** AP tomogram. **B** Computed tomogram. **C** Photograph made of lesion at surgery. This right paraspinal mass presented radiographic features of an extrapleural lesion. It shows sharp margin and obtuse angles at its base in two projections (*1*). Most localized paraspinal masses are neurogenic in origin. This mass was a neurilemoma

Venous Abnormalities

Dilated mediastinal veins produce an interesting variety of abnormal mediastinal contours above and below the aortic and the azygos arches [32, 86, 146]. These changes are discussed in the chapters on the supra-azygos areas (section 8.3) and on the supra-aortic area (section 6.2.2). An additional short discussion is included here because prominent azygos and hemiazygos veins in the paraspinal area so often produce shadows that distort the paraspinal line. These shadows can be smooth or lobulated.

A long, linear paraspinal venous shadow may be seen in azygos continuation of the inferior vena cava (see Fig. 8.26). In this condition congenital interruption of the infrahepatic portion of the inferior vena cava causes blood flow from the abdomen to be diverted into the azygos vein causing it to dilate and elongate. The enlarged vessel often protrudes laterally into the homolateral lung in a manner analogous to an elongated thoracic aorta. Hemiazygos continuation may show similar findings [157]; an example of this extremely rare anomaly is presented in Fig. 6.26. Another unusual variation is azygos continuation of a left inferior vena cava [45]. In this situation the dilated communication of the cava and the azygos vein may be seen as a more localized paraspinal mass on the left accompanying the prominent shadow of the azygos vein on the right.

When they are lobulated, paraspinal venous masses can simulate a number of other conditions, such as neurogenic tumor, lymphoma, enteric cyst, meningocele, paraspinal abscess, hematoma, and extramedullary hematopoesis, all of which should be considered in the differential diagnosis of a paraspinal mass lesion. Castellino et al. [20] have emphasized that dilated azygos and hemiazygos veins can produce lobulated masses in the paraspinal area bilaterally, that collateral blood flow can pass through the veins in either direction, and that such masses may change size with change in body position. Large lobulated venous shadows in the inferior paraspinal area can occur secondary to obstruction of the inferior vena cava and in patients with portal hypertension [32, 69, 74]

(Fig. 7.45). The radiologic diagnosis of mediastinal varices is supported by the finding of esophageal varices on a barium swallow. This association is not invariable (Fig. 7.45); in the 32 cases of mediastinal venous masses associated with portal hypertension, reported by Doyle et al. [32], esophageal varices were not demonstrated in one case and were of only minimal size in 14. The venous masses may impinge on the esophagus, producing extrinsic pressure defects (Fig. 7.45). Infrequently, rib notching is seen as a result of increased collateral blood flow through the intercostal veins [32]. Doyle et al. also state that at times widening of the paraspinal line in association with portal hypertension may be the result of edema of paraspinal soft tissues. Computed tomography with contrast enhancement is an excellent way to diagnose such venous abnormalities [41, 54]. Saks et al. [132] have described mediastinal abnormalities which may result from endoscopic injection therapy of esophageal varices.

Extramedullary Hematopoiesis

Extramedullary hematopoiesis is an unusual condition in which soft, bone marrow-like collections of tissue form focal tumors. This lesion most often presents as a lobulated mass or masses, frequently bilateral, in the paraspinal area between T-6 and T-12 [72, 145] (Fig. 7.46). Lowman et al. [92] have presented a case in which the masses were located in the upper paraspinal area. The condition is rare, only about 25 cases having been recorded in the literature up to 1969 [72]. It is extremely unusual to encounter a case in an individual younger than 20 years of age [145].

Extramedullary hematopoiesis is associated in most instances with some form of chronic hemolytic anemia, usually thalassemia or hereditary spherocytosis [145]. Papavasiliou [111] encountered five examples of the disease in 45 patients studied for thalassemia in Greece. Extramedullary hematopoiesis can also apparently develop in individuals with extensive marrow replacement by carcinoma or lymphoma [92]. However, in 25% of patients with extramedullary hematopoiesis no hematologic disease is

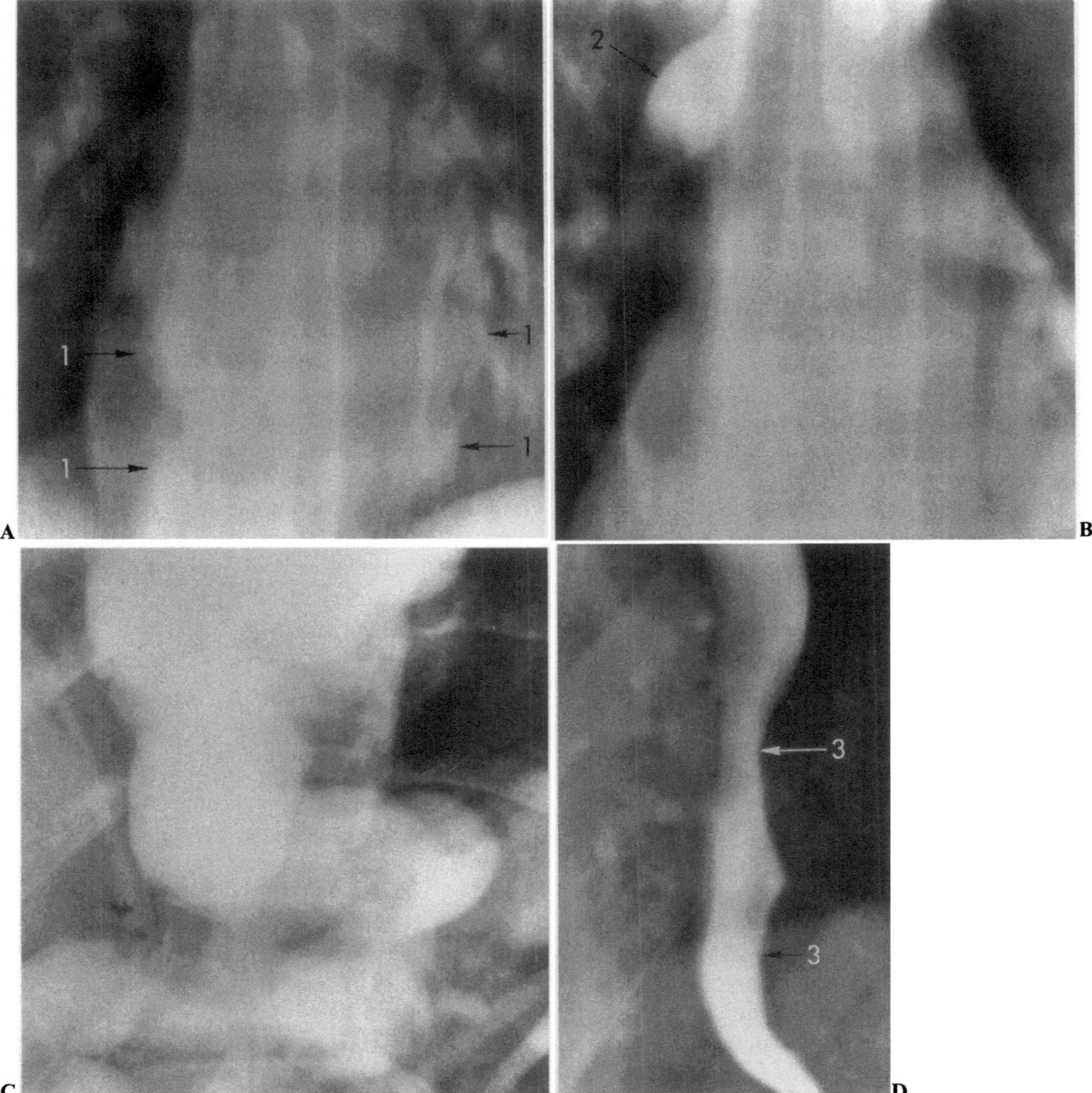

Fig. 45A–D. Mediastinal varices. **A** and **B** AP tomograms. **C** AP radiograph of venous phase from abdominal angiogram. **D** Right posterior oblique radiograph with barium in esophagus. In **A** bilateral lobulated masses (*1*) in patient with enlarged spleen caused lymphoma to be considered as possible diagnosis. Although mass shadows could not be made to change their config-uration with Valsalva's maneuver, large size of azygos vein (*2*) suggested possibility that this vessel was receiving increased flow through mediastinal varices. This was confirmed at angiography (**C**). Large venous masses impinge against esophagus (*3*), but in this patient, proven to have portal hypertension secondary to postnecrotic cirrhosis, esophageal varices were not present

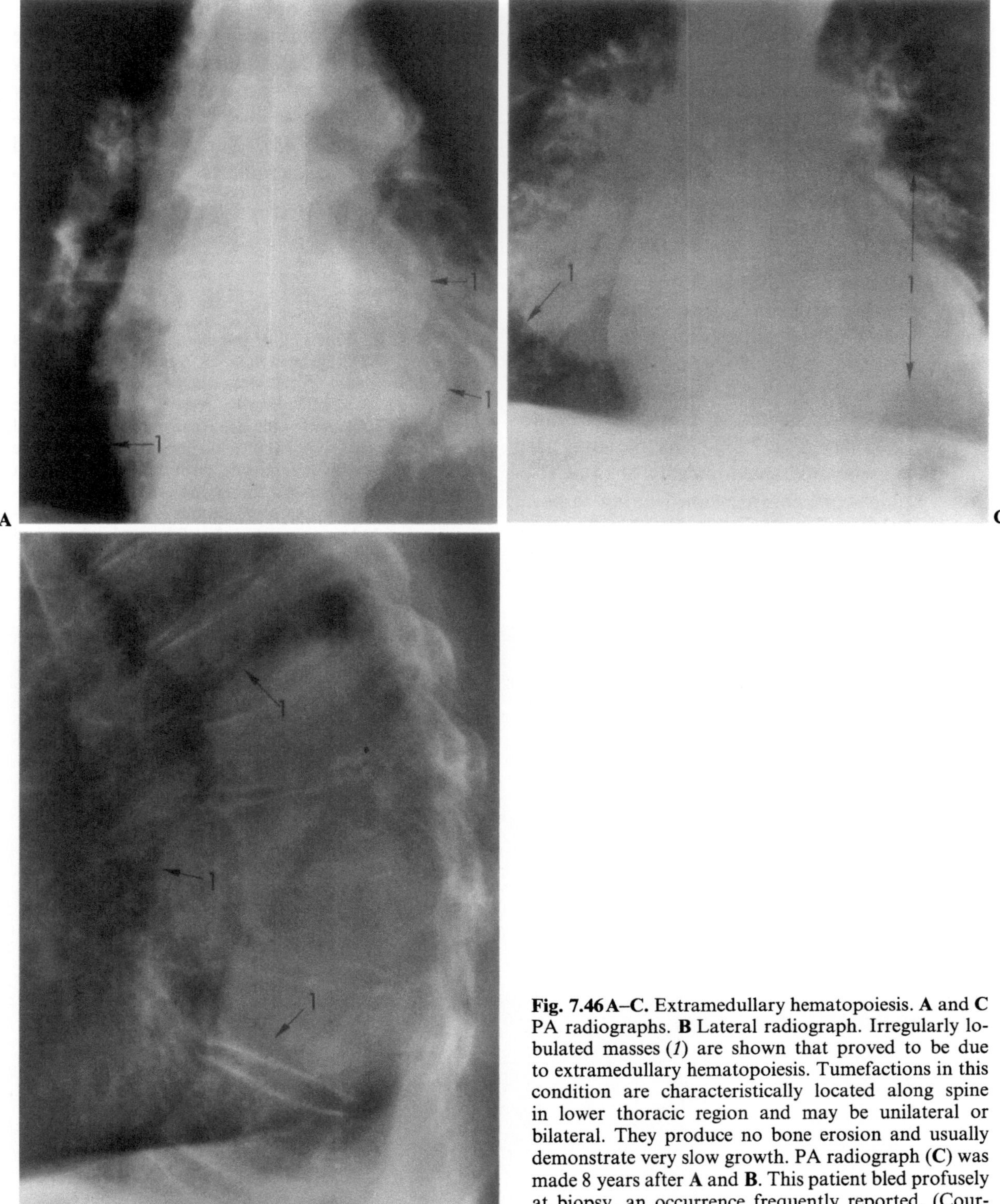

Fig. 7.46A–C. Extramedullary hematopoiesis. **A** and **C** PA radiographs. **B** Lateral radiograph. Irregularly lobulated masses (*1*) are shown that proved to be due to extramedullary hematopoiesis. Tumefactions in this condition are characteristically located along spine in lower thoracic region and may be unilateral or bilateral. They produce no bone erosion and usually demonstrate very slow growth. PA radiograph (**C**) was made 8 years after **A** and **B**. This patient bled profusely at biopsy, an occurrence frequently reported. (Courtesy G. Mitchell, Syracuse, NY)

found [145]; in some of these cases a family history of chronic hemolytic anemia can be elicited [72].

The pathogenetic mechanisms underlying the development of extramedullary hematopoiesis are obscure [2, 28, 138], as are the reasons for its predilection for the lower thoracic paraspinal area. One theory suggests that the process is an extension of heterotopic bone marrow from the intercostal veins [2, 109].

On radiographic examinations, extramedullary hematopoiesis produces bilateral, lobulated masses in the paraspinal area along the lower thoracic spine. They are slow growing (Fig. 7.46) and produce no bone erosion. They are ideally demonstrated with computed tomography [91] (see Fig. 7.53). The patients need not have associated splenomegaly or bone sclerosis. Spinal cord compression leading to paraparesis has been reported [64, 92, 109]. The process may simulate other paraspinal masses; one

reported case was operated upon with a preoperative diagnosis of neurogenic tumor [82]. The diagnosis should be established by open biopsy under direct vision since the masses are highly vascular and tend to bleed profusely when incised [82] (Fig. 7.46). Surgical excision and radiotherapy are the preferred methods of treatment [145].

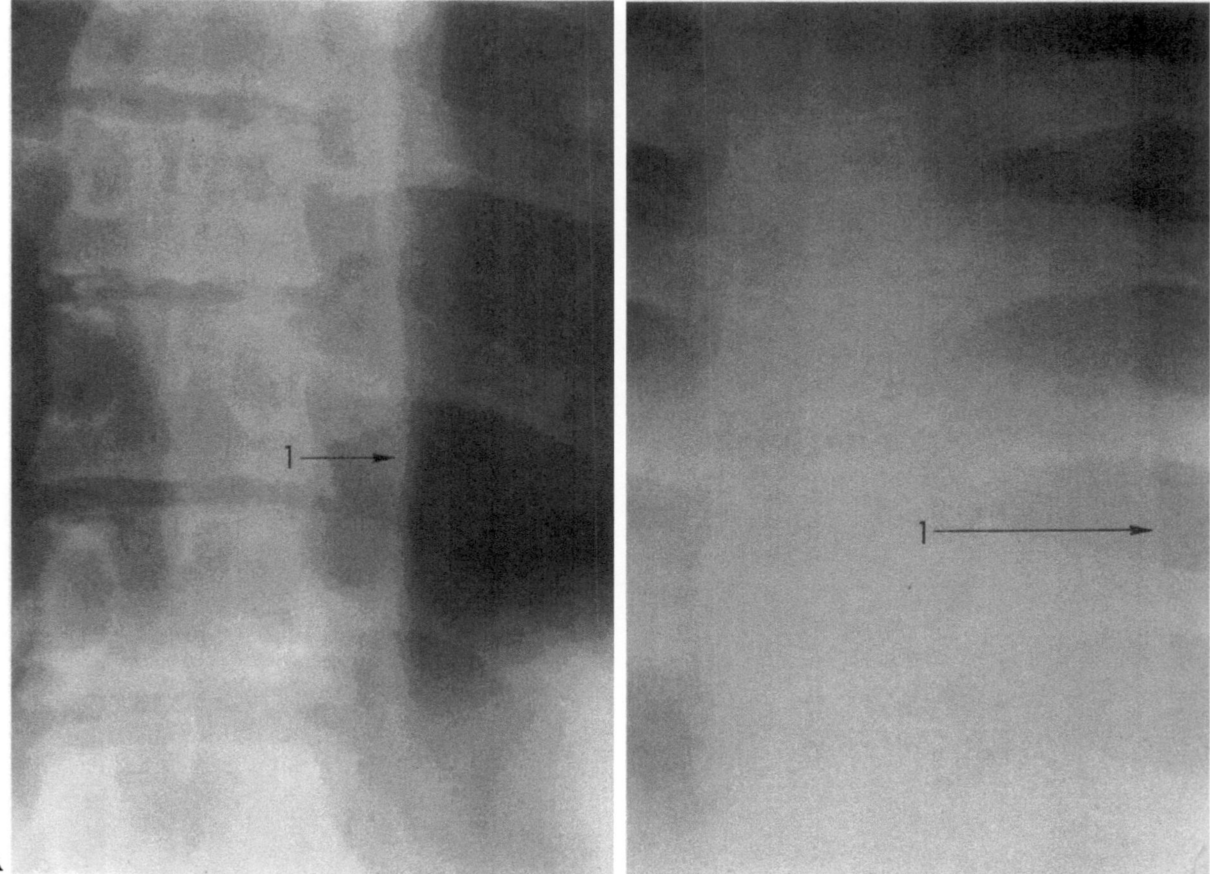

Fig. 7.47 A, B. Widening of paraspinal line in Cushing's syndrome (AP radiographs). In A normal paraspinal area is identified with distinct paraspinal line visible (1). Following period of high-dose steroid therapy, diffuse widening of paraspinal area has occurred and paraspinal line is far lateral. Note that it no longer seems to have radiolucency on its medial side, probably due to edema of paraspinal fat. Steroid therapy is well known to produce widening of upper mediastinum due to fat deposition; it should be appreciated that fat may be deposited in other extrapleural areas

A

B

Abnormal Fatty Infiltration

Widening of the anterior mediastinum and of the supra-azygos and supra-aortic areas by fatty infiltration secondary to Cushing's disease or high-dose steroid therapy is well known [12, 120] and has been reviewed in the section on the anterior mediastinum (see Figs. 5.24 and 5.25). The presence of a considerable quantity of fat in the paraspinal area provides an opportunity for widening of the paraspinal line in these conditions as well [148] (Fig. 7.47). Sometimes widening of extrapleural soft tissues adjacent to the ribs can be identified. These findings may be of help in radiologic differential diagnosis when large doses of steroids are being used in the treatment of lymphoma. Under these circumstances it may be difficult to determine whether widening of the anterior mediastinum or of the supra-aortic and supra-azygos areas is due to advancing lymphoma or steroid-induced fatty infiltration on plain radiographs. Widening of the paraspinal line or extrapleural soft tissues, if present, should favor steroid-induced fat deposition on a statistical basis. Computed tomographic examination easily resolves the dilemma [5, 33, 73].

The presence of considerable periaortic fat is a not infrequent normal mediastinal variant. It can, however, sometimes pose problems in the interpretation of chest radiographs. Several authors have measured the thickness of the aortic wall as the distance between contrast in the aorta and the adjacent lung or between intimal calcification and the lung [89, 141]. It has been said that this distance should not exceed 5 mm in normal individuals, and that, if it does, aortic dissection is likely. However, Price and Rigler [120] have reported three cases in which abundant periaortic fat interposed itself between the aorta and lung to produce measurements in excess of the stated normal values. This fact, of course, decreases the value of aortic wall measurement as a sign of aortic dissection. Localized collections of paraspinal fat presenting as paraspinal masses on plain films are not rare [53].

Pleural Effusion

Free pleural fluid will sometimes collect against the paraspinal soft tissues, displacing lung laterally and thus simulating widening of the paraspinal line on supine and sometimes erect radiographs [151]. When this occurs, the apparent widening is greater at the level of the diaphragm than it is above, since the triangular-shaped inferior pulmonary ligament binds the lung closer to the mediastinum at the hilar level than it does at the lung base [123] (see chapter 10). Decubitus radiographs will show the abnormality to be due to free fluid rather than to true paraspinal disease.

7.2.6 The Diaphragmatic Crura

7.2.6.1 Anatomic Considerations

Prior to the advent of computed tomography, the diaphragmatic crura received relatively little attention in the radiologic literature. In part, this was due to the fact that they are not often visible on conventional radiographs, although Whalen and Shaheen [159] point out that they may be outlined by extraperitoneal fat in some patients. The crura are, however, almost always identified on computed tomographic examinations; as a result they have now assumed greater significance in radiologic interpretation [17, 139].

The diaphragmatic crura form the anterior and lateral margins of the aortic hiatus in the diaphragm, an area bounded posteriorly by the body of the first lumbar vertebra [27] (Fig. 7.48). At their origins they are tendinous in nature and blend with the anterior longitudinal ligament of the vertebral column. The right crus is larger and longer than the left and arises from the anterior surfaces of the bodies and intervertebral fibrocartilages of the upper three lumbar vertebrae (Figs. 7.48, 7.49). Its sometimes strikingly fusiform appearance should not be mistaken for adenopathy on computed tomographic examinations (Fig. 7.49). The left crus stems from the upper two lumbar vertebrae only. The crura pass forward and medially to form an arch across the aorta (Figs. 7.48, 7.49).

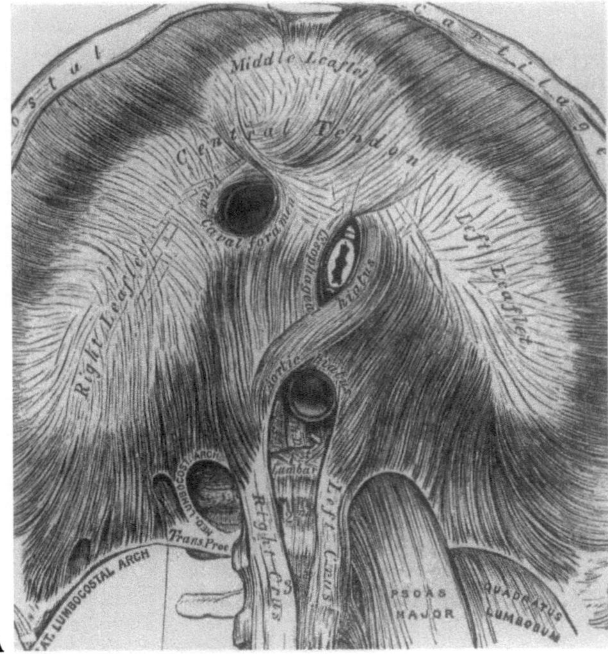
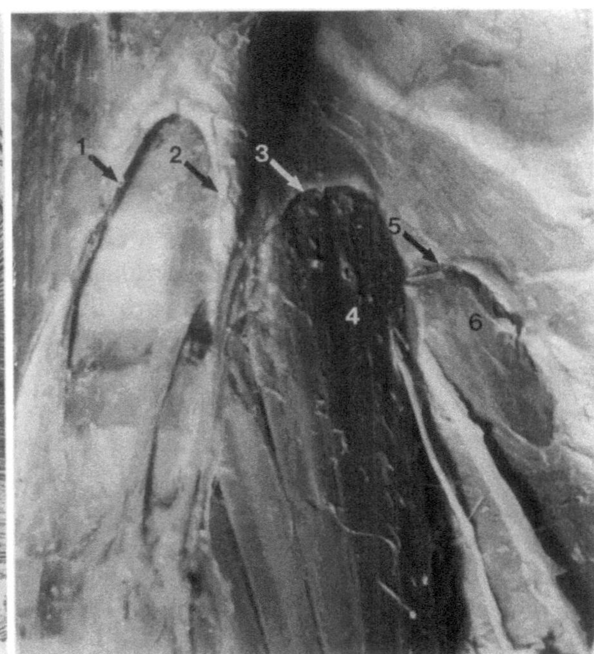

Fig. 7.48A, B. Anatomy of the diaphragmatic crura. **A** Inferior aspect of the diaphragm. **B** Photograph of the inferior aspect of the diaphragm from an anatomic specimen (the aorta has been removed). The aortic hiatus in the diaphragm is an osseoaponeurotic space behind the diaphragm formed by the right (*1*) and left (*2*) crural arches anterolaterally and the first lumbar vertebra posteriorly. On either side of the hiatus lie the medial lumbocostal arches (*3*) for passage of the psoas major muscles (*4*) and lateral to them are found the lateral lumbocostal arches (*5*) which are traversed by the quadratus lumborum muscles (*6*). These arches communicate the mediastinum with the posterior pararenal spaces of the abdomen. (**A** From [58])

The azygos vein, the hemiazygos vein, and the thoracic duct pass through this aperture with the aorta (Fig. 7.49). The demonstration of a dilated azygos vein in the aortic hiatus on computed tomograms is the ideal noninvasive way to diagnose azygos continuation of the inferior vena cava [54, 157] (see Fig. 8.26). Silverman et al. [143] have reported that exceptionally lung may be encountered in a retrocrural space. Apparently lung "herniates" into this position carrying the mediastinal pleura ahead of it.

Laterally, each crus is continuous with the medial lumbocostal arch or internal arcuate ligament, a tendinous arch in the fascia covering the psoas major muscle (Fig. 7.48). The lateral lumbocostal arch or external arcuate ligament encompassing the quadratus lumborum muscle is found lateral to the medial lumbocostal arch (Fig. 7.48).

7.2.6.2 Influence of Crura on Thoracoabdominal Extension of Tumor

Strictly speaking, the aortic hiatus is not an aperture in the diaphragm but an osseoaponeurotic opening behind the diaphragm and in front of the prevertebral fascia of the vertebral column [27]. The lumbar (lateral aortic) lymph nodes and the intestinal lymphatic trunks drain into the thoracic duct just below the hiatus. The importance of this area as an avenue for tumor spread is further enhanced by the fact that the posterior diaphragmatic lymph nodes lie on the back of the diaphragmatic crura.

Therefore, the hiatus and the lumbocostal arches, constitute avenues across which retroperitoneal disease processes extend from the abdomen into the thorax and vice versa; since the crura marginate the aortic hiatus and the medial aspect of the medial lumbocostal arch, they influence this spread of disease in a significant way. In turn, disease processes envelop and sometimes displace the crura.

Gray's Anatomy [27] states that the arch formed by the crura about the aorta is often poorly developed. On computed tomograms, however, it is one of the most consistently demonstrated of all normal anatomic landmarks (Fig. 7.49). On computed tomograms the arch formed by the crura resembles a croquet wicket leaning slightly to the left as it encompasses the aorta lying slightly to the left of the midline. The medial and lateral surfaces of each crus can usually be identified.

Computed tomography will commonly demonstrate evidence of retrocrural adenopathy [140]. Often, enlarged, discrete, nodes are seen (Fig. 7.51), but other signs of neoplastic disease crossing the aortic hiatus may be encountered. For example, since the crura are seen so often, failure to visualize them at computed tomography suggests their envelopment by disease (Figs. 7.50, 7.51, 7.53). More significant is the demonstration of only one crus (Fig. 7.51). A finding of major diagnostic importance is marked splaying of the crura, an appearance virtually pathognomonic of a solid mass crossing the aortic hiatus (Figs. 7.50, 7.53). Such a

finding also indicates unequivocally that the process is extrapleural in the thorax and retroperitoneal in the abdomen. The infra-aortic and infra-azygos areas of the mediastinum communicate freely with the posterior pararenal space of the abdomen [13, 100]. Knowledge of this anatomic fact helps to explain the rare situation in which pancreatic pseudocyst enters the mediastinum through the aortic hiatus [80, 142] (Fig. 7.52).

On occasion, masses may pass through the aortic hiatus and under the medial lumbocostal arch as well. When this occurs, computed tomograms may show a bilobate characteristic due to the extension of the disease through the apertures on either side of restraining influence of the medial crus. One lobe of the mass, that which crosses the aortic hiatus, is anterior and medial; the second, usually a smaller lobe, is posterior and lateral. Such a bilobate appearance at the diaphragmatic level is also virtually diagnostic of the retroperitoneal location of an abdominal mass (Fig. 7.53).

Felson has described a variation of the silhouette sign, which he has termed the "thoracoabdominal sign" [42]. Masses outlined by lung at their upper end, but silhouetted out inferiorly at the level of the diaphragm must lie in both the chest and abdomen (Fig. 7.54). An abnormal mediastinal contour, the lower end of which courses laterally as it approaches the diaphragm, suggests that the process is predominantly abdominal and that only the "tip of the iceberg" is being outlined by lung. The demonstration of such a finding, often minimal and requiring close scrutiny of well-penetrated films, may be the earliest radiographic evidence of an abdominal mass [42] (Fig. 7.54). Pathology revealing itself in such a manner is often extending into the thorax through the medial lumbocostal arch and sometimes through the aortic hiatus. Divergence of the inferior extent of the process from the spine is less marked when the disease lies more forward and passes through the aortic hiatus because of the restraining influence of the crura.

It is a rather frequent experience to see the paraspinal line deviate somewhat laterally as it approaches the diaphragm. Often it is difficult

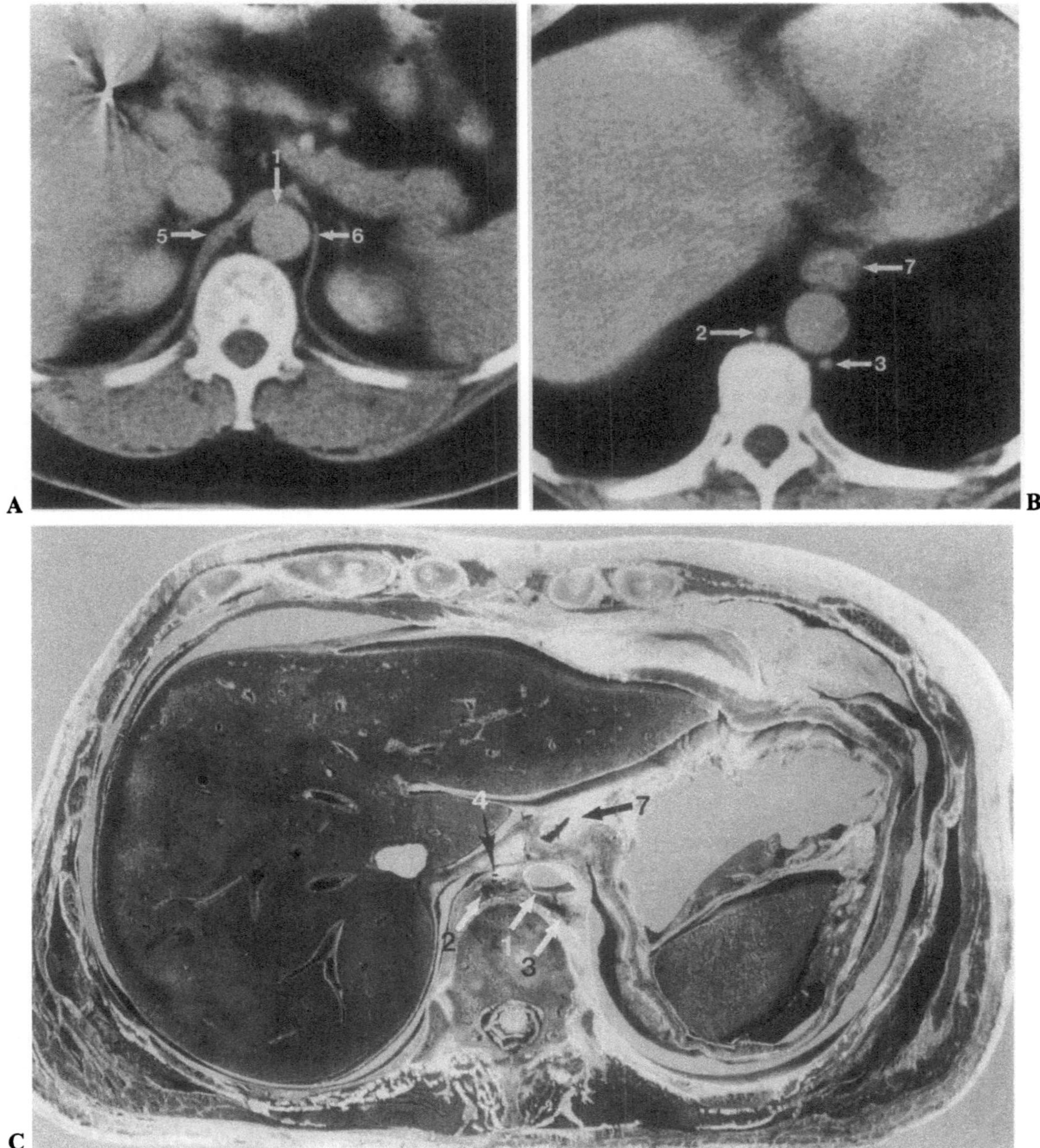

Fig. 7.49 A–C. Anatomy of the diaphragmatic crura as shown at computed tomography. **A** and **B** Computed tomograms. **C** Transverse body section. The crural arches encompass the aorta (*1*). The aortic hiatus is also traversed by the azygos vein (*2*), the hemiazygos vein (*3*) and the thoracic duct (*4*). The posterior diaphragmatic lymph nodes lie on the dorsal aspect of the crura (see Fig. 7.51). The right crus (*5*), as shown in **A**, is normally larger than the left (*6*) and, at times, may simulate an enlarged node. The esophageal hiatus (*7*) lies immediately anterior and somewhat to the left of the aortic hiatus

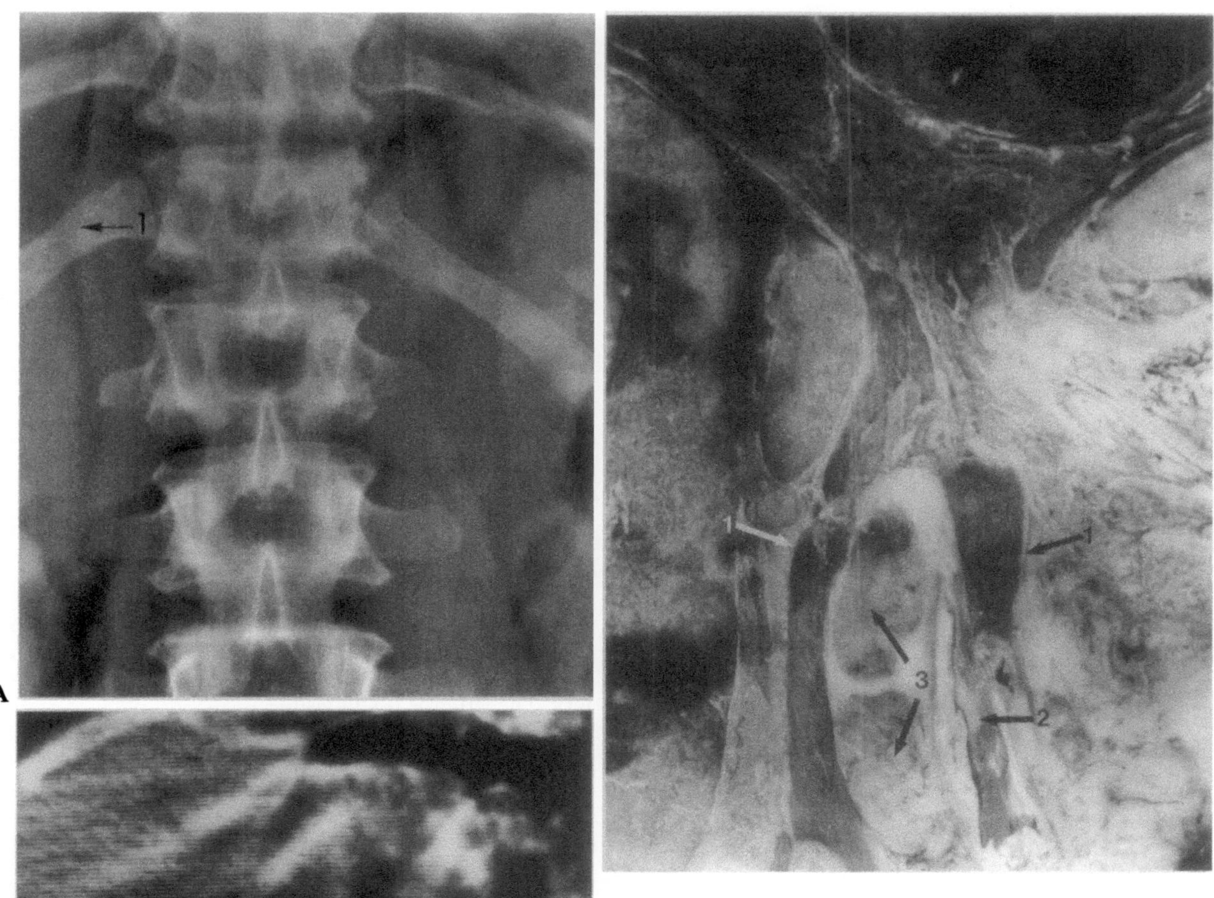

Fig. 7.50 A–C. Thoracoabdominal extension of tumor across the aortic hiatus. **A** AP radiograph. **B** Computed tomogram. **C** Coronal body section of a different patient. Tumor crossing the aortic hiatus can cause marked splaying of the crural arches (*1*). Note that in **B** the hiatus is expanded and, although the crura are still visible, the aorta is surrounded by tumor and cannot be seen. In **C** the aorta (*2*) is displaced to the left by enlarged lymph nodes (*3*)

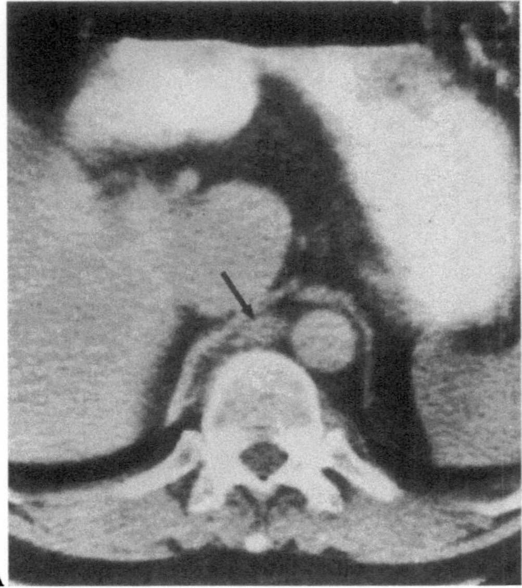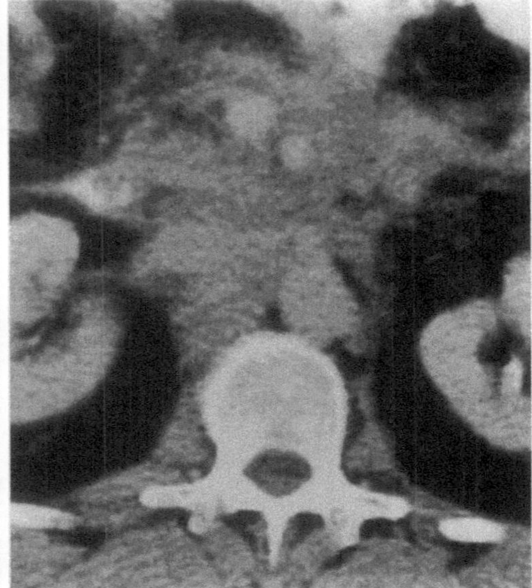

Fig. 7.51 A, B. Thoracoabdominal extension of tumor across the aortic hiatus. Computed tomograms. In this patient a single, retrocrural node (*arrow*) is seen in the upper portion of the aortic hiatus. Lower down (**B**) the outline of the right crus is obliterated by tumor which has extended forward to involve the root of the mesentery. The left crus is still visible

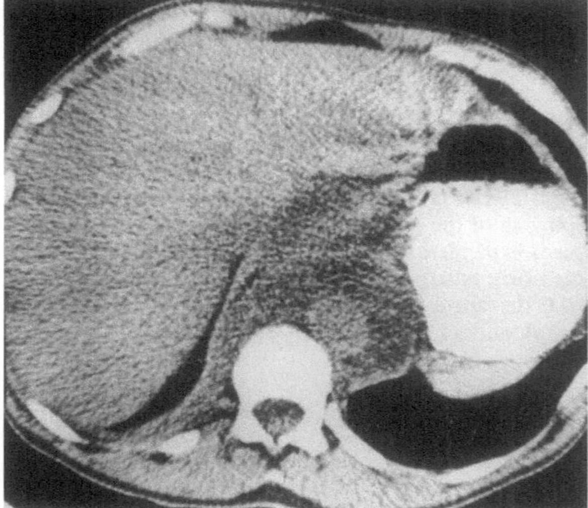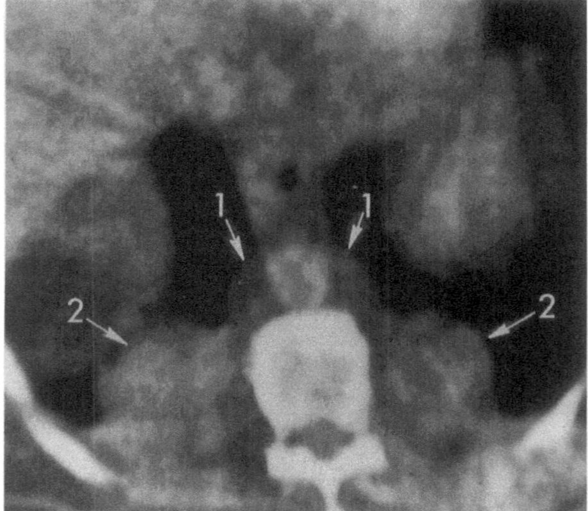

Fig. 7.52. Pancreatic pseudocyst crossing the aortic hiatus. Computed tomogram. Meyers [100] has demonstrated the pathway by which a pancreatic pseudocyst can migrate into the posterior pararenal space. Since this space communicates freely with the mediastinum across the aortic hiatus (see text), it would be expected that, rarely, a pseudocyst would be found crossing the hiatus into the mediastinum. (From [142])

Fig. 7.53. Thoracoabdominal extension of tumor across the aortic hiatus and the medial lumbocostal arches. This computed tomogram demonstrates splaying of diaphragmatic crura (*1*). Note that medial side of each crus cannot be visualized because normal fat in this area is replaced by tissue representing extramedullary hematopoesis. The process is also extending through medial lumbocostal arch on each side (*2*). This lobulated appearance, due to mass in aortic hiatus and in medial lumbocostal arches, is pathognomonic of retroperitoneal extension of tumor

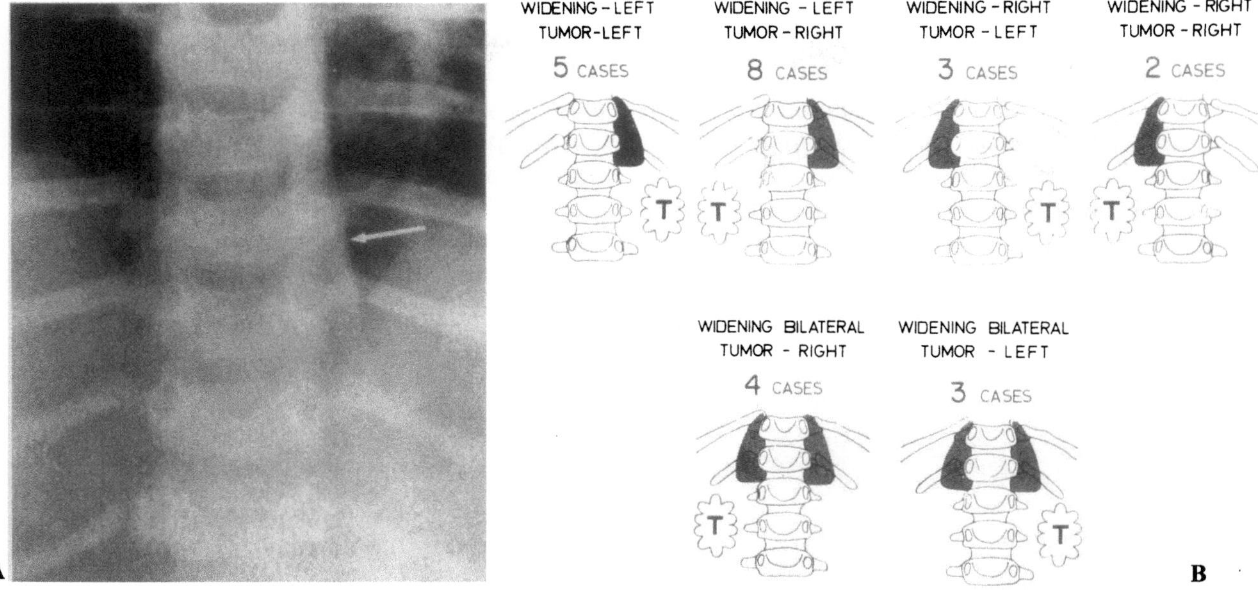

A   **B**

to exclude the possibility that this configuration of the paraspinal line reflects the cephalad edge of an abdominal mass. Eklof and Gooding [39] pointed out that this appearance was often a reflection of cephalad extension of tumor in children with neuroblastoma (Fig. 7.54). The configuration can, however, be a normal variant. Rarely, it is caused by the contact of left lower lobe with the extreme upper end of the psoas major muscle passing through the medial lumbocostal arch. Computed tomograms and, less often, plain films that show such a configuration extending in continuity with the psoas muscle in the abdomen suggest that the appearance is a normal variant. At times, fat in the aortic hiatus or medial lumbocostal arch will simulate the thoracoabdominal sign caused by tumor. Other radiographic examinations and careful follow-up with repeat radiographic studies will be necessary to exclude disease in many cases.

Fig. 7.54A, B. The thoracoabdominal sign. **A** AP radiograph. **B** Drawing. Felson [42] has described the thoracoabdominal sign. Masses outlined by lung at their upper end (*arrow*), but silhouetted out inferiorly at the level of the diaphragm must lie in both the chest and the abdomen. This sign is rather frequently seen in children with neuroblastoma; the experience of Eklof and Gooding [39] with 25 such cases is outlined in chart form in **B**. (**A** and **B** From [39])

7.2.6.3 The Crus Sign

At times, distinction of pleural fluid from ascites can be difficult on computed tomograms. Decubitus chest films or prone computed tomographic studies of course resolve the problem, but it is preferrable to make the distinction without resort to supplemental studies [62]. Dwyer [36] has pointed out an observation called the "displaced crus" or "crus sign" which aids in differentiation of pleural fluid from ascites. The terminology used is unfortunate since the crura are tendinous and are not altered by fluid above or below the diaphragm; it is the posterior muscular portions of the diaphragm arising from the crura which are displaced. Fluid above the diaphragm will widen the angle made by the posteromedial diaphragm and the crura while ascites will not (Fig. 7.55).

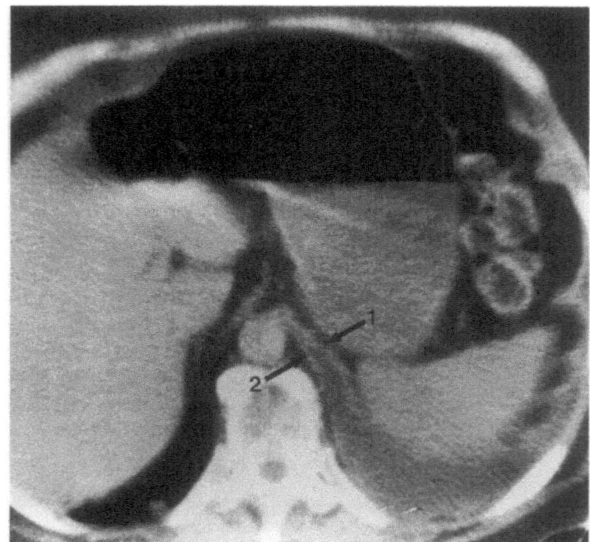

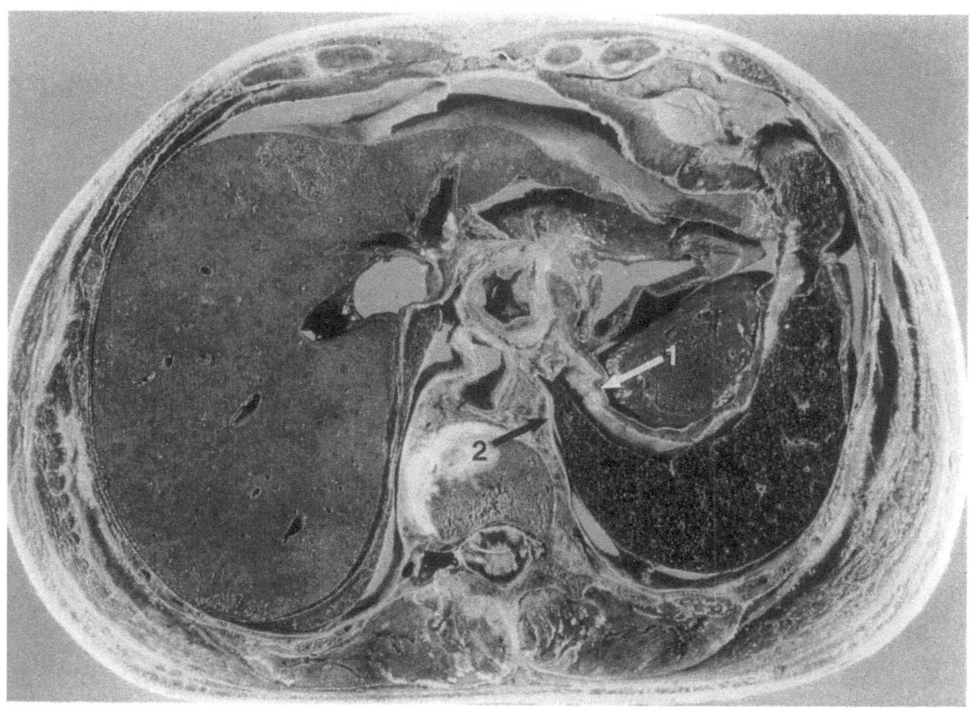

Fig. 7.55A, B. The crus sign. A Computed tomogram. B Transverse body section. The distinction of pleural fluid from ascites on computed tomograms can be difficult. The crus sign is helpful; fluid above the diaphragm will widen the angle made by the posteromedial aspect of the diaphragm (*1*) and the crura (*2*) while ascites will not

7.2.6.4 The Median Crus Syndrome (the Coeliac Artery Compression Syndrome)

Compression of the celiac artery by the diaphragmatic crura as they pass in front of the aorta is termed the "median crus syndrome." In most individuals the crura cross the aorta just above the origin of the celiac artery [127]. This relationship is variable. Angiography has shown that the angle made by the celiac artery with the aorta is more acute in inspiration. In expiration the celiac artery, like the other viscera, moves cephalad, and the angle made by the vessel with the aorta is more nearly 90° [37]. Expiration tends to bring the celiac artery into contact with the crura which compress its anterior aspect. If crus contact causes significant luminal narrowing, the median crus syndrome is thought by some observers to result. To relieve the condition, surgical division of the crural arch has been advocated [96]. The existence of this condition as a true clinical entity is, however, seriously doubted by many experts [150].

7.2.6.5 The Crura and Injury to the Thoracic Duct

Brown [15] has reported a case of traumatic rupture of the thoracic duct that he drained extrapleurally through the bed of the twelfth rib. He conjectured that laceration of the duct was caused by its impingement against the fixed and sharp crural arch resulting from hyperextension of the spine. A drawing of the surgical procedure in this case shows lateral bulging of the right crus of the diaphragm (Fig. 7.56), an abnormality that in this day might be demonstrated by computed tomography. Green [59] drew the same conclusion in a case of chylothorax resulting from child abuse.

Fig. 7.56. Laceration of the thoracic duct by blunt trauma. This drawing of surgical findings in patient with right chylothorax shows collection of chyle within aortic hiatus. It has been suggested that hyperextension injuries may cause thoracic duct to be torn by sharp edge of the crural arch. See Fig. 7.49. (Modified from [15])

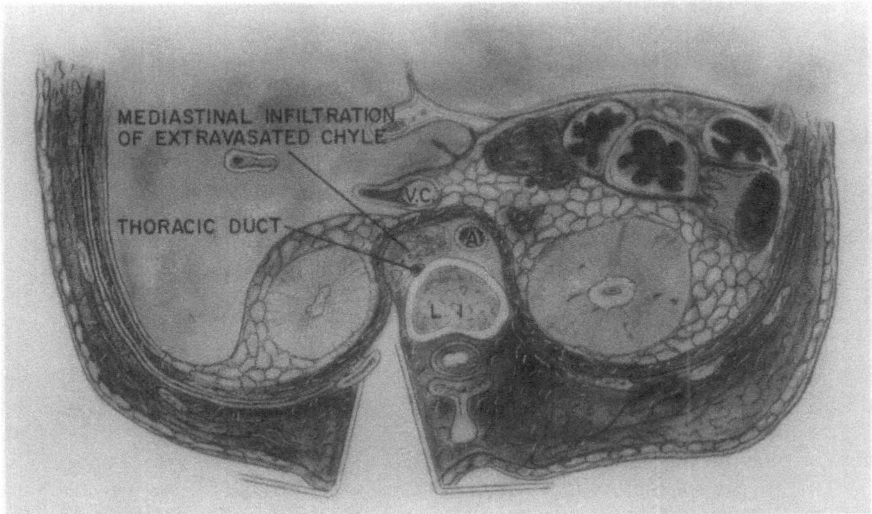

References

1. Alley RD, VanMierop LHS, Li EY, Jagdish KR, Kausel HW, Stranahan A (1966) Traumatic aortic aneurysm – four cases of graftless excision and anastomosis. Ann Thorac Surg 2:514–524
2. Ask-Upmark E (1945) Tumor simulating intrathoracic heterotopia of bone marrow. Acta Radiol 26:425–440
3. Baltaxe HA, Constable WC (1968) Mediastinal lymph node visualization in the absence of intrathoracic disease. Radiology 90:94–98
4. Barcia TC, Livoni JP (1983) Indications for angiography in blunt thoracic trauma. Radiology 149:639–642
5. Bein ME, Mancuso AA, Mink JH, Hansen GC (1978) Computed tomography in the evaluation of mediastinal lipomatosis. J Comput Assist Tomogr 2:379–383
6. Bennett BE, Cherry JK (1967) The natural history of traumatic aneurysms of the aorta. Surgery 61:516–523
7. Berne AS, Gerle RD, Mitchell GE (1969) The mediastinum – normal roentgen anatomy and radiologic techniques. Semin Roentgenol 4:4–21
8. Billing L (1946) On retrocardiac pulmo-pleural demarcation lines and their diagnostic significance. Acta Radiol 27:257–262
9. Birt AB, Connolly NK (1952) Traumatic chylothorax – a report of a case and a survey of the literature. Br J Surg 39:564–568
10. Blank N, Castellino RA (1972) Patterns of pleural reflections of the left superior mediastinum – normal anatomy and distortions produced by adenopathy. Radiology 102:585–589
11. Bobo WO, Billups WA, Hardy JB (1970) Boerhaave's syndrome: a review of six cases of spontaneous rupture of the esophaagus, secondary to vomiting. Ann Surg 172:1034–1038
12. Bodman SF, Condemi JJ (1967) Mediastinal widening in iatrogenic Cushing's syndrome. Ann Intern Med 67:399–403
13. Borlaza GS, Kuhns LR, Siegel RS, Rapp R (1979) The posterior pararenal space: an escape route for retrocrural masses. J Comput Assist Tomogr 3:470–473
14. Brailsford JF (1943) The radiographic posteromedial border of the lung, or the linear thoracic paraspinal shadow. Radiology 41:34–37
15. Brown AL (1937) Traumatic rupture of the thoracic duct with bilateral chylothorax and chylous ascites: new operation-report of a case. Arch Surg 34:120–128
16. Brownstein EG (1969) Spontaneous rupture of the distal thoracic esophagus. Med J Aust 1:849–852
17. Callen PW, Filly RA, Korobkin M (1978) Computed tomographic evaluation of the diaphragmatic crura. Radiology 126:413–416
18. Cammack K, Rapport RL, Paul J, Baird WC (1959) Deceleration injuries of the thoracic aorta. Arch Surg 79:244–251
19. Carey JP, Stemmer EA, Connolly JE (1969) Median arcuate ligament syndrome. Arch Surg 99:441–446
20. Castellino RA, Blank N, Adams DF (1968) Dilated azygous and hemiazygous veins presenting as paravertebral intrathoracic masses. N Engl J Med 278:1087–1091
21. Christoforidis A, Nelson SW (1957) Spontaneous rupture of the esophagus with emphasis on roentgenologic diagnosis. Am J Roentgenol 78:574–580
22. Cimmino CV (1956) The esophageal-pleural stripe on chest teleroentgenograms. Radiology 67:754–756
23. Cimmino CV (1965) A roentgenologic study in mediastinal anatomy afforded by air in the mid-esophagus – a normal finding but a potential source of diagnostic error. Am J Roentgenol Radium Ther Nucl Med 94:333–338
24. Cimmino CV (1961) Further notes on the esophageal-pleural stripe. Radiology 77:974–978
25. Cimmino CV (1985) Esophageal-pleural stripe: an update. Radiology 140:609–613
26. Cimmino CV, Snead LO (1965) The posterior mediastinal line on chest roentgenograms. Radiology 84:516–518
27. Clemente CD (1985) Anatomy of the human body by Henry Gray, 30th Am edn. Lea and Febiger, Philadelphia
28. Condon WB, Safarik LR, Elzi EP (1965) Extramedullary hematopoiesis simulating intrathoracic tumor. Arch Surg 90:643–647
29. Currarino G, Jackson JH (1970) Calcification of the ductus arteriosus and ligamentum Botalli. Radiology 94:139–142
30. Dalton CJ, Schwartz SS (1956) Evaluation of the paraspinal line in roentgen examination of the thorax. Radiology 66:195–200
31. Dodds WJ, Stewart ET, Vlymen WJ (1982) Appropriate contrast media for evaluation of esophageal disruption. Radiology 144:439–441
32. Doyle FH, Read AE, Evans KT (1961) The mediastinum in portal hypertension. Clin Radiol 12:114–129
33. Drasin GF, Lynch T, Temes GP (1978) Ectopic ACTH production and mediastinal lipomatosis. Radiology 127:610
34. Drinker CK, Yoffee JM (1941) Lymphatics, lymph and lymphoid tissue. Harvard University Press, Cambridge
35. Duffie ER, Moss AJ, Maloney JV (1962) Congenital pericardial defects with herniation of heart into the pleural space. Pediatrics 30:746–748
36. Dwyer A (1978) The displaced crus: a sign for distinguishing between pleural fluid and ascites on computed tomography. J Comput Assist Tomogr 2:598–599
37. Edwards AJ, Hamilton JD, Nichol WD (1970) Experiences with coeliac axis compression syndrome. Br Med J 1:342–345
38. Edwards EA, Malone PD, Collins JJ Jr (1972) Operative anatomy of the thorax. Lea and Febiger, Philadelphia

39. Eklof O, Gooding CA (1967) Paravertebral widening in cases of neuroblastoma. Br J Radiol 40:358–365

40. Ellis K, Leeds NE, Himmelstein A (1959) Congenital deficiencies in the pericardium – a review of two cases including successful diagnosis by plain roentgenography. Am J Roentgenol Radium Ther Nucl Med 82:125–137

41. Engel IA, Auh YH, Rubenstein WA, Sniderman K, Whalen JP, Kazam E (1983) CT diagnosis of mediastinal and thoracic inlet venous obstruction. AJR 141:521–526

42. Felson B (1973) Chest roentgenology. Saunders, Philadelphia

43. Fisher RG, Ward BE, Ben-Menachem Y, Maltox KL, Flynn TC (1982) Arteriography and the fractured first rib: too much for too little? AJR 138:1059–1062

44. Flaherty TJ, Wegner GP, Crummy AB, Francyk WP, Hipona FA (1969) Non-penetrating injuries to the thoracic aorta. Radiology 92:541–546

45. Floyd GD, Nelson WP (1976) Developmental interruption of the inferior vena cava with azygos and hemiazygos substitution. Radiology 119:55–57

46. Foley MJ, Ghahremani GG, Rogers LF (1982) Reappraisal of contrast media used to detect upper gastrointestinal perforations. Comparison of ionic water-soluble media with barium sulfate. Radiology 144:231–237

47. Fosburg RG, O'Sullivan JJ, As-Tye P, Bibbons JA, Oury JH (1974) Positive mediastinoscopy – an ominous finding. Ann Thorac Surg 18:346–356

48. Freed TA, Neal MP Jr, Vinik M (1968) Roentgenographic findings in extracardiac injury secondary to blunt chest automobile trauma. Am J Roentgenol Radium Ther Nucl Med 104:424–432

49. Garland LH (1942) The linear thoracic paraspinal shadow. Radiology 39:229

50. Garland LH (1943) The postero-medial pleural line. Radiology 41:29–33

51. Genereux GP (1983) The posterior pleural reflections. AJR 141:141–149

52. Gladnikoff H (1948) A radiographic study of the mediastinum in health and pulmonary carcinoma. Acta Radiol [Suppl] 73:1–87

53. Glickstein MF, Miller WT, Dalinka MK, Lally JF (1987) Paraspinal lipomatosis: a benign mass. Radiology 163:79–80

54. Godwin JD, Chen JTT (1986) Thoracic venous anatomy. AJR 147:674–684

55. Goldberg EM, Shapiro CM, Glicksman HS (1974) Mediastinoscopy for assessing mediastinal spread in clinical staging of lung carcinoma. Semin Oncol 1:205–215

56. Goldstein LA, Thompson WR (1982) Esophageal perforation: a 15 year experience. Am J Surg 143:495–503

57. Goorwitch J (1955) Traumatic chylothorax: a review of the literature and report of a case treated by mediastinal ligation of the thoracic duct. J Thorac Surg 29:467–479

58. Gray H (1974) Lewis WH (ed) Anatomy of the human body. Lea and Febiger, Philadelphia

59. Green HG (1980) Child abuse presenting as chylothorax. Pediatrics 66:620–621

60. Greendyke RM (1966) Traumatic rupture of the aorta – special reference to automobile accidents. JAMA 195:527–530

61. Griff LC, Griff RE (1968) Neuroblastoma – emphasis on mediastinal neuroblastoma. Am J Roentgenol Radium Ther Nucl Med 103:19–24

62. Halvorsen RA, Fedyshin PJ, Korobkin M, Thompson WM (1986) CT differentiation of pleural effusion from ascites. An evaluation of four signs using blinded analysis of 52 cases. Invest Radiol 21:391–395

63. Han SY, McElvein RB, Aldrete JS, Tishler JM (1985) Perforation of the esophagus: correlation of site and cause with plain film findings. AJR 145:537–540

64. Heffez DS, Sawaya R, Udvarhelyi GB, Mann R (1982) Spinal epidural extramedullary hematopoesis with spinal cord compression in a patient with refractory sideroblastic anemia. J Neurosurg 57:399–406

65. Heiberg E, Wolverson MK, Sundaram M, Shields JB (1983) CT in aortic trauma. AJR 140:1119–1124

66. Heilman RD, Collins VP (1963) Identification of laceration of the thoracic duct by lymphaniography – preoperative radiography of the traumatized thoracic duct. Radiology 81:470–472

67. Heitzman ER (1975) Roentgen anatomic correlations in the mediastinum. In: Margulis A, Gooding C (eds) Diagnostic radiology. University of California Press, Berkeley

68. Heitzman ER, Lane EJ, Hammack DB, Rimmler LJ (1975) Radiological evaluation of the aortic-pulmonic window. Radiology 116:513–518

69. Henrion J, Lebrec D, Nahum H, Ben-Hamou JP (1979) Pseudotumoral varices of the mediastinum in a case of portal hypertension. Gastroenterol Clin Biol 3:453–459

70. Heystraten FM, Rosenbusch G, Kingma LM, Lacquet LK (1986) Chronic posttraumatic aneurysm of the thoracic aorta: surgically correctable occult threat. AJR 146:303–308

71. Higgins CB, Mulder DG (1970) Mediastinal chyloma: roentgenographic sign of chylous fistula. JAMA 211:1188

72. Hochholzer L, Theros EG, Rosen SH (1969) Some unusual lesions of the mediastinum: roentgenologic and pathologic features. Semin Roentgenol 4:74–90

73. Homer MJ, Wechsler RJ, Carter BL (1978) Mediastinal lipomatosis. CT confirmation of a normal variant. Radiology 128:657–661

74. Ishikawa T, Tsukune Y, Ohyama Y, Fujikawa M, Sakuyama K, Fujii M (1980) Venous abnormalities in portal hypertension demonstrated by CT. AJR 134:271–276

75. Jahnke EJ Jr, Fisher GW, Jones RC (1964) Acute traumatic rupture of the thoracic aorta – report

of six consecutive cases of successful early repair. J Thorac Cardiovasc Surg 48:63–77

76. James AD, Montali RJ, Chaffee V, Strecker EP, Vessel K (1975) Barium or gastrographin: which contrast media for the diagnosis of esophageal tears? Gastroenterology 68:1103–1113

77. James EC, Ellwood RA (1974) Mediastinoscopy and mediastinal roentgenology: clinical correlation. Ann Thorac Surg 18:531–538

78. Jolles PR, Shin MS, Jones WP (1986) Aortopulmonary window lesions: detection with chest radiography. Radiology 159:647–651

79. Jolly PC, Hill LD, Lawless PA, West TL (1973) Parasternal mediastinotomy and mediastinoscopy. Adjuncts in the diagnosis of chest disease. J Thorac Cardiovasc Surg 66:549–556

80. Kirchner SG, Heller RM, Smith C (1977) Pancreatic pseudocyst of the mediastinum. Radiology 123:37–42

81. Kittredge RD (1983) Computed tomographic evaluation of the thoracic prevertebral and paravertebral spaces. CT 7:239–250

82. Knoblich R (1960) Extramedullary hematopoesis presenting as intrathoracic tumors. Cancer 13:463–467

83. LaBerge JM, Kerlan RK, Pogany AC, Ring EJ (1985) Esophageal rupture: complication of balloon dilatation. Radiology 157:56

84. Laforet EG (1965) Acute hypertension as a diagnostic clue in traumatic rupture of the thoracic aorta. Am J Surg 110:948–950

85. Lane EJ Jr, Whalen JP (1969) A new sign of left atrial enlargement: posterior displacement of the left bronchial tree. Radiology 93:279–284

86. Lane EJ, Heitzman ER, Dinn WM (1976) The radiology of the superior intercostal veins. Radiology 120:263–268

87. Lane EJ, Proto AV, Phillips TW (1976) Mach bands and density perception. Radiology 121:9–18

88. Lipchik EO, Robinson KE (1968) Acute traumatic rupture of thoracic aorta. Am J Roentgenol Radium Ther Nucl Med 104:408–412

89. Lodwick GW (1953) Dissecting aneurysms of thoracic and abdominal aorta: report of six cases, discussion of roentgenologic findings and pathologic changes. Am J Roentgenol Radium Ther Nucl Med 69:907–925

90. Loe RH (1946) Injuries of the thoracic duct. Arch Surg 53:448–455

91. Long LA Jr, Doppman JL, Nienhuis AW (1980) Computed tomographic studies of extramedullary hematopoesis. J Comput Assist Tomogr 4:67–70

92. Lowman RM, Bloor CM, Newcomb AW (1963) Roentgen manifestations of thoracic extramedullary hematopoiesis. Dis Chest 44:154–162

93. Lundevall J (1964) The mechanism of traumatic rupture of the aorta. Acta Pathol Microbiol Scand 62:34–46

94. MacFarlane JR, Holman CW (1972) Chylothorax. Am Rev Respir Dis 105:287–291

95. Madewell JE, Sobonya RE, Reed JC (1973) RPC from the AFIP-neurenteric cyst. Radiology 109:707–712

96. Marable SA, Milnar W, Beman FM (1966) Abdominal pain secondary to celiac artery compression. Am J Surg 111:493–495

97. Marnochka KE, Maglinte DDT (1985) Plain film criteria for excluding aortic rupture in blunt chest trauma. AJR 144:19–21

98. Marnochka KE, Maglinte DDT, Woods J, Goodman M, Peterson P (1984) Mediastinal-width/chest-width ratio in blunt chest trauma: a reappraisal. AJR 142:275–277

99. McClenathan JE, Brettschneider L (1965) Traumatic thoracic aortic aneurysms. J Thorac Cardiovasc Surg 50:74–82

100. Meyers MA (1982) Dynamic radiology of the abdomen. Normal and pathological anatomy, 2nd edn. Springer, Berlin Heidelberg New York

101. Michel L, Grillo H, Malt RA (1981) Operative and non-operative management of esophageal perforations. Ann Surg 194:57–63

102. Miller WS (1947) The lung, 2nd edn. Thomas, Springfield, IL

103. Molnar W, Pace WG (1966) Traumatic rupture of the thoracic aorta. Radiol Clin North Am 4:403–414

104. Morgan JR, Rogers AK, Forker AD (1971) Congenital absence of the left pericardium. Ann Intern Med 74:370–376

105. Naclerio EA (1957) The "V sign" in the diagnosis of spontaneous rupture of the esophagus (an early roentgen clue). Am J Surg 93:291–298

106. Neff C, Lawson DW (1985) Boerhaave syndrome: interventional radiologic management. AJR 145:819–820

107. Neuhauser EBD, Harris GBC, Berrett A (1958) Roentgenographic features of neurenteric cysts. Am J Roentgenol 79:235–240

108. Nogrady MB, Nemec J (1970) Partial congenital pericardial defect in childhood – report of four cases. J Can Assoc Radiol 21:116–119

109. Oustwani MB, Kurtides ES, Christ M, Ciric I (1980) Spinal cord compression with paraplegia in myelofibrosis. Arch Neurol 37:389–390

110. Panaro VA, Leslie ES (1965) Spontaneous rupture of the esophagus. Radiology 84:252–258

111. Papavasiliou CG (1965) Tumor simulating intrathoracic extramedullary hematopoesis – clinical and roentgenologic considerations. Am J Roentgenol Radium Ther Nucl Med 93:695–702

112. Parkinson J, Bedford DE (1936) The aortic triangle – a radiological landmark in the left oblique projection. Lancet 2:909–911

113. Parmley LF, Mattingly TW, Manion WC, Jahnke EJ Jr (1958) Nonpenetrating traumatic injury of the aorta. Circulation 17:1086–1101

114. Pate JW, Butterick OD, Richardsons RL (1968) Traumatic rupture of the thoracic aorta. JAMA 203:1022–1024

115. Pearson FG, Nelems JM, Henderson RD, Delarue NC (1972) The role of mediastinoscopy in the selection of treatment for bronchial carcinoma with involvement of superior mediastinal lymph nodes. J Thorac Cardiovasc Surg 64:382–390

116. Penn I (1962) Injuries of the cervical portion of the thoracic duct. Br J Surg 50:19–23

117. Pernkopf E (1963) Atlas of topographic and applied human anatomy, vol 2. Saunders, Philadelphia

118. Phillips LG, Cunningham J (1984) Esophageal perforation. RCNA 22:607–613

119. Pomerantz M, Herdt JRL, Rockoff SD, Ketcham AS (1963) Evaluation of the functional anatomy of the thoracic duct by lymphangiography. J Thorac Cardiovasc Surg 46:568–575

120. Price JE, Rigler LG (1970) Widening of the mediastinum resulting from fat accumulation. Radiology 96:497–500

121. Proto AV, Lane EJ (1977) Air in the esophagus: a frequent roentgen finding. Am J Roentgenol Radium Ther Nucl Med 129:433–440

122. Proto AV, Speckman JM (1979) The left lateral radiograph of the chest. Med Radiogr Photogr 55:30–74

123. Rabinowitz JG, Wolf BSW (1966) Roentgen significance of the pulmonary ligament. Radiology 87:1013–1020

124. Reed JC, Reeder MM (1974) Middle mediastinal lesion – topics in radiology, gamut. JAMA 230:891–892

125. Reed JC, Sobonya RE (1974) Foregut cysts in the thorax. Am J Roentgenol Radium Ther Nucl Med 120:851–860

126. Reed JC, Hallet KK, Feigin DS (1978) Neural tumors of the thorax: subject review from the AFIP. Radiology 126:9–17

127. Reuter SR (1971) Accentuation of celiac compression by the median arcuate ligament of the diaphragm during deep expiration. Radiology 102:561–564

128. Rigler LG (1929) The visualized esophagus in the diagnosis of the heart and aorta. Am J Roentgenol Radium Ther Nucl Med 21:563–571

129. Rigler L, Phelps KA (1930) Changes in the esophagus secondary to cardiac and aortic diseases. Arch Otolaryngol 11:188–191

130. Rogers LF, Puig AW, Dooley BN, Cuello L (1971) Diagnostic considerations in mediastinal emphysema: a pathophysiologic-roentgenologic approach to Boerhaave's syndrome and spontaneous pneumomediastinum. Am J Roentgenol Radium Ther Nucl Med 111:807–820

131. Rosenberger A, Abrams HL (1971) Radiology of the thoracic duct. Am J Roentgenol Radium Ther Nucl Med 111:807–820

132. Saks BJ, Kilby AE, Dietrich PA, Coffin LH, Krawitt EL (1983) Pleural and mediastinal changes following endoscopic injection therapy of esophageal varices. Radiology 149:639–642

133. Sanborn JC, Heitzman ER, Markarian B (1970) Traumatic rupture of the thoracic aorta – roentgen pathologic correlations. Radiology 95:293–298

134. Sealy WC (1974) Mediastinoscopy – does it have a place in the management of carcinoma of the lung? Ann Thorac Surg 18:433–436

135. Sefczek DM, Sefczek RJ, Deeb ZL (1983) Radiographic signs of acute traumatic rupture of the thoracic aorta. AJR 141:1259–1262

136. Seltzer SE, D'Orsi CJ, Kirshner R, DeWeese JA (1981) Traumatic aortic rupture: plain radiographic findings. AJR 137:1011–1014

137. Shafiroff BGP, Kan QY (1959) Cannulation of thoracic lymph duct. Surgery 45:814–819

138. Shaver RW, Clore FC (1981) Extramedullary hematopoiesis in myeloid metaplasia. AJR 137:874–876

139. Shin MS, Berland LL (1985) Computed tomography of retrocrural spaces: normal, anatomic variants and pathological conditions. AJR 145:81–86

140. Shin MS, Ho KJ, Witten DM (1981) Application of computed tomography in differential diagnosis of radiographic opacities in the lower thorax and upper abdomen. CT 5:519–528

141. Shuford WH, Sybers RG, Weens HS, Lindsay J Jr, Hurst JW (1969) Aortographic findings in dissecting aneurysm of aorta. Am J Cardiol 24:111–117

142. Siegelman SS, Copeland BE, Saba GP, Cameron JL, Sanders RC, Zerhouni E (1980) CT of fluid collections associated with pancreatitis. AJR 134:1121–1132

143. Silverman PM, Godwin JD, Korobkin M (1982) Computed tomographic detection of retrocrural air. AJR 138:825–827

144. Simeone JF, Deren MM, Cagle F (1981) Value of the left apical cap in the diagnosis of aortic rupture: a prospective and retrospective study. Radiology 139:35–37

145. Sorsdahl OS, Taylor PE, Noyes WD (1964) Extramedullary hematopoesis, mediastinal masses and spinal cord compression. JAMA 189:343–347

146. Steinberg I (1962) Demonstration of the hemiazygous veins in superior vena caval occlusion simulating mediastinal tumor. Am J Roentgenol Radium Ther Nucl Med 87:248–257

147. Stewart ET, Miller WN, Hogan WJ, Dodds WJ (1979) Desirability of roentgen esophageal examination immediately after pneumatic dilatation for achalasia. Radiology 130:589–591

148. Streiter ML, Schneider HJ, Proto AV (1982) Steroid-induced thoracic lipomatosis: paraspinal involvement. AJR 139:679–681

149. Symbas PN, Hatcher CR, Harlaftis N (1978) Spontaneous rupture of the esophagus. Ann Surg 187:634–640

150. Szilagyi DE, Rian RL, Elliot JP, Smith RF (1972) The coeliac artery compression syndrome. Does it exist? Surgery 72:849–863

151. Trackler RT, Brinker RA (1966) Widening of the left paravertebral pleural line on supine chest

roentgenograms in free pleural effusions. Am J Roentgenol Radium Ther Nucl Med 96:1027–1033

152. Van Pernis PA (1949) Variations in the thoracic duct. Surgery 26:806–809

153. Wales LR, Morishima MS, Reay D, Johansen K (1982) Nasogastric tube placement in acute traumatic rupture of the thoracic aorta: a postmortem study. AJR 138:821–823

154. Warwick R, Williams PR (1973) Gray's anatomy, 35th edn. Saunders, Philadelphia

155. Watne AL, Hatiboglu I, Moore GE (1960) A clinical and autopsy study of tumor cells in the thoracic duct lymph. Surg Gynecol Obstet 110:339–345

156. Webb WR, Gamsu G (1983) Computed tomography of the left retrobronchial stripe. JCAT 7:65–69

157. Webb WR, Gamsu G, Speckman JM, Kaiser JA, Federle MP, Lipton MJ (1982) Pictorial essay. Computed tomographic demonstration of mediastinal venous anomalies. AJR 139:157–161

158. Whalen JP, Lane EJ Jr (1969) Bronchial rearrangements in pulmonary collapse as seen on the lateral radiograph. Radiology 93:285–288

159. Whalen JP, Shaheen GA (1971) Visualization of subdiaphragmatic fat: aid in localizing of diaphragm. Br J Radiol 44:224–225

160. Wilson ES Jr (1969) Neurenteric cyst of the mediastinum. Am J Roentgenol Radium Ther Nucl Med 107:641–646

8 The Supra-azygos Area

8.1 General Anatomic Considerations

The supra-azygos area is that portion of the right side of the mediastinum extending cephalad from the azygos arch to the thoracic inlet. To understand the normal radiologic appearance of this region, a thorough understanding of the anatomy of the azygos vein and particularly the azygos arch is mandatory [48, 49].

The azygos vein begins opposite the first or second lumbar vertebral body, most often as a cephalad continuation of the right ascending lumbar vein and the right subcostal vein. Occasionally the vessel may be joined by a tributary from the right renal vein or from the inferior vena cava [27]. The ascending lumbar veins, lying anterior to the transverse processes of the lumbar vertebrae, communicate the four lumbar veins. Both ascending lumbar veins serve to connect the common iliac and pelvic veins with the azygos and hemiazygos systems. On the left, the ascending lumbar vein continues cephalad behind the left crus of the diaphragm as the hemiazygos vein (Fig. 8.2). The azygos vein continues upward, passing medial to the right crus of the diaphragm (Fig. 8.2) through the aortic hiatus into the thorax where it lies to the right of the descending aorta (Fig. 8.2). The azygos vein may at times pass lateral to the right crus of the diaphragm behind the internal arcuate ligament or may pass through one of the lesser apertures of the diaphragm, as may the hemiazygos vein. The accessory hemiazygos vein, descending behind the aorta, joins the hemiazygos vein at the T-8 or T-9 level; at this point the hemiazygos vein turns to the right, crossing in front of the vertebral bodies to meet the azygos vein (Figs. 8.1–8.3). The azygos vein then continues cephalad in a prevertebral course to the level of T-4 or T-5, where the vessel arches forward and slightly to the right, passing over the right upper lobe bronchus and the truncus anterior branch of the right pulmonary artery to terminate in the superior vena cava immediately above the pericardial reflection over that vessel (Figs. 8.3 and 8.4).

The azygos vein receives the fifth to the eleventh intercostal veins of the right side and the right subcostal vein (Fig. 8.4). The right superior intercostal vein drains the second, third, and fourth interspaces and terminates in the azygos vein as that vessel turns forward from the spine at the T-4 or T-5 level (Figs. 8.3 and 8.4). The right supreme intercostal vein carries blood from the first intercostal space and drains into the innominate vein. The right bronchial vein opens into the azygos vein near its termination.

An analogous drainage pattern exists on the left side. The hemiazygos vein receives the lower four of five intercostal veins and the subcostal vein. The accessory hemiazygos vein receives blood from the intercostal spaces between those drained by the hemiazygos vein and the left superior intercostal vein (Fig. 8.3). The correlated radiologic anatomy of the left superior intercostal vein, an important topic, is discussed in chapter 6. The left supreme intercostal vein carries blood from the first intercostal space and drains into the left innominate vein. The left bronchial veins terminate in the accessory hemiazygos vein or in the left superior intercostal vein.

The azygos arch can be visualized on most PA chest radiographs and the vessel is almost always identified for its entire course on computed tomograms. Its frequent visualization plus the intimate relationship of this vessel to

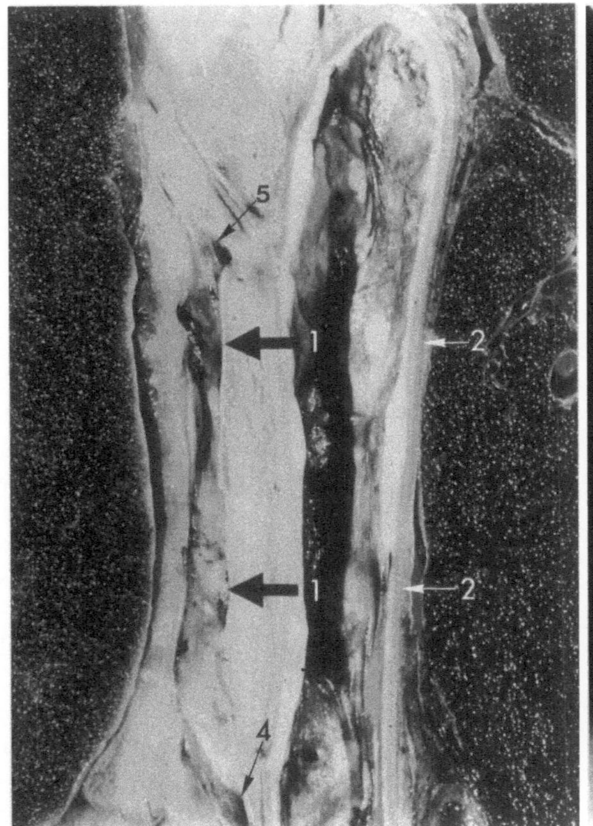

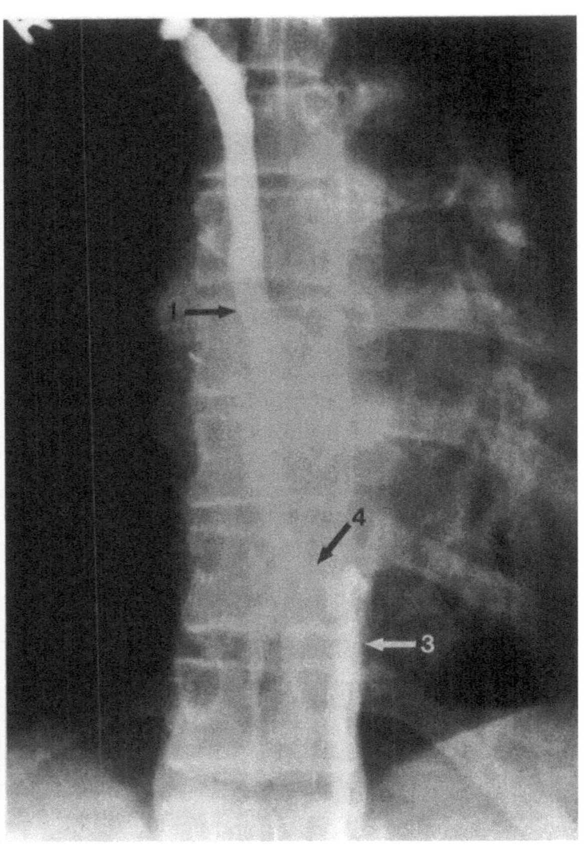

A   **B**

Fig. 8.1 A, B. Anatomy of azygos and hemiazygos venous systems. **A** Coronal body section. **B** AP azygogram. Azygos vein (*1*) ascends at right side of descending aorta (*2*). Hemiazygos vein (*3*) lies posterior to descending aorta and joins azygos vein at level of T-8, T-9, or T-10 (*4*). The AP azygogram clearly demonstrates communication between azygos vein (*1*) and hemiazygos vein (*3*). Hemiazygos vein enters thorax through aortic hiatus of diaphragm behind aorta and medial to left diaphragmatic crus. Apparently, in patient shown in **B**, major drainage through aortic hiatus is by way of left ascending lumbar vein to hemiazygos vein. At the level of T-4 or T-5 (*5*), azygos vein turns to right and forward from its prespinal location. (**A** From [48])

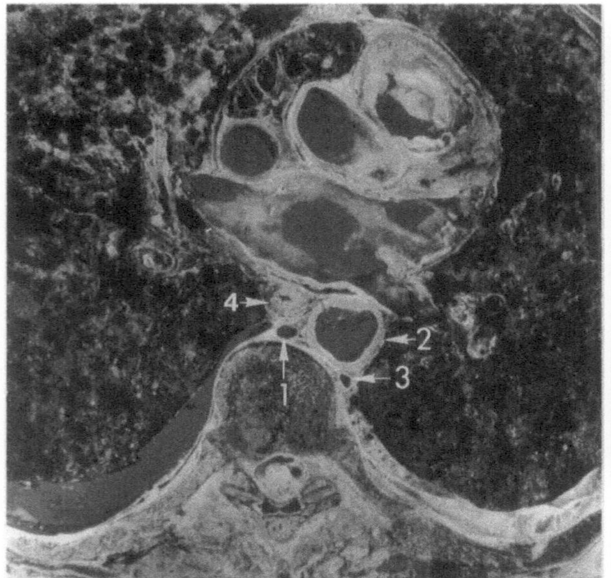

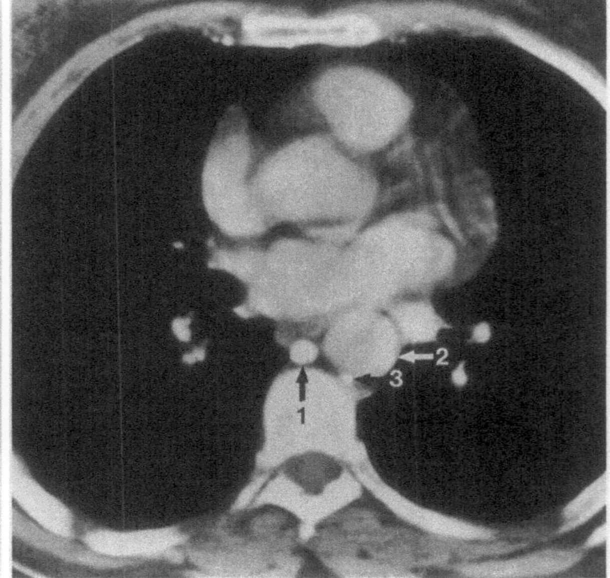

A   **B**

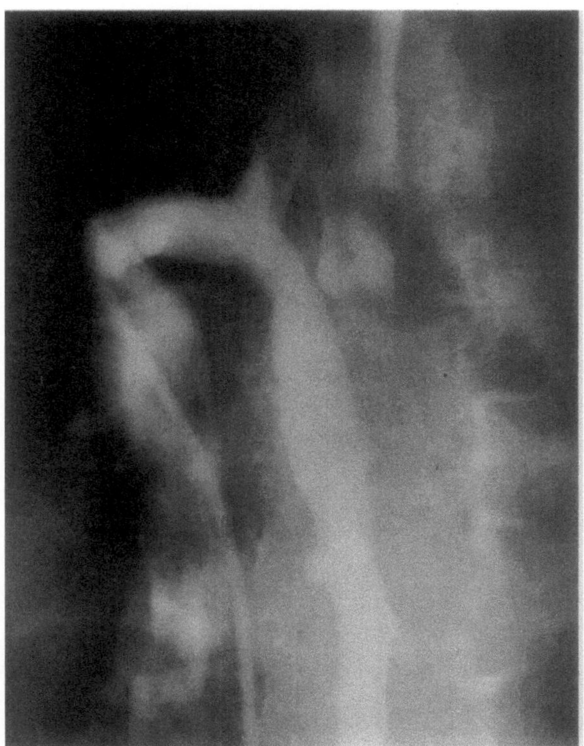

A

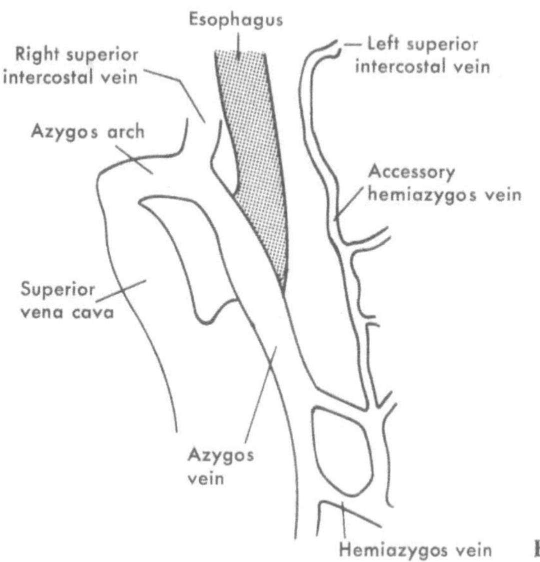

Fig. 8.3A, B. Anatomy of azygos and hemiazygos venous systems. **A** AP azygogram. **B** Diagrammatic representation of anatomy demonstrated in the azygogram. Azygos vein is continuation of right ascending lumbar vein and enters thorax through aortic hiatus in diaphragm. At level of T-8, T-9, or T-10, it receives hemiazygos vein from left side. Sometimes there is more than one communication. Hemiazygos vein enters thorax medial to left diaphragmatic crus and receives accessory hemiazygos vein, which in turn is joined by left superior intercostal vein in most individuals. Right superior intercostal vein joins azygos vein as that vessel begins to turn forward from its prespinal location. Note that azygos arch courses somewhat to right as it progresses forward to superior vena cava. (In this example deflection is accentuated because an enlarged azygos node was situated medial to arch)

<hr>

Fig. 8.2A, B. Anatomy of azygos and hemiazygos venous systems. **A** Transverse body section at level of diaphragm. **B** Computed tomogram with contrast enhancement. At the level of the aortic hiatus, the azygos vein (*1*) lies to the right of the aorta (*2*). The hemiazygos vein (*3*) traverses the aortic hiatus where it is situated posterior to the aorta. The azygos vein lies posterior to esophagus (*4*) and is frequently separated from it in living subjects by air in azygoesophageal recess

most of the structures in the posterior part of the mediastinum, the right upper mediastinum, and the right hilum, makes an understanding of the anatomy of the azygos vein and its pleural reflections a vital key to analysis of the radiographic appearance of the right side of the mediastinum. Despite this fact, the normal radiologic anatomy of this important mediastinal landmark has received relatively little attention in the literature. Most previous radiologic publications concerning the azygos vein have placed major emphasis on congenital variation in the azygos system [1], and on dilatation of the azygos vein in acquired disease [39, 57]. Older articles [7, 53, 86, 92] emphasized the technique and application of azygography, an examination now rarely, if ever, performed. In 1942, Lachman [60] compared the appearances of the posterior boundaries of the lungs and pleura in the cadaver with roentgenograms of living persons and pointed out the intimate relationship of the right posterior lung and pleura to the azygos vein.

The azygos vein and, particularly, the azygos arch predicate the position of the posterior right mediastinal pleura and of the lung that lies

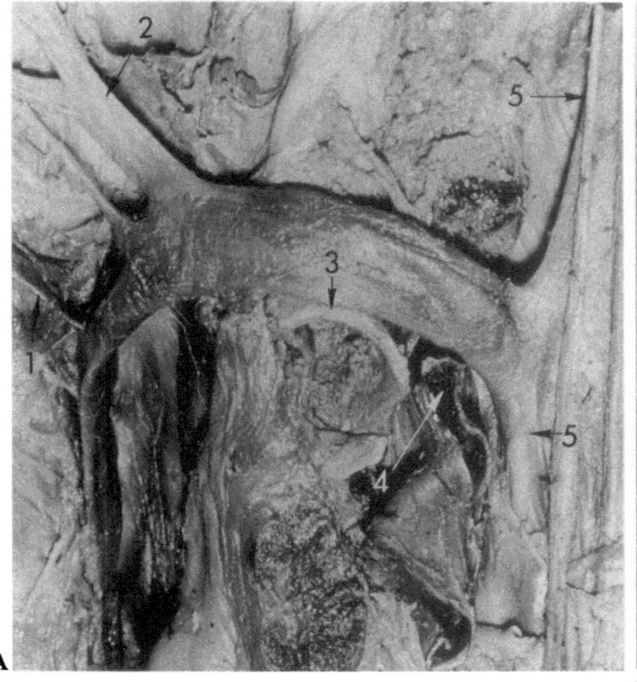

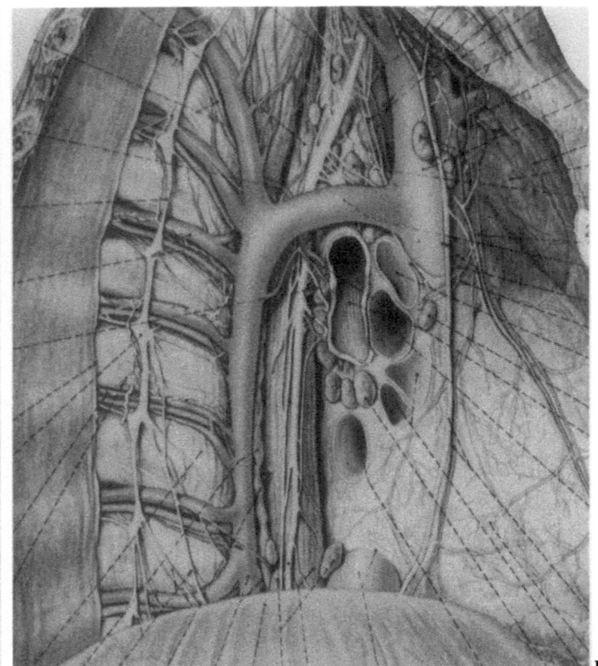

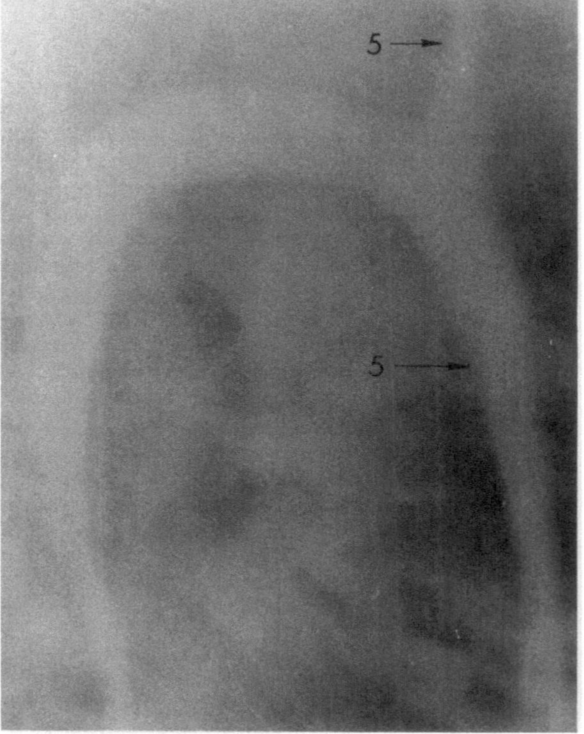

Fig. 8.4A–C. Anatomy of azygos and hemiazygos venous systems; the azygos arch. **A** Right side of mediastinum with mediastinal pleural removed. **B** Structures of right side of mediastinum. **C** Lateral azygogram. Ascending portion of azygos vein receives some of right posterior intercostal veins (*1*). As it turns forward and to right from its prespinal location, it is also joined by right superior intercostal vein (*2*) (see also Fig. 8.30). Azygos arch crosses right upper lobe bronchus (*3*) and truncus anterior branch of right pulmonary artery (*4*) on its way to join superior vena cava (*5*). (**A** From [48]; **B** from [80])

against this portion of the pleura [48, 49]. The resulting interfaces produce a number of normal landmarks that are extremely helpful in the roentgen evaluation of the mediastinum. Some of these landmarks are readily recognized and produce no difficulties in interpretation. Others, almost as easily visualized, have received little attention in the literature and can be misconstrued as evidence of mediastinal tumor or other abnormality.

8.2 The Azygos Arch

As the azygos vein passes forward from the level of T-4 or T-5, it grooves the right lung (Fig. 8.5). This intimate contact with air-containing lung renders the arch visible on plain radiographs and especially on overpenetrated films, conventional tomograms, and computed tomograms. The anterior portion of the arch just behind its point of entry into the superior vena cava is visible on many chest examinations. It lies superior and lateral to the point of origin

of the right main bronchus from the trachea. This portion of the arch is often called the "azygos vein," although it represents only a small segment of this vessel. It is interesting that Felson [35] could identify this portion of the azygos arch in only 24% of 400 well-penetrated chest radiographs.

Many years ago, Stauffer et al. [99] described the radiographic appearance of the normal azygos vein. There are significant variations in the configuration of the anterior portion of the azygos arch as it appears on radiographs. These shapes can be described as round, oval, pearshaped, and so on (Fig. 8.6) and are dependent upon the size of the anterior arch and the inti-

Fig. 8.5. Anatomy of azygos venous system. Medial surface of right lung, hardened in situ. Impressions made by azygos vein on medial surface of right lung are clearly shown in this specimen. Groove produced by azygos arch as it progresses forward to join superior vena cava is well demonstrated above structures of right lung root. Above azygos arch and behind superior vena cava, lung is free to extend deeply into mediastinum. (From [28])

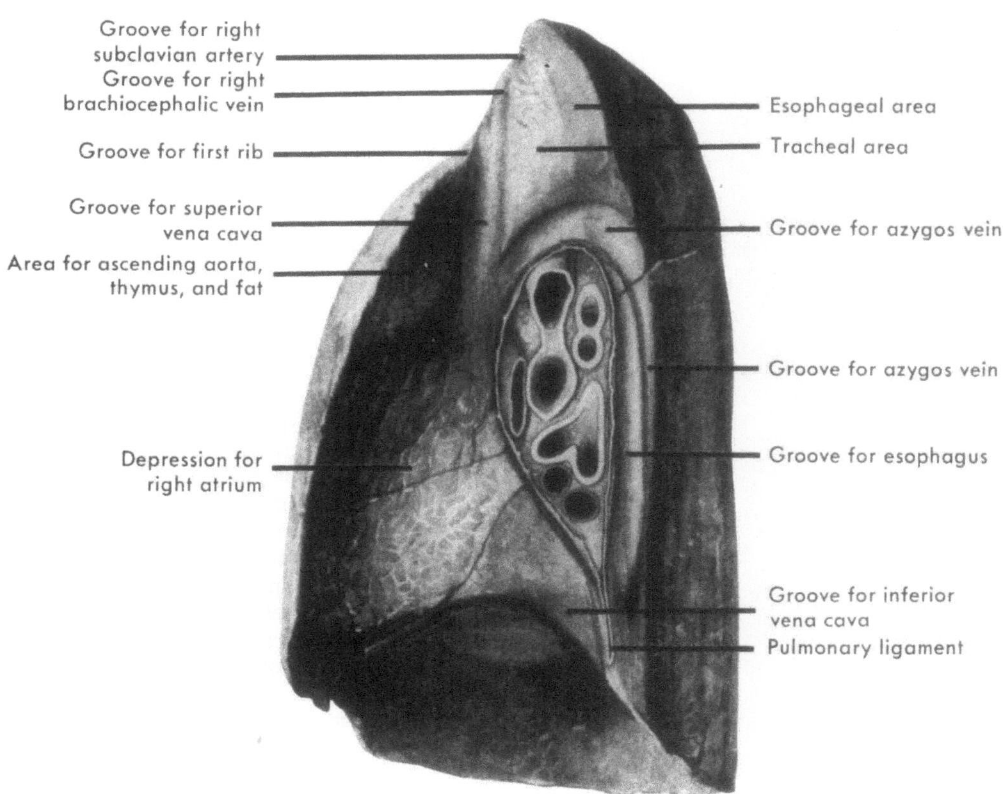

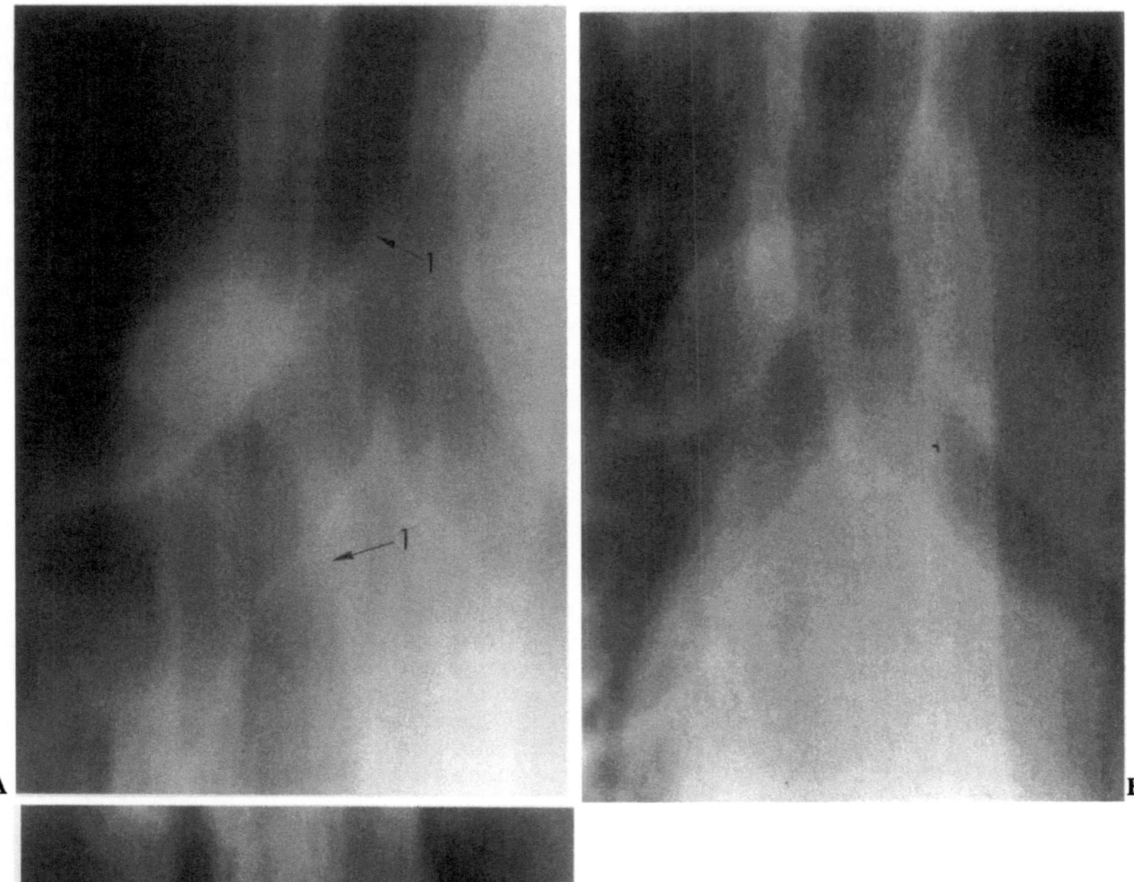

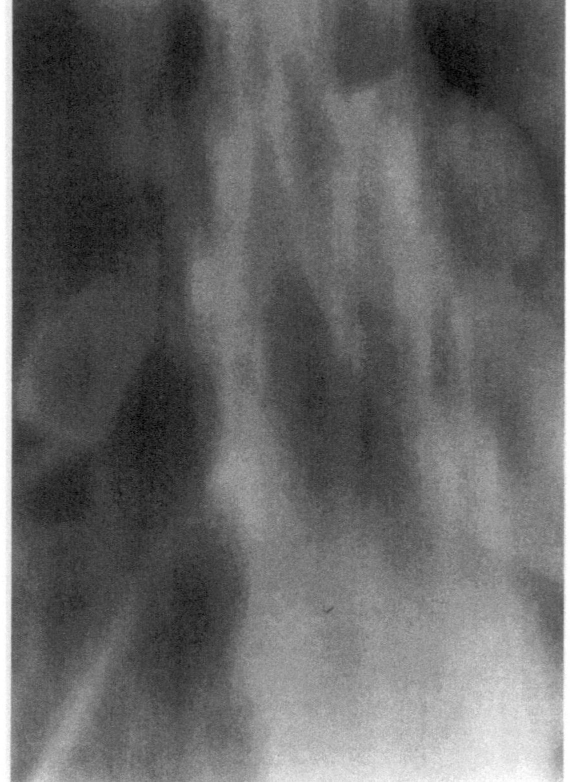

Fig. 8.6 A–C. Configuration of anterior aspect of azygos arch on AP radiographs. AP tomograms through plane of trachea. Anterior portion of azygos arch lies lateral to trachea and right main bronchus, above take-off of right upper lobe bronchus. Considerable variation in its configuration can be encountered; here, round, oval, and "teardrop" shapes are demonstrated. When shadow presents acute angles with trachea as shown in **A** and when mediastinal recesses (*1*) subtend from this structure (an appearance demonstrated in **A** and **B**) other differential considerations such as nodal enlargement can be virtually excluded. (**A** From [49])

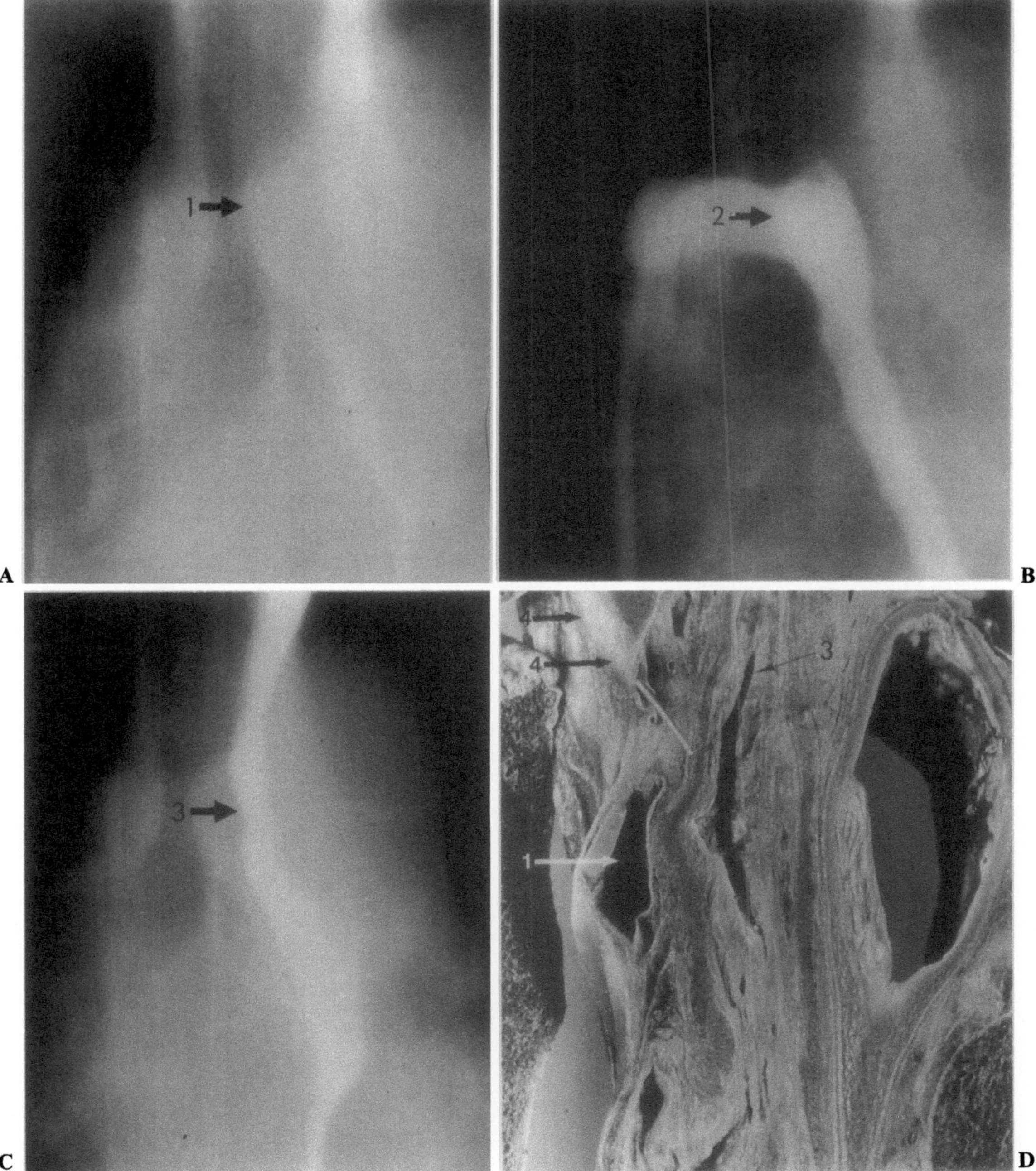

Fig. 8.7A–D. Radiographic anatomy of azygos arch. Posterior turn of azygos arch–azygos "knob." **A** AP tomogram. **B** AP azygogram. **C** AP tomogram with barium in esophagus. **D** Coronal body section through level of esophagus. Posterior turn of azygos vein as it deflects forward and to right from its prespinal location can often be identified through air column of trachea (*1*). It is outlined by lung on its right side. Azygogram clearly shows elliptical configuration of right side of this posterior turn (*2*). Barium-filled esophagus is in intimate contact with left side of posterior turn of azygos vein and is often impressed upon by vessel (*3*). Coronal body section (**D**) demonstrates posterior turn of azygos vein (*1*) about to be joined by the right superior intercostal vein (*4*). A wire has been placed in the latter vessel. The posterior turn of the azygos vein is outlined on its right lateral side by superior segment of right lower lobe; its left lateral side is in intimate contact with esophagus (*3*). Posterior turn of azygos arch is analogous to posterior turn of aortic arch. Each is outlined on its lateral side by lung; each is in intimate contact on its medial side with esophagus. Posterior turn of aortic arch is sometimes termed aortic "knob." Visualization of azygos knob by virtue of its contact with esophagus should not be misconstrued as a node or mass. (**A–C** From [48])

macy of the pleural reflections over them [5, 30]. If the combined visceral and mediastinal pleurae are closely applied to the vein, its shadow appears round or oval, often demonstrating acute angles with the pleurae at its base (Fig. 8.6 A). Such an appearance is so characteristic of the anterior arch that other differential considerations, such as nodal enlargement or other mediastinal mass, can be virtually excluded.

The posterior portion of the azygos arch lying in a prespinal position can also be occasionally identified on overpenetrated frontal radiographs and tomograms (Fig. 8.7). This portion of the arch is rendered visible by virtue of its contact with the aerated superior segment of the right lower lobe. Opacification of the superi-

or segment by disease will cause the outline of the posterior portion of the azygos arch to be lost. The elliptical shadow produced by this portion of the azygos vein should not be misconstrued as a node or a mass. At times it is possible to see the whole arch, the anterior part, the posterior part, and the portion in between (Fig. 8.8). The arch may adopt a somewhat downward course with its anterior portion at a lower level than its posterior part (Fig. 8.8).

Austin and Thorsen [5] have studied the appearance of the azygos arch on conventional tomograms made in the frontal projection and distinguished five variant patterns. The two most common types were: (a) the inferior margin of the arch crossed posterior to the right main bronchus; and (b) the inferior margin of the arch crossed posterior to the left main bronchus and extended behind the trachea above the carina.

The posterior turn of the azygos arch bears a close relationship to the esophagus, which lies to the left of the vein and slightly anterior to it. As it courses forward, the arch often contacts the esophagus and sometimes indents it to pro-

Fig. 8.8 A, B. Radiographic anatomy of azygos arch. **A** AP tomogram, **B** AP tomogram with barium in esophagus. At times entire azygos arch can be seen on AP tomograms (*1*). Posterior aspect of arch (*2*) is frequently identified as being higher than anterior aspect of arch (*3*). This may be due to projection but also can be result of some inferior deflection of arch as it progresses anteriorly. Note marked azygos "imprint" (*4*)

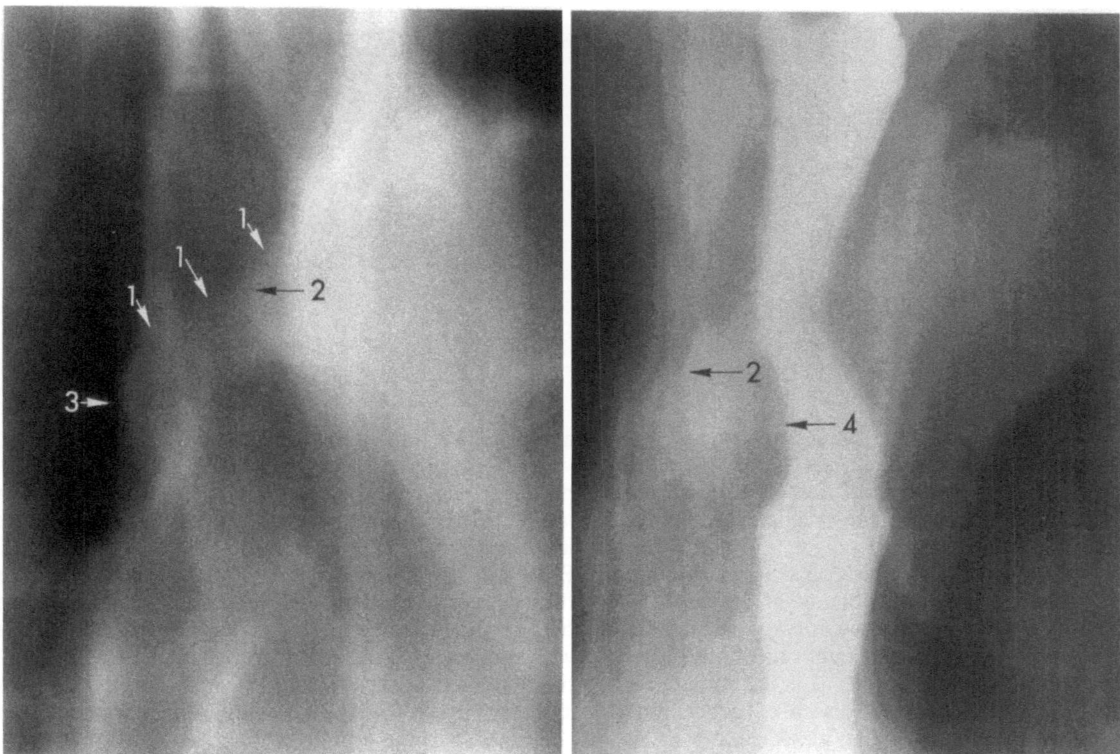

duce a defect that has been called the "azygos imprint" [48]. The imprint can frequently be seen very well on frontal radiographs (Figs. 8.7 and 8.8), but because the arch courses along the right posterolateral aspect of the esophagus (Fig. 8.9), the most prominent indentation is usually encountered in the right anterior oblique or left posterior oblique projections (Fig. 8.9). Likewise, this impression should not be mistaken on radiographs for a node or a mass.

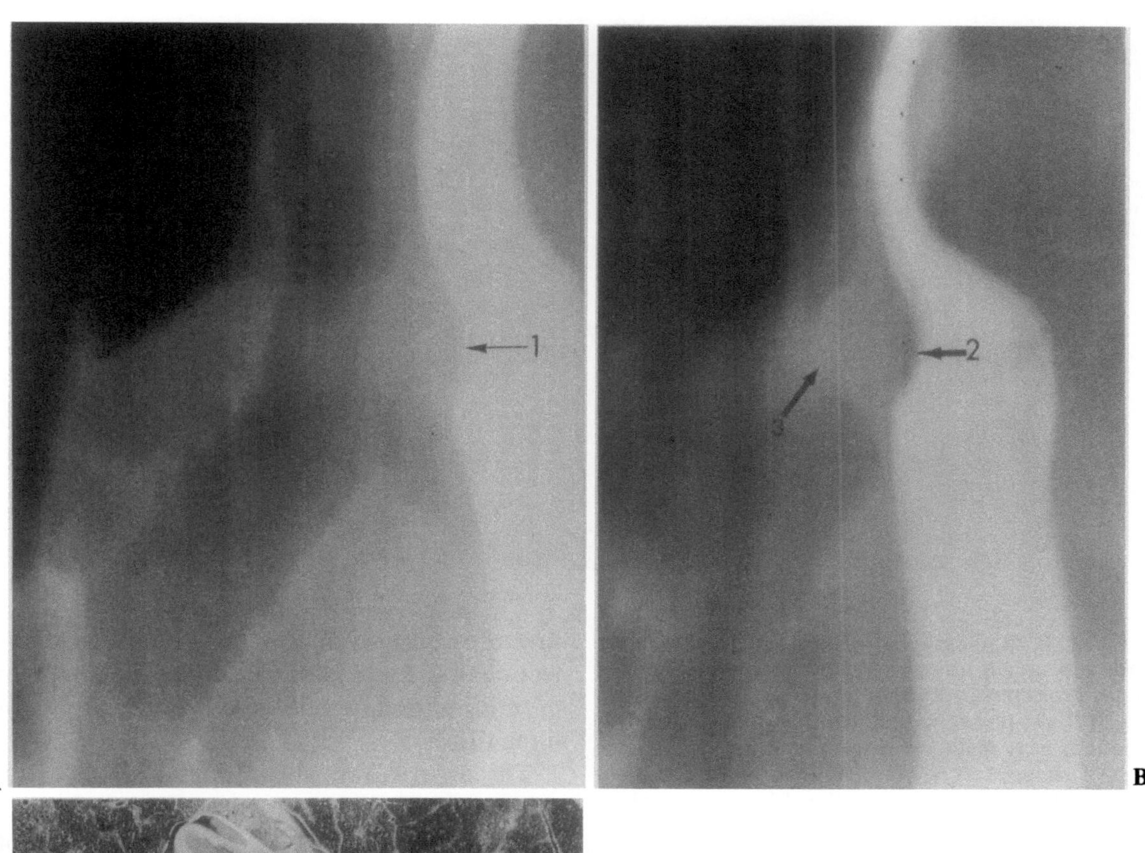

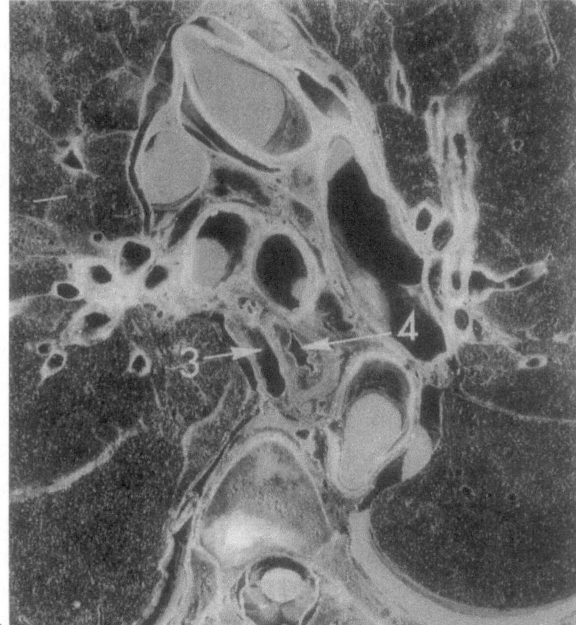

Fig. 8.9A–C. Radiographic anatomy of azygos arch. Appearance in right anterior oblique and left posterior oblique projections. A AP tomogram with barium in esophagus. B Left posterior oblique tomogram on same patient also with barium in esophagus. C Coronal body section through level of azygos arch. Azygos imprint (1) seen in AP tomogram (A) is sometimes better visualized and appears deeper in left posterior oblique or right anterior oblique projections (2). This is due to fact that azygos arch (3) grooves right posterolateral aspect of esophagus (4) as it courses forward. Although there is rarely a need to demonstrate azygos arch in this projection, imprint on esophagus is frequently encountered on esophograms and should not be misconstrued as extrinsic defect caused by node or mass. Note that in A entire azygos arch can be seen. (B From [48])

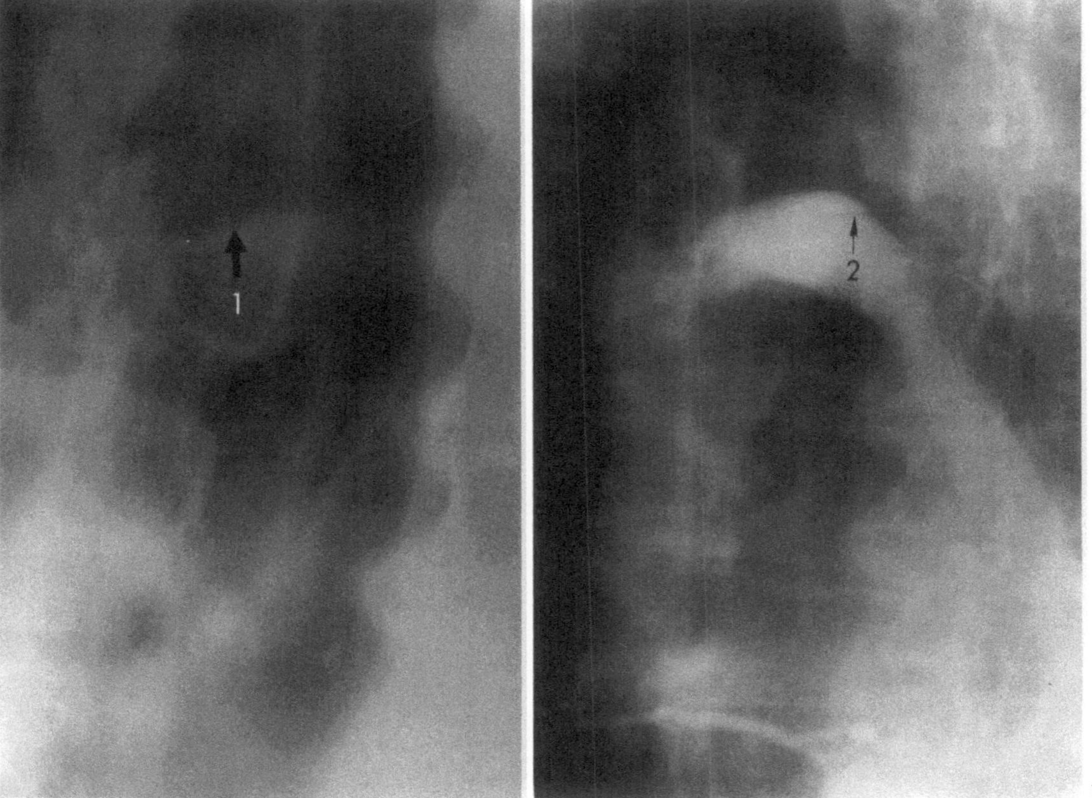

Fig. 8.10A, B. Radiographic anatomy of azygos arch. Appearance in left anterior oblique and right posterior oblique projections. **A** Right posterior oblique tomogram. **B** Right posterior oblique azygogram. These examinations were made on same patient. Entire superior aspect of superior azygos arch (*1*) can be seen in right posterior oblique tomogram outlined by air in mediastinal recess cephalad of azygos arch. Appearance of azygos arch in left anterior oblique and right posterior oblique projections is analogous to appearance of aortic arch that is "opened up" in these projections. Note appearance of valves in azygos vein (*2*). In contrast to pulmonary veins, which do not have valves, azygos vein contains valves

As the azygos arch extends anteriorly and to the right across the mediastinum, its orientation is in a plane similar to that of the aortic arch: the aortic arch courses posteriorly to the left; the azygos arch anteriorly to the right. Both are seen "end on" in RAO and LPO projections (Fig. 8.9), and each is "opened up" to be seen in profile in LAO and RPO views (Fig. 8.10). Demonstration of the azygos arch on oblique views is rarely of diagnostic value in the interpretation of chest radiographs, but an appreciation of the appearance of the arch in these projections can be helpful to obviate the possibility of misinterpretation of these shadows on oblique films.

The azygos and aortic arches share certain other similarities. The posterior turn of each is outlined on its lateral aspect by lung, and both impinge against the esophagus on their medial side (Fig. 8.7). Since the posterior turn of the aortic arch is commonly referred to as the aortic "knob," the posterior turn of the azygos arch can be called the azygos "knob" [48].

The appearance of the azygos arch on lateral radiographs has received only limited mention in the literature [48, 63, 83]. Its configuration in this projection must be appreciated to avoid mistaking the back of the azygos knob as a node or a mass. The ability to see the azygos arch on lateral radiographs is dependent upon the deep intrusion of lung into the mediastinum around the arch. The posterior portion of the right mediastinal pleura is reflected cephalad and caudad from the azygos arch like a sheet draped over a clothesline (Fig. 8.6). As a result, two

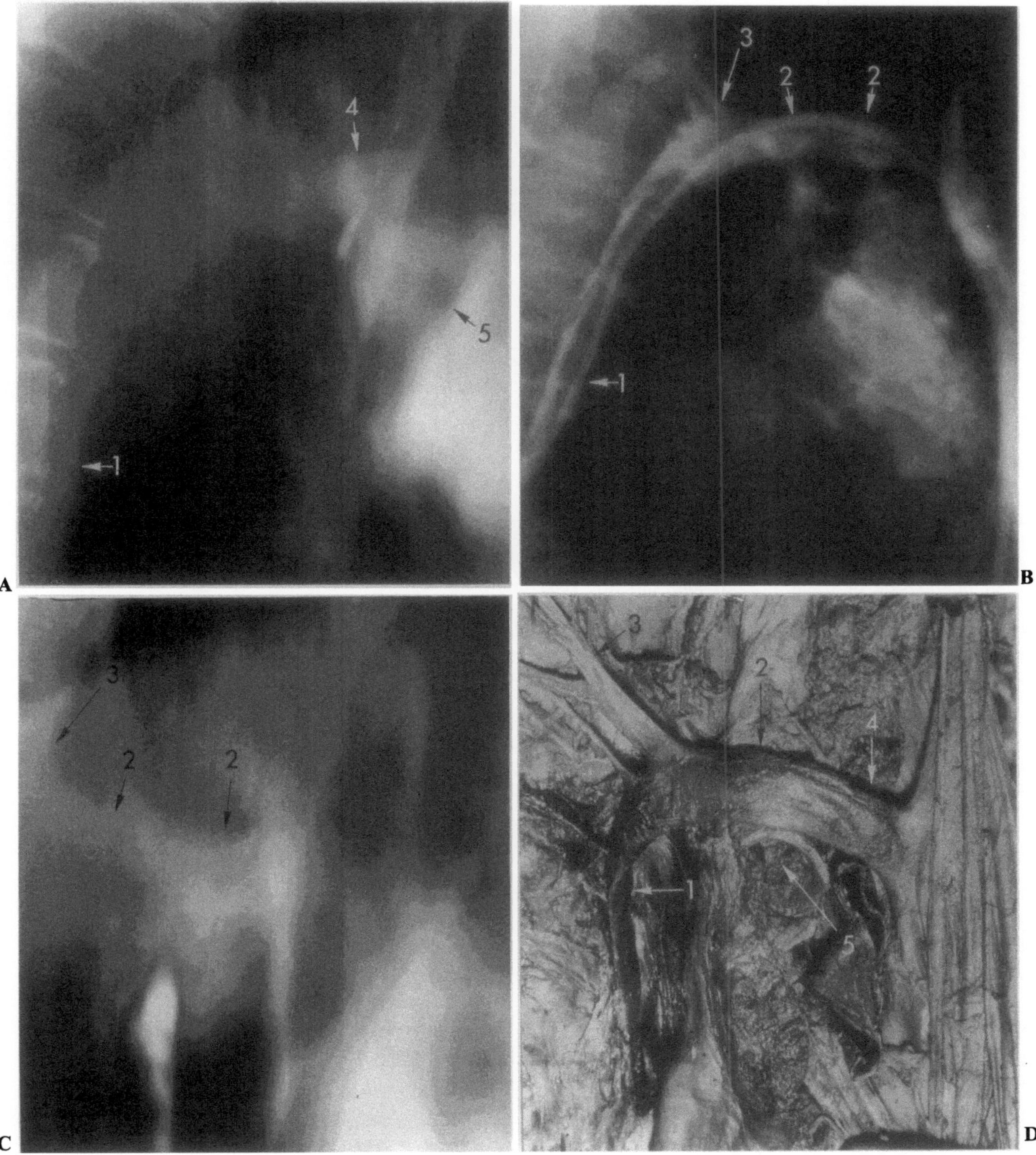

Fig. 8.11A–D. Radiographic anatomy of azygos arch (lateral projection). **A** and **C** Lateral tomograms. **B** Lateral azygogram of same patient. **D** Right side of mediastinum with mediastinal pleura removed. Azygos arch can be identified on plain lateral radiographs and tomograms when arch deeply grooves right lung. Ascending portion of azygos vein (*1*) can be seen outlined by lung anterior to it. Two lateral tomograms at different levels of cut combine to demonstrate entire superior surface of azygos arch (*2*). Posterior portion is seen to receive right superior intercostal vein (*3*) outlined by lung anterior to it. Anterior portion of arch (*4*) can be seen coursing forward above right upper lobe bronchus (*5*). (**A** From [47])

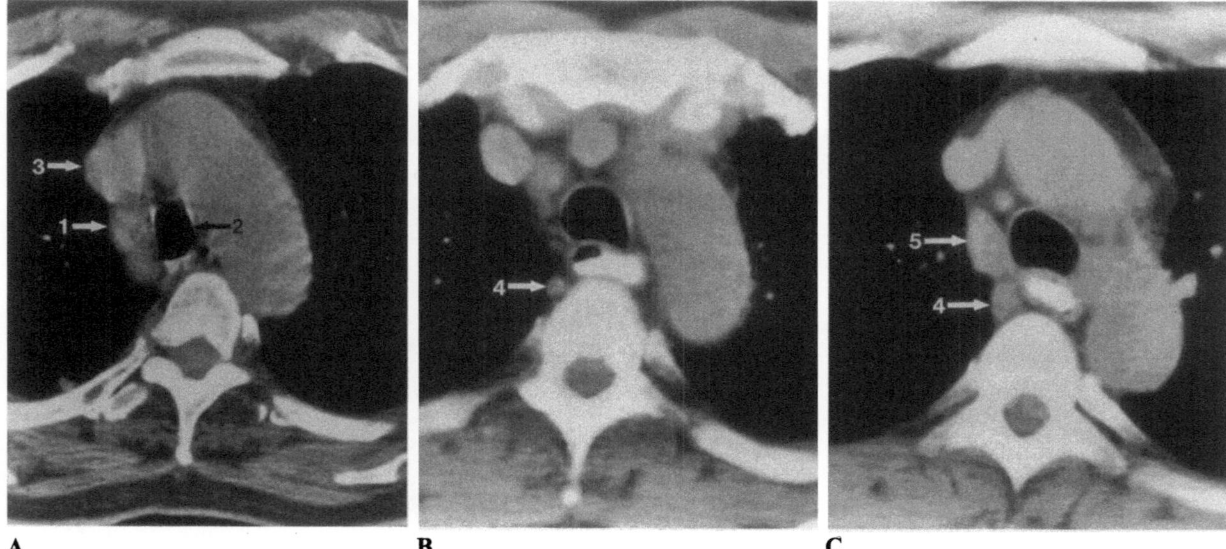

Fig. 8.12 A–C. Radiographic anatomy of azygos arch (computed tomograms). Computed tomography often nicely demonstrates azygos arch (*1*) as it courses along right lateral side of trachea (*2*) to join superior vena cava (*3*). Note that lung inserts itself behind azygos "knob." When interpreting computed tomography one should be careful not to mistake normal shadow of azygos arch for widened right paratracheal stripe. This pitfall can be avoided by carefully noting level of section. In **B** the right superior intercostal vein (*4*) can be seen approaching the posterior turn of the azygos arch and in **C** joins the arch. Undulations of the arch may be imaged in a fashion to suggest adenopathy (*5*)

deep mediastinal recesses are formed. The caudad reflection of the pleura extends medially in front of the azygos vein and in contiguity with the esophagus. This latter intrusion into the posterior mediastinum, termed the "azygoesophageal recess," will be discussed in detail in chapter 9. The cephalad sweep extends medially behind the superior vena cava and in front of the right superior intercostal vein (Fig. 8.11). The extension of lung deep into the mediastinal recesses above and below the azygos arch can produce a prominent ridge of mediastinal soft tissue between the two; this ridge, the azygos arch, can be seen on standard lateral radiographs but is more often identified on lateral tomograms and computed tomograms. On such examinations the confluence of the shadows of the ascending portion of the azygos vein and

the descending course of the right superior intercostal vein can often be seen outlined by lung extending anterior to them (Figs. 8.11 and 8.12). The shadow of the azygos arch can be seen running anteriorly from this confluence between the cephalad recess above and the azygoesophageal recess below (Fig. 8.11). However, the azygos arch is not commonly seen on lateral radiographs unless the recesses above or below the azygos arch are exceptionally deep. The arch is seen immediately above the right upper lobe bronchus, much as the left pulmonary artery is seen passing above the left upper lobe bronchus. The entry of the azygos arch into the back of the superior vena cava may be identified (Fig. 8.11).

In some patients a considerable volume of lung intrudes itself almost directly posterior to the azygos arch as it deflects forward from the spine (Figs. 8.12 and 8.13). In these cases the posterior portion of the azygos arch (the azygos knob) may be visualized on lateral films or lateral tomograms as a semicircular density marginated by lung posteriorly (Fig. 8.13). The shadow is seen in a position slightly behind the trachea immediately above or slightly behind the shadow of the right upper lobe orifice. This demonstration of the normal azygos arch on the lateral view should not be misinterpreted as a mediastinal node or mass. When it is difficult to determine on frontal radiographs whether a promi-

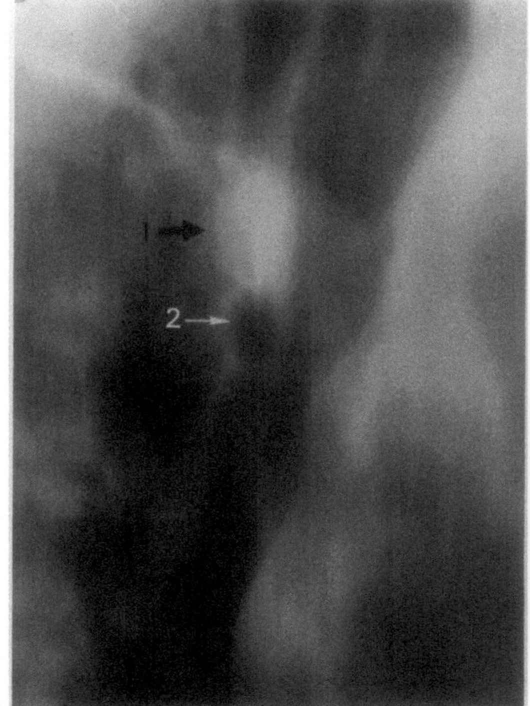
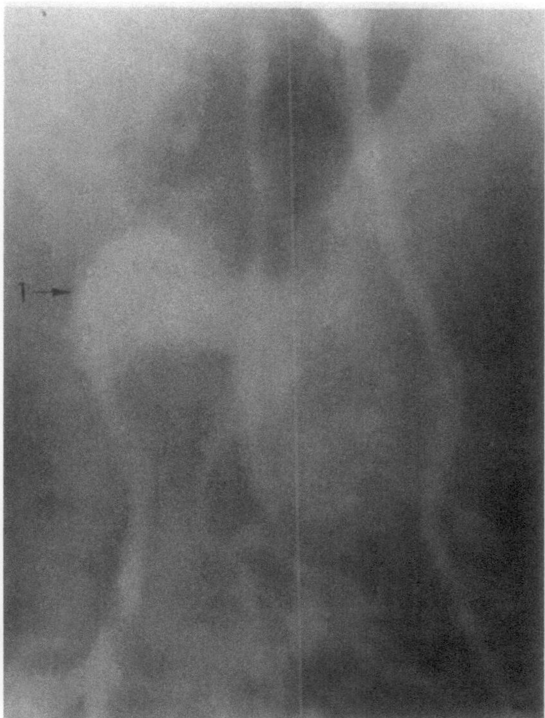
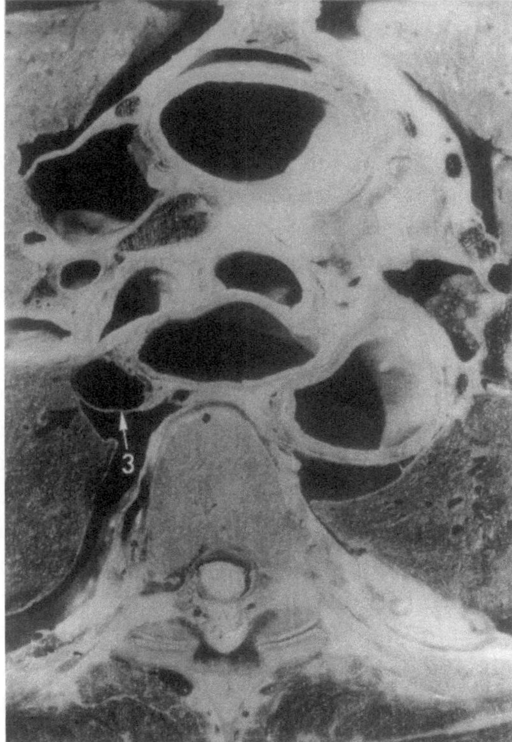

Fig. 8.13 A–C. Radiographic anatomy of azygos arch (lateral projection). **A** Lateral tomogram. **B** Cross-table lateral azygogram on same patient. **C** Transverse body section through posterior turn of azygos arch. In some individuals, plain lateral radiographs and lateral tomograms will demonstrate posterior turn of azygos arch, azygos knob, as a rounded shadow (*1*) projected behind plane of trachea and above shadow of right upper lobe bronchus (*2*). Lateral azygogram confirms that rounded shadow represents posterior turn of azygos vein. Shadow should not be mistaken for node or mass. Note that lateral tomogram made with patient lying on left side shows azygos knob to be situated quite forward of spine, whereas lateral azygogram made supine shows knob to be superimposed on anterior aspect of vertebral bodies. This change in position of mediastinal structures relative to spine is graphic evidence of mobility of mediastinal structures with change in body position. Although azygos knob is prespinal structure, it may be demonstrated on lateral films as in **A** because it lies slightly to right of midline, permitting lung to insert itself behind posterior turn of vein (*3*). Compare **C** with Fig. 8.12. (**A** From [48])

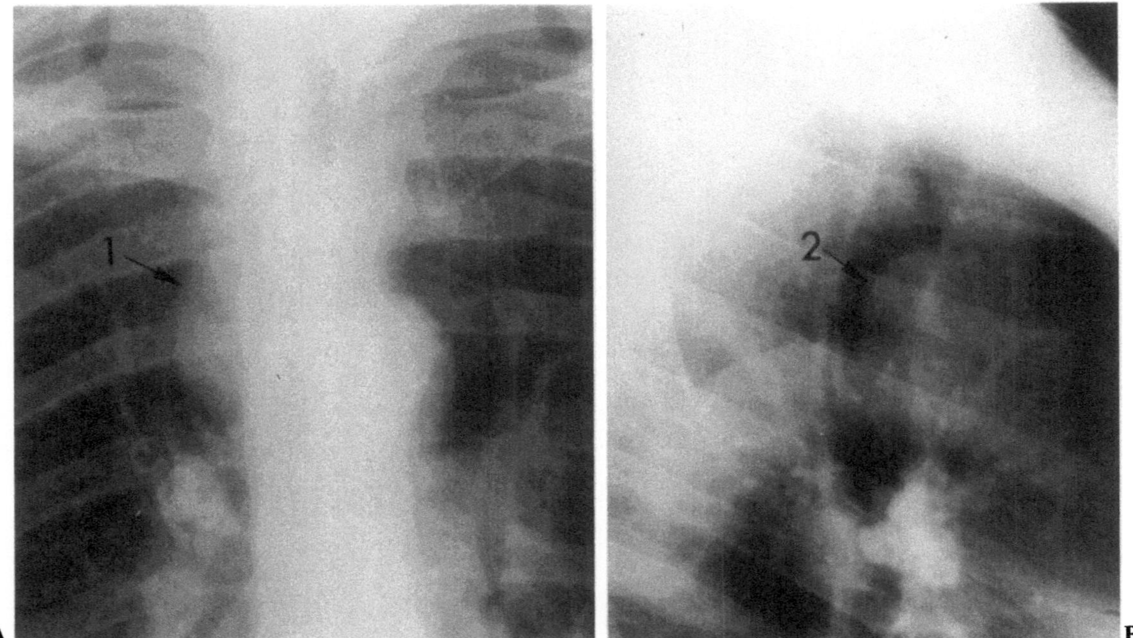

Fig. 8.14A, B. Position of enlarged azygos node contrasted with position of azygos arch. A PA radiograph. B Lateral radiograph. Prominent rounded structure shown in right side of mediastinum (1) could conceivably be considered to represent aneurysmal dilation of azygos vein. Lateral film, demonstrating posterior aspect of this shadow through air-filled trachea (2), proves that shadow cannot represent azygos vein, the posterior turn of which would have to be demonstrated posterior to plane of trachea. The mass, located in position of azygos node in two projections, should have been considered to represent enlargement of node. At surgery azygos node was found to be involved by metastatic tumor

nent shadow lateral to the origin of the right main bronchus from the trachea is produced by the azygos arch or an enlarged azygos node, identification of the density on the lateral film distinguishes between the two possibilities. An enlarged azygos node will lie at the junctions of the azygos arch with the superior vena cava, anterior to the plane of the trachea, whereas the posterior turn of a prominent azygos arch will lie posterior to the plane of the trachea (Figs. 8.13 and 8.14).

Since the mediastinal recesses above and below the azygos arch frequently extend across the midline in front of the spine, the lung in these recesses can provide contrast to demon-

strate on lateral radiographs the thickness of the soft tissues between the anterior surfaces of the thoracic vertebral bodies and the lung. Thus, a prespinal line analogous to the paraspinal line can sometimes be identified above the azygos arch or below it [48]. When the prespinal line is visible, it can be analyzed radiographically in a manner similar to the analysis of the paraspinal line. Because the prespinal line is more often visible below the azygos arch than above it, it will be discussed further in chapter 9.

The azygos arch can be seen on all computed tomograms. Sometimes it is seen in one level of section only; in other patients it may be seen on two sections. Commonly the right superior intercostal vein can be seen as it enters the posterior portion of the arch (Fig. 8.12). Landay [61] has noted that the arch could be seen interposed between lung and the posterior wall of the right main or right upper lobe bronchus on 9% of computed tomograms. Since these portions of the airway are normally contacted by lung, soft tissue density seen in this location should raise the question of tumor; to avoid error, variant appearances of the position of the azygos vein must be appreciated.

Smathers et al. [97] have presented a review of the appearance of the azygos arch on computed tomograms. They have emphasized that the anterior portion of the arch may take a "dip" before entering the superior vena cava. When this variant occurs the anterior portion of the arch may be imaged as a round or oval shadow behind the superior vena cava and may mimic a lymph node (Fig. 8.12). Knowledge of this variation in the appearance of the anterior azygos arch should lead to the performance of a contrast-enhanced scan which will confirm the shadow to be a vessel.

8.2.1 Congenital Displacement of the Azygos Arch

The arch of the azygos vein is displaced from its normal position by two relatively common anomalies: the azygos lobe and right aortic arch.

8.2.1.1 The Azygos Lobe

The azygos lobe is a common anomaly occurring in 0.4%–1.0% of individuals [14]. The right posterior cardinal vein represents the embryonic source of the azygos arch. In early fetal life the right lung apex lies medial to this vein. Normally, it migrates over the top of the lung to reach its usual position [98]. Although the exact embryologic events leading to the development of the azygos lobe are unknown, it is apparent that the anomaly results from persistence of some right lung medial to the evolving azygos arch [15]. Instead of passing over the top of the right upper lobe, the cardinal vein penetrates the lobe carrying parietal and visceral pleura ahead of it. The lobe is therefore not a supernumerary one but merely a partially subdivided right upper lobe [45]. The amount of lung tissue interposed medial to the right posterior cardinal vein determines the size of the lobe. In an analysis of 12 cases from the literature, Boyden [15] concluded that the azygos lobe was aerated by branches from either the apical or posterior segmental bronchi of the right upper lobe and that smaller lobes were supplied by one of these branches. He stated "the azygos vein descends

erratically into the substance of the lung in such a way as to bend and separate branches of a given segment." Whether this fact explains the occasional instances of abnormal perfusion and ventilation of azygos lobes demonstrated at isotopic scanning is conjectural [82]. The arterial supply to the azygos lobe in general follows the bronchial supply; independent arterial supply is rare [26].

The azygos arch, "trapped" between medial and lateral portions of the right upper lobe, has a characteristic "teardrop" configuration superior and lateral to its usual position (Fig. 8.15). It is suspended from the dome of the thorax by a double fold of visceral and parietal pleura termed the "mesoazygos" [45] (Fig. 8.15). The enclosed azygos vein can often be identified on lateral radiographs as well because it is totally surrounded by aerated lung (Fig. 8.17). On such radiographs the lung confined by the mesoazygos can be seen to lie behind the superior vena cava and anterior to the right superior intercostal vein (Fig. 8.17). This anatomic arrangement is depicted in cross section in Fig. 8.15. The termination of the azygos arch in the superior vena cava is at a higher level in patients with azygos lobes than it is in normal subjects [98]. On radiographs the most superior portion of the azygos fissure is posterior and in contact with the posterior chest wall at a point called the "parietal trigone" [35] (Figs. 8.15–8.17). At this point, the azygos vein may simulate a pulmonary nodule on computed tomograms [98] (Fig. 8.16).

Speckman et al. [98] have emphasized that computed tomography is an ideal modality to demonstrate the relationships of the azygos lobe to the right side of the mediastinum. They found the superior vena cava to be elliptical in shape in many patients with an azygos lobe. The long axis of the ellipse was oriented such that its anterior aspect lay to the left, its posterior portion to the right. The azygos lobe intruded deeply behind the cava often outlining its left or medial side. In most patients studied by them, the azygos lobe was situated both anterior and posterior to the trachea. The anterior tracheal wall could be seen in five of nine lateral chest radiographs they studied. The esophagus was often found at the left side of the trachea (Fig. 8.17).

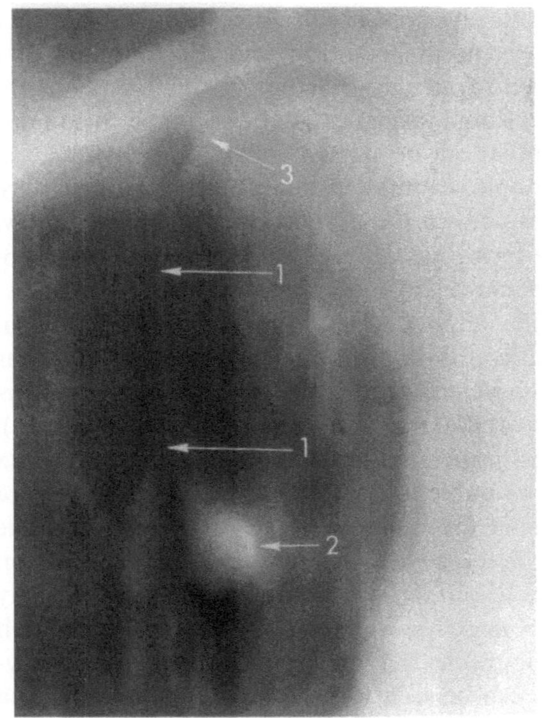

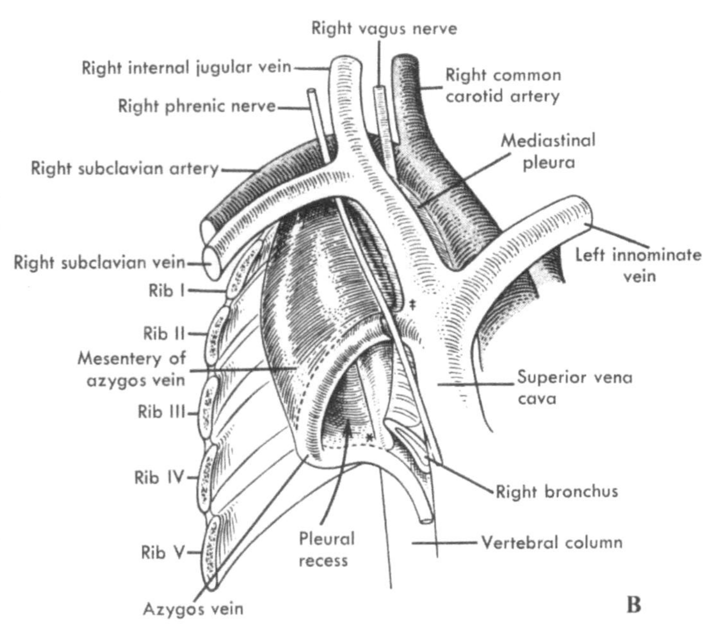

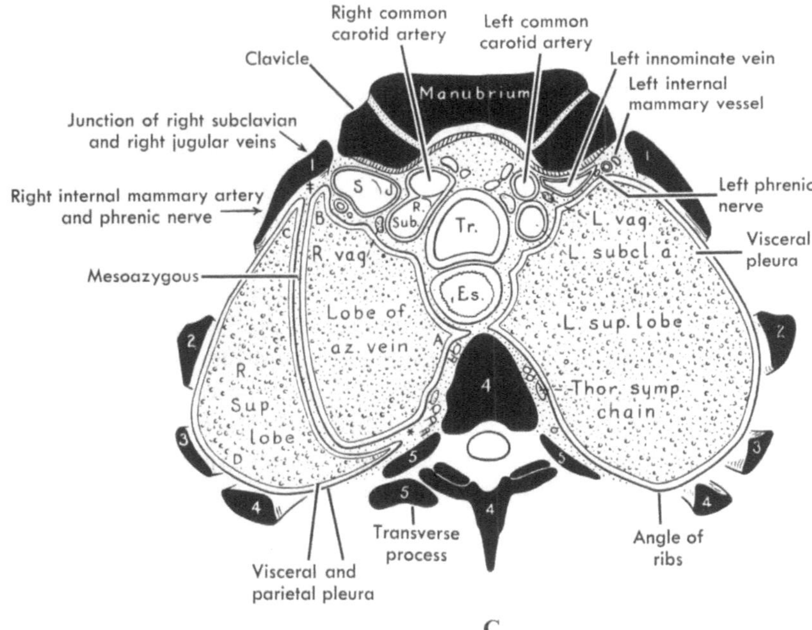

Fig. 8.15 A–C. Congenital displacement of azygos arch. The azygos lobe. **A** AP tomogram. **B** Azygos fissure viewed from anterior aspect. **C** Transverse body section depicting azygos lobe. Azygos fissure, a double fold of visceral and parietal pleura (*1*), encompasses azygos vein, which adopts characteristic "teardrop" configuration at inferior aspect of fissure (*2*). Most superior portion of azygos fissure is posterior and medial, in contact with posterior chest wall at point called "parietal trigone" (*3*). (Area of parietal trigone is *starred* in **C**). (**A** Courtesy G. Tricomi, Rome, Italy. **B** and **C** From [15])

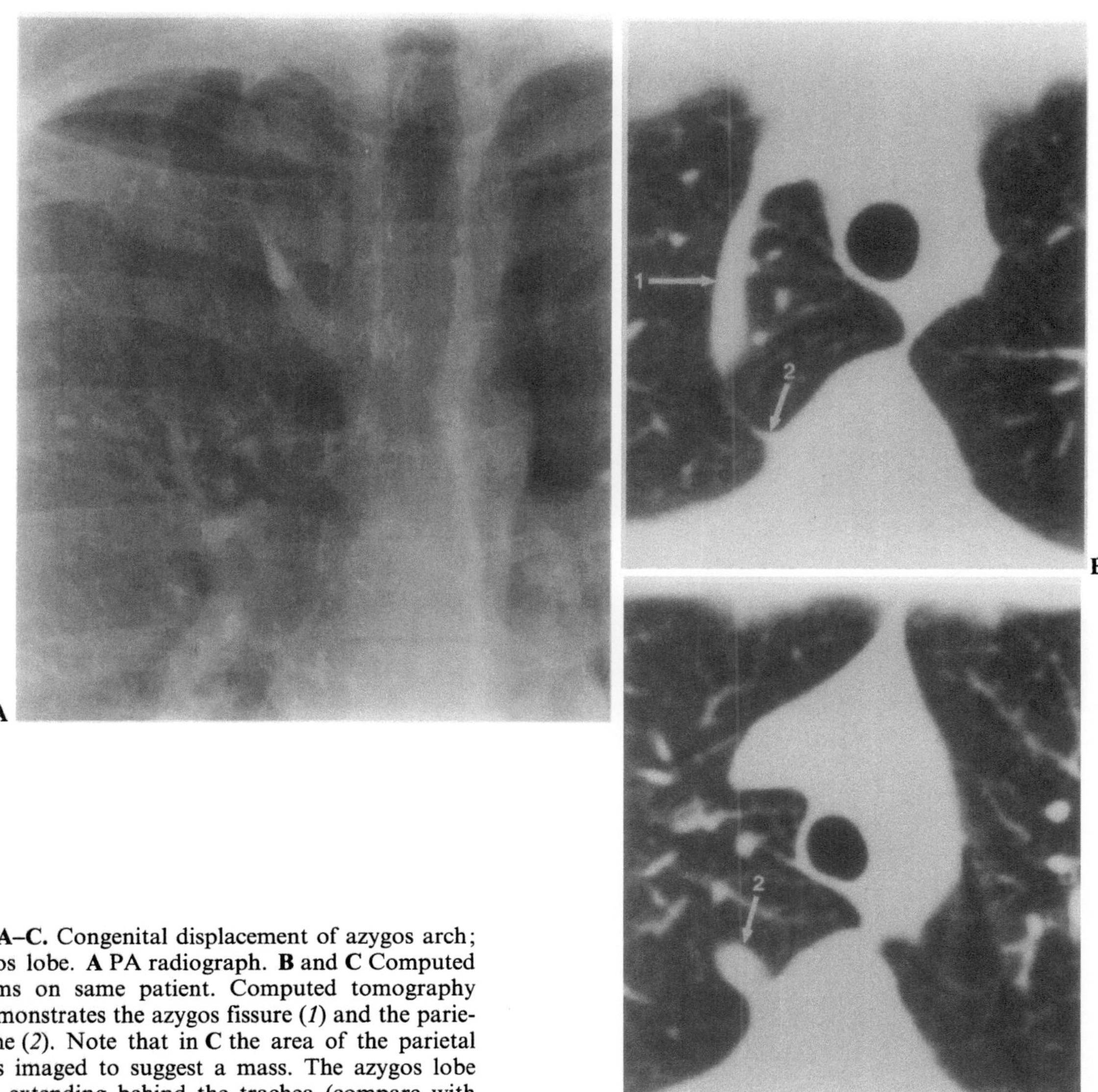

Fig. 8.16A–C. Congenital displacement of azygos arch; the azygos lobe. **A** PA radiograph. **B** and **C** Computed tomograms on same patient. Computed tomography nicely demonstrates the azygos fissure (*1*) and the parietal trigone (*2*). Note that in **C** the area of the parietal trigone is imaged to suggest a mass. The azygos lobe is shown extending behind the trachea (compare with Fig. 8.15) but can extend anterior to it as well

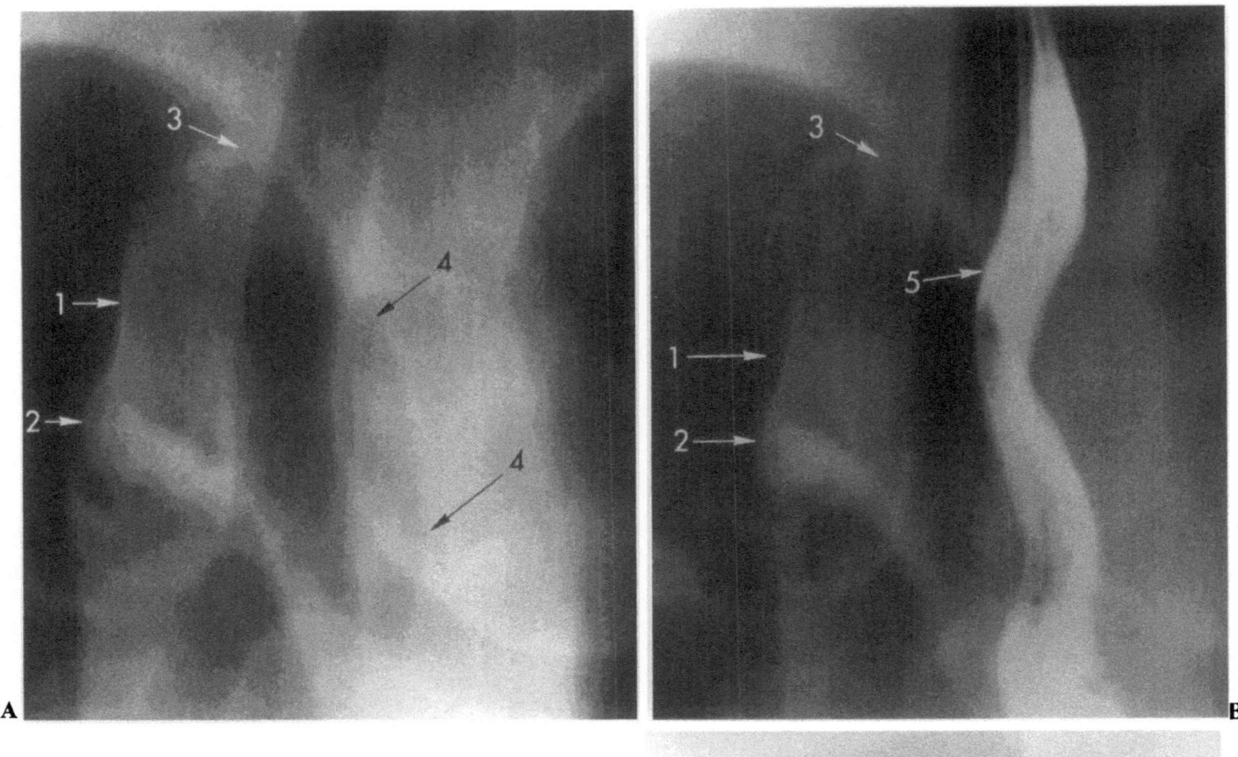

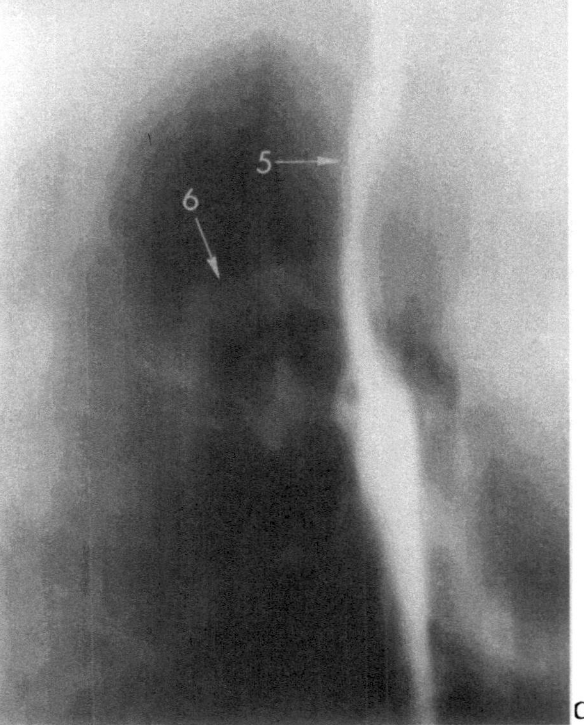

Fig. 8.17 A–C. Congenital displacement of azygos arch; the azygos lobe. **A** AP tomogram. **B** AP tomogram with barium in esophagus. **C** Lateral tomogram with barium in esophagus. Azygos fissure (*1*), azygos vein (*2*), and parietal trigone (*3*) are clearly demonstrated. Note deep medial extension of azygos lobe (*4*) against mediastinum. This intrusion of azygos lobe can be seen extending behind esophagus (*5*) which lies to the left side of the trachea. Because of envelopment of azygos vein by lung, shadow of vein is usually very clearly demonstrated on plain lateral radiographs or tomograms (*6*)

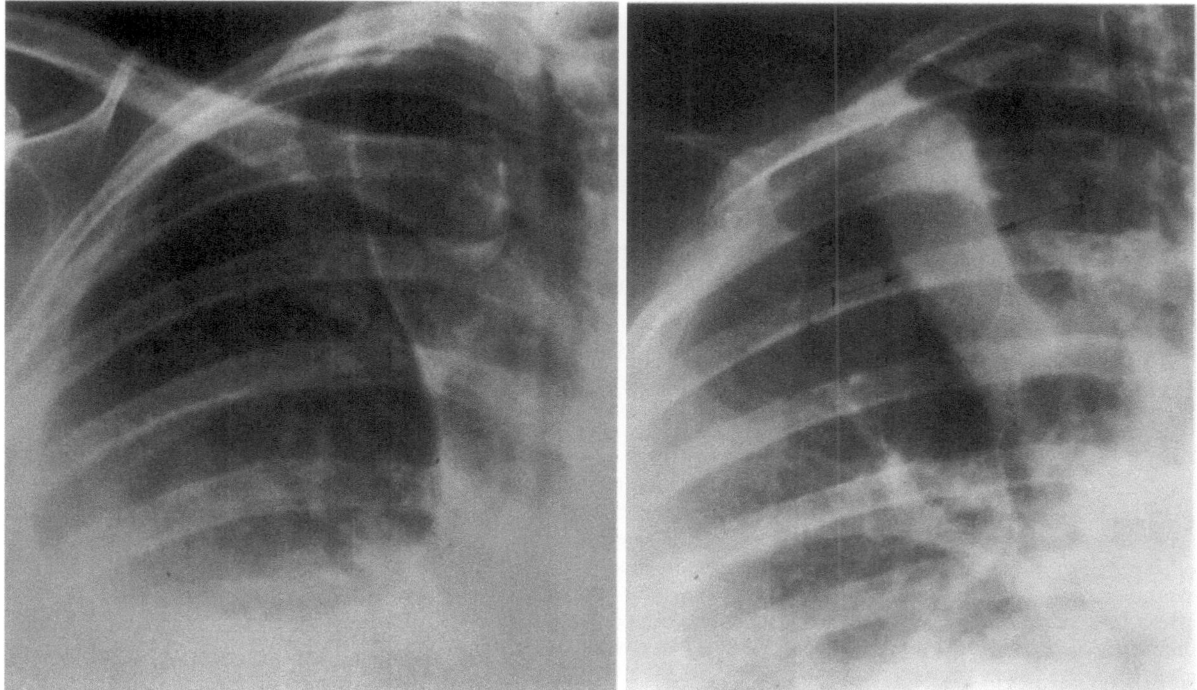

Fig. 8.18A, B. Azygos fissure; pleural effusion (PA radiographs). Although azygos fissure is composed of double layer of visceral and parietal pleurae, it should be recalled that space between each of apposed layers of visceral and parietal pleura is in communication with general pleural cavity and may contain air or fluid in cases of pneumothorax or pleural effusion (*1*). In these two films made a few days apart, fluid has widened fissure, forcing two visceral pleural components against lung. Extrapleural fluid also can enter fissure by extending between apposed parietal pleurae. (Courtesy E. Carsky, Syracuse, NY)

The space between the visceral and parietal pleurae in the azygos fissure communicates with the general pleural space and may contain air or fluid in cases of pneumothorax or pleural effusion (Fig. 8.18). Goebel [43] has described a case in which lung was identified medial to the right brachiocephalic vein on computed tomography, a situation analogous to an azygos lobe. He termed this variant the "lobe" of the right brachiocephalic vein.

8.2.1.2 The Right Aortic Arch

When the aortic arch is left sided, the azygos arch is constant in position lateral to the angle formed by the origin of the right main bronchus from the trachea. The one exception to this statement is found in cases of azygos lobe. However, in cases of right-sided position of the aortic arch the aorta is interposed between the trachea and the superior vena cava. Since the anterior azygos arch terminates in the superior vena cava, it is carried laterally with the cava and,

Fig. 8.19. Congenital displacement of azygos arch; right aortic arch (AP radiograph). In patients with right aortic arch, azygos arch must swing laterally around right side of descending aorta to reach superior vena cava. In this example, anterior portion of azygos arch (*1*) is seen lateral to right side of calcified descending aorta extending inferiorly from right aortic arch. Separation of azygos arch from its usual position against right lateral wall of trachea (*2*) has been said to be a finding supportive of diagnosis of right aortic arch when other appearances are equivocal [38]

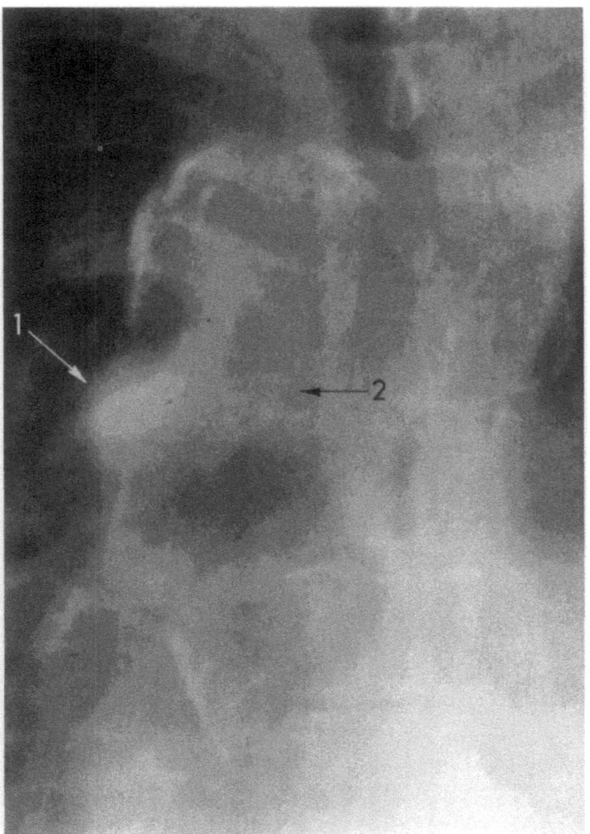

as pointed out by Fishbone [38], is displaced from its normal position against the trachea (Fig. 8.19). Although a right-sided aortic arch is ordinarily readily identified in adults, its diagnosis in children and particularly infants may be difficult. If the azygos vein is seen to be separated from the trachea, the possibility of right-sided aortic arch should be considered [38].

8.3 The Prominent Azygos Vein

The azygos arch can be enlarged in a number of conditions. In order to determine "how big is too big" several studies of its size in normal subjects have been undertaken [30, 34, 35, 39, 57, 104]. A standard method of measurement was used in all of these investigations. The diameter of the anterior portion of the azygos arch was used to judge the size of the azygos vein; for this purpose a line perpendicular to the wall of the right main bronchus and extending to the most convex portion of the arch was measured (Fig. 8.20). In 1952, Fleischner and Udis [39] stated that the maximum diameter of the azygos arch measured perpendicular to the right main bronchus was 6 mm. Subsequently, Keats et al. [57] studied the appearance of the azygos arch on conventional erect PA radiographs and stated that in normal persons the maximum diameter using the same method of measurement was 7 mm. Felson [34, 35] states that in his series of normal patients the diameter of the azygos arch never exceeded 1 cm. Wishart [104] has provided such measurements for children, and Doyle et al. [30] have given the range of normal arch diameter for supine tomographic studies. In the review of Doyle et al., the normal vein width for a 73.6 kg individual examined supine was 14.2 mm; one standard deviation represented 2.6 mm. In the final analysis, the absolute size of the arch is much less significant to diagnosis than is change in size over time.

The anterior portion of the azygos arch can sometimes be difficult to distinguish from an enlarged node. As previously mentioned, a shadow with acute angles at its base is almost

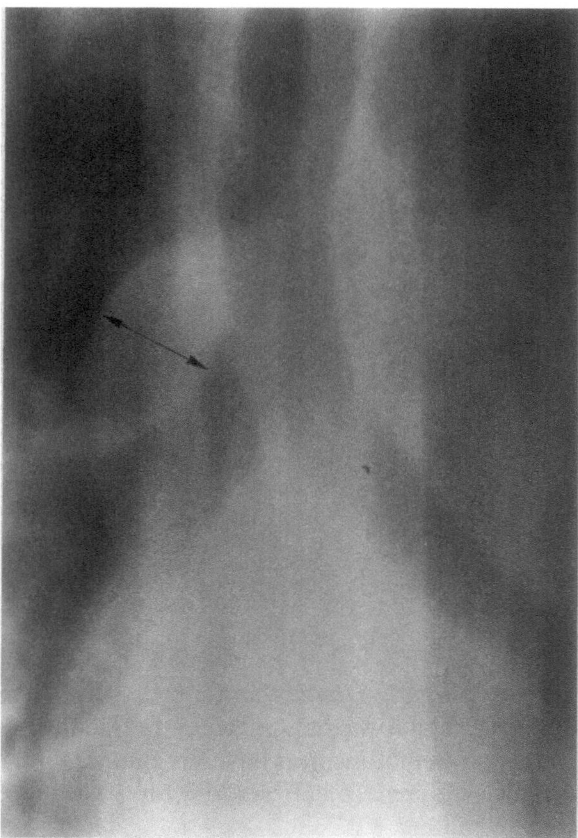

Fig. 8.20. Measurement of size of azygos vein (AP tomogram). Standard measurement of azygos vein is achieved by determining distance from midpoint of arc of azygos vein against lung perpendicular to wall of right main bronchus (*arrow*). It should be appreciated that this dimension represents diameter of anterior portion of azygos arch. Standards are available for PA radiographs and for AP tomograms (see text)

Fig. 8.21 A, B. Azygos arch; effect of Valsalva's maneuver. **A** AP tomogram with barium in esophagus. **B** AP tomogram made during Valsalva's maneuver. Change in configuration of shadow thought to be azygos arch during Valsalva's maneuver proves shadow to be compressible, and therefore not a solid mass. Valsalva's maneuver, reducing venous return and cardiac output while increasing intrathoracic pressure, causes azygos arch to flatten (*1*) or diminish in size

▽

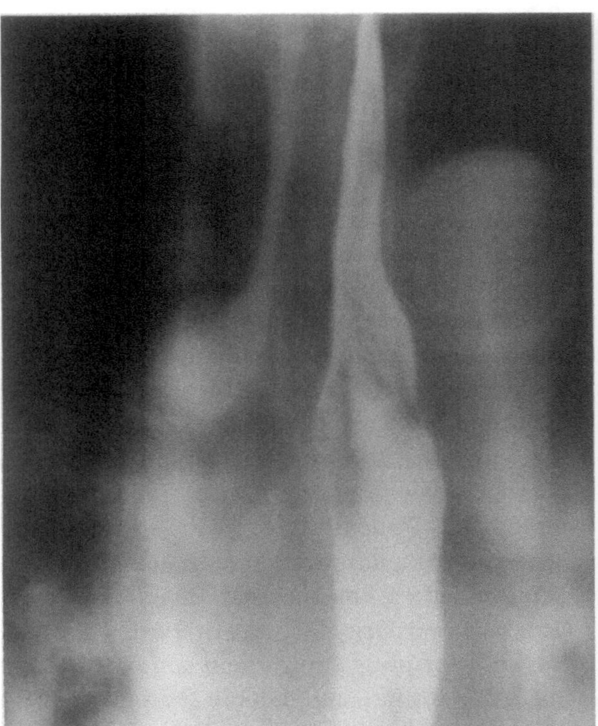

A

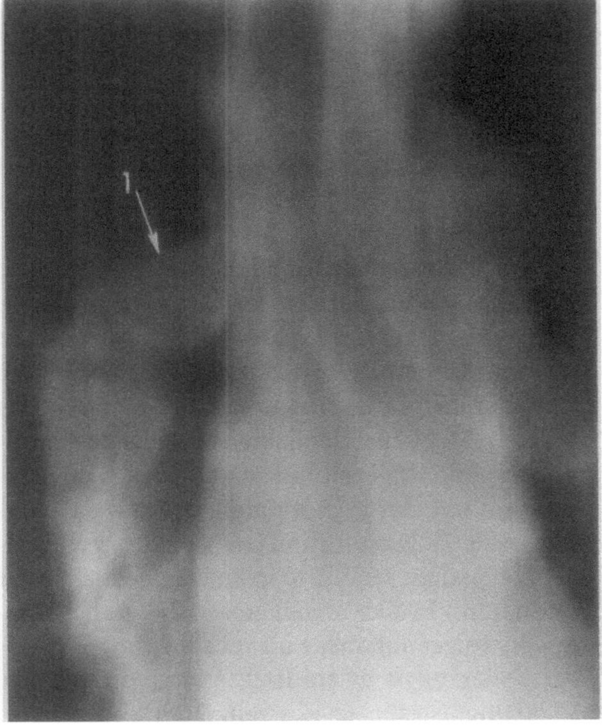

B

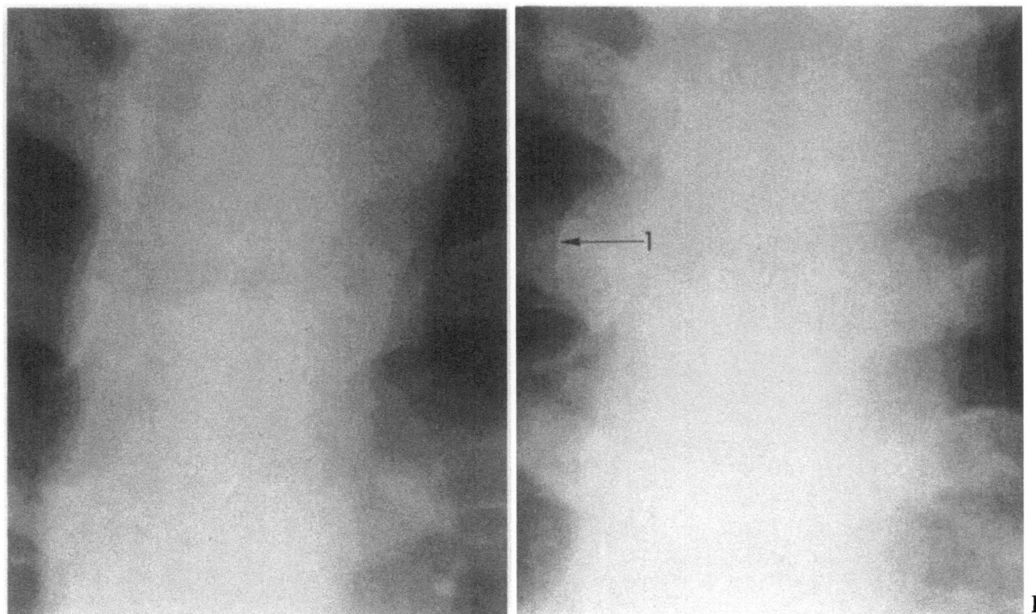

Fig. 8.22 A, B. Azygos arch; effect of recumbency (PA radiographs). Azygos vein is often seen to be larger in recumbent position than in erect position. In **A** azygos arch is not visible, whereas in **B** it is quite prominent (*1*). Change in configuration from erect to recumbent position can be used to prove that shadow in question is not solid mass. When comparing such films one should take into account fact that erect films are usually made at 72 inches (183 cm), whereas recumbent films are usually made AP at shorter distances, a technique causing anteriorly placed structures to be magnified

invariably the vein (Fig. 8.6A). If the density is situated in the characteristic location behind the trachea on the lateral view, it is the vein (Fig. 8.13). Frequently, however, one must resort to films made with change in intrathoracic pressure or body position to clarify the problem. Valsalva's maneuver increases pressure in the thorax and reduces venous return; the azygos vein diminishes in size under these conditions (Fig. 8.21). Müller's maneuver results in the opposite physiologic situation and causes the azygos vein to enlarge. Both maneuvers are accomplished in full inspiration. In Valsalva's maneuver the patient strains to exhale against a closed glottis; in Müller's maneuver the patient attempts to get still more air into the lungs, usually by sucking or by sniffing. A simple expedient to distinguish the azygos vein from a solid mass

is to compare a recumbent film with an erect one. A shadow that enlarges in recumbency after proper allowances have been made for geometric differences between the films is the azygos vein (Fig. 8.22).

8.3.1 Aneurysmal Dilatation of the Azygos Arch

Rarely, the azygos arch may achieve very large size, as great as 2–3 cm in diameter, without associated disease [67] (Fig. 8.23). This condition, commonly termed "aneurysmal dilatation of the azygos vein," is idiopathic and may be thought of as a normal variant; more often it is considered to be a congenital abnormality. There are no reported cases of rupture of such aneurysmal dilatations, and apparently the condition is entirely benign. However, one should be somewhat wary of the very large azygos vein since traumatic aneurysms of the arch having a more serious portent do occur, although very rarely [35]. Patients have been operated upon under the assumption that a dilated azygos vein represented a mediastinal mass lesion [18]. Rockoff and Druy [87] have reported a case in which a tortuous azygos vein simulated a mass on both frontal and lateral radiographs. The differential diagnosis is usually easily resolvable

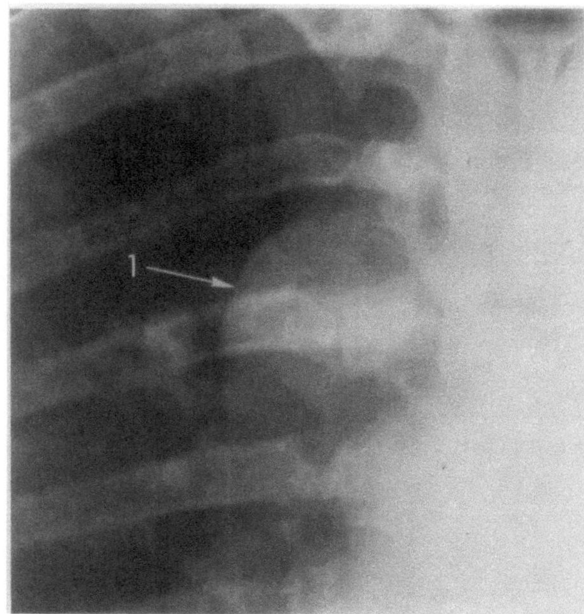

Fig. 8.23. Aneurysmal dilation of azygos vein (PA radiograph). Exceptionally azygos arch is very large (*1*) without known cause. Such a situation, known as "aneurysmal dilatation of azygos vein," is a benign condition; rupture is not known to occur. One should keep in mind, however, that rarely an aneurysm of the azygos vein may develop following trauma; in this situation rupture apparently can occur [35]

by simple radiologic methods if the possibility of aneurysmal dilatation or tortuosity of the azygos vein is considered. Decrease in size of the structure or flattening of its lateral aspect during Valsalva's maneuver proves the lesion to be vascular (Fig. 8.21). In addition it is often possible to demonstrate that the lesion becomes larger when the patient is recumbent than when erect, providing evidence that the mass is not solid in character (Fig. 8.22).

8.3.2 Azygos Vein Enlargement Secondary to Increased Right Ventricular Pressure

The azygos vein may dilate in any cardiovascular abnormality that produces increased pressure within the right ventricle and the superior vena cava. Any of the conditions in which an elevated right heart pressure is the result of an increase in postcapillary pulmonary resistance may show enlargement of the azygos vein. Its enlargement in left ventricular failure has probably received the most attention in the literature [57] (Fig. 8.24). Unfortunately, the studies

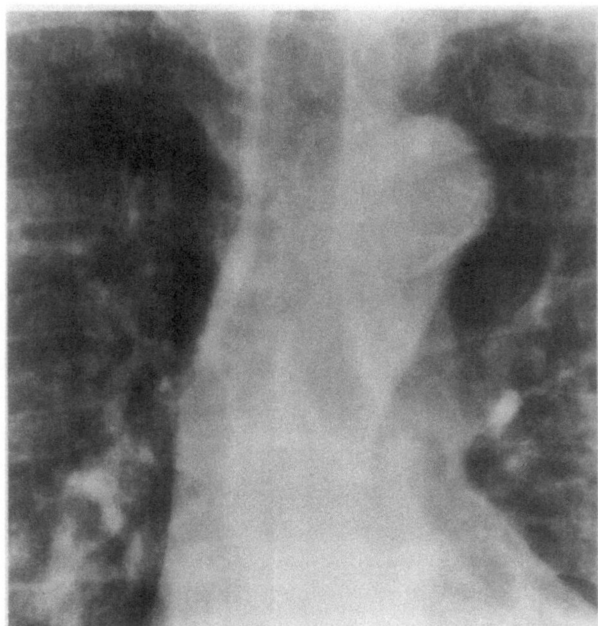

A

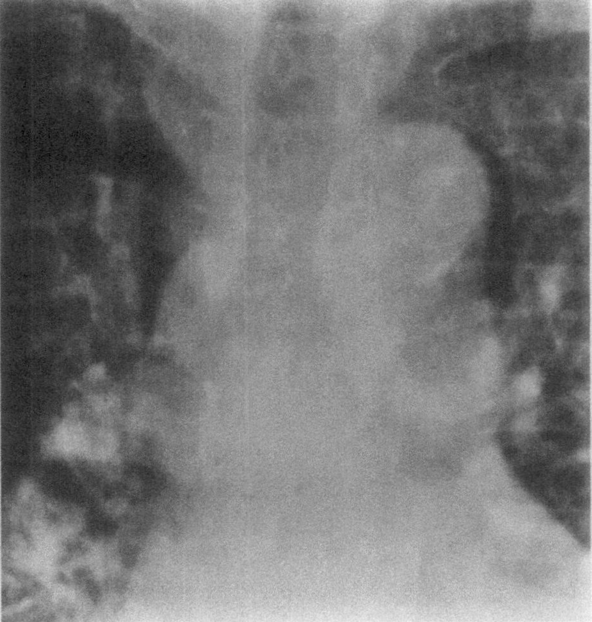

B

Fig. 8.24A, B. Enlargement of the azygos vein in left ventricular failure. PA radiographs. In **A** the azygos arch is flattened, in **B**, made during a period of left ventricular failure, the azygos arch is distended. The change is the result of increased pressures in the right side of the heart secondary to pulmonary venous hypertension. Enlargement of the azygos arch is a helpful clue to the diagnosis of left ventricular failure if other causes for pulmonary hypertension can be excluded

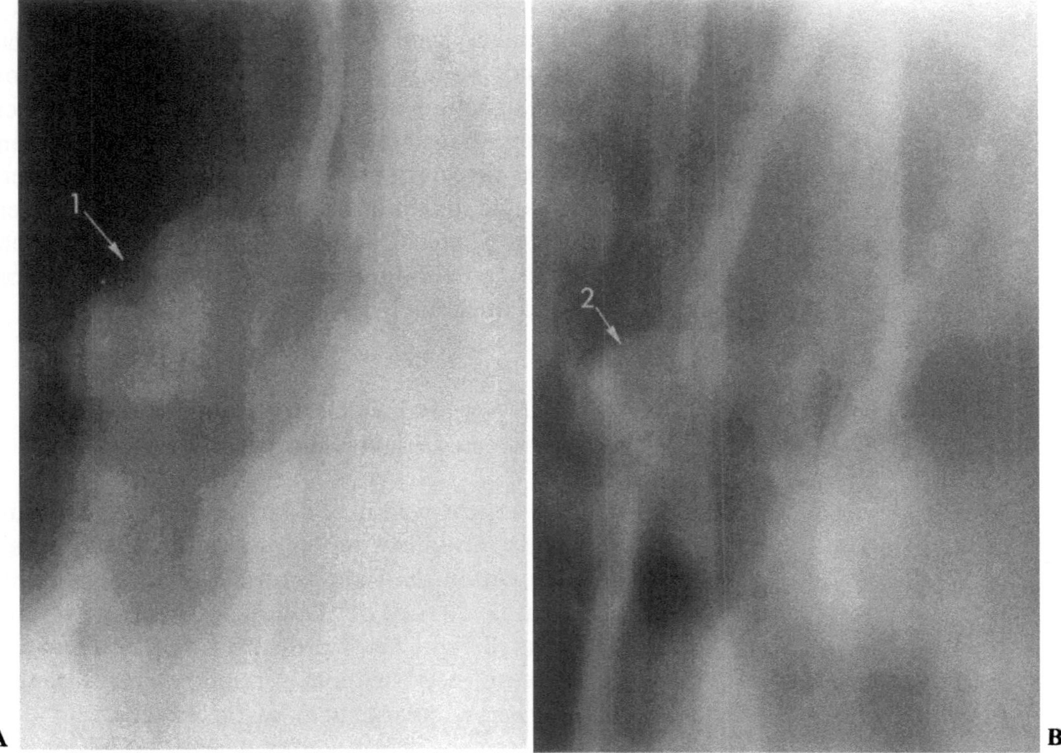

Fig. 8.25A, B. Increase in size of azygos arch secondary to chronically elevated right ventricular pressure (Pickwickian syndrome). **A** AP tomogram. **B** Lateral tomogram. Azygos arch may dilate secondary to chronic increase in pressure in right heart. Marked increase in size of anterior part of azygos arch (*1*) is shown in **A**. Prominence of posterior portion of azygos arch is seen in characteristic position posterior to trachea (*2*). In these patients with marked obesity, chronic cor pulmonale develops, apparently due to peripheral pulmonary vasoconstriction secondary to alveolar hypoventilation

thus far reported give no indication of the statistical frequency of azygos dilatation in left ventricular failure. We have seen many instances of rather marked pulmonary venous hypertension and pulmonary edema unassociated with dilatation of the azygos vein, even though it is a virtual certainty that in some of the patients right ventricular pressures were high.

The azygos vein also enlarges in a wide variety of disorders that cause an increase in precapillary pulmonary resistance. These conditions can be acute or chronic (Fig. 8.25). Enlargement of the azygos vein can be particularly helpful in the diagnosis of constrictive pericarditis, which almost always causes nonspecific radiographic findings. In such cases the likelihood of increased right ventricular pressure suggested by a prominent azygos arch or one which has increased in size on serial radiographic studies may well lead to definitive diagnositc procedures. Pulmonary thromboembolic disease also presents difficult challenges for the clinician and radiologist. Most deaths due to pulmonary embolism occur in patients in whom the diagnosis was not suspected and therefore not treated. A retrospective study of this problem by Hildner and Ormond [51] revealed that the correct diagnosis was made in only 40% of cases despite utilization of all diagnostic methods short of pulmonary angiography. In those difficult cases that require pulmonary embolism and myocardial infarction to be entertained in the differential diagnosis, the radiographic finding of a prominent azygos arch, suggestive of acute cor pulmonale, should cause thromboembolism to be considered the likely diagnosis if left ventricular failure can be excluded. When studying a single radiograph or a series of roentgenograms, it should be kept in mind that films made on very ill patients are often made supine and that the azygos arch enlarges in the supine position. It should also be emphasized that an azygos arch of normal size does not necessarily mean that the right ventricular pressures are normal. Despite these limitations, careful analysis of the azygos arch can be a worthwhile index to judge elevation of pressures in the right ventricle. Milne et al. [70, 71] and Pistolesi et al. [81] have expanded upon this theme in a series of articles discussing "the vascular pedicle of the heart" and the azygos vein in the normal subject and in patients with a variety of acquired cardiovascular problems.

8.3.3 Azygos Vein Enlargement Due to Increased Blood Flow Through It

Enlargement of the azygos vein caused by an increase in blood flow through it can result from anomalies of the azygos or hemiazygos systems, from obstruction of the superior or inferior vena cava, and from pregnancy. The most frequently encountered congenital anomaly producing increased flow in the azygos system is azygos continuation of the inferior vena cava [1, 2, 3, 11]. In this condition the infradiaphragmatic interruption of the cava causes divergence of blood through the azygos system, which dilates in compensation. The condition should be considered on plain films when the azygos arch and the ascending portion of the azygos vein are dilated in the absence of known caval obstruction (Fig. 8.26). The condition should also be suspected when an enlarged azygos arch and ascending azygos vein are seen with abnormal thoracic or abdominal situs (Fig. 8.26). Of 32 cases reviewed by Anderson et al. [3], situs was normal in 18 and abnormal in 14. Elliott et al. [32] reported eight cases having discordant position of the aortic arch and gastric air bubble (that is, the gastric air bubble and aortic arch were demonstrated to be on opposite sides of the body rather than on the same side); azygos continuation of the inferior vena cava was present in all. Azygos continuation may be isolated and benign, but more often it is associated with a variety of congenital cardiac defects. Azygos

continuation is readily diagnosed by inferior vena cavography (Fig. 8.26), but this study has been supplanted by computed tomography which establishes the diagnosis in a noninvasive manner [16, 21, 102] (Fig. 8.26).

Dilatation of the azygos system due to increased flow can be acquired when obstruction of systemic venous return through conventional channels leads to divergence of blood flow into the azygos and hemiazygos veins [10, 33, 42, 52]. Obstruction of the superior vena cava may be the result of thrombosis (Fig. 8.27) or obstruction by tumor invasion or compression (Fig. 8.28). Exceptionally, mediastinal fibrosis may cause its occlusion. Etiologic considerations in superior vena caval syndrome have been reviewed by Engel et al. [33] and by Parish et al. [78]. With caval obstruction the venous return from the head and upper extremities follows alternate venous pathways through the mediastinum and the chest wall, ultimately draining into the azygos and hemiazygos vein [75] (Figs. 8.27 and 8.28). This additional flow of blood from the head and upper extremities is added to the usual azygos blood flow, and the azygos system dilates as a consequence. On chest films, these dilated veins may produce abnormal mediastinal contours unilaterally or bilaterally (see Figs. 6.27 and 8.27) and are usually well demonstrated at computed tomography [10, 33] (Fig. 8.28 C). McMurdo et al. [69] have discussed the value of magnetic resonance imaging in the diagnosis of mediastinal venous occlusion. Collateral blood flow through the left superior intercostal vein may produce a rounded prominence sometimes called the aortic "nipple" at the lateral margin of the aortic knob [13, 62, 66, 76] (see Figs. 6.23 and 6.24). On occasion, collateral flow may involve the upper esophageal veins, producing on esophograms serpiginous filling defects that have aptly been termed "downhill varices" [36, 93] (see Fig. 6.28). A further discussion of the radiographic abnormalities produced by these collateral venous channels is included in the chapters on the supra-aortic and infra-aortic areas (chapters 6 and 7).

A similar sequence of events can result from obstruction of the inferior vena cava [18]

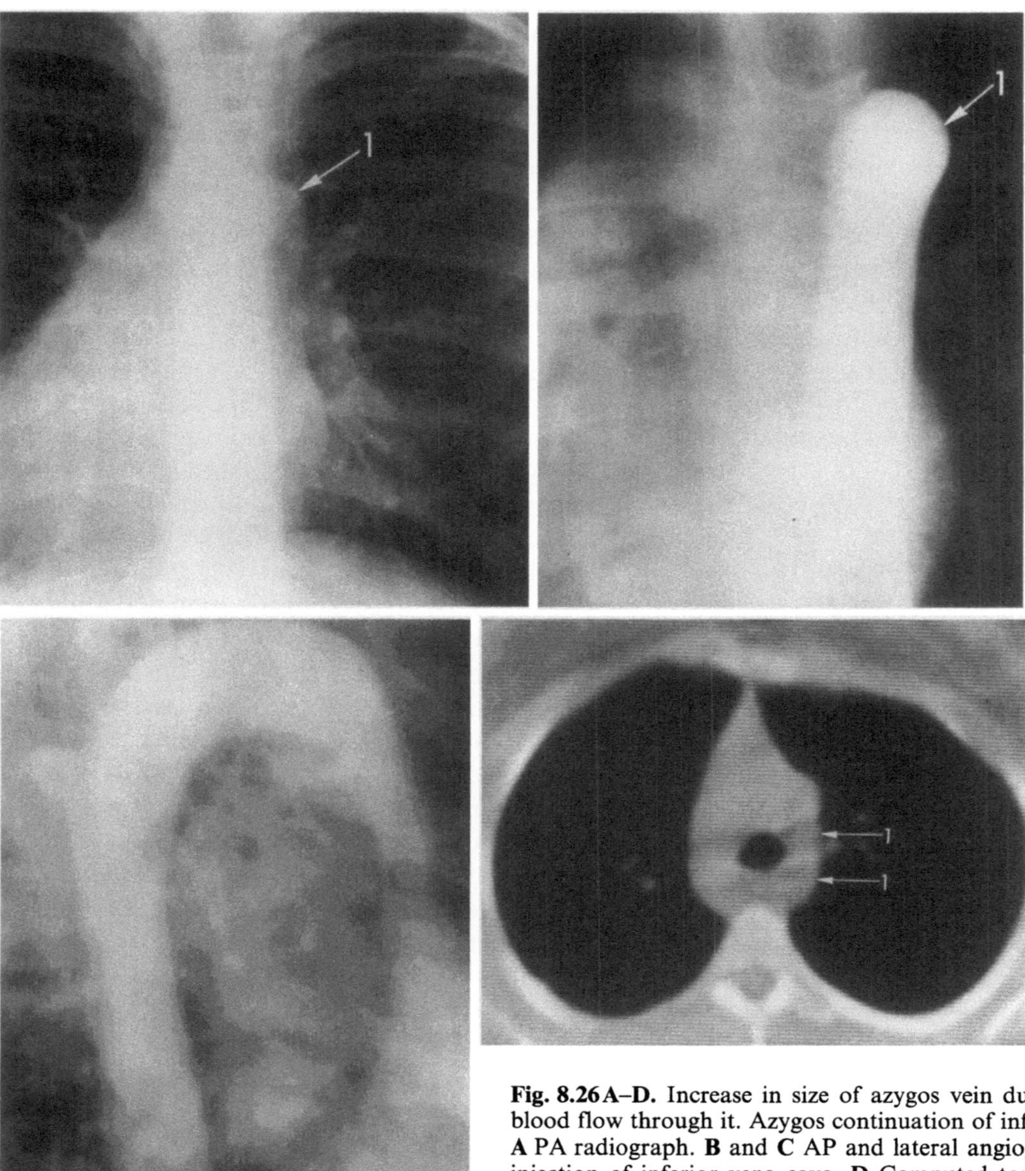

Fig. 8.26A–D. Increase in size of azygos vein due to increase in blood flow through it. Azygos continuation of inferior vena cava. **A** PA radiograph. **B** and **C** AP and lateral angiograms following injection of inferior vena cava. **D** Computed tomogram. In this patient with dextrocardia, azygos arch is extremely prominent (*1*). Note also that ascending portion of azygos vein is extremely dilated due to fact that vessel is handling all of venous return from abdomen. Characteristic "candy cane" appearance of dilated azygos vein on lateral azygogram is also demonstrated. (**B** From [46])

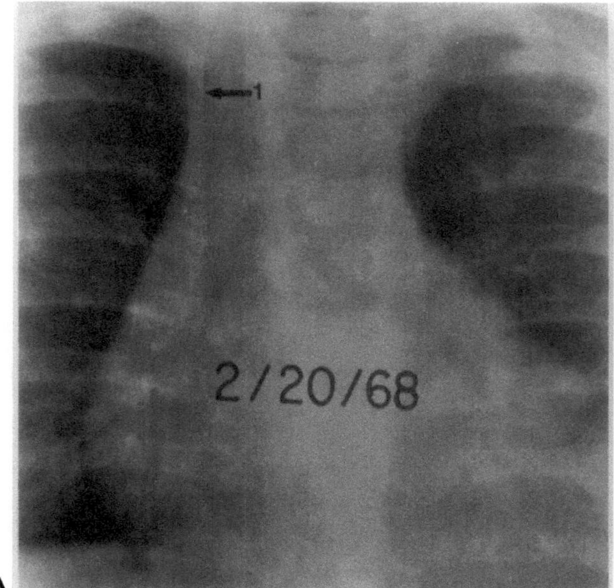
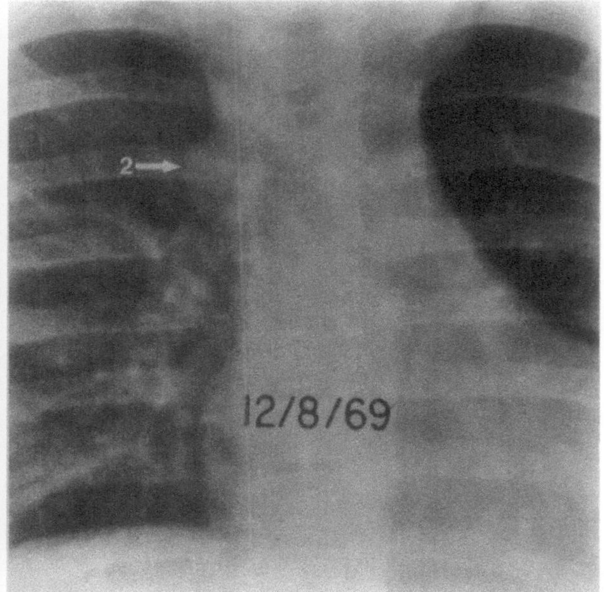
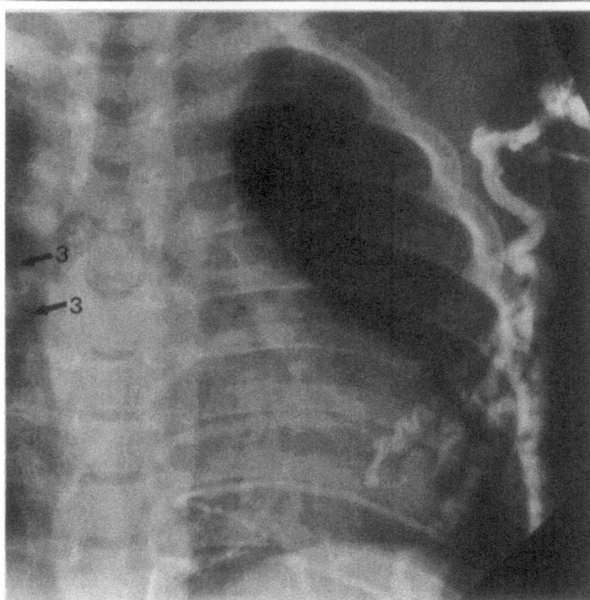

Fig. 8.27 A–C. Increase in size of azygos vein due to increase in blood flow through it. Collateral blood flow. **A** and **B** PA radiographs. **C** AP angiogram following injections of veins of left arm. In this child with hydrocephalus, a Spitz-Holtzer valve (*1*) was placed with its tip in right atrium. Child developed superior vena caval syndrome due to thrombosis of superior vena cava and innominate veins 22 months later. Marked dilatation of azygos arch is shown (*2*); dilatation of ascending portion of azygos vein, which has buckled against right lung, is also apparent (*3*). Dilatation of ascending portion of azygos vein may cause this portion of vessel to buckle into homolateral chest where its contact with lung causes it to be visualized in manner analogous to demonstration of tortuous descending aorta. Significant dilatation of ascending portion of azygos vein occurs only as result of increased blood flow through it. This portion of vessel does not dilate appreciably as result of increased pressure in right side of heart. Following injections of veins of left arm, collateral blood flow can be seen feeding into intercostal veins on left, which in turn empty into hemiazygos and azygos systems. (From [46])

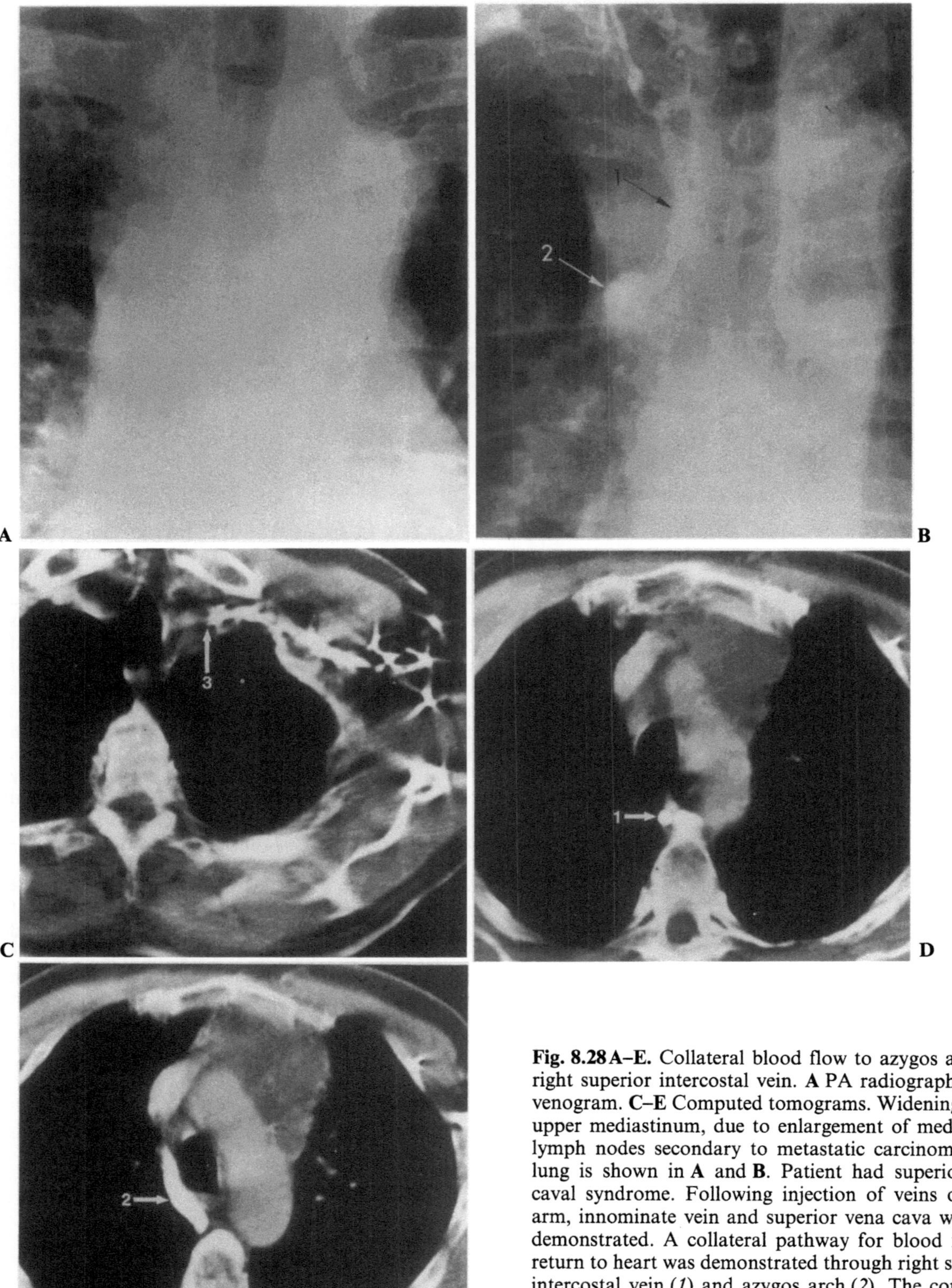

Fig. 8.28A–E. Collateral blood flow to azygos arch via right superior intercostal vein. **A** PA radiograph. **B** AP venogram. **C–E** Computed tomograms. Widening of the upper mediastinum, due to enlargement of mediastinal lymph nodes secondary to metastatic carcinoma from lung is shown in **A** and **B**. Patient had superior vena caval syndrome. Following injection of veins of right arm, innominate vein and superior vena cava were not demonstrated. A collateral pathway for blood flow to return to heart was demonstrated through right superior intercostal vein (*1*) and azygos arch (*2*). The computed tomograms (**C**), made on another patient with superior vena caval syndrome secondary to bronchogenic carcinoma, show that this is often an ideal noninvasive way to investigate such patients. Actually, as shown in **C**,

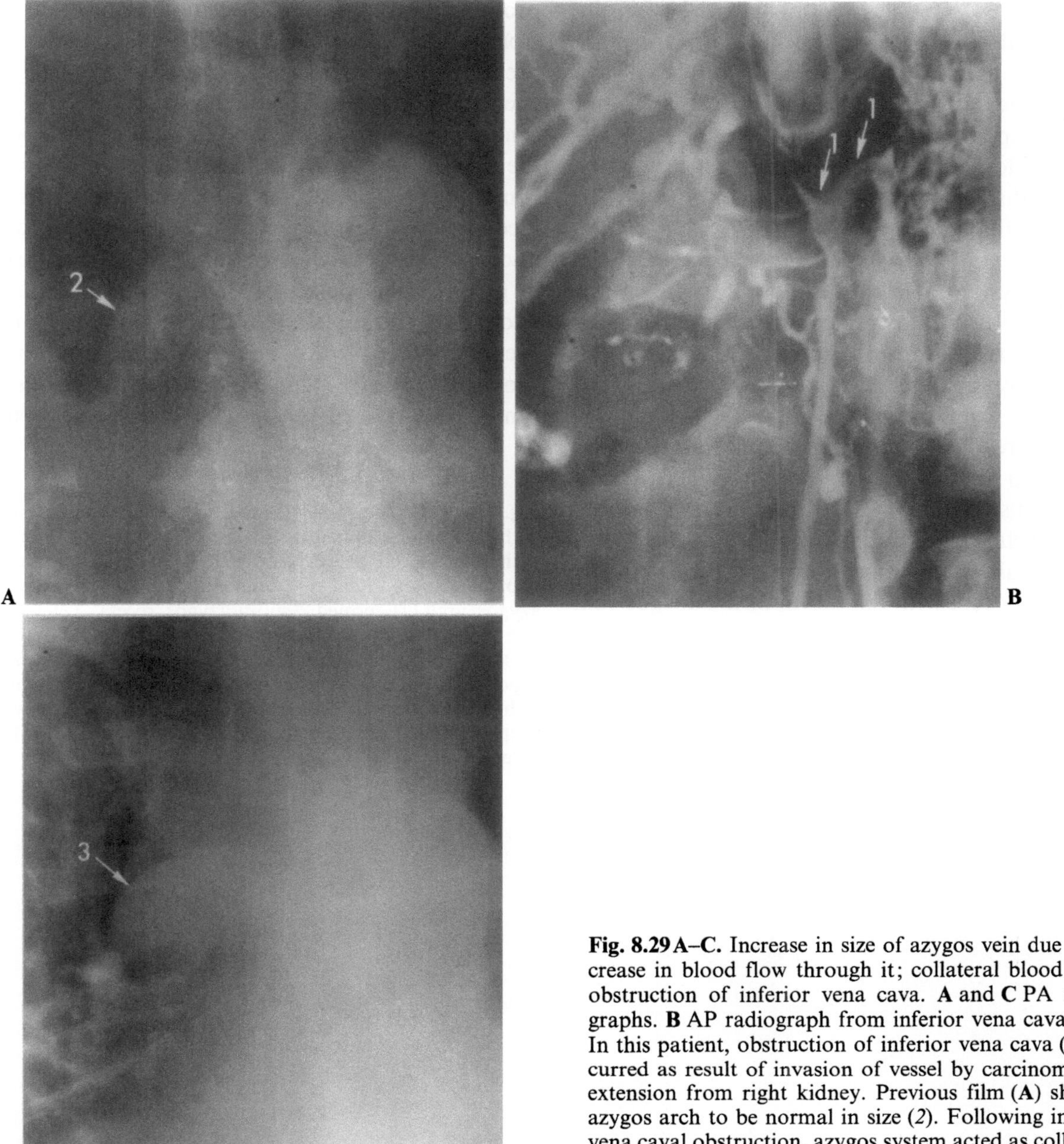

Fig. 8.29 A–C. Increase in size of azygos vein due to increase in blood flow through it; collateral blood flow; obstruction of inferior vena cava. **A** and **C** PA radiographs. **B** AP radiograph from inferior vena cavagram. In this patient, obstruction of inferior vena cava (*1*) occurred as result of invasion of vessel by carcinomatous extension from right kidney. Previous film (**A**) showed azygos arch to be normal in size (*2*). Following inferior vena caval obstruction, azygos system acted as collateral pathway for venous return to heart, and azygos arch became markedly dilated (*3*). (Courtesy H. Shulman, Toronto, Ontario, Canada)

the left brachiocephalic vein (*3*) is obstructed by the large neoplastic mass in the anterior mediastinum shown in **D** and **E**. Extensive collateral circulation is evident in the left chest wall returning contrast through the right superior intercostal vein (*1*) and the azygos vein (*2*). However, sometimes the precise point of obstruction may be difficult to demonstrate at computed tomography

(Fig. 8.29). The abnormal mediastinal contours that result are found in the inferior paraspinal area and may be smooth [96] or lobulated [18]. Sometimes they achieve impressive size and length, apparently because of the volume of diverted blood flow and because such flow must course through the total length of both the azygos and the hemiazygos veins.

Ferris et al. [37] have emphasized that the azygos system acts as an alternate pathway of venous return following complete or partial surgical interruption of the inferior vena cava. Occasionally the dilated azygos system can be seen on plain chest roentgenograms following this procedure. The azygos and hemiazygos systems may also dilate in the presence of portal venous hypertension [50, 52]. Obstruction of the hepatic veins (the Budd-Chiari syndrome) may also result in divergence of blood through the azygos system with dilatation of the azygos vein and arch [30]. Keats [57] has reported that in pregnancy the azygos arch may dilate to a diameter of 15 mm, presumably secondary to the hypervolemia occurring in the pregnant state.

Occasionally, it is possible to distinguish the prominent azygos vein due to increased flow from enlargement associated with increased pressure in the right heart on the basis of plain chest radiographs. With increased flow the ascending portion of the azygos vein as well as the azygos arch may be dilated; this dilatation is manifest on chest films as an abnormal interface between the lung and mediastinum produced by the dilated ascending azygos vein as it grooves the posterior lung [46] (Figs. 8.26 and 8.27). This interface is analogous to the impression made on the lung by a dilated or tortuous descending aorta. Enlargement of the ascending portion of the azygos vein is not seen

Fig. 8.30 A, B. Supra-azygos recess. **A** AP tomogram with barium in esophagus. **B** Right side of mediastinum with mediastinal pleura removed. Lung intrudes into two recesses in right side of mediastinum: one above azygos arch (*1*) termed "supra-azygos recess" (*2*) and one below azygos arch termed "azygoesophageal recess" (*3*). At anterior margin of supra-azygos recess is superior vena cava (*4*); at posterior limit of recess is right superior intercostal vein (*5*) and spine. Potentially, deepest portion of recess is region behind esophagus (*6*). (**A** and **B** From [48])

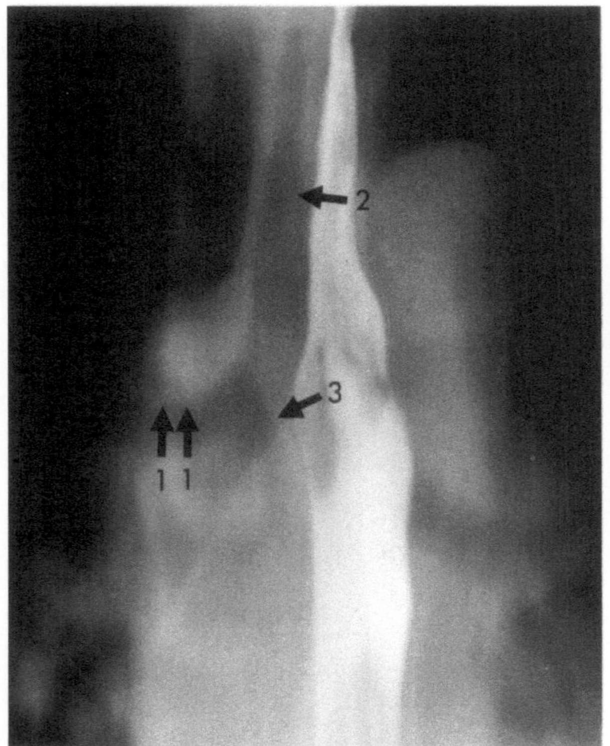

A

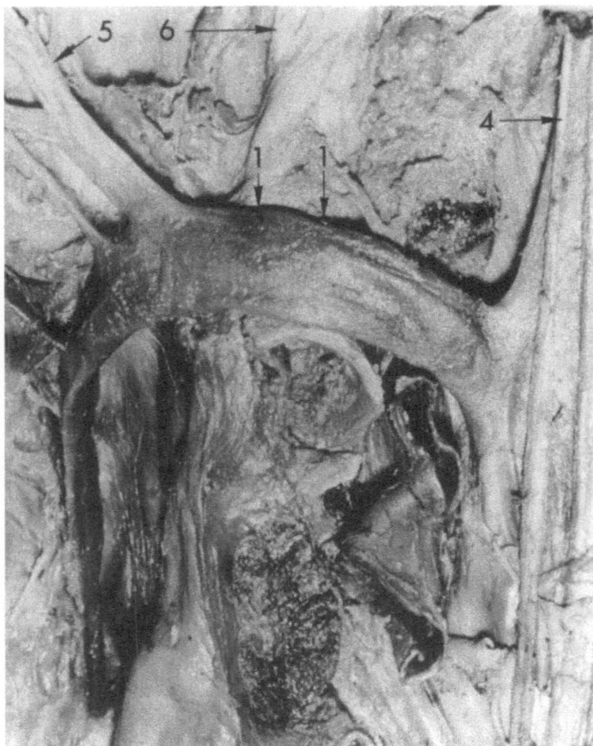

B

in pregnancy, probably because the increase in blood flow is not sufficiently great. In our experience, enlargement of the ascending portion of the azygos vein does not occur as a result of elevated pressures in the right heart, even if this elevated pressure is prolonged and severe.

8.4 The Supra-azygos Recess

It has been mentioned previously that lung commonly intrudes deeply into the mediastinum over the azygos arch to produce an air-filled space termed the "recess cephalad of the azygos arch" or the "supra-azygos recess." This space, containing right upper lobe anteriorly and right lower lobe behind (Figs. 8.30 and 8.31), extends from the superior vena cava backward to the right superior intercostal vein and the spine (Fig. 8.30). As would be anticipated, it is deepest in those patients with emphysema and in those with loss of volume of the left lung. Infrequently the recess is accentuated in cases of collapse of the right upper lobe due to the fact that the displaced right upper lobe bronchus carries the azygos arch upward and somewhat laterally into the lung.

It is often stated that the right lung makes contact on its medial side with the structures in the supra-azygos area to produce six interfaces, which are from front to back: the anterior junction line, the margin of the superior vena cava, the right paratracheal line, the paraesophageal stripe, the posterior junction line, and the paraspinal line (Fig. 8.31). The anterior junction line represents the anterior contact of the right and left visceral and parietal pleurae. These pleural leaves also mark the lateral boundaries of the anterior mediastinum. For

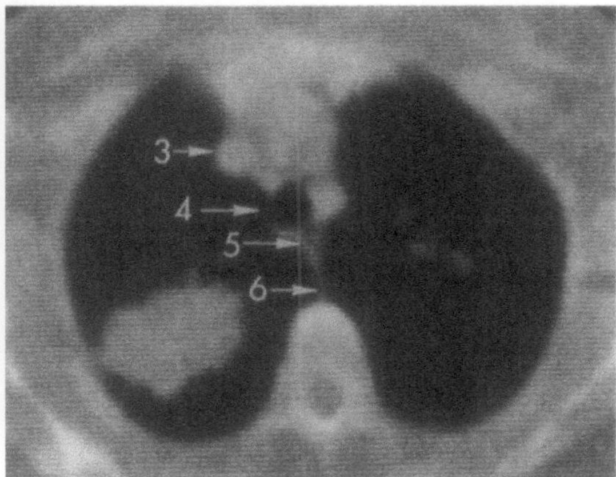

Fig. 8.31 A, B. Supra-azygos recess. Interfaces made by lung in supra-azygos recess with structures in supra-azygos area. Transverse body section (**A**) and computed tomogram through supra-azygos area (**B**) above transverse plane through level of azygos arch. Right lung makes six major interfaces with mediastinal pleura from front to back. Most anterior of these is anterior junction line (*1*), whereas most posterior is paraspinal line (*2*). Between these two, right lung in supra-azygos recess produces interfaces with four structures, which are from front to back superior vena cava (*3*), trachea (*4*), esophagus (*5*), and left lung to produce the posterior junction line (*6*). Note that at times lung in supra-azygos recess can insert itself not only against lateral wall of superior vena cava and trachea, but can also contact posterior wall of these two structures. Lesion in right upper lobe is carcinoma. Clearcut delineation of normal mediastinal interfaces excludes gross right paratracheal adenopathy at this level

A   B

this reason the anterior junction line is discussed in the chapter on the anterior mediastinum (chapter 5). The paraspinal line is produced by the contact of the paraspinal soft tissues and lung, not in the supra-azygos recess but behind it. The correlated radiographic anatomy of the paraspinal line will be covered only briefly in this section; a more comprehensive discussion is included in chapter 7. The ensuing comments will be concerned with the correlated radiographic anatomy of the remainder of the mediastinal interfaces that are produced by lung in the supra-azygos recess. Individual variation in mediastinal configuration and depth of the recess in different coronal planes is great; as a result, not all of the interfaces are seen in every patient.

8.4.1 The Superior Vena Cava and Related Supra-azygos Vessels

In its position at the anterior limit of the supra-azygos recess, the superior vena cava commonly grooves the right lung, which lies lateral and often posterior to it (Figs. 8.31 and 8.32). This interface can be identified correctly on frontal films when its margin becomes continuous with the border of the right atrium. Sometimes it can be seen on lateral radiographs as a linear shadow anterior to the trachea, with convexity directed forward and merging inferiorly with the anterior aspect of the azygos arch (Fig. 8.32).

As the great vessels become ectatic in later life, the superior vena cava is frequently displaced further into the right lung by the dilated and tortuous ascending aorta that lies medial to it. When this occurs, it can at times be difficult to distinguish the displaced caval shadow from right upper lobe parenchymal disease, including atelectasis, and from significant mediastinal pathology [31]. On other occasions, a buckled or widened ascending aorta may contact lung anterior to the cava, again simulating disease (Fig. 8.33); an ectatic innominate [20] or right subclavian artery bulging laterally behind the cava and the right innominate vein may do the same thing. Although the distinction between vascular prominence in the right supra-

azygos area and disease is often difficult, the configuration of the upper portion of the shadow may be of great help. On conventional frontal radiographs the upper margin of the shadow caused by great vessels fades off imperceptibly at the level of the clavicle, although it is seen clearly lower down due to the fact that at this higher level the vessels impinge more on the anterior aspect of the lung than they do on its medial side (see chapter 4). It is true that anterior mediastinal masses may cause the same appearance (the cervicothoracic sign), but the distinction between vessel ectasia and an anterior mediastinal mass can usually be made with a lordotic view. This projection, better demonstrating the course of the right subclavian artery and vein in profile, will often show the characteristic arcuate course of these vessels over the anteromedial aspect of the right upper lobe (see Fig. 4.21).

The utilization of computed axial tomography of the thorax makes the distinction of prominent great vessels from pathologic conditions simple (Fig. 8.31). The innominate artery is normally not visible on conventional radiographs due to its central position within the mediastinum. Sometimes an ectatic innominate artery may simulate a supra-azygos neoplasm [20]. The point of origin of the vessel from the aortic arch lies medial to the superior vena cava and in front of the trachea (Fig. 8.34). An impression produced by this vessel on the anterior trachea wall can sometimes be identified on lateral chest radiographs in infants [12, 100].

Anomalous origin of the left pulmonary artery from the right pulmonary artery may cause stridor in infants [55, 103]. The anomalous vessel swings around the right side of the trachea just above the carina to pass between the trachea and esophagus. The tracheal compression produces stridor; the impression upon the esophagus can be seen on an esophogram. In infants the shadow of the anomalous vessel per se cannot be seen on plain radiographs. However, one proven case in an asymptomatic adult demonstrated a rounded shadow not unlike a prominent azygos vein lying against the trachea above the right upper lobe bronchus on frontal radiographs [56].

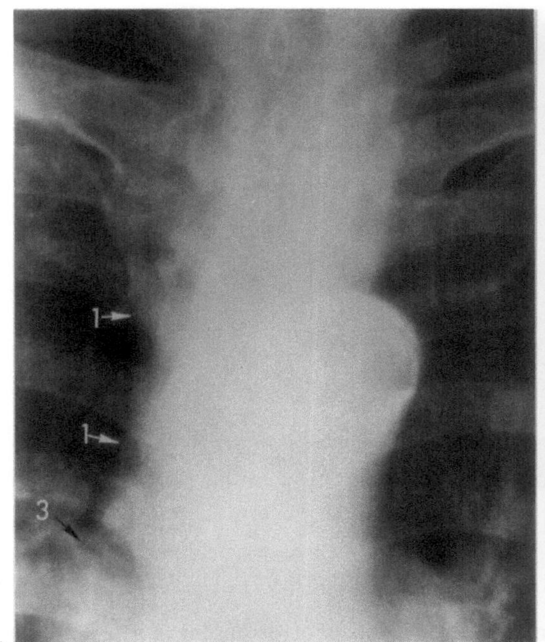

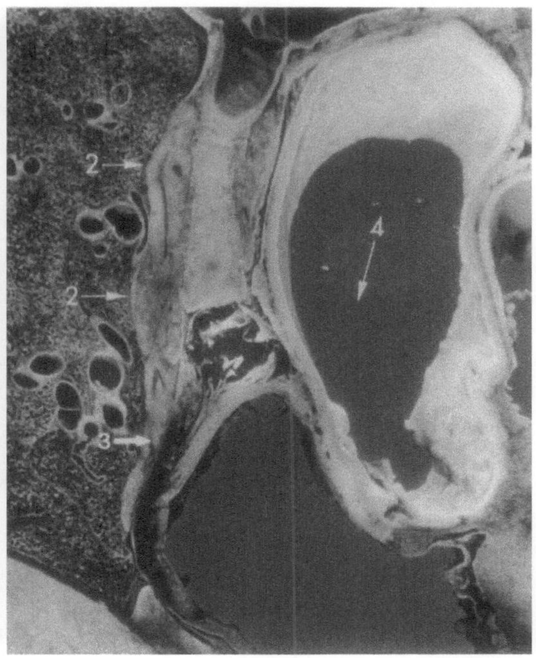

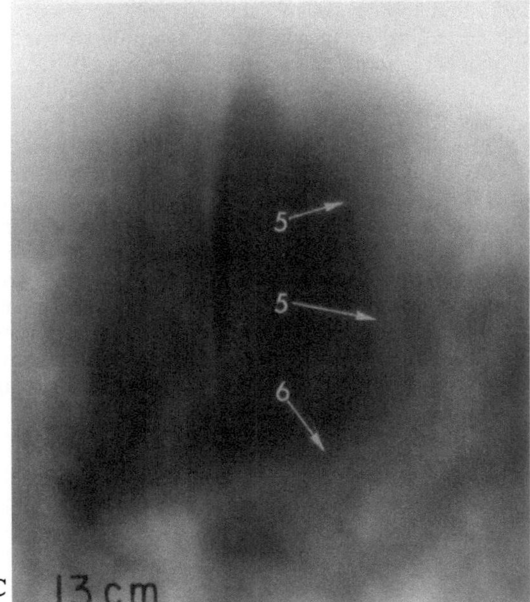

Fig. 8.32 A–C. Superior vena cava. **A** PA radiograph. **B** Coronal body section through superior vena cava. **C** Lateral tomogram. Superior vena cava is identified in high percentage of PA radiographs as shadow in right supra-azygos area having lateral concavity (*1*) or convexity (*2*). At its cephalad extent, superior venal shadow merges with that of right innominate vein coursing across anterior aspect of right upper lobe. Its lower margin becomes continuous with lateral edge of the right atrium (*3*). Position of ascending aorta (*4*), lying medial to superior vena cava and in intimate contact with it, frequently causes superior cava to be displaced laterally when ascending aorta is dilated. When lung inserts itself deeply into supra-azygos recess the posterior wall of the superior vena cava is often identified on lateral films as arcuate shadow with convexity directed forward (*5*) (see Figs. 8.30). Lower margin of caval shadow can be seen to merge with shadow of azygos arch (*6*). (**C** From [48])

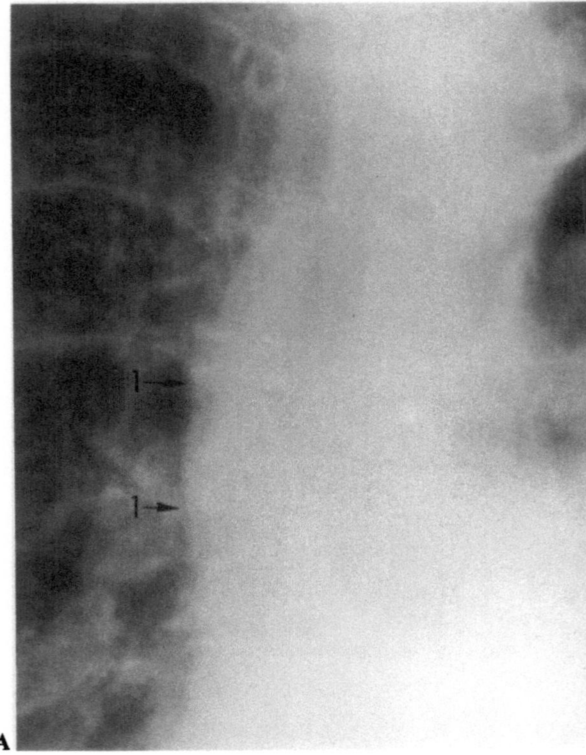

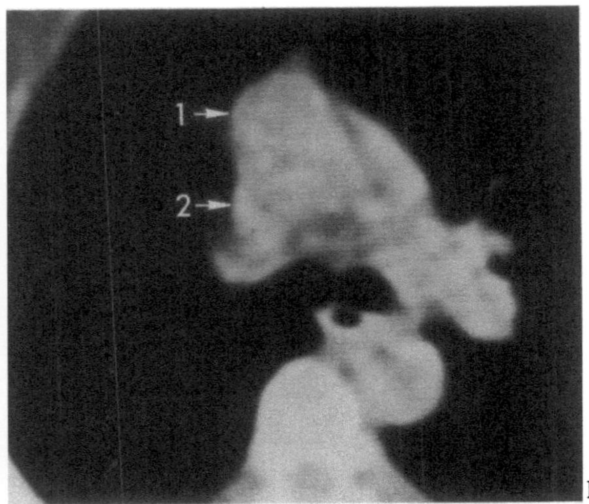

Fig. 8.33A, B. Contact of ascending aorta with right lung anterior to superior vena cava. A PA radiograph. B Computed tomogram of same patient. At times, an ectatic ascending aorta will buckle laterally to contact right lung (*1*) anterior to superior vena cava (*2*)

Fig. 8.34A, B. Relationship of innominate artery to trachea. A Coronal body section through superior vena cava. B Computed tomogram. From its point of origin, innominate artery (*1*) crosses immediately in front of trachea (*2*). In infants and young children, innominate artery may produce impression on anterior tracheal wall. Vessel continues behind superior vena cava (*3*) to give origin to right subclavian artery (*4*) and right common carotid artery (*5*). The computed tomogram also shows the left innominate vein (*6*), the left common carotid artery (*7*), and the left subclavian artery (*8*)

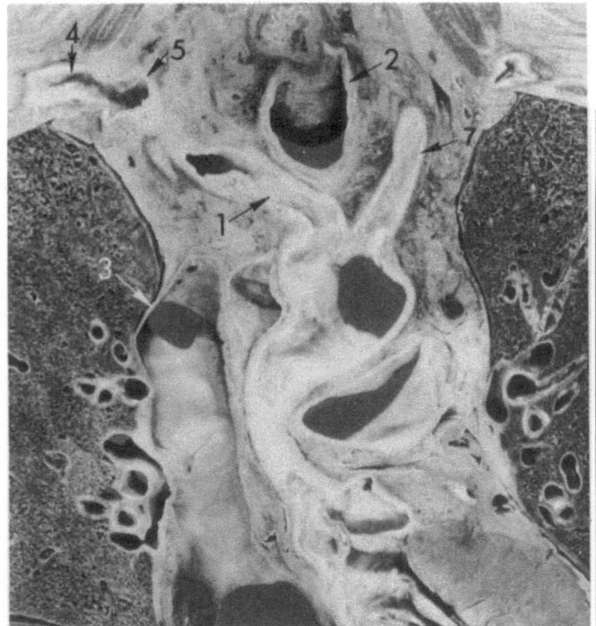

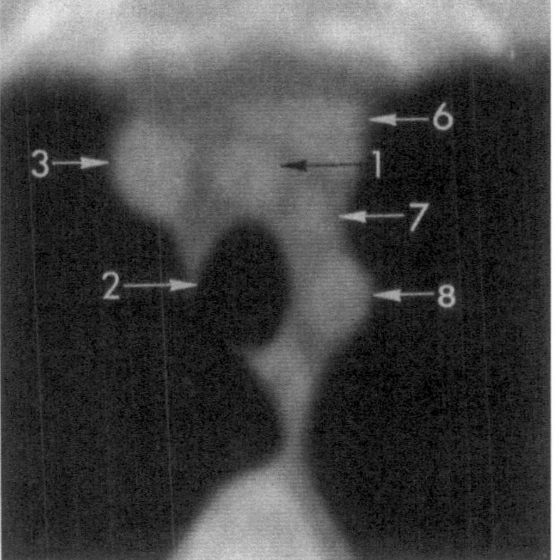

8.4.2 The Right Paratracheal Line

Disease processes involving the trachea are frequently overlooked on plain chest radiographs [40, 54]. For reasons that are not clear, this large air-filled structure, usually clearly visible on well-penetrated frontal and lateral films, is too often looked at in a cursory manner or ignored altogether. Tracheal contours outlined by intraluminal air and by surrounding lung should be inspected carefully in all patients, especially those with stridor.

8.4.2.1 Anatomic Considerations

The contact of lung in the supra-azygos recess with the right lateral wall of the trachea produces the right paratracheal line (Figs. 8.31, 8.35, and 8.37). Felson [35] found the line to be visible in 63% of patients. Bachman [6] identified it in 43%. Our own evaluation, derived from a study of randomly selected computed axial tomograms of the chest, showed the lung in contact with the lateral tracheal wall in 82%.

Apparently in the remainder of the patients, areolar tissue, fat, and small lymph nodes were interposed between the lung and the trachea. Savoca et al. [90] have found the line to be present much more frequently; it was identified in 94% of their 1200 cases. The normal width of the paratracheal line did not exceed 4 mm in their series. It is obvious that when making determinations of the line thickness on frontal films one should measure above the azygos arch. One should not make the mistake of measuring the arch itself. This admonition is totally unnecessary if determinations are made on frontal radiographs; it is a greater potential source of error if the evaluation is made from isolated computed axial tomographic sections (see Fig. 8.12).

When considering the significance of an abnormal paratracheal line, it should be borne in mind that the measurement reflects the thickness of the visceral and mediastinal pleurae, the tracheal wall, and the soft tissues in between.

Fig. 8.35 A, B. Right paratracheal line. **A** AP tomogram. **B** Computed tomogram through supra-azygos area. Lung commonly contacts right lateral tracheal wall to produce right paratracheal line (*1*). Interface between lung and trachea is not, however, seen as fine line in all patients (see Fig. 8.36). Changes in thickness of line on serial radiographic examinations or localized changes in thickness of line are more significant than absolute measurements made from single film. On PA radiographs it is possible to confuse lateral edge of superior vena cava (*2*) anterior to trachea for lateral edge of paratracheal line thus creating false impression of thickening of line

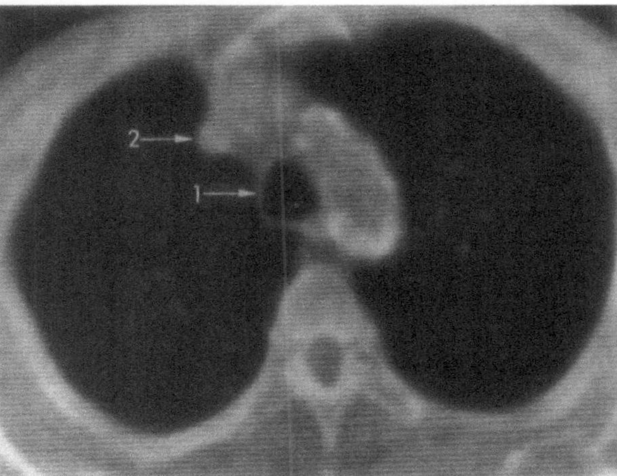

A   B

Thus it has been of help in evaluating pleural thickening, tracheal carcinoma and other tracheal pathology, and mediastinal disease. One problem in evaluating the paratracheal line on PA radiographs involves being sure that the lung-mediastinal interface that appears to be the lateral edge of the paratracheal line is actually in the same coronal plane as the trachea. Bachman and Teixidor [6] have pointed out that at times this interface may be lung against superior vena cava well forward of the trachea (Fig. 8.35). Computed tomograms eliminate this problem.

Is a paratracheal line wider than 4 mm always pathologic? Despite the findings of Savoca et al., it is felt that this opinion cannot be justified. Anatomic variation, causing separation of the lung and trachea in 37% of Felson's cases [35], 57% of Bachman and Teixidor's [6], and 18% of our own normal patients requires this conclusion. On computed axial tomograms of randomly selected patients the distance between the lung in the supra-azygos recess and the trachea can always be measured and often exceeds 4 mm. Furthermore it is an anatomic fact that normal mediastinal fat may infiltrate the mediastinum, separating its contents from lung (Fig. 8.36). These statements are not meant

to imply that the concept of the paratracheal line has no value; localized thickening of the line and change in its thickness on serial examinations are highly important observations often leading to significant diagnoses.

A posterior tracheal line, analogous to the right paratracheal line, can be seen on many lateral radiographs [6, 83, 94]. The line is produced by contact of the posterior tracheal wall with lung in the supra-azygos recess (Fig. 8.37). In some patients the esophagus lies immediately behind the trachea, but in other individuals the esophagus lies to the left of the sagittal plane of the trachea, permitting lung to contact a portion of or all of the posterior tracheal wall (Fig. 8.37). The fact that the posterior tracheal wall is flat (Fig. 8.37) and is oriented in a true coronal plane aids in its visualization on lateral radiographs. In the series of 200 patients studied by Bachman and Teixidor [6], the posterior tracheal line was visible in 91% of patients and was identified more than twice as frequently as the right paratracheal line. The normal thickness of the line did not exceed 4 mm. Proto and Speckman [83] identified the line in 45% of pa-

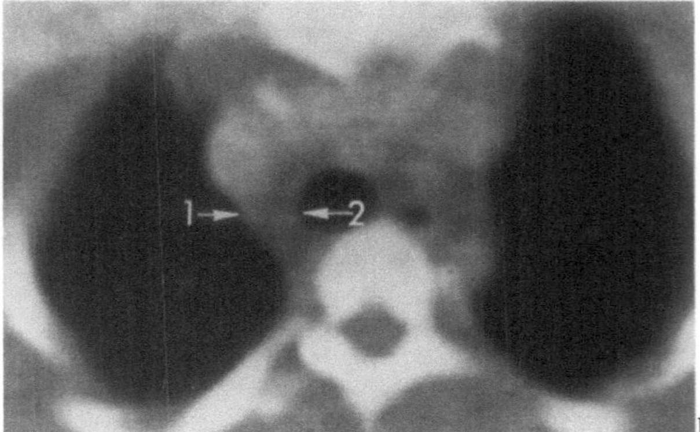

Fig. 8.36A, B. Widening of right paratracheal line due to physiologic fat deposition. **A** Coronal body section. **B** Computed tomogram through supra-azygos area. Physiologic deposition of fat in mediastinum can increase distance between right lung (*1*) and right tracheal wall (*2*). In computed tomogram this distance is almost equivalent to tracheal diameter. No disease was present in this patient, but computed tomography demonstrated considerable fat throughout mediastinum. It is felt that absolute measurements of thickness of right paratracheal line are of little clinical significance

A   B

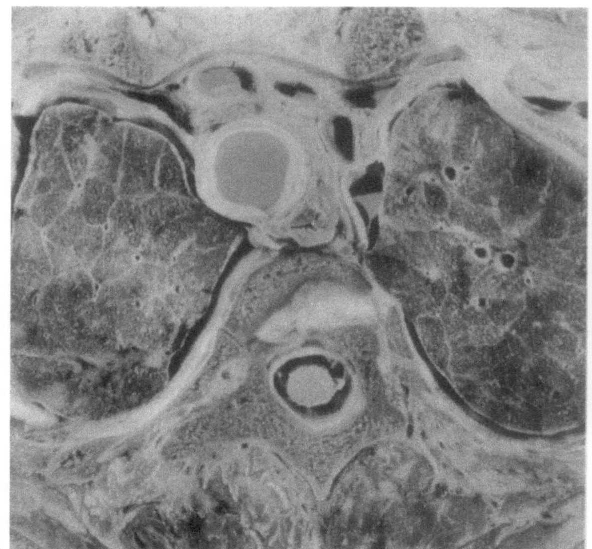

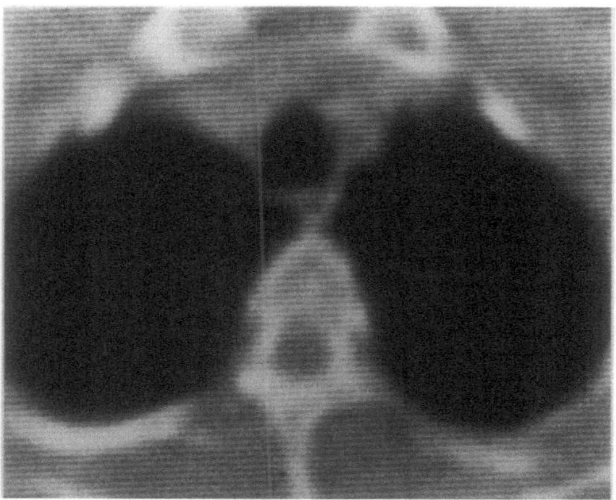

Fig. 8.37 A, B. Retrotracheal line. **A** Transverse body section. **B** Computed tomogram at same level. Lung commonly inserts itself behind the right side of the posterior wall of the trachea. Since posterior tracheal wall is flat, presence of lung behind part or all of its posterior surface often allows posterior tracheal wall to be identified on lateral radiographs. Concept of retrotracheal line can be used in interpretation of chest radiographs in manner analogous to use of concept of right paratracheal line. Changes on serial films are more significant than measurements made from a single radiograph

tients; in their series the thickness of the line varied from 1 to 5.5 mm. The line is somewhat more frequently seen on left lateral films made with the right chest rotated slightly forward of the left [8]. Kormano and Yajana [59] have provided a study comparing the appearance of the posterior paratracheal line on lateral chest films with computed tomography. In our smaller series of observations made from computed axial tomograms the line could be demonstrated in 52% of cases.

At times the posterior tracheal line represents not a lung-tracheal interface but the soft tissue stripe between the air-filled trachea and the air-filled esophagus [77] (Fig. 8.37). Although in the latter anatomic situation the stripe represents the combined thickness of the posterior tracheal wall and the anterior esophageal wall, the diagnostic implications are the same.

Diseases causing opacification of the medial portion of the right upper lobe and mediastinal abnormality will cause obliteration or distortion of the line. Bachman and Teixidor [6] point out that loss of the line in patients with left upper lobe pathology indicates mediastinal involvement. Since the left upper lobe itself cannot contribute anatomically to the formation of the posterior tracheal line, obliteration of the line must be due to mediastinal disease if the right upper lobe is aerated. Putman et al. [84] have

discussed thickening of the line in association with esophageal carcinoma (Fig. 8.38). Saks et al. [89] have emphasized that, infrequently, the posterior paratracheal line is thickened following sclerotherapy for esophageal varices.

Lung visualized posterior to the trachea on lateral films outlines an area that has been called the "aortic triangle" [79] the "retrotracheal triangle" [85], and the "retrotracheal space" [94]. This radiolucent zone is bounded by the trachea in front, the spine behind, the aortic arch below, and the thoracic inlet above. The radiolucency is produced by air in both lungs; the posterior tracheal wall is outlined by right lung; the aortic arch, by left lung. Air is excluded from the space by pulmonary disease and by mediastinal abnormality. Vascular anomalies such as right aortic arch [9] and aberrant right subclavian artery, esophageal pathology, and posterior lesions such as posterior goiter will distort the area [85]. The space is best visualized on high-kilovolt radiographs and films made with the arms hyperextended as when attempting to touch the elbows behind the back [94].

Proto and Speckman [83] identified an anterior paratracheal line in 16% of lateral radiographs; its thickness varied from 1–2.5 mm. A wide variety of pathological conditions can alter the supra-azygos recess and the paratracheal and retrotracheal lines; some of them are discussed in the chapter on the thoracic inlet (chapter 4). The abnormality most commonly encountered is right paratracheal adenopathy.

8.4.2.2 Enlargement of Right Tracheobronchial Lymph Nodes

The right tracheobronchial lymph nodes lie lateral to the trachea extending downward to the origin of the right main bronchus (Fig. 8.39). According to Cahan et al. [17], the right tracheobronchial nodes lie in a niche, the boundaries of which are as follows: in front, the superior vena cava; behind, the right anterolateral surface of the trachea; above, the subclavian artery; below, the azygos arch; and medially, the arch of the aorta. Laterally, the niche is closed by the mediastinal pleura. Rouviere [88] states that three to six nodes make up the right tracheobronchial chain (Fig. 8.39). In 1983, a new classification of mediastinal lymph nodes

was proposed by the American Thoracic Society [101]. In this system the right paratracheal nodes are divided into two groups. "Right upper paratracheal nodes," given the designation "2R," are defined as being nodes to the right of the midline of the trachea, between the intersection of the caudal margin of the innominate artery with the right side of the trachea and the apex of the lung. "Right lower paratracheal nodes," given the designation "4R," are defined as being nodes to the right of the midline of the trachea, between the cephalic border of the azygos vein and the intersection of the caudal margin of the innominate artery with the right side of the trachea. The lowermost of the right paratracheal nodes are sometimes referred to as the "nodes of the azygos arch" [64], and the largest and most inferior of these nodes is the azygos node (Fig. 8.39). This node lies medial to the anterior portion of the azygos arch, which swings around the lower pole of the node (Figs. 8.39 and 8.45). The azygos node is variable in position and may be found somewhat more forward, medial to the superior vena cava.

Fig. 8.38 A, B. Retrotracheal disease. Carcinoma of the esophagus. **A** Lateral radiograph. **B** Computed tomogram. In **A** the retrotracheal space (see text) demonstrates increased density and the trachea is displaced forward. Note the separation of the tracheal air column and the nasogastric tube. The computed tomogram (**B**) also clearly demonstrates the large retrocarinal mass displacing the airway anteriorly. Again note the separation of the airway and the nasogastric tube

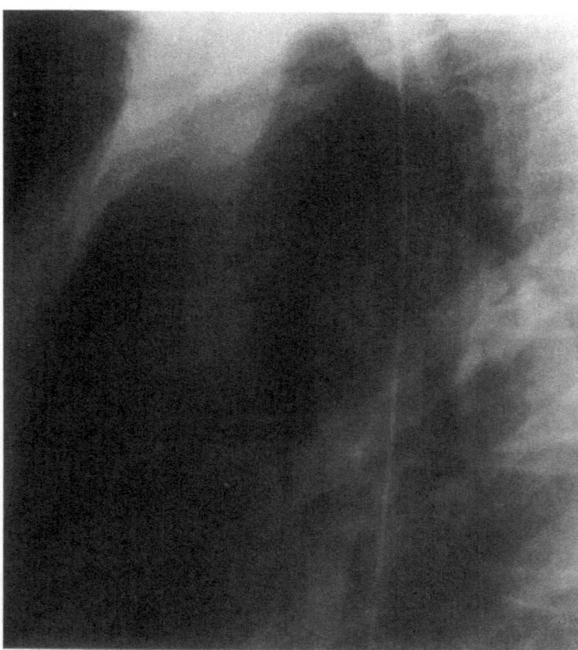

A

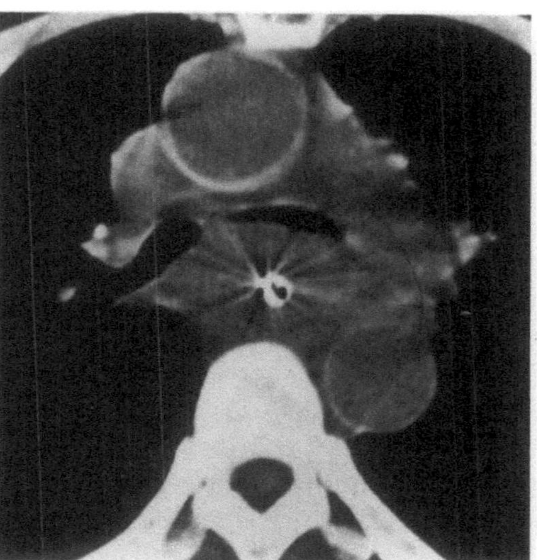

B

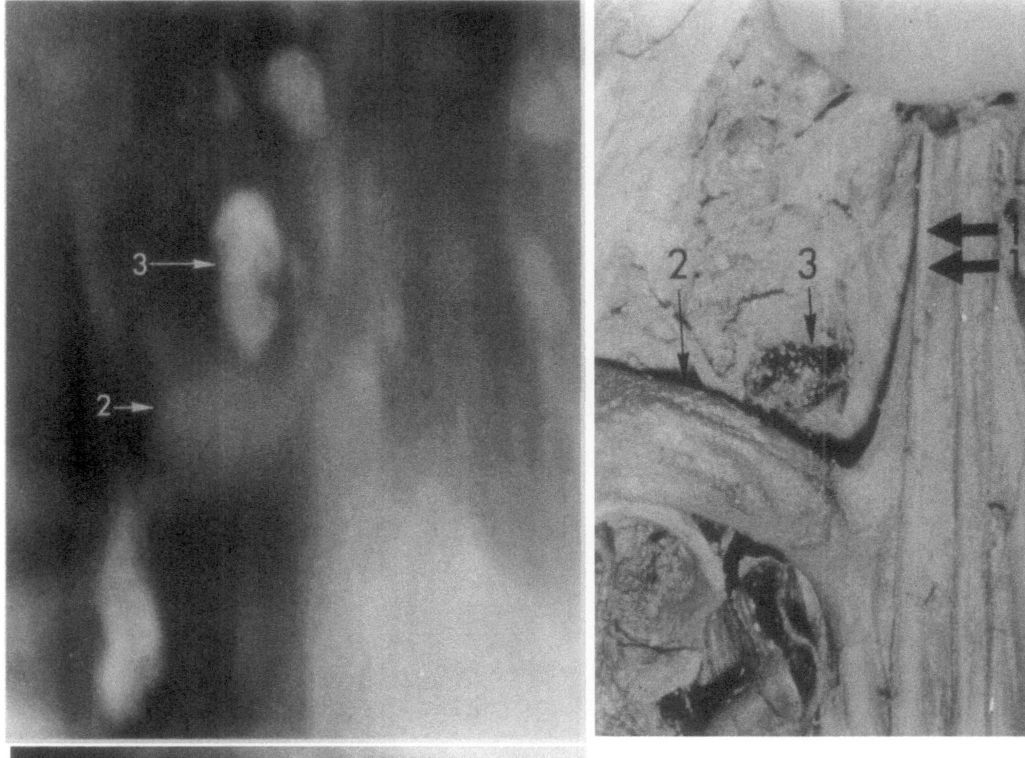

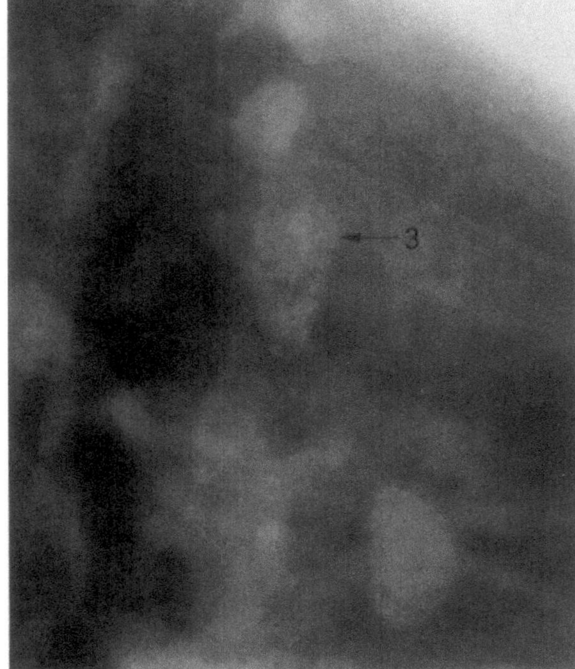

Fig. 8.39 A–C. Anatomy of right upper and lower paratracheal nodes. Upper and lower groups. **A** AP tomogram. **B** Lateral radiograph. **C** Right side of mediastinum with mediastinal pleura removed. Right paratracheal nodes, usually three to six in number, lie behind superior vena cava (*1*) along anterolateral margin of trachea. They are situated above azygos arch (*2*) and extend upward to the apex of the lung. Radiographs demonstrate contrast material in right paratracheal nodes following lymphangiography, a not uncommon occurrence. The azygos node is the largest and most inferior of nodes in right tracheobronchial chain. It is situated along anterolateral aspect of trachea immediately above right upper lobe bronchus. Its lower pole is crossed laterally by azygos arch. Note position of azygos node (*3*) medial to azygos arch (*2*). (**C** From [48])

The right tracheobronchial group of nodes drains the right lung and, by way of the subcarinal nodes, the left lower lobe as well. Rouviere's early demonstration of this point [88] has been confirmed by Nohl [73, 74], McCort and Robbins [68], and by Goldberg et al. [44]. It should be realized that contralateral nodal involvement can also occur as the result of neoplasms of the right lung [44]. Contralateral involvement without ipsilateral nodal disease is not uncommon with tumors of the left lung, but is rare with neoplasms of the right lung [44]. A more complete discussion of mediastinal lymph node size and its significance in roentgen diagnosis is included in chapter 3.

The right tracheobronchial node group is in immediate contact with the right mediastinal pleura; hence the usual radiographic finding encountered when adenopathy is present is exclusion of lung from the supra-azygos recess. The resulting impression made by the nodal mass on the lung may be smooth (Figs. 8.41, 8.43) or lobulated (Fig. 8.40). The paratracheal line may be widened. In patients with deep supra-azygos recesses, the intimate contact of lung and mediastinum makes it hard for nodes to remain hidden. In patients with more shallow recesses, even rather large nodes may be present without obvious abnormality on plain radiographs. As in most areas of radiology, comparison of serial film examinations, if available, is often the most significant step leading to early diagnosis. Even subtle changes should be viewed with utmost suspicion.

Schnyder and Gamsu [91] described the appearance of normal azygos node or nodes as seen in the pretracheal, retrocaval space at computed tomography. Nodes were identified in 88% of normal subjects. More than one node was identified in 30% of scans. Only 3% of normal nodes exceeded 11 mm in diameter.

Computed tomography is an ideal examination for the study of right paratracheal adeno-

pathy (Fig. 8.41). Muller et al. [72] studied 98 patients and compared plain film findings with computed tomographic appearances. In 36 patients with paratracheal nodes greater than 15 mm in diameter, plain films showed:

1. Widening of the right paratracheal stripe in 31%
2. Enlargement of the azygos node in 42%
3. Lateral convexity of the superior vena cava in 47% and
4. Increased density in the region of the superior vena cava in 83%

A pitfall to be avoided in the diagnosis of enlargement of the azygos node at computed tomography is to mistake a prominent transverse sinus of the pericardium for an enlarged node [4, 65] (Fig. 8.42). There is a minor semantic problem over whether the pericardial sinus posterior to the aortic root should be considered transverse or superior [4, 65]. Pernkopf [80] designates this portion of the pericardial space as "transverse sinus." The distinction of the transverse sinus from a lymph node is readily made if the density can be seen to be-

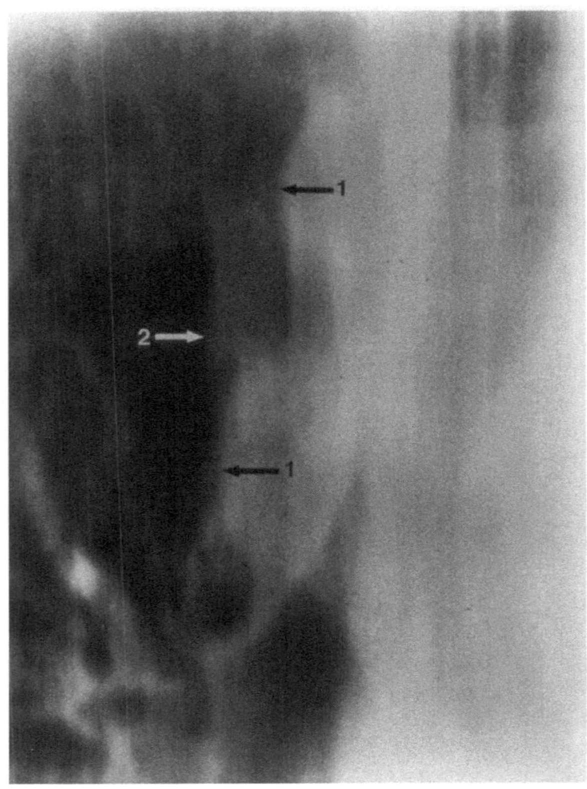

Fig. 8.40. Right paratracheal adenopathy (AP tomogram). Characteristically, enlargement of right paratracheal nodes produces lobulated abnormalities (*1*). Right paratracheal line is often irregularly widened; superior vena cava may be displaced to right (*2*)

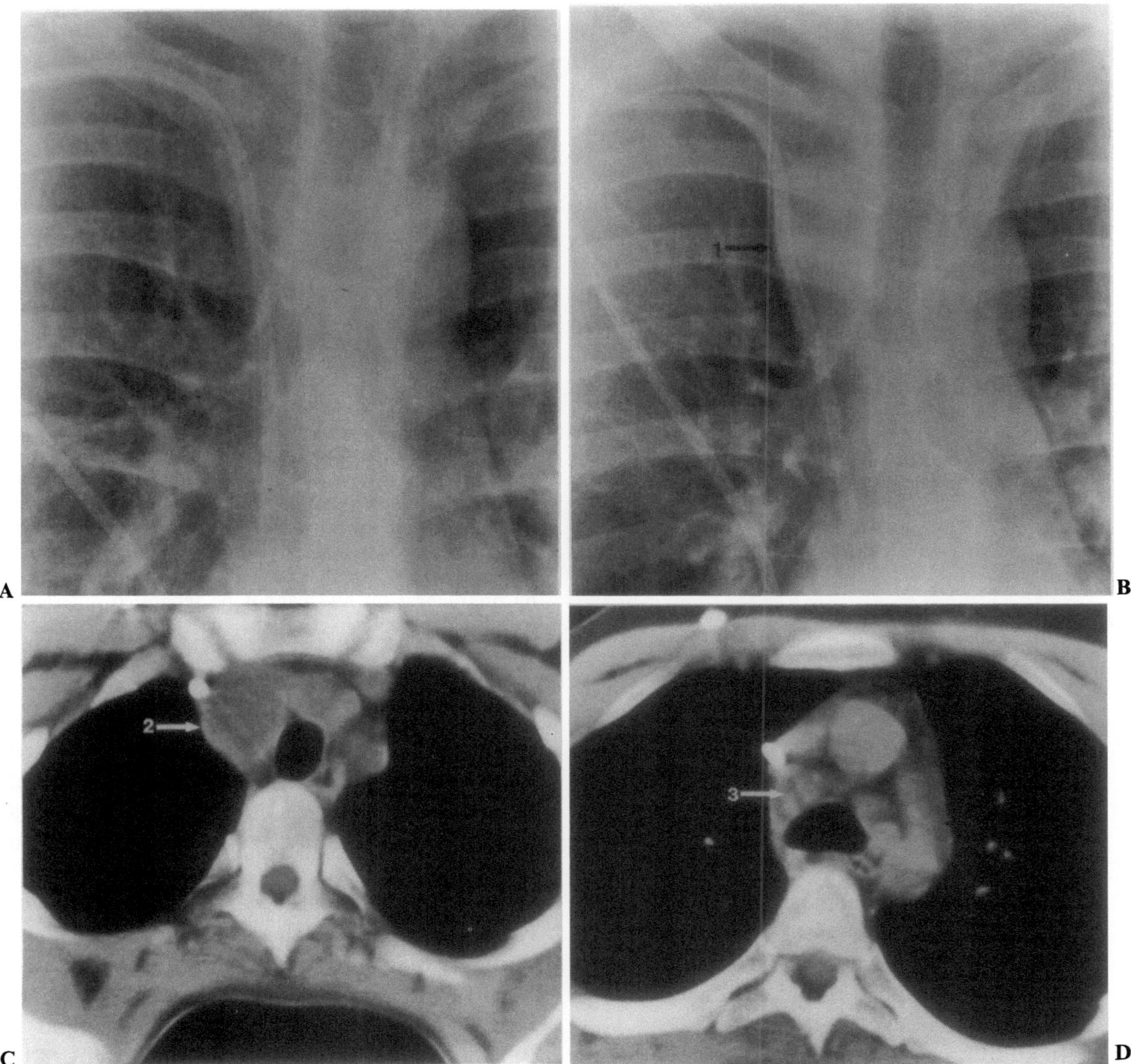

Fig. 8.41 A–D. Right paratracheal adenopathy. Computed tomography. **A** and **B** PA radiographs made 10 weeks apart. **C** and **D** Computed tomograms. In **B** a right paratracheal mass is clearly shown. The right paratracheal stripe is markedly widened. Note the displacement of the superior vena cava identified by the presence of the Hickman catheter passing through it. The vena presents a localized convex bulge against the right lung (*1*) in contrast to its normally smooth contour. Large upper paratracheal node or nodes (*2*) and smaller lower paratracheal nodes are well shown on the computed tomograms (*3*). The upper mass has a low density center and is probably necrotic

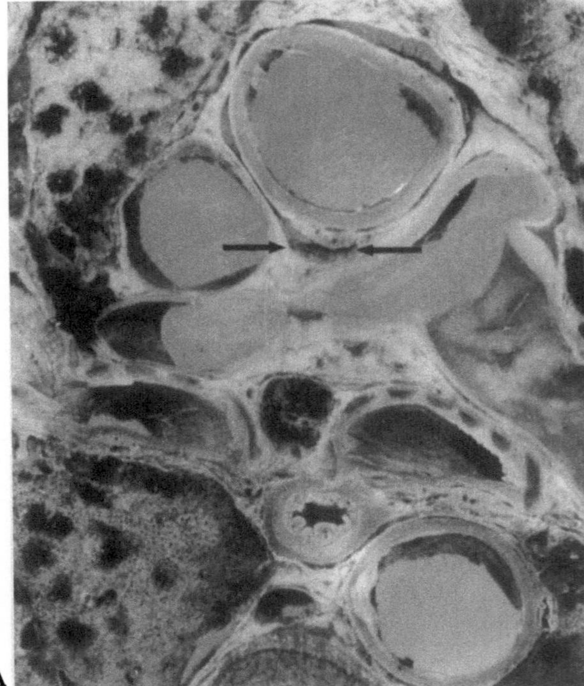

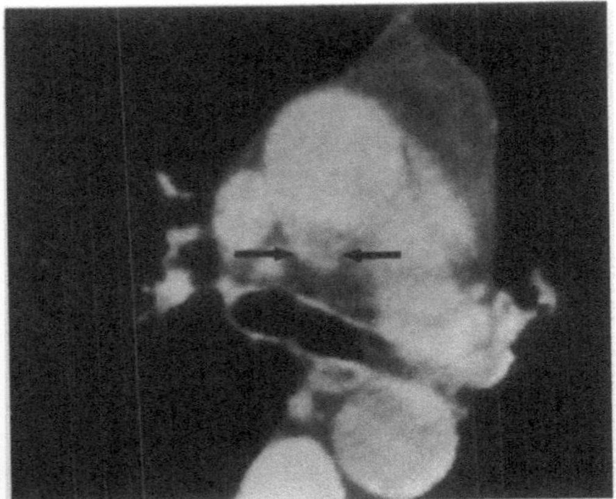

Fig. 8.42 A, B. The transverse sinus of the pericardium. A Transverse body section. B Computed tomogram. The prominent or distended transverse sinus of the pericardium can present as a soft tissue density (*arrows*) behind the ascending aorta and anterior to the trachea. It may simulate a pretracheal node. An enlarged pretracheal node is usually surrounded circumferentially by fat. An elliptical density, which is outlined on its posterior aspect by pretracheal fat and cannot be separated anteriorly from the aorta, is likely to be the transverse sinus of the pericardium

come continuous with the superior sinus. The margins of an enlarged node can usually be seen in their entirety; the shadow of the transverse sinus often has a sharply defined posterior border directed dorsally but no sharp anterior margin can be found behind the aortic root (Fig. 8.42). A prominent transverse sinus due to pericardial effusion is usually associated with distended superior sinus. At times a prominent superior sinus can be mistaken for an anterior mediastinal mass [95].

In addition to the comments just made, some specific anatomic details must be reviewed because of their importance to the radiographic diagnosis of right paratracheal adenopathy. A key point in the anatomy of this area, which has been emphasized repeatedly in this section, is that lung in the supra-azygos recess enters into this space *above* the azygos arch. Figure 8.43 depicts a case in which failure to appreciate this simple point led to an incorrect diagnosis. The elliptical shadow in the angle of origin of the right main bronchus from the trachea was thought to be a prominent azygos vein, even though a part of the shadow projected above the line that represented lung in the supra-azy-

gos recess. Under no anatomic circumstance could the azygos arch have been projected above this line. The density in question turned out to be an enlarged azygos node projecting upward into the supra-azygos recess medial to the azygos arch.

Another principle, vital to evaluation of lymphadenopathy in this portion of the mediastinum, is that the azygos arch is always situated lateral to the azygos node (Fig. 8.39). A convenient way to keep this relationship in mind is to recall that in those cases in which right radical pneumonectomy and mediastinal lymph node dissection is performed, the azygos arch must be sacrificed to allow access to the tracheobronchial lymph nodes and to facilitate their removal en bloc [17] (Fig. 8.44 C). Figure 8.44 shows a mass that was erroneously called an "enlarged azygos node" despite the visualization of the azygos arch well to the left of the lateral margin of the abnormal shadow, a finding that makes this diagnostic consideration an anatomic impossibility. This mass was actually situated posteriorly in the right upper lobe.

Since the azygos arch terminates in the superior vena cava, it follows that lateral displacement

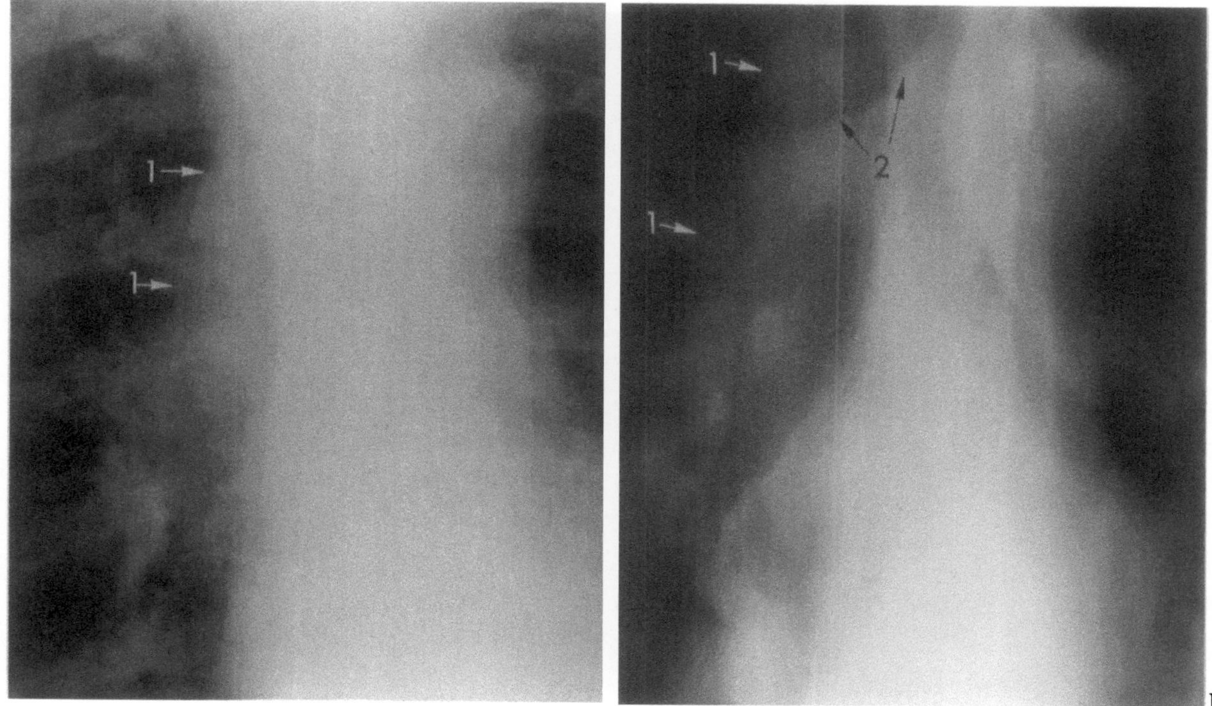

Fig. 8.43 A, B. Right paratracheal adenopathy. **A** PA radiograph. **B** AP tomogram. In this patient, widening of supra-azygos area was thought to be due to nodal enlargement or to prominent great vessels. AP tomogram was interpreted as proving that prominent shadow (*1*) was azygos vein. This, in fact, could not be the case anatomically, since shadow extends well above line representing lung in supra-azygos recess (*2*) and azygos arch must lie below this line. Abnormality represented an azygos node, enlarged by tumor, projecting upward within arc of azygos arch

of the azygos arch will cause the cava, to which it is attached, to be displaced laterally as well (Figs. 8.41, 8.45, 8.46). Figure 8.45 shows the azygos arch stretched around an azygos node enlarged by metastatic bronchogenic carcinoma. Under these circumstances the lateral edge of the displaced superior vena cava can often be identified as a straight interface projecting inferiorly. This is a usual finding in patients with right paratracheal adenopathy and should not be misinterpreted as caudal extension of the pathologic process. The arch itself is stretched and flattened from side to side and therefore cannot usually be identified on plain films or tomograms as shadow lateral to the nodal mass.

The superior vena cava can be focally as well as generally deviated by enlargement of right tracheobronchial lymph nodes. Figure 8.46 shows a minimal lateral bulge of the lower portion of the superior vena cava. Since this prominence was clearly of the cava, which could be followed cephalad in its typical configuration, it was initially dismissed as being of little clinical significance. When an earlier film subsequently became available for comparison and showed no such bulge, the patient was explored, and an azygos node, involved by metastatic tumor, was found lying medial to the cava at the level of the local caval prominence. A similar case is shown in Fig. 8.41.

It is important to reiterate that lateral radiographs sometimes permit a distinction to be made between a prominent azygos vein and an enlarged azygos node when the appearance of the frontal radiograph causes both possibilities to be entertained. The shadow of the enlarged node is seen well forward of the tracheal air column (see Fig. 8.14), whereas the posterior turn of a prominent azygos arch is always behind the plane of the trachea (see Figs. 8.13 and 8.25).

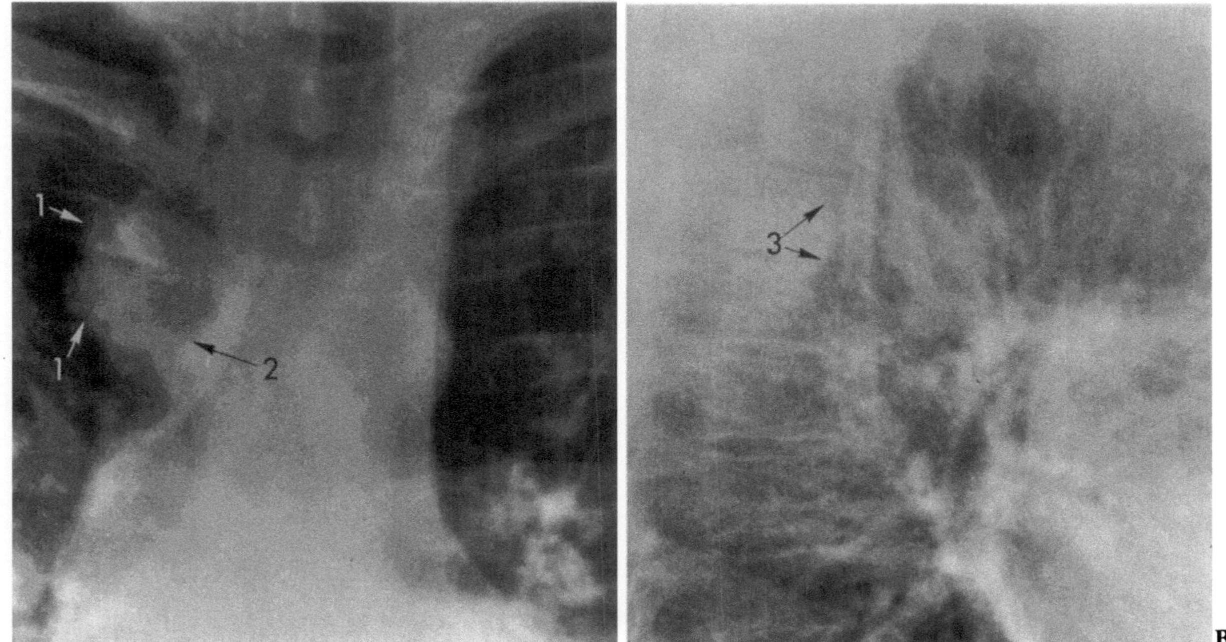

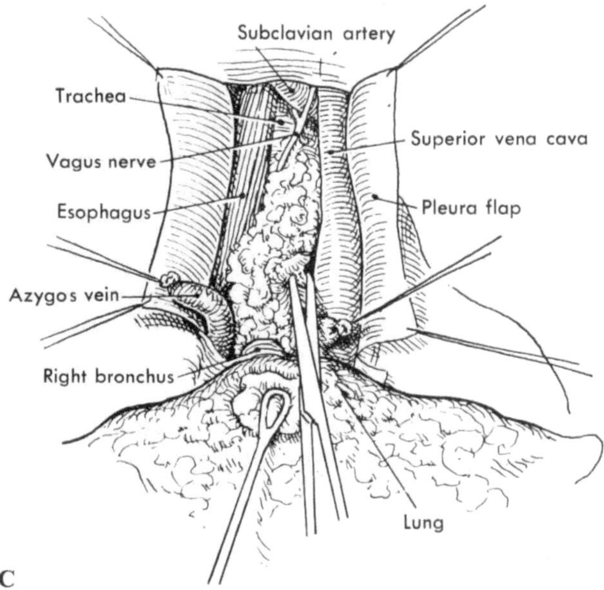

Fig. 8.44 A–C. Right paratracheal adenopathy. **A** and **B** PA and lateral radiographs. **C** Right side of mediastinum showing approach to dissection of right paratracheal nodes as part of right radical pneumonectomy. PA and lateral radiographs of this patient show irregular mass (*1*) which was interpreted as enlarged azygos node. This could not be the case anatomically because shadow of azygos arch (*2*) is seen to lie medial to it. If mass represented enlarged azygos node, azygos arch would have to lie lateral to node. In fact, mass is seen to lie posteriorly on lateral view (*3*) and proved to be right upper lobe bronchogenic carcinoma. A convenient way to remember relationship of azygos arch to azygos node is to recall that to approach right paratracheal nodes surgically, azygos vein must be sacrificed (**C**). (**C** From [17])

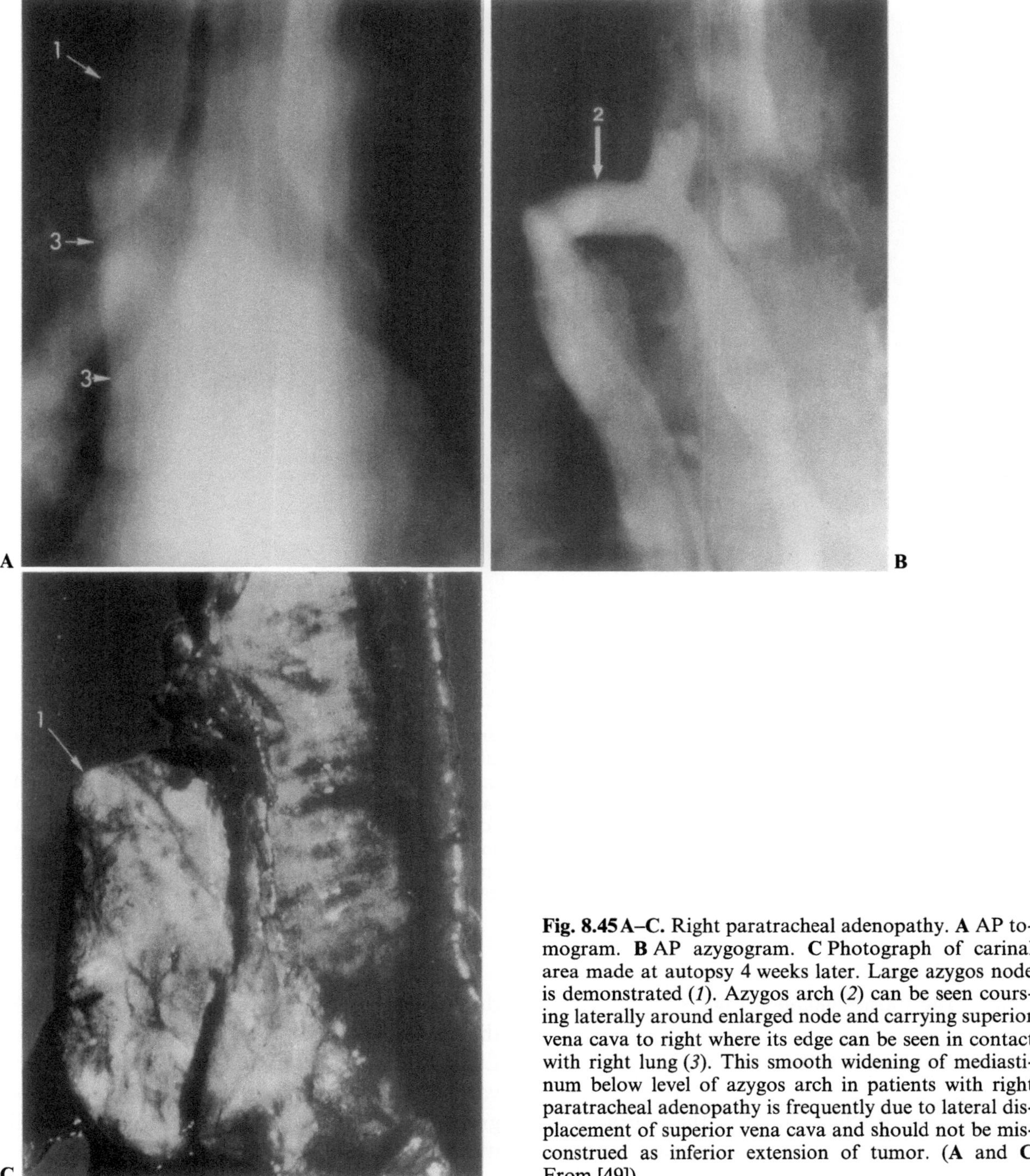

Fig. 8.45 A–C. Right paratracheal adenopathy. **A** AP tomogram. **B** AP azygogram. **C** Photograph of carinal area made at autopsy 4 weeks later. Large azygos node is demonstrated (*1*). Azygos arch (*2*) can be seen coursing laterally around enlarged node and carrying superior vena cava to right where its edge can be seen in contact with right lung (*3*). This smooth widening of mediastinum below level of azygos arch in patients with right paratracheal adenopathy is frequently due to lateral displacement of superior vena cava and should not be misconstrued as inferior extension of tumor. (**A** and **C** From [49])

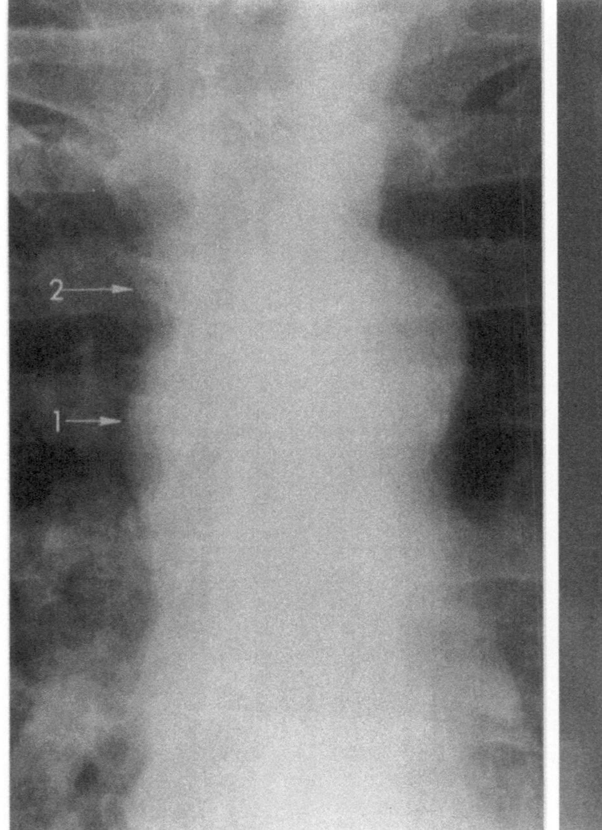

A

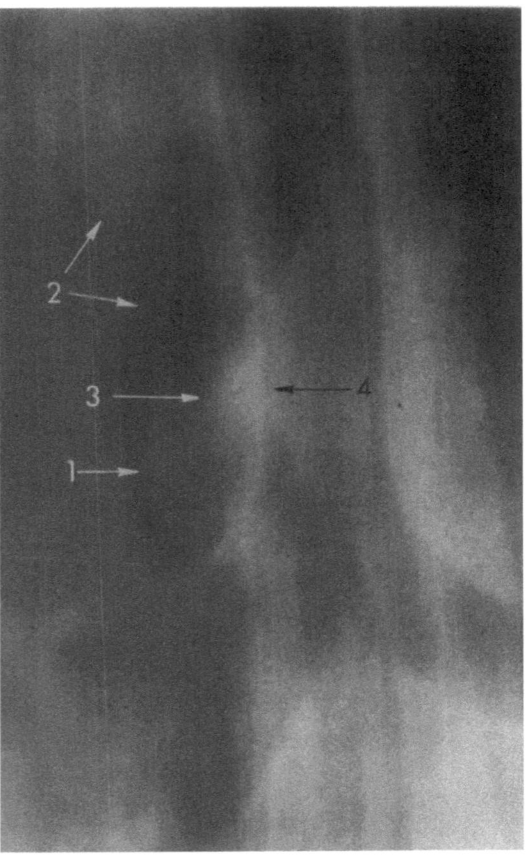

B

Fig. 8.46 A, B. Right paratracheal adenopathy. **A** AP radiograph. **B** AP tomogram. Minimal bulge in supra-azygos area (*1*) was considered suspect in this patient with known metastases to brain. Tomogram was interpreted as showing that prominence was due to a localized bulge in the configuration of the inferior portion of superior vena cava since margin of shadow continued cephalad in course highly characteristic for superior vena cava and right innominate vein (*2*). Furthermore, configurations of anterior and posterior parts of azygos arch (*3* and *4*) were thought to be normal. At surgery, an enlarged azygos node involved by metastatic tumor was found. It displaced the superior vena cava laterally creating a localized convexity in caval contour. Such a configuration should be considered strongly suggestive of disease. Compare with Fig. 8.41

8.4.3 The Paraesophageal Line

8.4.3.1 Anatomic Considerations

Behind the trachea, lung in the supra-azygos recess may contact the right lateral esophageal wall to produce the paraesophageal line (Fig. 8.47). Although the work of Lachman [60] and Knutsson [58] laid the anatomic groundwork for an understanding of the line on radiographs, it is interesting that it was misinterpreted by several authors prior to the paper by Cimmino in 1956 [22]. In the following decade, Cimmino [23] and Cimmino and Snead [25] pro-

duced other important papers concerned with the paraesophageal line and its variations. Later, Cimmino compared his plain film observations with those drawn from computed tomograms [24]. A review of these publications is well worthwhile and provides an instructive insight into the evolution of the author's thinking about plain film study of the mediastinum. Gladnikoff [41] found this line to be present in one-third of his cases. Other than this work, there are no good statistical studies concerning the frequency of visualization of this line.

When lung in the supra-azygos recess contacts an esophagus that contains barium or is

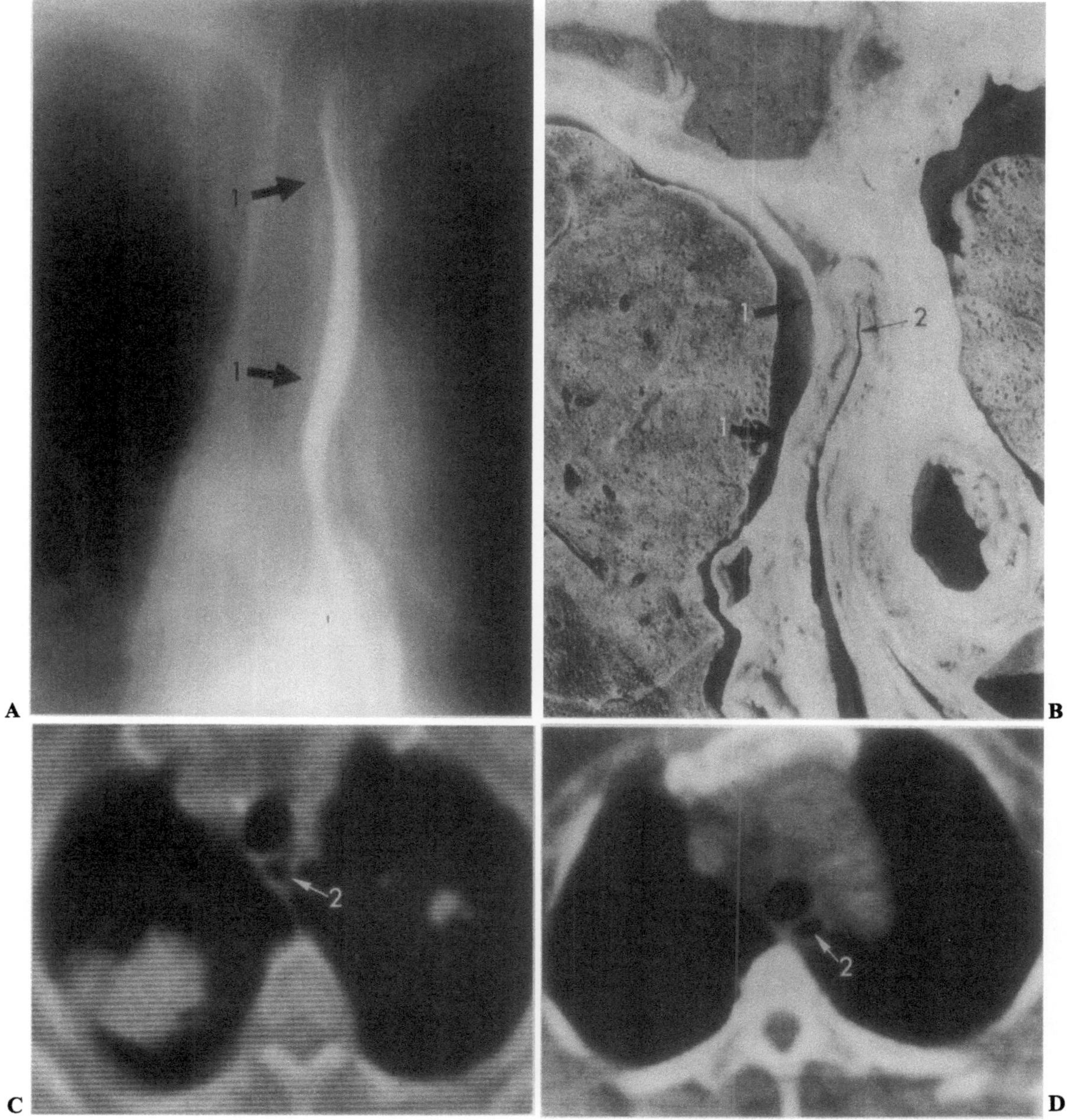

Fig. 8.47 A–D. Paraesophageal line. **A** AP tomogram with barium in esophagus. **B** Coronal body section. **C** and **D** Computed tomograms. Lung in supra-azygos recess (*1*) on occasion will contact esophagus (*2*) to produce paraesophageal line, sometimes called "pleuroeso-phageal stripe." In **C** each lung contacts the air-filled esophagus. Relationship of right lung to right lateral wall of esophagus is quite variable; in **D** right lung and esophagus are not in contact. (**B** From [49])

air filled at this level, it is possible to see a soft-tissue stripe between the two (Fig. 8.47). Just as lung in the supra-azygos recess may or may not contact the right tracheal wall, it may or may not touch the esophageal wall. Estimation of esophageal wall thickness on this basis is therefore risky. Like the paratracheal lines, the paraesophageal line is useful in the evaluation of pleural disease, esophageal disease, and mediastinal pathology between the lung and mediastinum; localized changes and changes in contour seen on serial film examinations are more important than determinations of the line thickness on a single radiograph. The right lung may contact the esophagus below the azygos arch as well as above it. In general the lower portion of the pleuroesophageal line has greater radiologic significance than does its upper part. For this reason a discussion of the line in greater depth will be reserved for the chapter concerning the infra-azygos area (chapter 9).

8.4.3.2 Achalasia

When the esophagus is dilated, as in achalasia, it contacts the right lung more intimately than when it is not dilated. In most instances it indents the right lung rather deeply, producing on frontal radiographs an abnormal, gently undulating mediastinal contour often extending from the thoracic inlet to the diaphragm on the right side (Fig. 8.48). The inferior portion of this abnormal line sometimes lies lateral to the right heart border (Figs. 8.48, 8.49), but is sometimes seen through it. No condition other than dilata-

tion of the esophagus will produce this long undulating contour, but the diagnosis is further strengthened if the abnormal contour bulges laterally above and below the azygos arch (Fig. 8.48). Since the azygos arch is situated lateral to the esophagus, dilatation of the esophagus will bring it into intimate contact with the azygos arch on its right side (Figs. 8.47 and 8.48). The arch then "tethers" the esophagus, which may balloon out above and below it (Figs. 8.48, 8.49, and 8.50). This appearance is apparently not common in achalasia; in our material it occurred in only two of ten cases.

Fig. 8.48 A, B. Supra-azygos mass resulting from achalasia. A PA radiograph. B AP radiograph. Dilatation of esophagus secondary to achalasia is usually identified as undulating shadow seen in infra-azygos and supra-azygos areas (1). Frequently shadow of right atrium (2) is seen superimposed on dilated esophagus. In some patients with achalasia, dilated esophagus appears to be tethered by azygos arch, which swings around its right lateral aspect (3). In other patients with this condition, this feature is not seen, apparently due to fact that azygos arch has been stretched by dilated esophagus

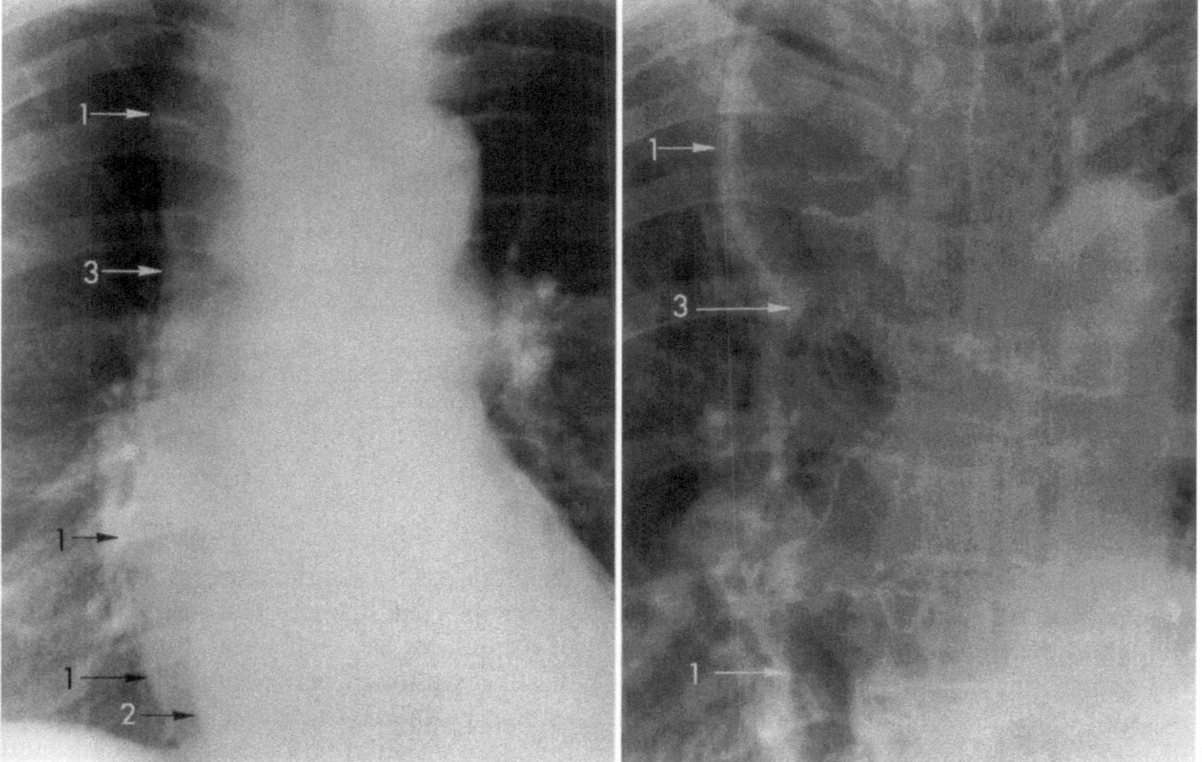

A   B

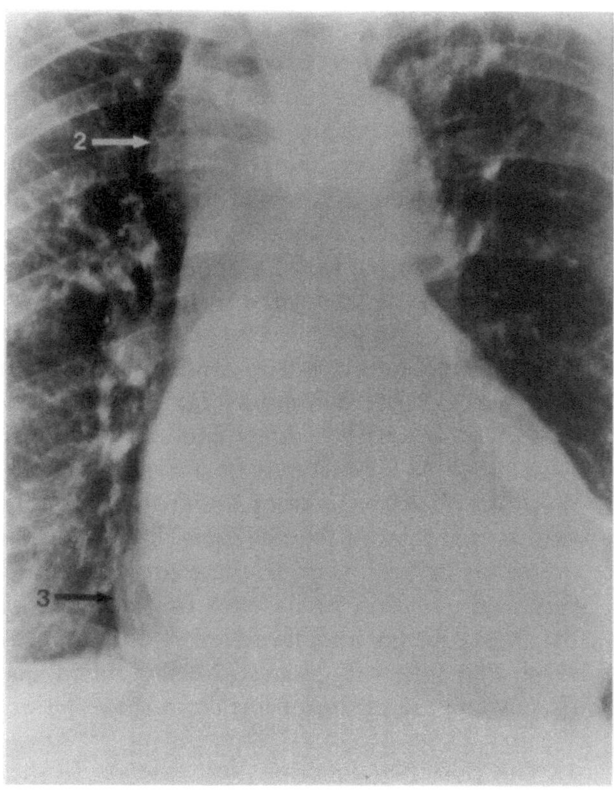

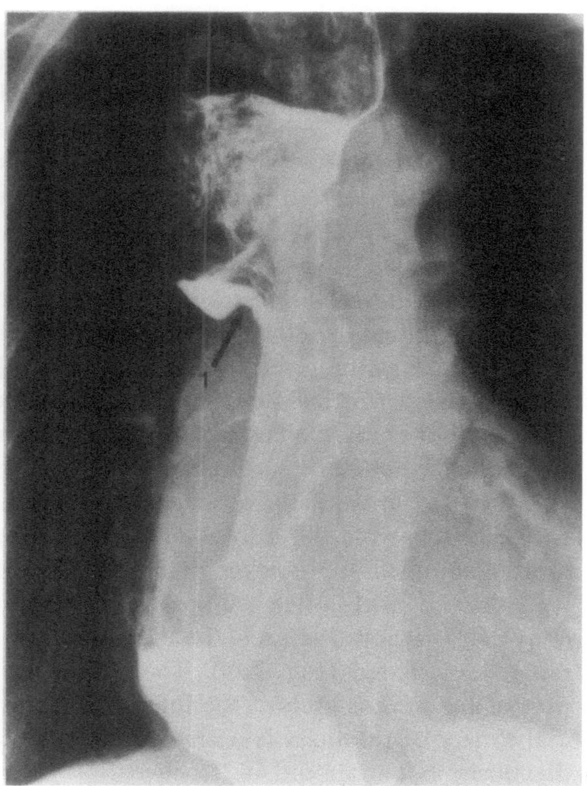

A

B

Fig. 8.49 A, B. Supra-azygos mass resulting from Chagas disease. **A** PA radiograph. **B** PA radiograph with barium in esophagus. In some patients with esophageal dilatation, here occurring as the result of Chagas disease, tethering of esophagus by azygos arch (*1*) causes esophagus to dilate markedly above arch, producing striking rounded mass in supra-azygos area (*2*). Dilatation of esophagus in infra-azygos area (*3*) may at times be much less prominent than in the supra-azygos area. (Courtesy Tufik Bauab, Rio Prieto, Brazil)

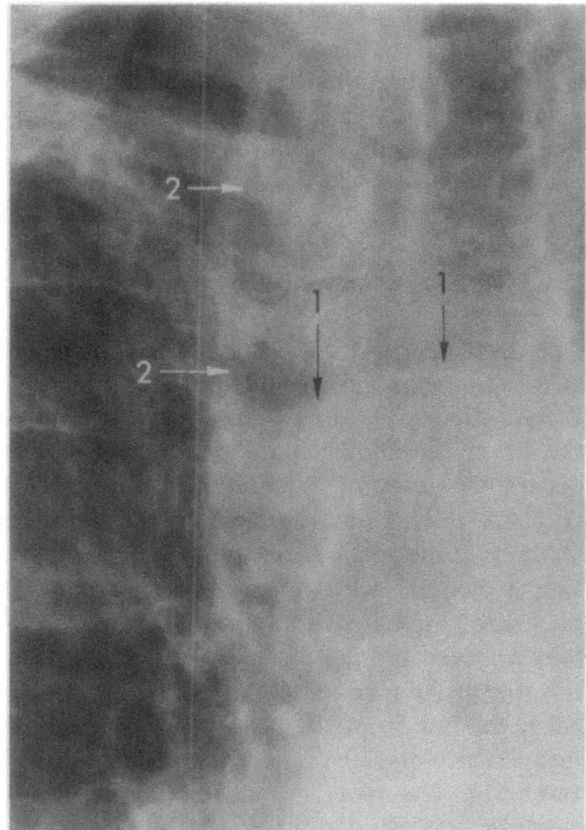

Fig. 8.50. Achalasia (AP radiograph). Exceptionally, air in esophagus that is markedly dilated as result of achalasia can be seen to outline superior surface of azygos arch (*1*) as dilated, air-filled esophagus (*2*) extends into supra-azygos area above arch

In both of these cases the esophagus was markedly dilated. In several other patients with marked esophageal dilatation the azygos arch did not tether the esophagus. In some patients a mild azygos imprint was evident; in others, no defect at all was produced. Apparently, in these cases the gradual dilatation of the esophagus stretched the azygos arch to the point that it produced no visible impression. The esophagus was significantly tethered by the azygos arch in six of 14 cases reported by Chasen et al. [19]. Their article is worthwhile reading to review the general subject of mediastinal impressions on the dilated esophagus.

In two of our cases the esophagus was markedly dilated above the azygos arch, producing a large rounded supra-azygos mass that could be confused with other supra-azygos lesions (Fig. 8.49). Below the arch the esophagus was much less dilated (Fig. 8.49). The demonstration of the azygos arch at the inferior and medial aspect of the mass is a clue to the correct diagnosis, but it should be recalled that other supra-azygos masses, for example, intrathoracic goiter, may be similarly limited at their lower end by the arch. The demonstration of an air-fluid level in the supra-azygos mass suggests the correct diagnosis and should lead to the performance of a barium swallow to confirm the presence of achalasia.

8.4.4 The Posterior Junction Line

The deepest portion of the supra-azygos recess is usually behind the esophagus (see Fig. 8.4). In fact, this is the only point at which lung in the recess can contact the left lung. When this occurs, the posterior junction line is formed [25] (Fig. 8.51). This line represents a combination of the visceral and parietal pleurae of the right side in contact with the visceral and parietal pleurae of the left. Although it is composed of four apposed layers of pleura, it is paper thin; this fine linear appearance can be used to distinguish the line from the right pleuroesophageal stripe which usually is thicker [25] (Figs. 8.47 and 8.51). The pleurae forming the posterior junction line are continuous behind, with the

pleura covering the paraspinal soft tissues; anteriorly they divide to encompass the esophagus. These pleural layers can then properly be called the "mesentery" of the esophagus (Fig. 8.51).

Radiographically, the posterior junction line may appear as a long sickle-shaped curve with convexity directed to the left (as may the pleuroesophageal stripe), with its upper extent diverging over the lung apices and its lower limit separating to encompass the azygos arch on the right and the posterior aortic arch on the left (Fig. 8.51). More commonly its midportion is a straight line with a direct caudal orientation (Fig. 8.51). At times it may be difficult to distinguish the posterior junction line from the anterior junction line on frontal films. Oblique films are rarely helpful, since in these projections the posterior junction line is not in the plane of the X-ray beam and is therefore infrequently seen. The following points are helpful in distinguishing the posterior line from the anterior:

1. The posterior junction line extends further cephalad. Since the thoracic inlet is a plane inclined upward from front to back, the lungs can contact one another at a higher level behind the esophagus than they can anteriorly. The cephalad extent of the anterior junction line reaches only the sternoclavicular notch (see Figs. 5.3 and 5.4).
2. The upper portion of the anterior junction line subtends off the innominate veins, deviating slightly to the left as it progresses caudally to diverge about the heart (see Figs. 5.3 and 5.4).
3. The upper portion of the posterior junction line subtends off the lung apices, progressing in a straight caudal direction to diverge over the azygos and aortic arches (Fig. 8.51).

Exceptionally, the posterior junction line can be used radiologically to localize pulmonary processes that "silhouette out" the line. It is distorted by mediastinal disease and especially by esophageal abnormality. Serial films showing change are again of most diagnostic help, but local disruptions of the line also can be useful in arriving at a correct radiographic interpretation.

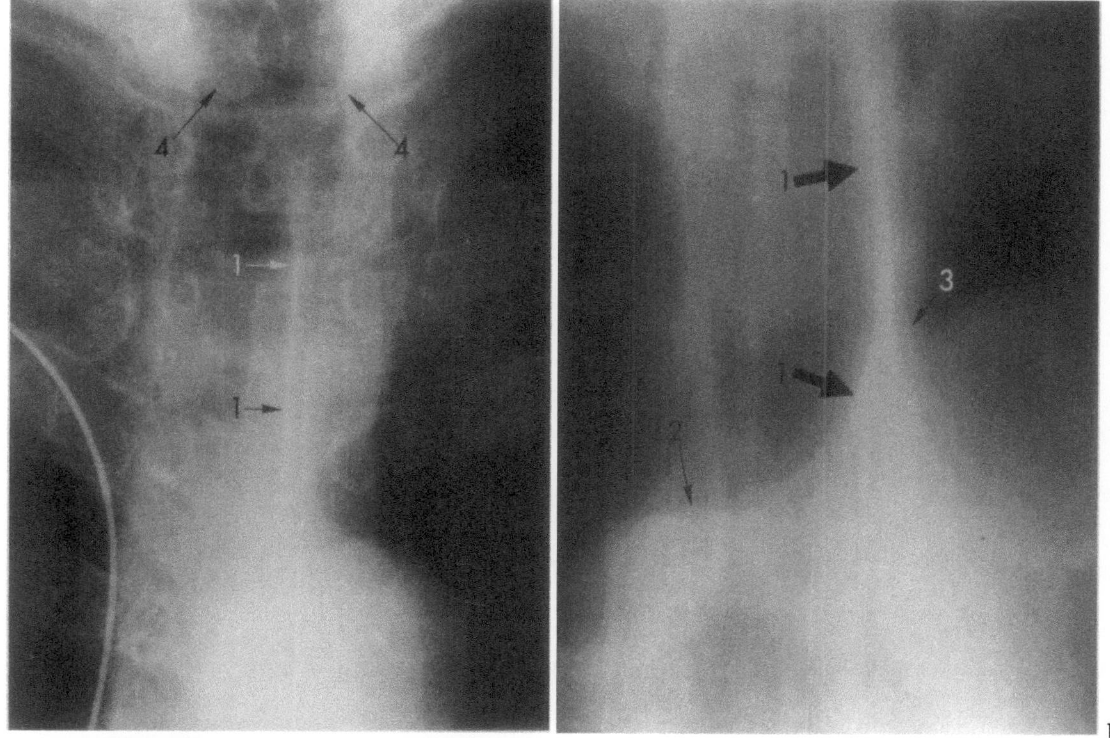

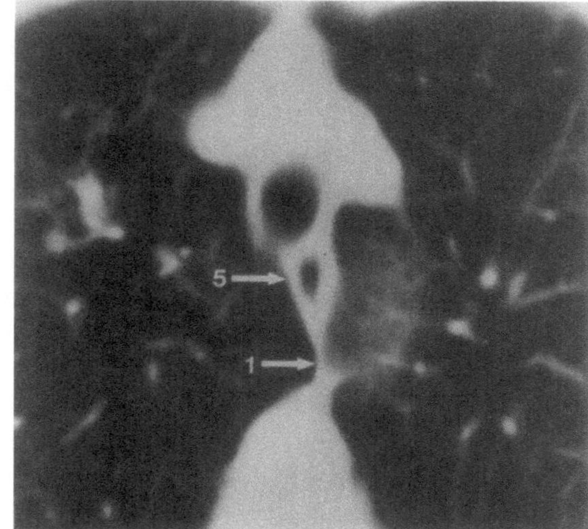

Fig. 8.51 A–C. Posterior junction line. **A** PA radiograph. **B** AP tomogram. **C** Computed tomogram. Posterior junction line (*1*), representing contact of right and left lungs behind esophagus is thus composed of four layers of pleura. Posterior junction line usually is straight vertical line (**A**) or bows slightly to the left (**B**). Inferiorly line is seen to deflect over azygos arch on right (*2*) and aortic arch on left (*3*). Superiorly line is seen to deflect over apex of each lung (*4*). Anteriorly leaves of posterior junction line diverge to encompass esophagus (*5*), posterior junction line is therefore sometimes called "mesentery" of esophagus. (**B** From [49])

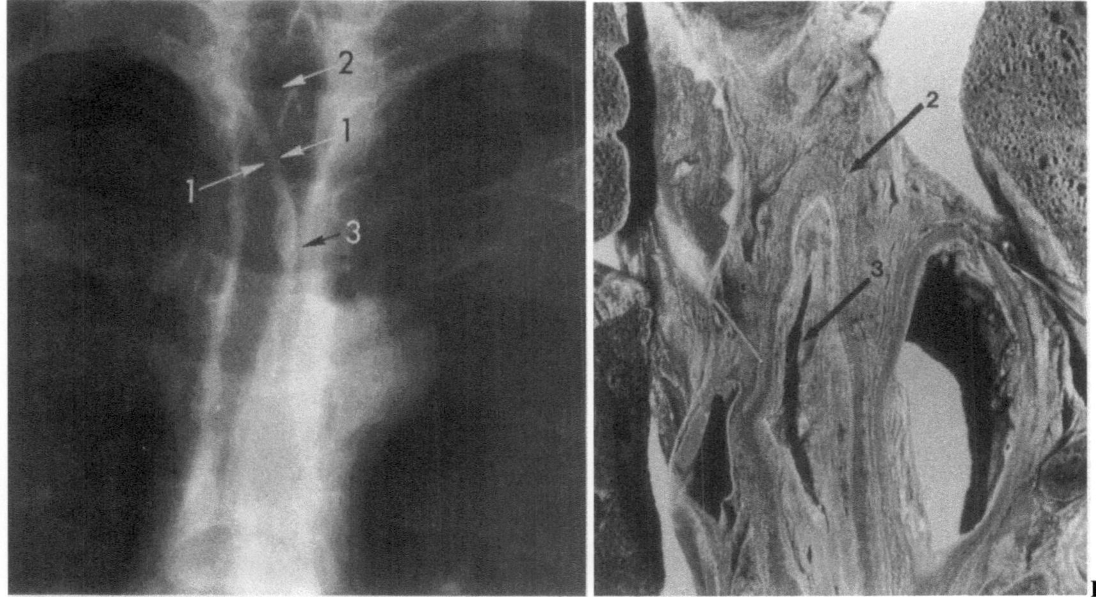

Fig. 8.52 A, B. Posterior junction line. **A** PA radiograph. **B** Coronal body section. Occasionally reflection of pleura from lung apex medially to become posterior junction line appears as stripe of density with radiolucency on either side (*1*). Lateral radiolucency is, of course, lung. Some of radiolucency medial to line may at times be produced by gas in esophagus, but more commonly it is due to fat (*2*) about esophagus (*3*). (Courtesy E. Buonocore, Knoxville, TN)

In some patients the reflections of the pleura off the lung apices appear as radiolucent lines rather than as lung-mediastinal interfaces as they approach one another to form the posterior junction line (Fig. 8.52). The medial radiolucency can be attributed to gas in the esophagus in some cases. More often, the medial radiolucency is caused by periesophageal prespinal fat (Fig. 8.52).

When lung intrudes deeply behind the esophagus and especially when it contacts lung from the other side, air in lung provides contrast that allows visualization of the prespinal soft tissues. The soft-tissue stripe lying between the lung and the anterior margins of the vertebral bodies has been termed the "prespinal line" [48]. The line is interrupted by the posterior turn of the azygos arch and right superior intercostal vein extending downward to join the arch (see Fig. 8.11). The line will be discussed in greater detail in chapter 9.

8.5 The Paraspinal Line

Behind the lung in the supra-azygos recess the right lung contacts the paraspinal soft tissues to produce the paraspinal line, a narrow soft-tissue stripe paralleling the spine from apex to diaphragm. This line is much less prominent and is less often visible on the right than on the left. This fact is usually attributed to the left-sided position of the descending aorta, which causes the interface of the posterior left lung with the paraspinal tissues to lie in a true sagittal plane. In support of this contention is the observation of Dalton and Schwartz [29] that the right paraspinal line is more prominent with right aortic arch and descending aorta. The paraspinal line discussed in greater detail in chapter 7.

References

1. Abrams HL (1957) The vertebral and azygous venous systems and some variations in systemic venous return. Radiology 69:508–526
2. Abrams HL (1983) Abrams angiography. Vascular and interventional radiology, 3rd edn. Little and Brown, Boston
3. Anderson RC, Adams P, Burke B (1961) Anomalous inferior vena cava with azygous continuation (infrahepatic interruption of the inferior vena cava). J Pediatr 59:370–383
4. Aronberg D, Peterson RR, Glazer HS, Sagel SS (1984) The superior sinus of the pericardium: CT appearance. Radiology 153:489–492
5. Austin JHM, Thorsen MK (1981) Normal azygous arch: retrotracheal visualization on frontal chest tomograms. AJR 137:1205–1208
6. Bachman AL, Teixidor HS (1975) The posterior tracheal band: a reflector of local superior mediastinal abnormality. Br J Radiol 48:352–359
7. Bachman AL, Ackerman W, Macken K (1961) Azygography – its value in mediastinal adenopathy and tumors. Ann Surg 153:344–356
8. Bachman DM, Ellis K, Austin JHM (1978) The effect of minor degrees of obliquity on the lateral chest radiograph. Radiol Clin North Am 16:465–485
9. Baron RL, Gutierrez FR, Sagel SS, Levitt RG, McKnight RC (1981) CT of anomalies of the mediastinal vessels. AJR 137:571–576
10. Bechtold RE, Wolfman NT, Karstaedt N, Choplin RH (1985) Superior vena caval obstruction: detection using CT. Radiology 157:485–487
11. Berdon WE, Baker DH (1968) Azygous continuation of the inferior vena cava. Am J Roentgenol Radium Ther Nucl Med 104:452–457
12. Berdon WE, Baker DH, Bordiuk J, Mellins R (1969) Innominate artery compression of the trachea in infants with stridor and apnea. Radiology 92:272–278
13. Berk RN (1964) Dilatation of the left superior intercostal vein in plain film diagnosis of chronic superior vena cava obstruction. Radiology 83:419–423
14. Boyden EA (1952) The distribution of bronchi in gross anomalies of the right upper lobe, particularly lobes subdivided by the azygous vein and those containing pre-eparterial bronchi. Radiology 58:797–807
15. Boyden EA (1955) Segmental anatomy of the lungs – a study of the patterns of the segmental bronchi and related pulmonary vessels. McGraw-Hill, New York
16. Breckenridge JW, Kinlaw WB (1980) Azygos continuation of the inferior vena cava. CT appearance. J Comput Assist Tomogr 4:392–397
17. Cahan WG, Watson WL, Pool JL (1951) Radical pneumonectomy. J Thorac Surg 22:449–473
18. Castellino RA, Blank N, Adams DF (1968) Dilated azygous and hemiazygous veins presenting as paravertebral intrathoracic masses. N Engl J Med 278:1087–1091
19. Chasen MH, Rugh KS, Shelton DK (1984) Mediastinal impressions on the dilated esophagus. Radiol Clin North Am 22:591–605
20. Christensen EE, Landay MJ, Dietz GW, Brinley G (1978) Buckling of the innominate artery simulating a right apical lung mass. AJR 131:119–123
21. Churchill RJ, Wesby G III, Marsan RE, Moncada R, Reynes CJ, Love L (1980) Computed tomographic demonstration of anomalous inferior vena cava with azygous continuation. J Comput Assist Tomogr 4:398–402
22. Cimmino CV (1956) The esophageal-pleural stripe on chest teleroentgenograms. Radiology 67:754–756
23. Cimmino CV (1961) Further notes on esophageal-pleural stripe. Radiology 77:974–978
24. Cimmino CV (1981) The esophageal-pleural stripe: an update. Radiology 140:609–613
25. Cimmino CV, Snead LO (1965) The posterior mediastinal line on chest roentgenograms. Radiology 84:516–518
26. Civetta JM, Daggett WM (1968) The azygous lobe – clinical implications and an unusual variant. J Thorac Cardiovasc Surg 56:430–434
27. Clemente CD (1985) Gray's anatomy, 30th Am edn. Lea and Febiger, Philadelphia
28. Cunningham DJ (1972) In: Romanes GJ (ed) Textbook of anatomy, 11th edn. Oxford University Press, London
29. Dalton CJ, Schwartz SS (1956) Evaluation of the paraspinal line in roentgen examination of the thorax. Radiology 66:195–200
30. Doyle FH, Read AE, Evans KT (1961) The mediastinum in portal hypertension. Clin Radiol 12:114–129
31. Drasin E, Sayre RW, Castellino RA (1972) Nondilated superior vena cava presenting as a superior mediastinal mass. J Can Assoc Radiol 23:273–274
32. Elliott LP, Jae KL, Amplatz K (1966) Roentgen classification of cardiac malposition. Invest Radiol 1:17–28
33. Engel IA, Auh YH, Rubenstein WA, Sniderman K, Whalen JP, Kazam E (1983) CT diagnosis of mediastinal and thoracic inlet venous obstruction. AJR 141:521–526
34. Felson B (1967) Letter from the editor. Semin Roentgenol 2:323
35. Felson B (1973) Chest roentgenology. Saunders, Philadelphia
36. Felson B, Lessure AP (1964) "Downhill" varices of the esophagus. Dis Chest 46:740–746
37. Ferris EJ, Vittingarga FJ, Byrne JJ, Nabseth DC, Shapiro JH (1967) The inferior vena cava after ligation and plication. Radiology 89:1–10
38. Fishbone G (1970) The azygous vein in right aortic arch. Radiology 96:45–46
39. Fleischner FG, Udis SW (1952) Dilatation of the azygous vein. Am J Roentgenol Radium Ther Nucl Med 67:569–575

40. Fleming RJ, Medina J, Seaman WB (1962) Roentgenographic aspects of tracheal tumors. Radiology 79:628–635

41. Gladnikoff H (1948) A radiographic study of the mediastinum in health and pulmonary carcinoma. Acta Radiol [Suppl] 73:1–87

42. Godwin JD, Chen JTT (1986) Thoracic venous anatomy. AJR 147:674–684

43. Goebel N (1983) The "lobe" of the right brachiocephalic vein. CT-Sonographie 3:146–148

44. Goldberg EM, Shapiro CM, Blicksman HS (1974) Mediastinoscopy for assessing mediastinal spread in clinical staging of lung carcinoma. Semin Oncol 1:205–215

45. Gruenfeld GE, Gray SH (1941) Malformations of the lung. Arch Pathol 31:392–407

46. Heitzman ER (1973) Radiologic appearance of the azygos vein in cardiovascular disease. Circulation 47:628–634

47. Heitzman GR (1975) Roentgen anatomic correlations in the mediastinum. In: Margulis AR, Gooding CA (eds) Diagnostic radiology. University of California Press, Berkeley

48. Heitzman ER, Scrivani JV, Martino J, Moro J (1971) The azygos vein and its pleural reflections. I Normal roentgen anatomy. Radiology 101:249–258

49. Heitzman ER, Scrivani JV, Martino J, Moro J (1971) The azygos vein and its pleural reflections. II Applications in the radiological diagnosis of mediastinal abnormality. Radiology 101:259–266

50. Henrion J, Lebrec D, Nahum H, Ben-Hamou JP (1979) Pseudotumor varices of the mediastinum in a case of portal hypertension. Gastroenterol Clin Biol 3:453–459

51. Hildner FJ, Ormond RS (1967) Accuracy of the clinical diagnosis of pulmonary embolism. JAMA 202:567–576

52. Ishikawa T, Tsukune Y, Ohyama Y, Fujikawa M, Sakuyama K, Fufii M (1980) Venous abnormalities in portal hypertension demonstrated by CT. AJR 134:271–276

53. Janower ML, Dreyfuss JR, Skinner DB (1966) Azygography and lung cancer. N Engl J Med 275:803–808

54. Janower ML, Grillo HC, MacMillan AS Jr, James AE (1970) The radiological appearance of carcinoma of the trachea. Radiology 96:39–43

55. Jue KL, Raghib G, Amplatz K, Adams P, Edwards JE (1965) Anomalous origin of the left pulmonary artery from the right pulmonary artery. Report of 2 cases and review of the literature. Am J Roentgenol Radium Ther Nucl Med 95:598–610

56. Kale MK, Rafferty RE, Carton RW (1970) Aberrant left pulmonary artery presenting as a mediastinal mass. Report of a case in an adult. Arch Intern Med 125:121–125

57. Keats TE, Lipscomb GE, Betts CS III (1968) Mensuration of the arch of the azygous vein. Radiology 90:990–994

58. Knuttson F (1955) Mediastinal pleura. Acta Radiol 43:265–275

59. Kormano MJ, Yajana J (1980) Posterior tracheal band: correlation between computed tomography and chest radiography. Radiology 136:689–694

60. Lachman E (1942) Comparison of the posterior boundaries of the lungs and pleura as demonstrated on the cadaver and on the roentgenogram of the living. Anat Rec 83:521–542

61. Landay M (1983) Azygous vein abutting the posterior wall of the right main and upper lobe bronchi: a normal CT variant. AJR 140:461–462

62. Lane EJ, Heitzman ER, Dinn WM (1976) The radiology of the superior intercostal veins. Radiology 120:263–268

63. Leigh TF, Weens HS (1959) The mediastinum. Thomas, Springfield, ILL

64. Leszczynski SZ (1972) Purulent and fibrous mediastinitis – radiological diagnosis. Polish Medical Publishers, Warsaw

65. Levy-Ravetch M, Auh YH, Rubenstein WA, Whalen JP, Kazam E (1985) CT of the pericardial recesses. AJR 144:707–714

66. MacDonald CJ, Castellino RA, Blank N (1970) The aortic "nipple." The left superior intercostal vein. Radiology 96:533–536

67. Magbitang MH, Hayford FC, Blake JM (1960) Dilated azygous vein simulating a mediastinal tumor. N Engl J Med 263:598–600

68. McCort JJ, Robbins LL (1951) Lymph node metastases in carcinoma of lung. Radiology 57:339–360

69. McMurdo KK, deGeer G, Webb WR, Gamsu G (1986) Normal and occluded mediastinal veins: MR imaging. Radiology 159:33–38

70. Milne ENC, Pistolesi M, Miniati M, Guintini C (1984) Vascular pedicle of the heart and the vena azygos. I The normal subject. Radiology 152:1–8

71. Milne ENC, Imray TJ, Pistolesi M, Miniati M, Guintini C (1984) Vascular pedicle of the heart and the vena azygos. III In trauma – the "vanishing" azygos. Radiology 153:25–31

72. Muller NL, Webb WR, Gamsu G (1985) Paratracheal lymphadenopathy: radiographic findings and correlation with CT. Radiology 156:761–765

73. Nohl HC (1956) An investigation into the lymphatic and vascular spread of carcinoma of the bronchus. Thorax 11:172–185

74. Nohl HC (1962) The spread of carcinoma of the bronchus. Year Book Medical Publishers, Chicago

75. Okay NH, Bryk D (1969) Collateral pathways in occlusion of the superior vena cava and its tributaries. Radiology 92:1493–1498

76. Pagniez B, Denies JL, DuPuis C, Remy J (1975) The left superior intercostal vein. J Radiol Electrol Med Nucl 56:285–298 (in French)

77. Palayew MJ (1979) The tracheo-esophageal stripe and the posterior tracheal band. Radiology 132:11–13

78. Parish JM, Marschke RF, Diness DE, Lee RE (1981) Etiologic considerations in the superior vena caval syndrome. Mayo Clin Proc 56:407–413

79. Parkinson J, Bedford DE (1936) The aortic triangle. Radiological landmark in the left oblique projection. Lancet 2:909–911

80. Pernkopf E (1963) Atlas of topographical and applied human anatomy, vol 2. Saunders, Philadelphia

81. Pistolesi M, Milne ENC, Miniati M, Giuntini C (1984) Vascular pedicle of the heart and the vena azygos. II Acquired heart disease. Radiology 152:9–17

82. Polga JP, Drum DE (1972) Abnormal perfusion and ventilation scintigrams in patients with azygos fissures. J Nucl Med 13:633–636

83. Proto AV, Speckman JM (1980) The left lateral radiograph of the chest, part 1. Med Radiogr Photogr 56:38–64

84. Putman CE, Curtis AM, Westfried M, McLoud TC (1976) Thickening of the posterior tracheal stripe: a sign of squamous cell carcinoma of the esophagus. Radiology 121:533–536

85. Raider L (1973) The retrotracheal triangle. Chest 63:835–838

86. Ranniger K (1968) Retrograde azygography. Radiology 90:1097–1104

87. Rockoff SD, Druy EM (1982) Tortuous azygous arch simulating a pulmonary lesion. AJR 138:577–579

88. Rouviere H (1932) Anatomie des lymphatiques de l'homme. Masson, Paris

89. Saks BJ, Kilby AE, Dietrich PA, Coffin LH, Kranitt EL (1983) Pleural and mediastinal changes following endoscopic injection therapy of esophageal varices. Radiology 149:639–642

90. Savoca CJ, Austin JHM, Goldberg HJ (1977) Widening of the right paratracheal stripe. Radiology 122:295–301

91. Schnyder PA, Gamsu G (1981) CT of the pretracheal retrocaval space. AJR 136:303–308

92. Schwartz S, Handel J, Candel S (1959) Azygography. Radiology 72:338–343

93. Sheiner NM, Palayew MJ (1969) "Downhill" esophageal varices in superior vena caval obstruction. Can Med Assoc J 100:961–964

94. Shields JB, Holtz S (1976) The retrotracheal space. Radiology 120:19–23

95. Shin MS, Jolles PR, Ho K-J (1980) CT evaluation of distended pericardial recess presenting as a mediastinal mass. J Comput Assist Tomogr 10:860

96. Shuford WH, Weens HS (1958) Azygous vein dilatation simulating mediastinal tumor. Am J Roentgenol Radium Ther Nucl Med 80:225–230

97. Smathers RL, Buschi AJ, Pope TL, Brenbridge AN (1982) Pictorial essay. The azygous arch: normal and pathologic CT appearance. AJR 139:477–483

98. Speckman JM, Gamsu G, Webb WR (1981) Alterations in CT mediastinal anatomy produced by an azygous lobe. AJR 137:47–50

99. Stauffer HM, Labree J, Adams FH (1951) The normally situated arch of the azygous vein: its roentgenologic identification and classification. Am J Roentgenol Radium Ther Nucl Med 66:353–360

100. Strife JL, Baumel AS, Dunbar JS (1981) Tracheal compression by the innominate artery in infancy and childhood. Radiology 139:73–75

101. Tisi GM, Friedman PJ, Peters RM, Pearson G, Carr D, Lee RE, Selawry O (1983) Clinical staging of primary lung cancer. Am Rev Resp Dis 127:659–664

102. Webb WR, Gamsu G, Speckman JM (1982) Pictorial essay: computed tomographic demonstration of mediastinal venous anomalies. AJR 139:157–161

103. Wittenborg MH, Tantiwongse T, Rosenberg BF (1956) Anomalous course of left pulmonary artery with respiratory obstruction. Radiology 67:339–345

104. Wishart DL (1972) Normal azygous vein width in children. Radiology 104:115–118

105. Yajana J (1980) The posterior tracheal band and recurrent esophageal carcinoma. Radiology 136:615–618

9 The Infra-azygos Area

9.1 General Anatomic Considerations

The portion of the mediastinum to be considered in this chapter lies below the azygos arch and behind the right side of the anterior mediastinum. The anatomy of the azygos arch has been reviewed in detail in chapter 8. The coronal plane marking the anterior boundary of the infra-azygos area passes through the superior vena cava. Along the anterior aspect of the infra-azygos area, lung contacts heart in front of the right inferior pulmonary ligament. The configurations produced by the contact of lung with the right atrium are well known and will not be discussed further. The appearances of the contact of lung with the left atrium and left pulmonary veins will be considered later in this chapter. It is the purpose of this chapter to correlate radiologic appearances with the anatomy and pathology of the structures situated between the azygos arch and the posterior aspect of the heart: the esophagus, the ante-esophageal spaces, and the right paraspinal area.

The anatomy of the infra-azygos area is predicated to a considerable degree on the course of the lower portion of the esophagus. Knutsson [24] quotes Poirier as stating that below the level of the azygos and aortic arches there are bilateral ante-esophageal and retroesophageal pouches into which lung intrudes against the mediastinum. The ante-esophageal recesses lie along the posterolateral borders of the heart (Fig. 9.4); Poirier states that they are 2–3 cm in height and that their bases lie on the diaphragm. He feels that they are of no consequence, although lung in the right-sided ante-esophageal pouch provides contrast that permits visualization of the posterior wall of the inferior vena cava on lateral radiographs (Fig. 9.5). The left ante-esophageal recess seems to have no practical radiologic significance.

The retroesophageal pouch on the right side, sometimes referred to as the "space of the Holzknecht," is of major importance to radiologic interpretation, a fact first emphasized by Lachman in 1942 [25] (Figs. 9.1, 9.2). He compared the appearances of the posterior boundaries of the lungs and pleurae in the cadaver with roentgenograms in living man and pointed out the intimate relationship of the right posterior lung and pleura to the azygos vein. The azygoesophageal recess lies lateral or posterior to the esophagus and in front of the spine and the ascending portion of the azygos vein. It is bordered above by the azygos arch, lying at the T-4 or T-5 level, and extends caudally to the diaphragm (Figs. 9.1 and 9.2). Heiss, also quoted by Knutsson [24] states that the recess extends only as far down as T-10, presumably inferring that the descending aorta excludes lung from the recess below this level. The descending aorta progresses downward on the left side of the spine, but begins to turn forward at about the T-10 level. By the time it reaches T-12, it lies along the left anterolateral aspect of the spine as it passes through the aortic hiatus in the diaphragm. It has been our experience with computed tomograms that the azygoesophageal recess can be seen extending all the way down to the diaphragm in many patients and that the descending aorta infrequently intrudes into it. However, when an elongated descending aorta buckles into the right lower chest rather than the left, the recess is significantly compromised at its lower extent (Fig. 9.3). This aortic intrusion has been misdiagnosed as a right inferior mediastinal mass lesion [48].

Lachman [25] credits Merkel with being the first observer to identify the crista pulmonis,

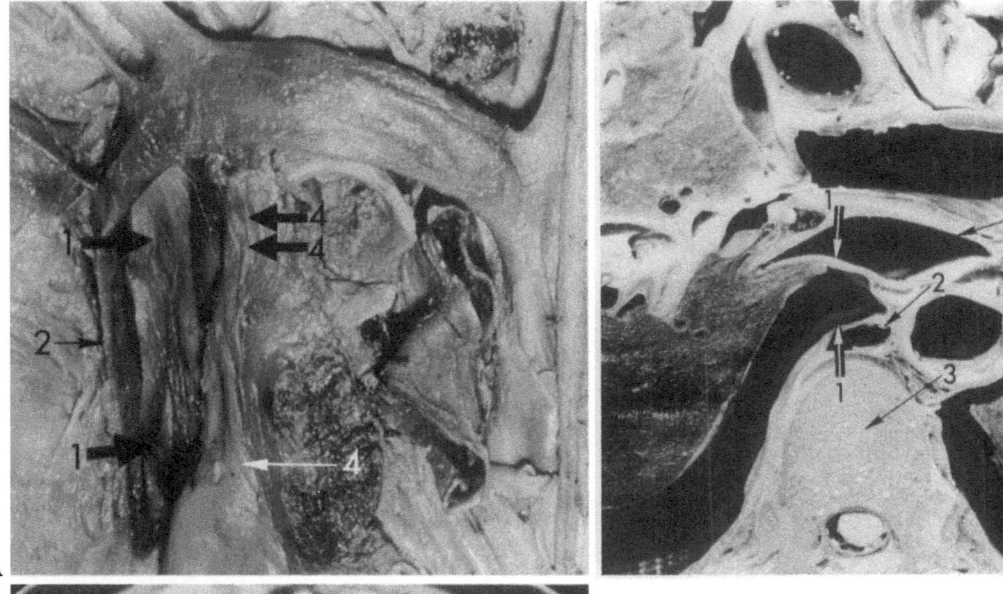

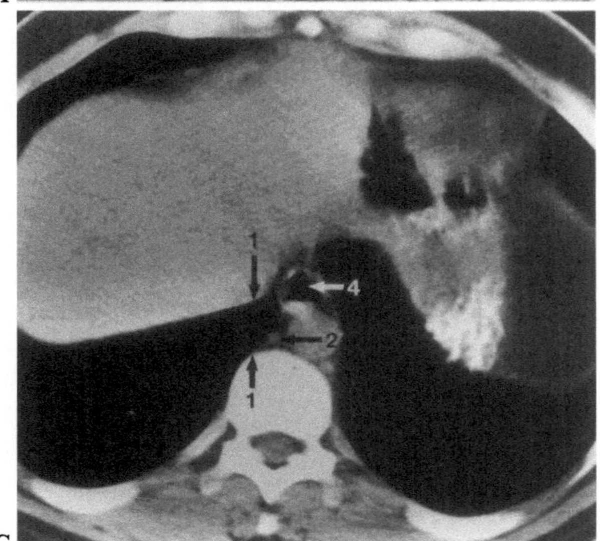

Fig. 9.1 A–C. Anatomy of the azygoesophageal recess. **A** Right side of mediastinum with mediastinal pleura removed. **B** Transverse body section. **C** Computed tomogram. Azygoesophageal recess, sometimes called "space of Holzknecht," is often not well demonstrated in dissecting room specimens but is identified commonly in living subjects (**C**). Cadaver preparation clearly shows azygoesophageal recess (*1*) lying in intimate relationship to the azygos vein (*2*) and spine (*3*) posteriorly, and esophagus (*4*) anteriorly. In patient shown on computed tomogram the esophagus lies to left of recess. Space often extends well to left of midline. (**A** From [21])

a crest extending along the posteromedial surface of the right lower lobe (Figs. 9.8, 9.9) as being the portion of lung which inserts into the azygoesophageal recess. The crista pulmonis in the azygoesophageal recess provides an excellent contrast material that permits evaluation of most structures along the posterior aspect of the right side of the mediastinum. For this reason the azygoesophageal recess has great clinical and radiologic relevance [21, 22]. It is interesting that this important anatomic area is not depicted at all in many standard textbooks of anatomy, presumably because it is seen poorly or not at all in the postmortem state. Lachman [25] has used this fact to emphasize the point that anatomy displayed in the cadaver is not always representative of the normal anatomic situation in life and that radiography is an important adjunct to the study of anatomy.

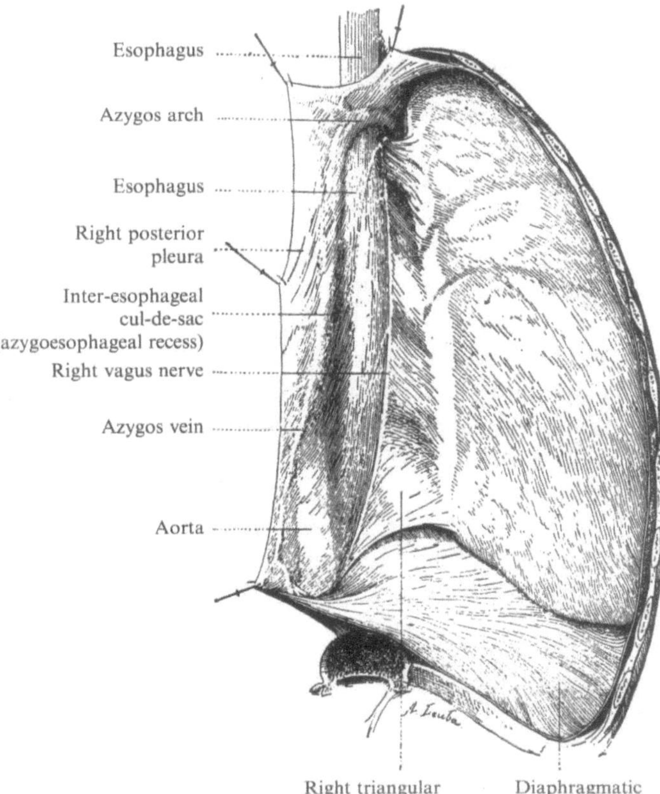

Fig. 9.2. Anatomy of the azygoesophageal recess. This drawing shows azygoesophageal recess as viewed from behind. Right mediastinal pleura, which would lie along spine, has been drawn to left showing azygoesophageal recess (here called the "cul-de-sac inter. oesoph.") opened like a book. (From [25])

Fig. 9.3 A, B. Buckling of left descending aorta into right hemithorax. **A** PA radiograph. **B** Computed tomogram. PA radiograph shows descending aorta with its upper portion lying to left of midline (*1*). When it is tortuous, the descending aorta commonly buckles prominently into left lung. Occasionally, it may intrude into right lung to appear as right retrocardiac mass (*2*). Such an appearance should not be mistaken for pathologic process. Computed tomogram made on this patient at level of inferior pulmonary veins shows that the aorta has swung to right side (*2*). Note that some left lower lobe has continued to follow aorta to right, outlining its left lateral aspect

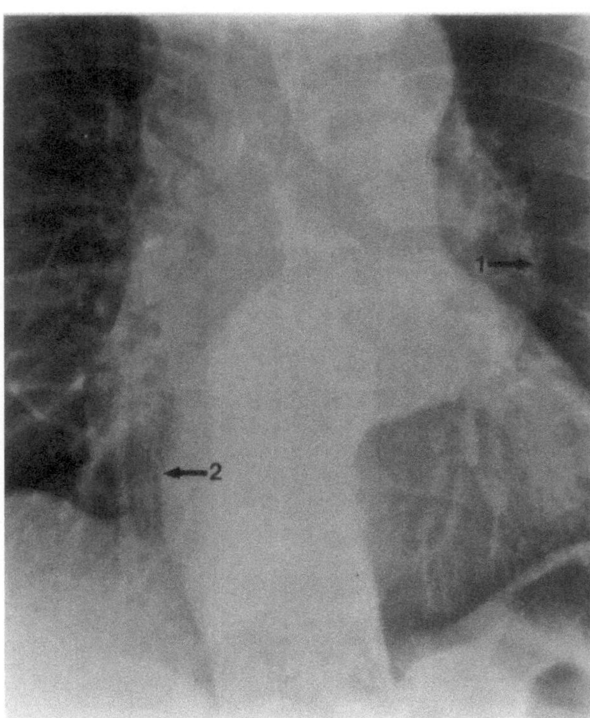

A

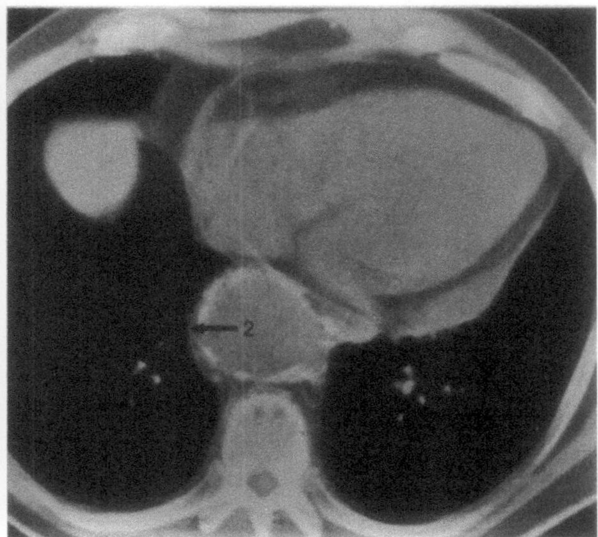

B

9.2 The Inferior Vena Cava

Behind the posterior pericardium and in front of the coronal plane of the esophagus the right lung below the azygos arch is in contact with only the right atrium and the inferior vena cava (Fig. 9.4). The cava is outlined on radiographs by lung in the right ante-esophageal recess. Rarely, the anterior wall of the lower esophagus may be in contact with lung in the ante-esophageal recesses (see Fig. 9.5).

Also a rare occurrence is the presence of lung anterior to the inferior vena cava, producing an anatomic situation referred to as "isolation" of the inferior vena cava [51] (Fig. 9.6). Tonkin et al. [51] have described five cases in which ante-esophageal lung "isolated" the inferior vena cava. On lateral radiographs of patients with this anatomic variant, the inferior vena cava may appear as a mass; at times its anterior surface may be almost horizontal and may simulate an air-fluid level [51].

The interface made by lung and the inferior vena cava is directed obliquely forward as the vessel passes upward from the caval foramen to the right atrium. The cava angulates forward at the diaphragm, sometimes to a marked degree [13]. Its supradiaphragmatic contour, visible on lateral radiographs because of contact with lung behind it, may adopt straight line configuration but more often shows a gentle curve with concavity directed posteriorly (Fig. 9.7). The shadow of the inferior vena cava is not present in patients with azygos continuation of the inferior vena cava, a condition in which the

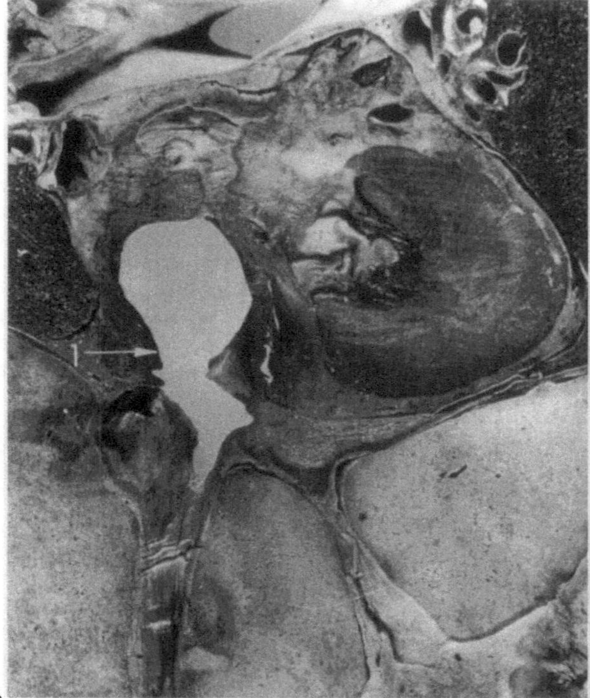

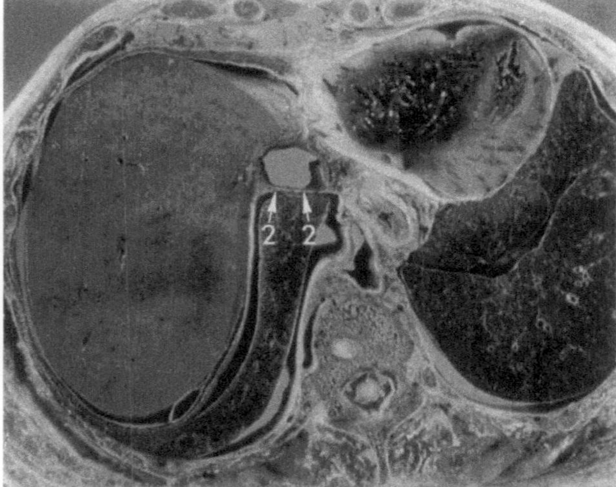

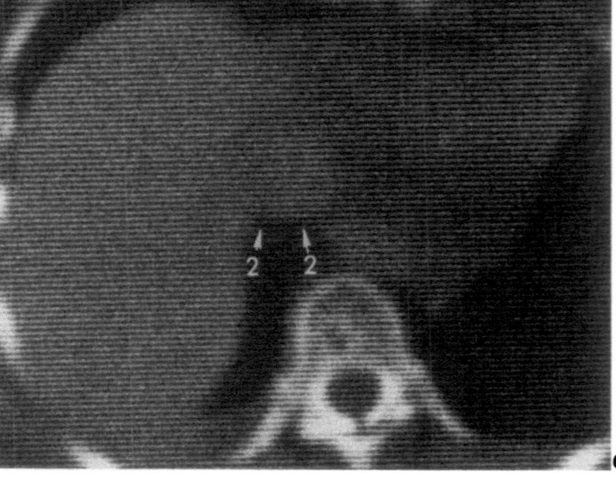

Fig. 9.4A–C. Inferior vena cava. **A** Coronal body section. **B** Transverse body section. **C** Computed tomogram made post mortem on cadaver shown in **B**. Right lower lobe is in contact with lateral border of upper portion of inferior vena cava (*1*), and lung in the right ante-esophageal recess contacts its posterior wall (*2*). Therefore, inferior vena cava is commonly identified in cardiophrenic angle on PA and lateral radiographs

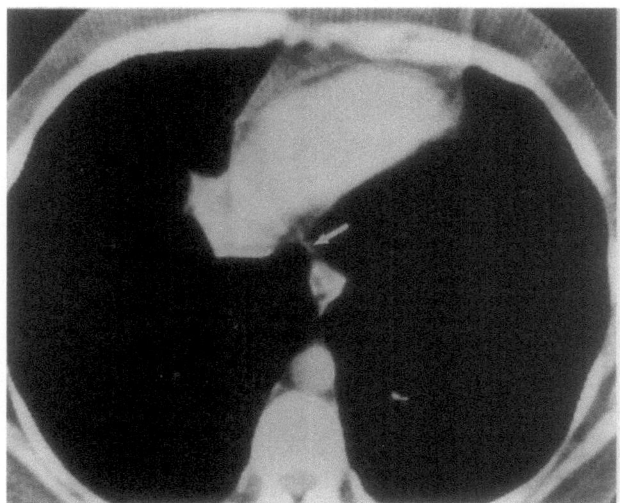

Fig. 9.5. Ante-esophageal recesses. Computed tomogram. Ante-esophageal recesses are rarely seen on computed tomograms. They lie immediately behind the heart and extend inferiorly to the diaphragm. They are of little consequence; lung in the right ante-esophageal recess provides contrast permitting visualization of the posterior wall of the inferior vena cava (see Fig. 9.4). In this patient, the two lungs meet in front of the esophagus to create a pre-esophageal line (*arrow*)

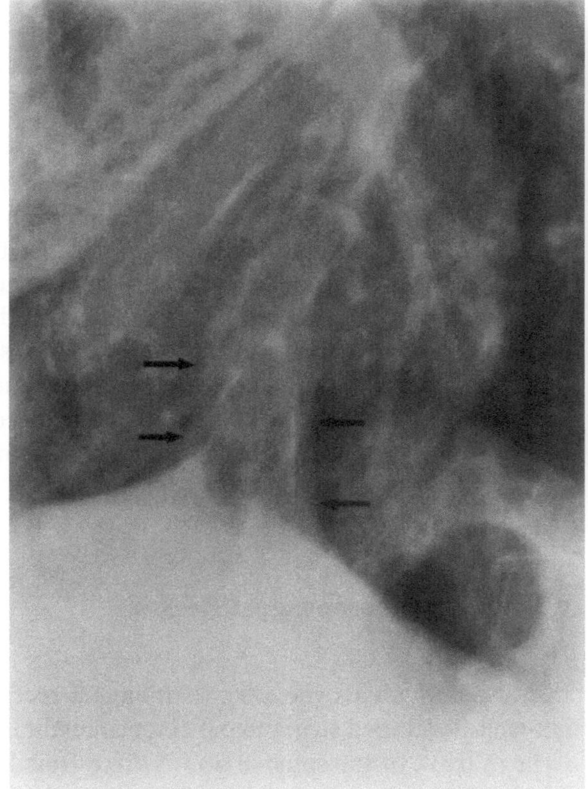

A

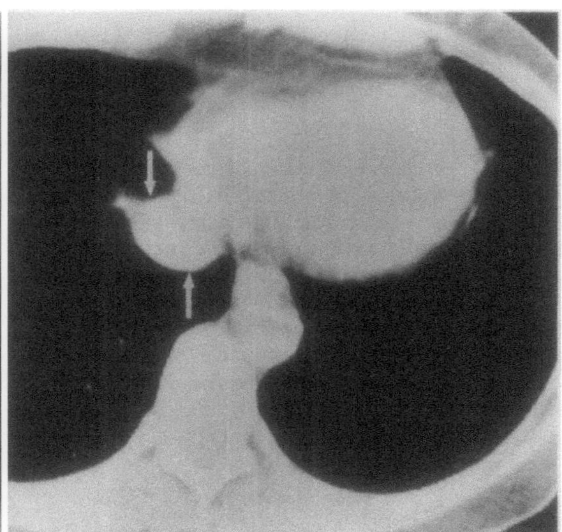

B

Fig. 9.6A, B. "Isolation" of the inferior vena cava. **A** Lateral radiograph. **B** Computed tomogram. Rarely, lung may outline the anterior surface of the inferior vena cava as well as its posterior aspect, thereby "isolating" the vessel. On lateral films this occurrence usually results in a band-like, vertically oriented density (*arrows*). Occasionally, a mass may be simulated

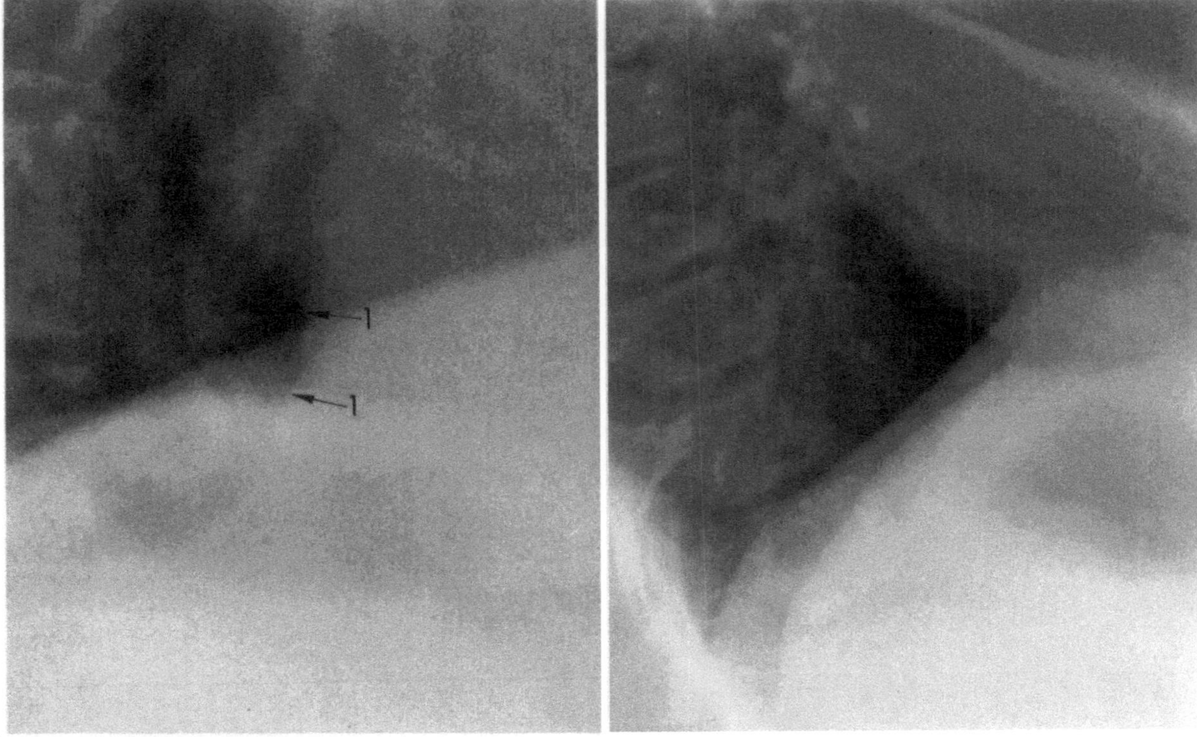

A   **B**

Fig. 9.7A, B. Absence of shadow of inferior vena cava in azygos continuation. **A** Normal lateral radiograph. **B** Radiograph from patient with proven azygos continuation. Normal configuration of lung in ante-esophageal recess outlining posterior wall of inferior vena cava (*1*) is not encountered in patients with azygos continuation (**B**). Absence of shadow of inferior vena cava on lateral radiographs is sign supportive of diagnosis of azygos continuation and should require an arm vein to be used for venous entry into heart when this diagnosis is suspected ED

infrahepatic portion of the cava is absent (Fig. 9.7). Failure to visualize this segment of the cava on lateral radiographs, especially in cyanotic patients with abnormalities of abdominal situs, is an important clue to this diagnosis [23]. The observation is of further significance since it should cause an arm vein, rather than a leg vein to be used for catheterization [23].

Doppman [13], Doppman et al. [14], and Rubinson et al. [45] have shown that the inferior vena cava does not narrow significantly with Valsalva's maneuver. They state that venous collapse with Valsalva's maneuver is due to the passage of blood from a high-pressure to a low-pressure chamber and claim that during this maneuver the thoracic and abdominal cavities may be regarded as one uniform pressure compartment. Therefore, response to Valsalva's maneuver cannot be used to determine whether a shadow visualized on lateral radiographs in the posterior cardiophrenic angle is the inferior vena cava or not, although such response can be used to identify the azygos arch and superior vena cava.

9.3 The Azygoesophageal Recess

In most individuals the azygoesophageal recess is a well-developed structure; it extends medially to lie in front of the spine in about three-fourths of cases [27]. Lund and Lien [27] studied the depth of the azygoesophageal recess on computed tomograms. The recess extended across the midline in most older patients, but did so much less frequently in individuals below age 50. In general the recess was deeper at its

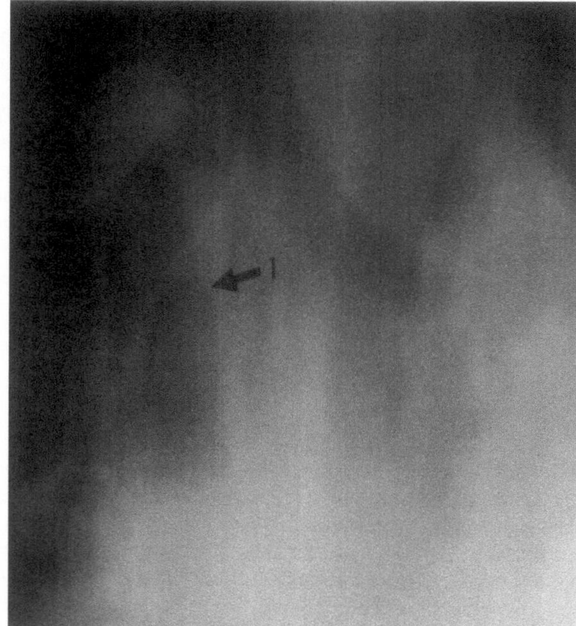

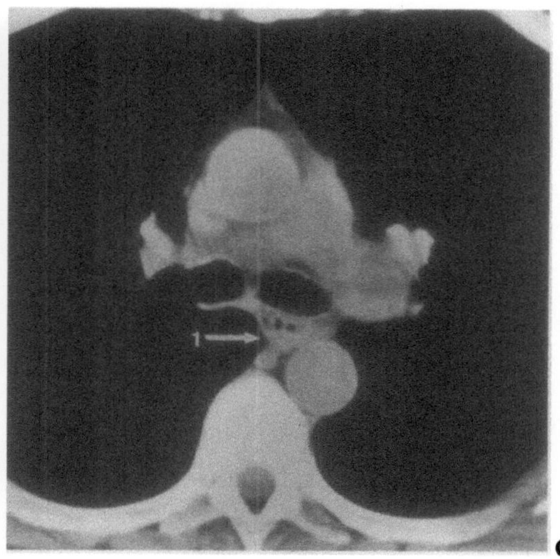

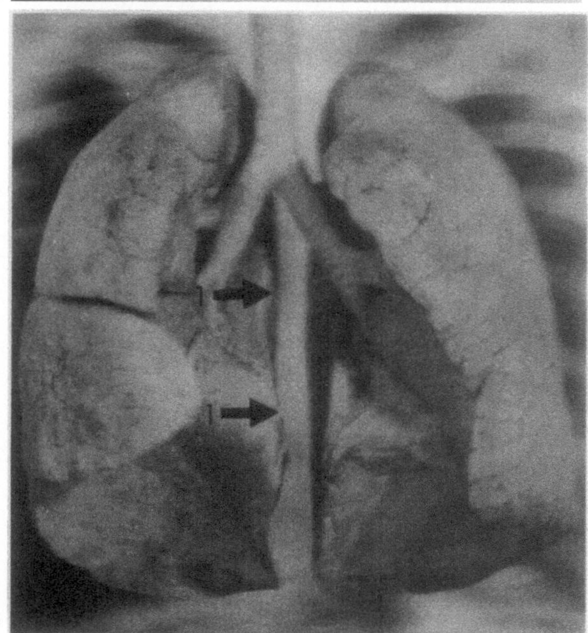

Fig. 9.8 A–C. Normal radiographic anatomy of the azygoesophageal recess. **A** AP tomogram. **B** Frontal photograph of anatomic specimen superimposed on chest roentgenogram. **C** Computed tomogram. Portion of lung that inserts itself into azygoesophageal recess is crista pulmonis (*1*) of right lower lobe. Note that lung extends to left of midsagittal plane and is in close proximity to left lower lobe. Note also intimate relationship of right lung to posterior aspect of right main bronchus, right upper lobe bronchus, and intermediate bronchus as well as to immediate subcarinal area. (**B** Courtesy B. Sills, New York, NY. From [19])

inferior extent than it was higher up. The recess deepens in full inspiration and, according to Lachman [25], in the erect position. It is more prominent in thoracic kyphosis and in emphysema.

The recess can often be visualized on standard PA radiographs of the chest and it is seen very frequently on overpenetrated AP views and conventional tomograms. Its medial boundary be-

low the azygos arch is readily recognized on frontal radiographs as a smooth arc with convexity directed to the left, extending caudad from the azygos arch (Fig. 9.8). Convexity directed to the right immediately below the azygos arch on frontal radiographs is never normal.

Onitsuka [37] has reported that, on computed tomograms, the upper portion of the recess may at times show a convex configuration directed

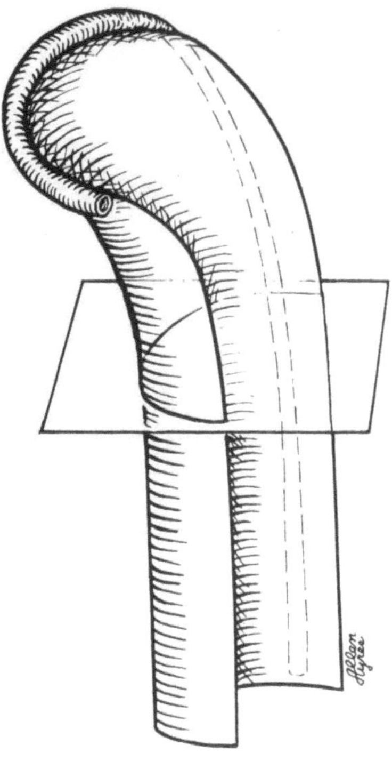

◁ **Fig. 9.9.** Normal radiographic anatomy of the azygoesophageal recess; drawing. On frontal radiographs, the upper portion of the azygoesophageal recess presents an arcuate configuration with convexity directed to the left. Convexity to the right is always abnormal (see Fig. 9.10). Although the axial or transverse outline of recess is usually U shaped with convexity directed to the left, sometimes the convexity in cross section is directed to the right. As this drawing demonstrates, such an anatomic variation still results in the recess always having a convexity directed to the left on frontal radiographs (see text)

Fig. 9.10 A, B. Normal radiographic anatomy of the azygoesophageal recess. AP tomograms. Crista pulmonis lying in depths of azygoesophageal recess makes arcuate interface with mediastinum in infra-azygos area. At times the convexity, directed to left, is rather deep (*1*) and at other times rather shallow (*2*). This interface does not normally present a convexity directed to right; such an appearance should raise strong suspicion of presence of pathologic process

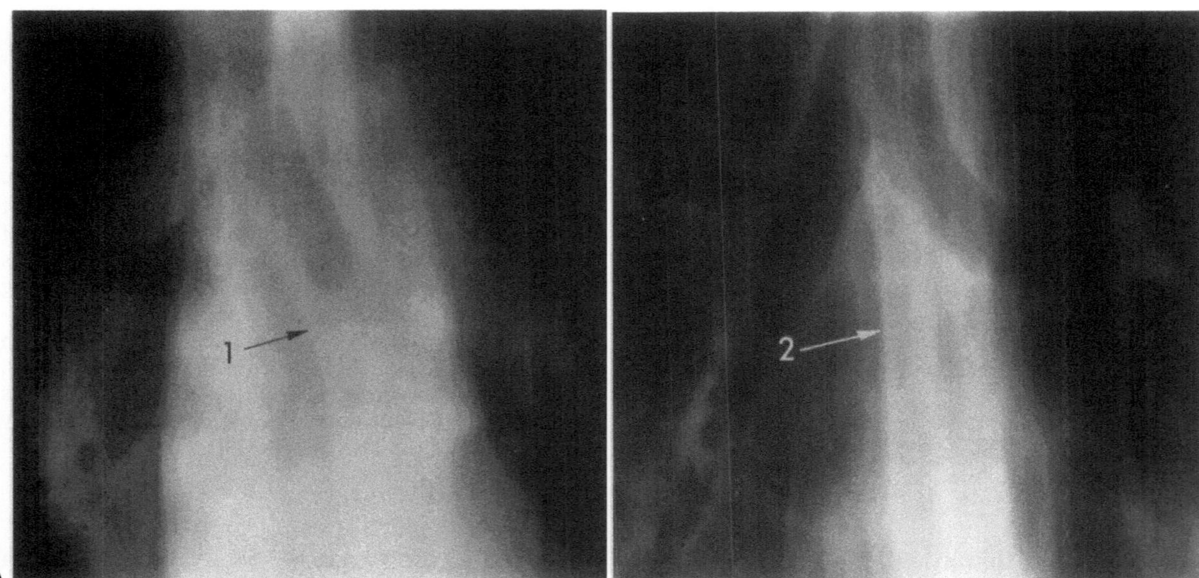

A   B

to the right. This observation was not made in Lund and Lien's [27] series of normal computed tomograms. We agree with Onitsuka [37] that, occasionally, normal computed tomograms show a mild convexity of the upper portion of the recess directed to the right; the appearance simulates minimal subcarinal adenopathy. Although the axial or transverse outline of recess is usually U shaped with convexity directed to the left, sometimes the convexity in cross section is directed to the right. These observations do not negate the statement that the normal azygoesophageal recess immediately below the azygos arch never presents a convexity to the right on frontal films (Fig. 9.9). To clarify this point consider Fig. 9.9. If a garden hose were laid out in the shape of an inverted letter J, it would have a convexity directed to the left when viewed from the front. If the hose were cut across (as with computed tomography) its right lateral margin would present a convexity directed to the right. On frontal radiographs, the convex configuration directed to the left may be either a gentle curve or a deeply rounded one (Fig. 9.10). Local irregularities in this curvature or any reversal in the curvature from convex to concave should suggest mediastinal pathology. At the level of the inferior pulmonary veins, the recess is more shallow (less deep from front to back) than elsewhere and the lung mediastinal interface at this point is often less sharp. Occasionally, minimal right-sided convexity of the recess is encountered at the level of the inferior pulmonary veins. Differences in the depth of the azygoesophageal recess produce a number of variations in the relationship of the lung and esophagus (Fig. 9.12).

9.3.1 The Right Pleuroesophageal Stripe

Early in his studies of the radiologic appearances of the interface between lung and the mediastinum posteriorly, Cimmino [7–9] pointed out that the lung makes intimate contact with the esophagus in many patients. He used the term "pleuroesophageal stripe" for this interface. Since Cimmino's original description, it has been thought by many observers that the right lateral wall of the esophagus is in contact with lung in every individual. In fact this relationship has been considered so constant that it has been suggested that the shadow between the line and the barium-coated esophageal mucosa could be used as an index of esophageal wall thickness [38]. In actuality the relationship of the esophagus to lung in the azygoesophageal recess is variable [9, 27]. Although the concept of the pleuroesophageal stripe can be justified on anatomic grounds in most patients (Fig. 9.11), in other individuals with a poorly developed recess the lung may not contact the esophagus at all (Figs. 9.12–9.14). In those cases the arcuate line subtended from the azygos arch and overlying the lower thoracic spine is not the pleuroesophageal stripe at all, but merely lung in the azygoesophageal recess; the esophagus may actually lie quite far to the left of the line [9, 27]. Since this relationship of lung and esophagus is inconstant, it is suggested that the use of the line to predict the position of the esophagus is unwise. For similar reasons, there is a potential pitfall in the use of the concept to estimate the thickness of the esophageal wall (Figs. 9.13, 9.14). If the stripe is seen to parallel perfectly the barium- or air-filled esophagus, separated from the lumen by 2 or 3 mm, a conclusion that the thickness of the esophageal wall is normal is probably justified. Similarly, localized changes in the stripe also have diagnostic significance. Utilization of this concept to estimate esophageal wall thickness under other circumstances, however, should be approached with caution.

In many patients, lung in the azygoesophageal recess lies not against the right lateral wall of the esophagus, but rather against its right posterolateral aspect (Figs. 9.12 and 9.15) or posterior surface (Fig. 9.12). Therefore, when lung does touch the esophagus, the radiographic demonstration of this point of contact is dependent upon film projection. The pleuroesophageal stripe can be demonstrated to best advantage in frontal projections in most individuals, in right anterior oblique or left posterior oblique projections in some patients, and in lateral projections in a few cases. It is worth reemphasizing that the crista pulmonis of the right lower lobe

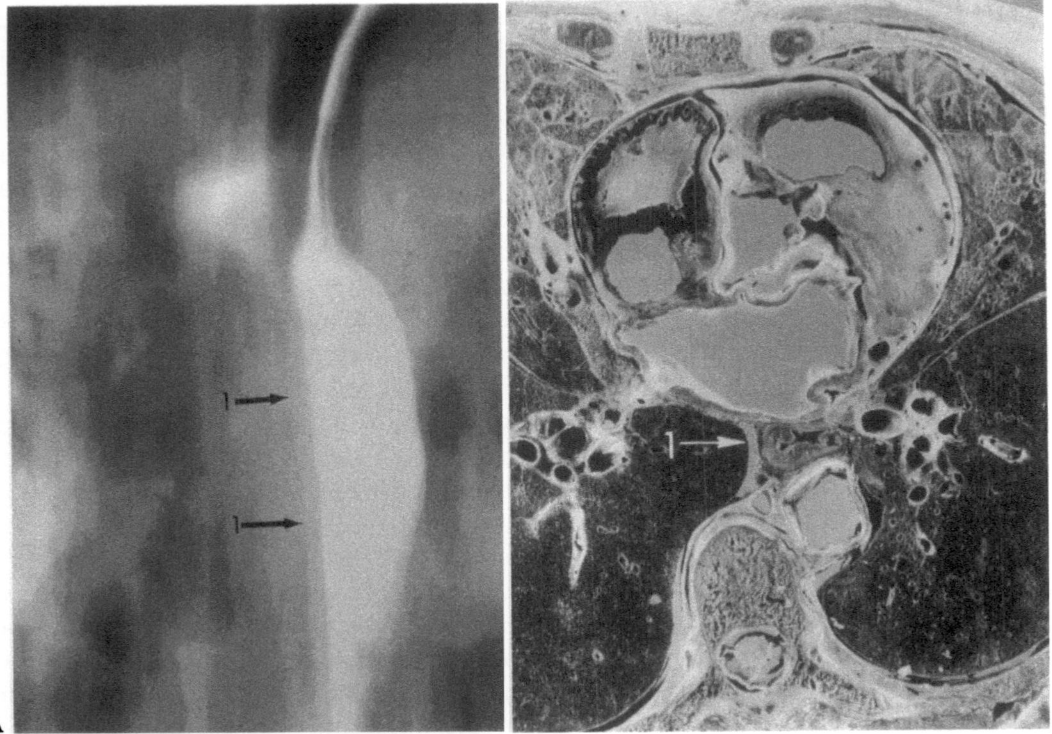

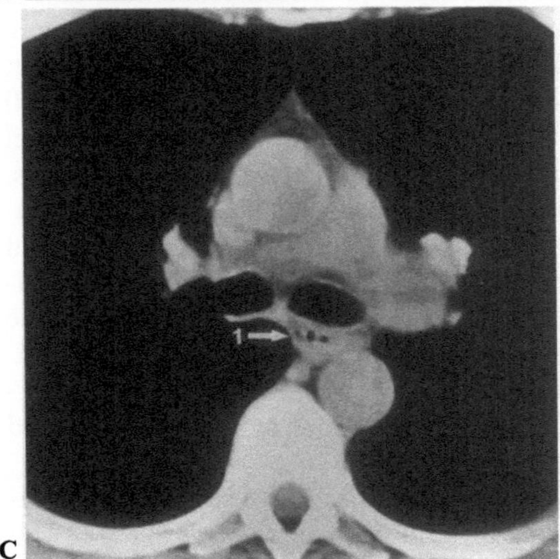

Fig. 9.11A–C. Pleuroesophageal stripe. **A** AP tomogram. **B** Transverse body section. **C** Computed tomogram. In many patients, crista pulmonis of right lower lobe filling azygoesophageal recess contacts wall of esophagus through mediastinal pleura (*1*). This relationship, although present in a high percentage of individuals, is not invariable. For this reason it is felt that use of this line to predict position of esophagus or use of line in conjunction with presence of air or barium in esophageal lumen to predict thickness of esophageal wall is unwise. Changes in line on serial radiographic examinations or localized changes in line are felt to be more significant. (**A** From [21])

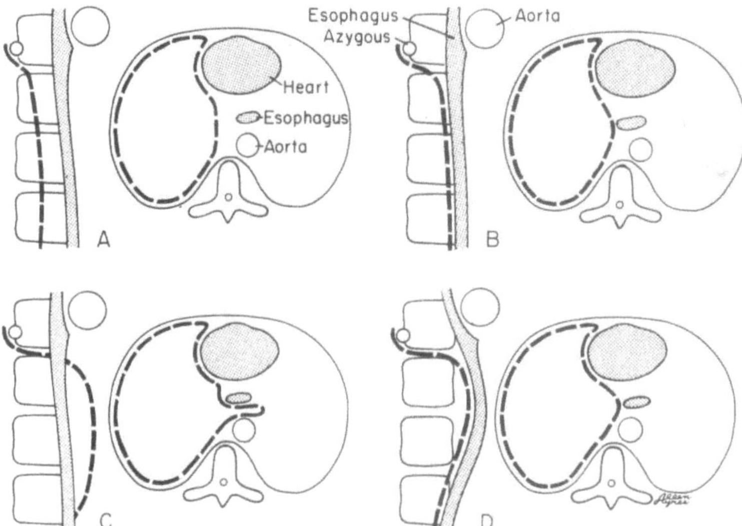

Fig. 9.12 A–D. Variability in relationship of right lower lobe to esophagus. This drawing shows in diagrammatic fashion relationship of right lung to esophagus in frontal and transverse projections. In **A** a very shallow azygoesophageal recess does not allow lung to contact esophagus. In **B** a deeper azygoesophageal recess permits their approximation. In **C** a very deep azygoesophageal recess extends behind esophagus to lie well to left of esophagus. In **D** the esophagus lies well to left of midline, and azygoesophageal recess follows esophagus, remaining in contact with it

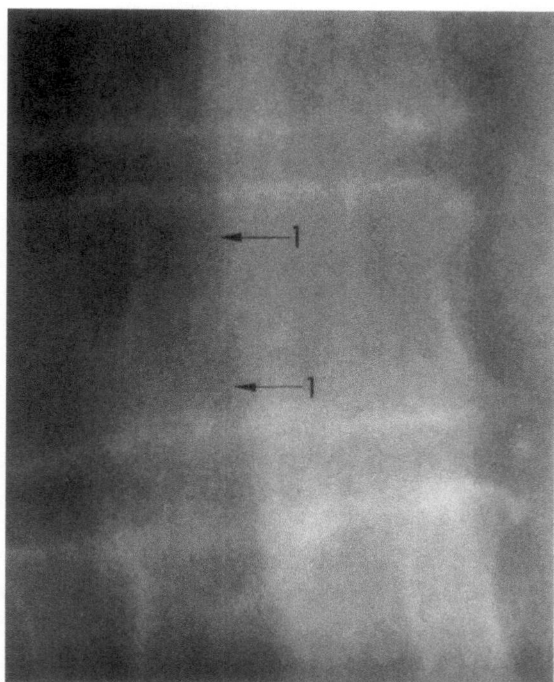

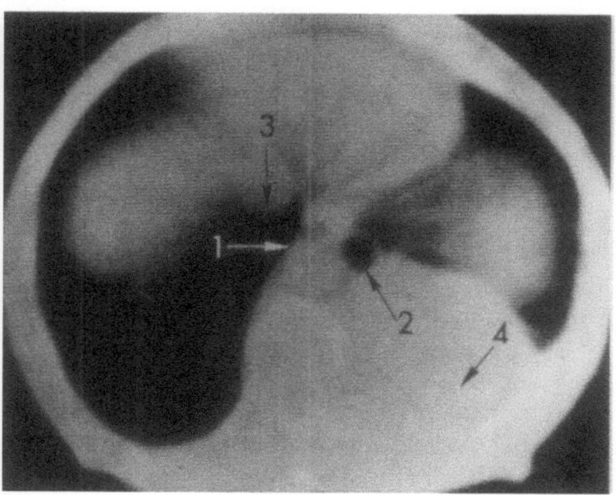

Fig. 9.13 A, B. Failure of right lung to contact esophagus. **A** AP radiograph. **B** Computed tomogram. AP radiograph clearly shows lung lying in front of spine in azygoesophageal recess (*1*). In this patient, the fact that point of contact of right lung with mediastinum is quite removed from air-filled esophagus (*2*) is shown clearly on computed tomogram. The inferior vena cava is well shown (*3*). A large bronchogenic carcinoma is present in left lower lobe (*4*)

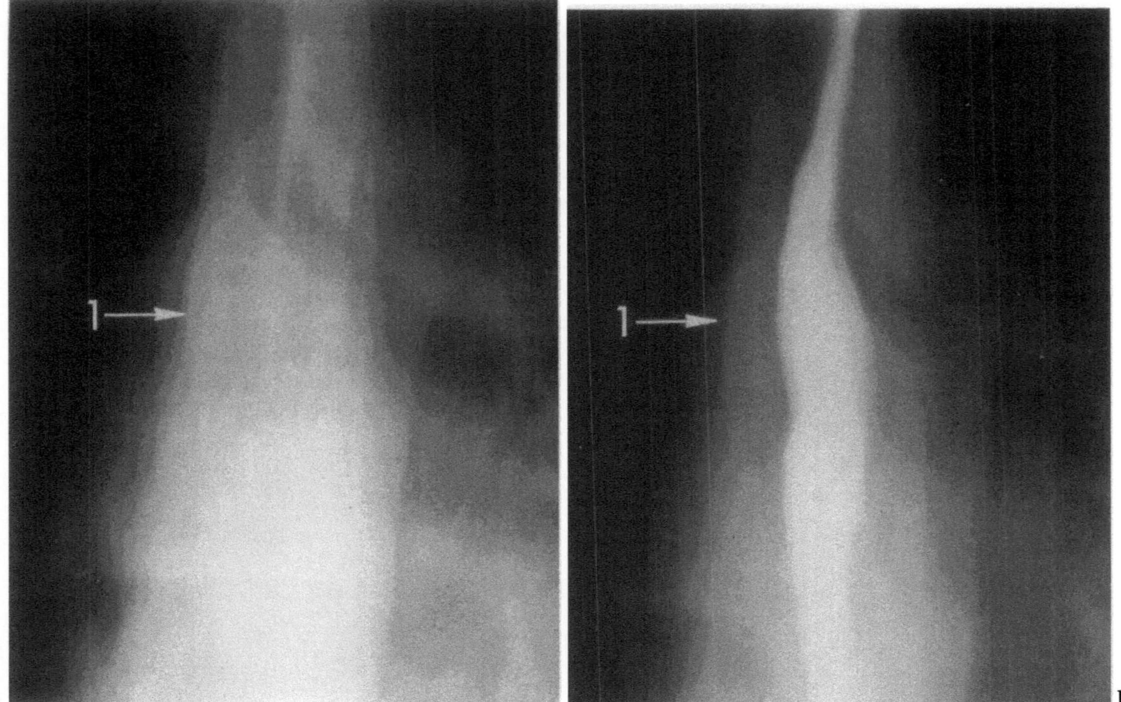

Fig. 9.14A, B. Failure of right lung to contact esophagus. A AP tomogram. B AP tomogram with barium in esophagus. In this patient, lung in azygoesophageal recess (1) lies considerably to right of barium-filled esophagus. These structures were apparently separated by presence of intervening nodes that were found at mediastinoscopy. Esophageal wall was normal

may extend into the azygoesophageal recess in front of the ascending portion of the azygos vein and behind the esophagus. Not infrequently, this portion of the lung extends further to the left than either the azygos vein or esophagus (Fig. 9.12). The depth of the recess is, therefore, only indirectly predicated on the position of these two structures.

At times, if the esophagus is particularly left sided or has been deviated to the left by an ectatic aorta, lung in the azygoesophageal recess will follow the esophagus, continuing to lie just to its right. In such instances the upper portion of the recess will lie immediately behind the tracheal bifurcation, allowing the demonstration of the exterior surface of the posterior wall of each major bronchus on conventional lateral tomograms (Figs. 9.16 and 9.17) or computed to-

mograms (Fig. 9.17). Similarly, the posterior wall of the right upper lobe bronchus is always identified on normal computed tomograms. Proto and Speckman [41] identified the posterior wall of the right main and intermediate bronchi in 95% of normal lateral chest radiographs; Bachman and Teixidor [1] were able to identify the posterior wall of the bronchus intermedius in 97% of conventional lateral chest radiographs. Proto and Speckman [41] found that the range of thickness of the posterior wall of the intermediate bronchus in normal subjects was 0.5–3.0 mm. Schnur et al. [47] have discussed thickening of the wall in a variety of disease states. Further comment on the diagnostic significance of thickening of the central bronchial walls is made in chapter 10.

The anterior aspect of the recess may intrude itself under the carina allowing visualization of the exterior surface of the medial wall of each major bronchus (Fig. 9.17), a finding originally noted by Gladnikoff [16]. The exterior wall of the medial aspect of the right main bronchus is much more commonly visualized than the left. Often, one can trace the outer wall of the right main bronchus and exceptionally the left main

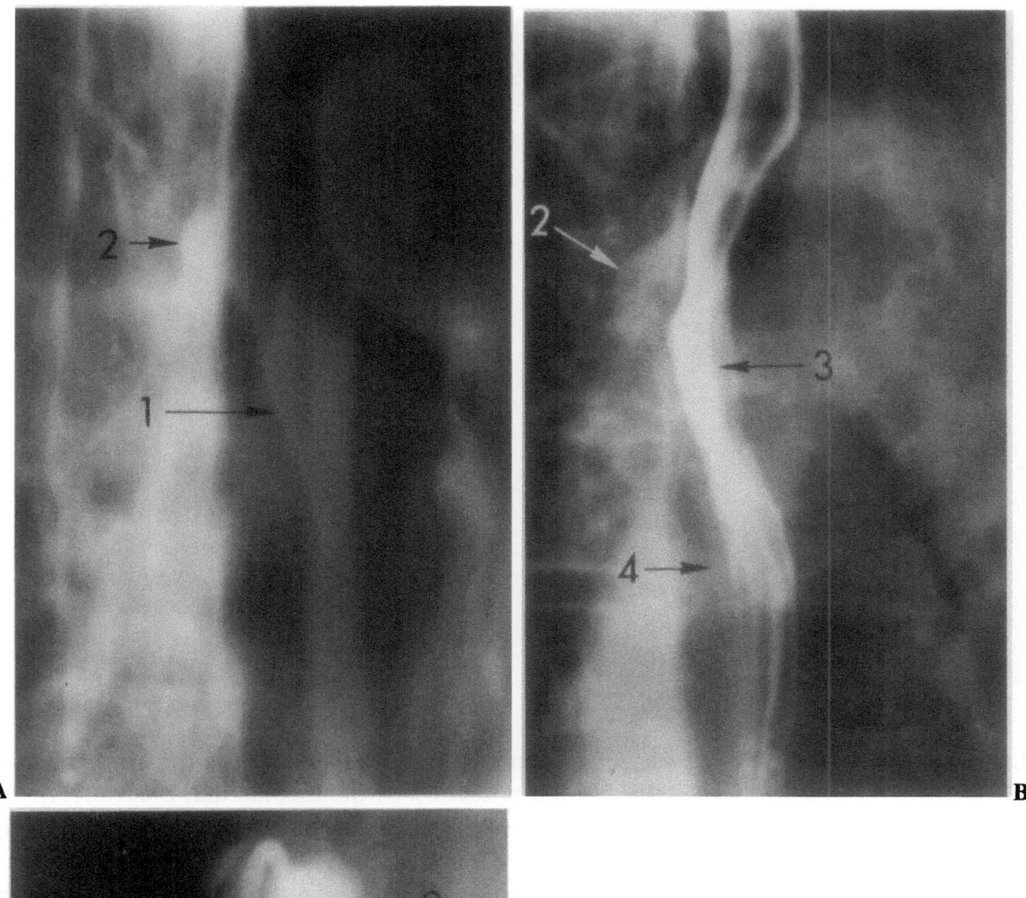

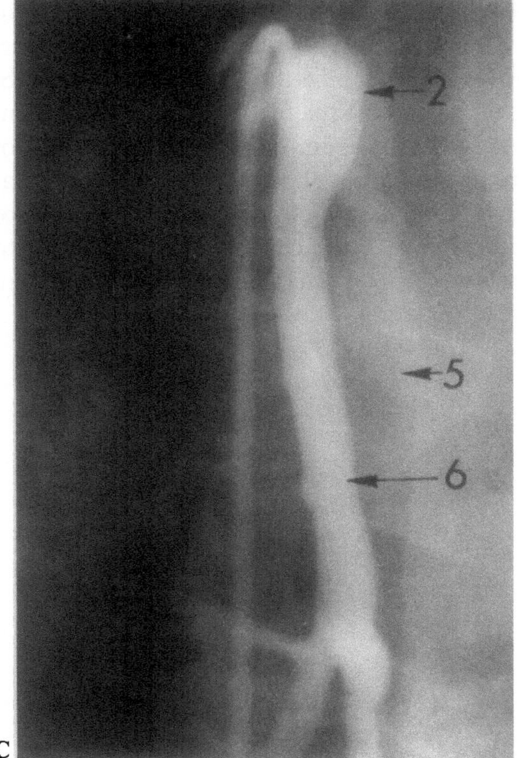

Fig. 9.15A–C. Relationship of right lower lobe to esophagus. **A** Left posterior oblique tomogram. **B** Right anterior oblique radiograph with barium in esophagus. **C** Left posterior oblique radiograph from azygogram. Lung enetering azygoesophageal recess (*1*) under azygos arch (*2*) may contact right posterolateral wall of esophagus (*3*). Under these circumstances, right pleuroesophageal stripe (*4*) is seen most clearly in oblique radiographs (**B**). Less often, stripe is best identified on lateral radiographs when anatomic situation is as depicted in Fig. 9.12C. Lung in azygoesophageal recess can be seen in **C** (*5*), behind esophagus and in front of azygos vein (*6*). (**A** From [21])

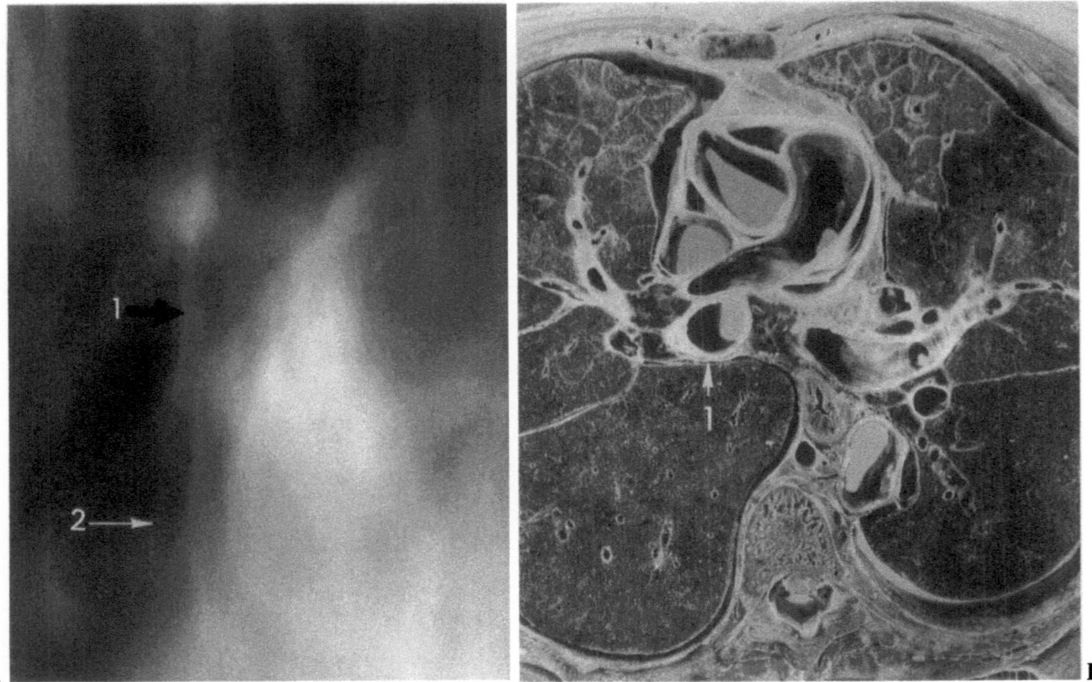

Fig. 9.16A, B. Lung in azygoesophageal recess outlining inferior and posterior walls of major bronchi. **A** Lateral tomogram. **B** Transverse body section. Lung in upper aspect of azygoesophageal recess is invariably in contact with posterior wall of right upper lobe bronchus and in most patients with posterior aspect of right main bronchus as well. This allows visualization of posterior wall of right main bronchus (*1*) and sometimes permits visualization of outer aspect of intermediate bronchus as well (*2*). (See also Fig. 9.8 B.) (**A** From [21])

bronchus proximal to the point where the caudal reflection of the mediastinal pleura from the azygos arch crosses. The outer wall of the bronchus cannot be seen beyond the point of deepest extension of lung into the recess due to the absence of air against the bronchus to provide contrast (Fig. 9.17). From a study of computed tomograms, Muller et al. [33] have concluded that in many patients the contrast demonstration of the outer wall of the central bronchi is due to contrast provided by mediastinal fat rather than by air in lung.

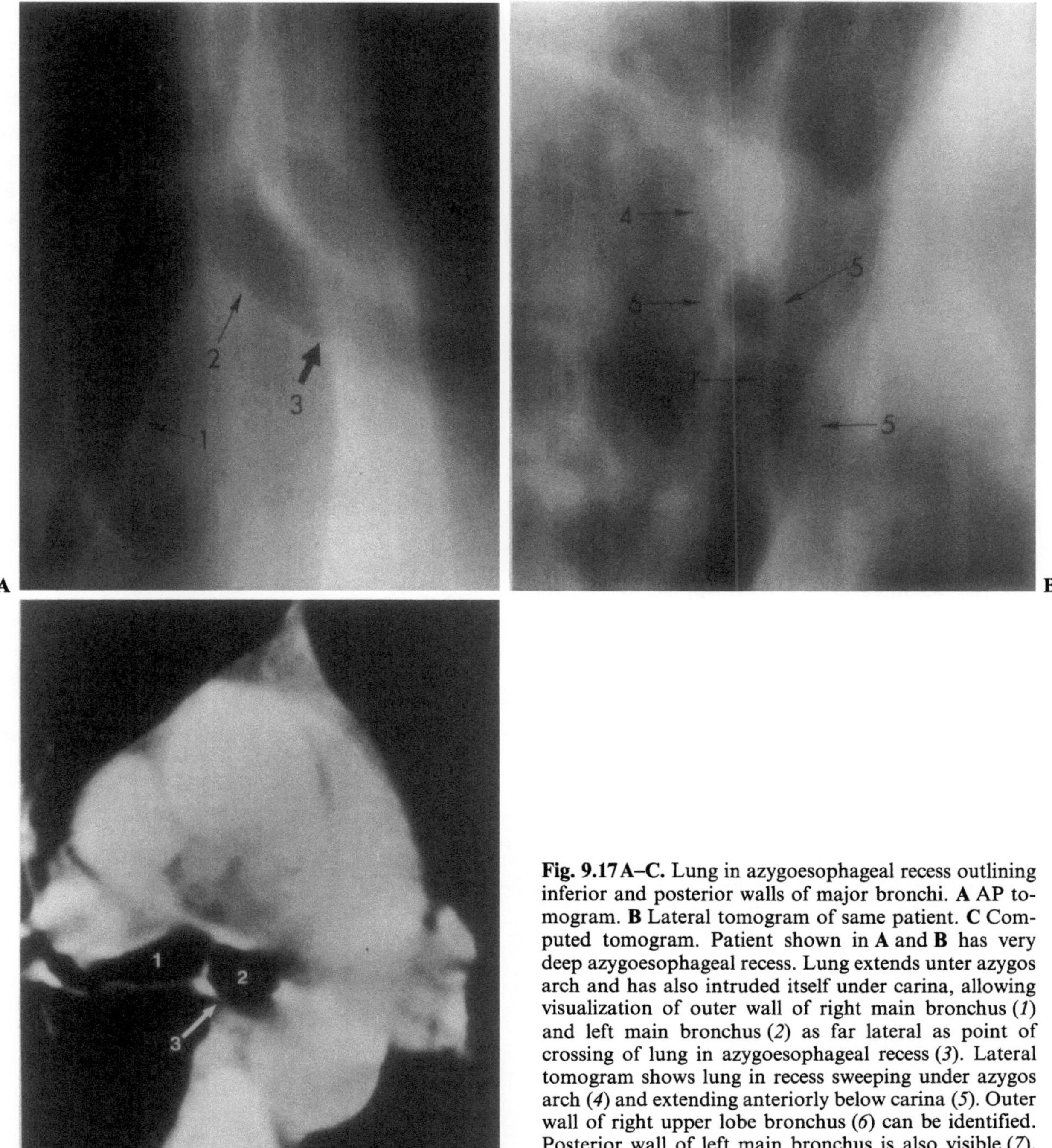

Fig. 9.17A–C. Lung in azygoesophageal recess outlining inferior and posterior walls of major bronchi. **A** AP tomogram. **B** Lateral tomogram of same patient. **C** Computed tomogram. Patient shown in **A** and **B** has very deep azygoesophageal recess. Lung extends unter azygos arch and has also intruded itself under carina, allowing visualization of outer wall of right main bronchus (*1*) and left main bronchus (*2*) as far lateral as point of crossing of lung in azygoesophageal recess (*3*). Lateral tomogram shows lung in recess sweeping under azygos arch (*4*) and extending anteriorly below carina (*5*). Outer wall of right upper lobe bronchus (*6*) can be identified. Posterior wall of left main bronchus is also visible (*7*). Similar anatomic arrangement is shown in **C**. (**A** From [21])

9.3.2 The Posterior Junction Line

Lung in the depths of the azygoesophageal recess may extend behind the esophagus to contact the left lower lobe. The resulting interface is termed the "posterior junction line" [10, 21] (Fig. 9.18). The left lower lobe contributes to the formation of the line by extending medially in front of the descending aorta. Like its counterpart, cephalad of the azygos and aortic arches, the caudal portion of the posterior junction line represents the right visceral and parietal pleurae meeting the left visceral and parietal pleurae. The right and left pleural components sweep forward off the paraspinal soft tissues, contact one another to form the line, and diverge to encompass the esophagus. Like its cephalad counterpart, the posterior junction line below the level of the azygos and aortic arches also can be considered the "mesentery" of the esophagus. At their upper extent the sheets of pleura that form the posterior junction line separate as they sweep under and around the azygos arch on the right and the aortic arch on the left. The posterior junction line is rarely visible below T-10 due to the prespinal position of the descending aorta, which prevents the left lung from extending to the right at this level.

It has been mentioned several times before that the crista pulmonis in the azygoesophageal recess is visible on frontal radiographs as an arcuate line overlying the spine and subtending inferiorly from the azygos arch. At times, lung in the recess contacts the esophagus to produce the pleuroesophageal stripe. On other occasions, it contacts only fat and connective tissue under the mediastinal pleura. In still other individuals, it extends behind the esophagus to contact the left lung to produce the posterior junction line.

9.3.3 Disease Distorting the Azygoesophageal Recess

9.3.3.1 Subcarinal Lymph Node Enlargement

The lymph nodes situated beneath the tracheal bifurcation are usually included with the tracheobronchial group of nodes and are sometimes called simply the "bronchial nodes." More often they are termed the "subcarinal

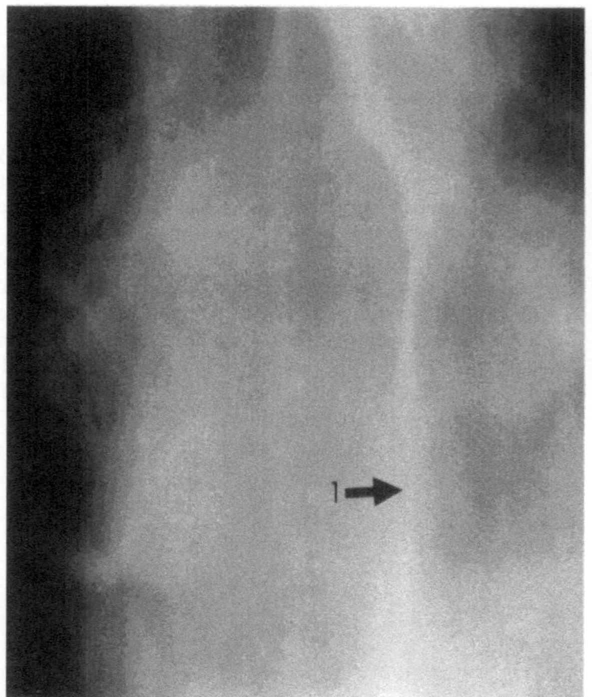
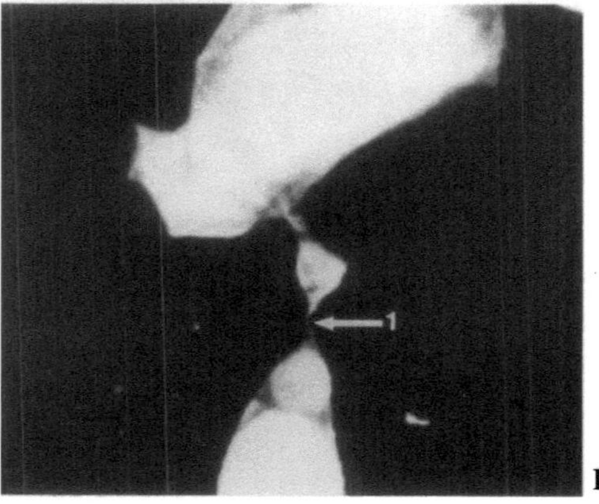

Fig. 9.18A, B. Posterior junction line. **A** AP tomogram. **B** Computed tomogram. Lung in azygoesophageal recess can in some individuals contact left lung behind esophagus to produce posterior junction line (*1*). Crista pulmonis of right lower lobe in azygoesophageal recess is contacted by posteromedial aspect of left lower lobe in preaortic location. (**A** From [19])

nodes." The recent American Thoracic Society reclassification of the mediastinal nodes left the subcarinal node designation unchanged [50]. These nodes, commonly three to five in number, are enclosed in a connective tissue envelope and are found below the carina slightly posterior to the coronal plane of the trachea [2, 5, 35, 36] (Fig. 9.19). They drain both lower lobes, the right middle lobe, and the posterior mediastinum. Their efferents communicate with the right tracheobronchial lymph node chain and less frequently with the left tracheobronchial lymph node chain. This group of nodes is straddled by the main bronchi, which lie to its left and right sides. Anteriorly the nodes are in relationship to the right pulmonary artery above and the upper aspect of the left atrium below. Behind them is the esophagus (Fig. 9.19).

Since the subcarinal nodes are confined by relatively fixed structures anteriorly and laterally, their enlargement, when involved by disease, is primarily posteriorly. Subcarinal nodal en-

largement commonly causes impressions on the medial surface of the main bronchi; splaying of the carina by subcarinal adenopathy may occur (Fig. 9.20). Displacement of the barium-filled esophagus posteriorly and to the left is a rather constant finding if the nodes are enlarged to any significant degree (Fig. 9.21). The nodal mass and the esophagus lying immediately in front of the cephalad portion of the azygoesophageal recess both intrude into the recess, displacing lung posteriorly (Fig. 9.21). This finding is particularly evident when the recess

Fig. 9.19 A, B. Subcarinal lymph nodes. **A** Right side of mediastinum with pleura removed. **B** Transverse body section. Subcarinal nodes, commonly three to five in number, are enclosed in connective tissue packet (*1*). Nodes lie immediately in front of esophagus (*2*) and upper portion of azygoesophageal recess (*3*) and are intimately related to posterior wall of right pulmonary artery (*4*) at its point of origin. Note again the intimate relationship of right lung to posterior wall of right main bronchus (*5*). (**A** From [21])

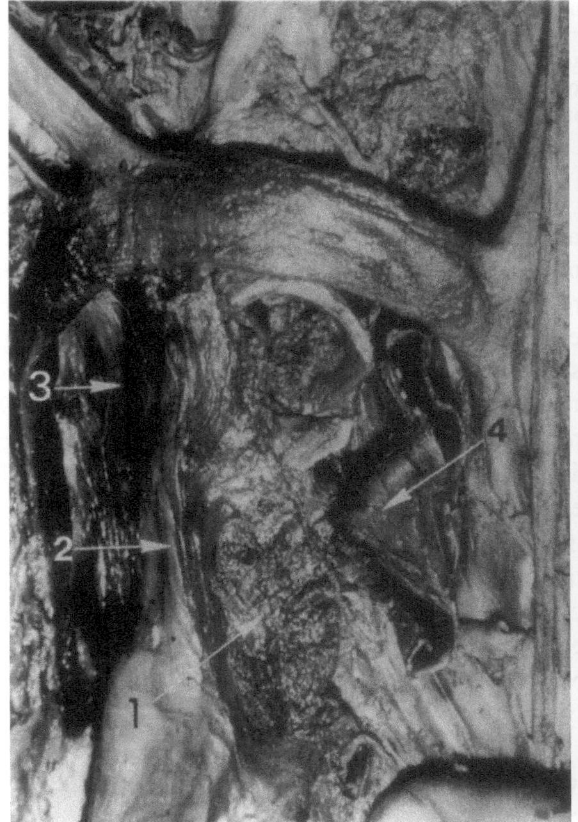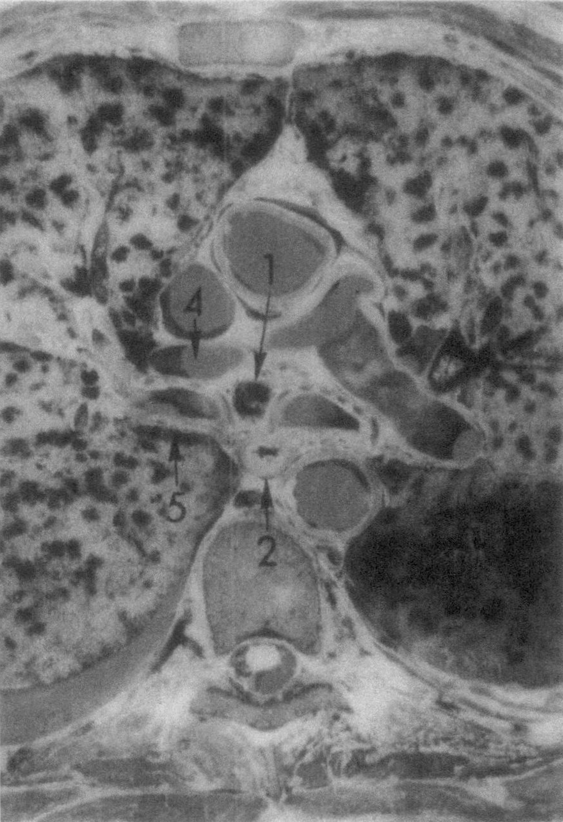

A   B

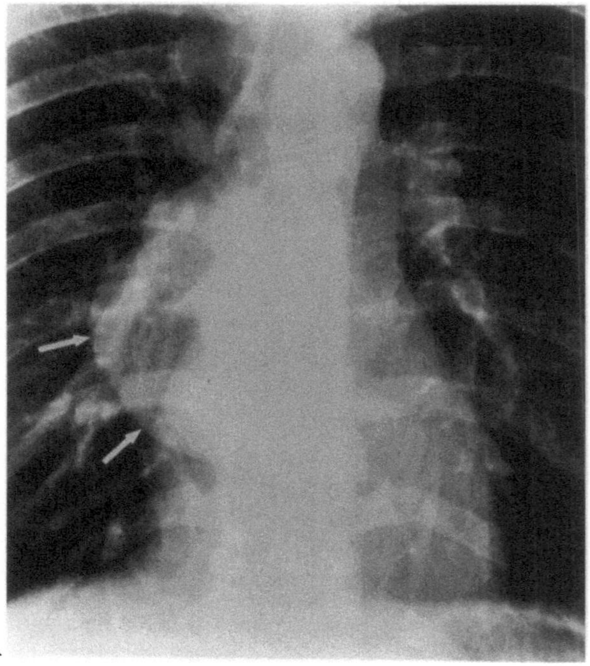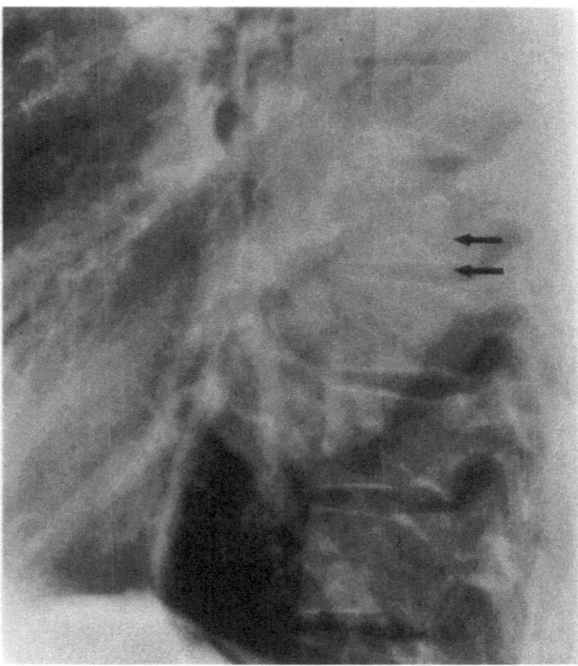

Fig. 9.20 A, B. Enlargement of subcarinal lymph nodes. **A** PA radiograph. **B** Lateral radiograph. Isolated massive enlargement of subcarinal nodes is unusual but not rare. As shown in this case, extension to the right against the azygoesophageal recess (*single arrows*) allows the mass to be demonstrated. The recess is flattened from front to back (*double arrows*). Predominant extension to the right is probably due to the left sided position of the descending aorta. (Case courtesy G. Matthew, Chicago, IL)

was initially deep. The impression of the nodal mass flattens the upper part of the recess from front to back. Since this makes the recess more shallow above than it is below, the line representing the most medial portion of the recess on frontal films is visualized only faintly superiorly although it is well defined below, where a greater depth of lung mediastinal interface is presented to the X-ray beam (Fig. 9.22). Muller et al. [33] have emphasized that an increase in subcarinal opacity on frontal radiographs is a common finding in subcarinal adenopathy occurring in 40% of patients with nodal enlargement in their study. This observation was more frequent than the visualization of abnormality in the contour of the azygoesophageal recess.

As the nodal mass enlarges, it intrudes into the recess causing more and more lung displace-

ment. In cross section the azygoesophageal recess usually has a U-shaped configuration open only to the right. (An exception is shown in Fig. 9.9.) When lung is extruded from the recess by nodal pressure, it is displaced in the only direction it is permitted to go, that is, to the right. The resultant impression of the nodal mass on the extruded lung is often lobulated (Fig. 9.21), but frequently presents a smooth convex contour directed inferiorly and to the right (Figs. 9.20, 9.22). Remember that the usual appearance of the upper portion of the azygoesophageal recess on frontal radiographs is just the opposite: the interface of lung and mediastinum causes a convex contour directed upward and to the left (see Figs. 9.8 and 9.10). Any straightening or reversal of this curve should be viewed with suspicion, and a lobulated appearance should be considered strongly indicative of a mass in the subcarinal area. Statistically, this will most often turn out to represent enlarged lymph nodes.

A normal-appearing azygoesophageal recess does not exclude subcarinal adenopathy since proved nodal masses 1.5 cm in diameter have failed to alter the configuration of the recess on PA radiographs [33]. Muller et al. [33] studied 30 patients in whom computed tomograms

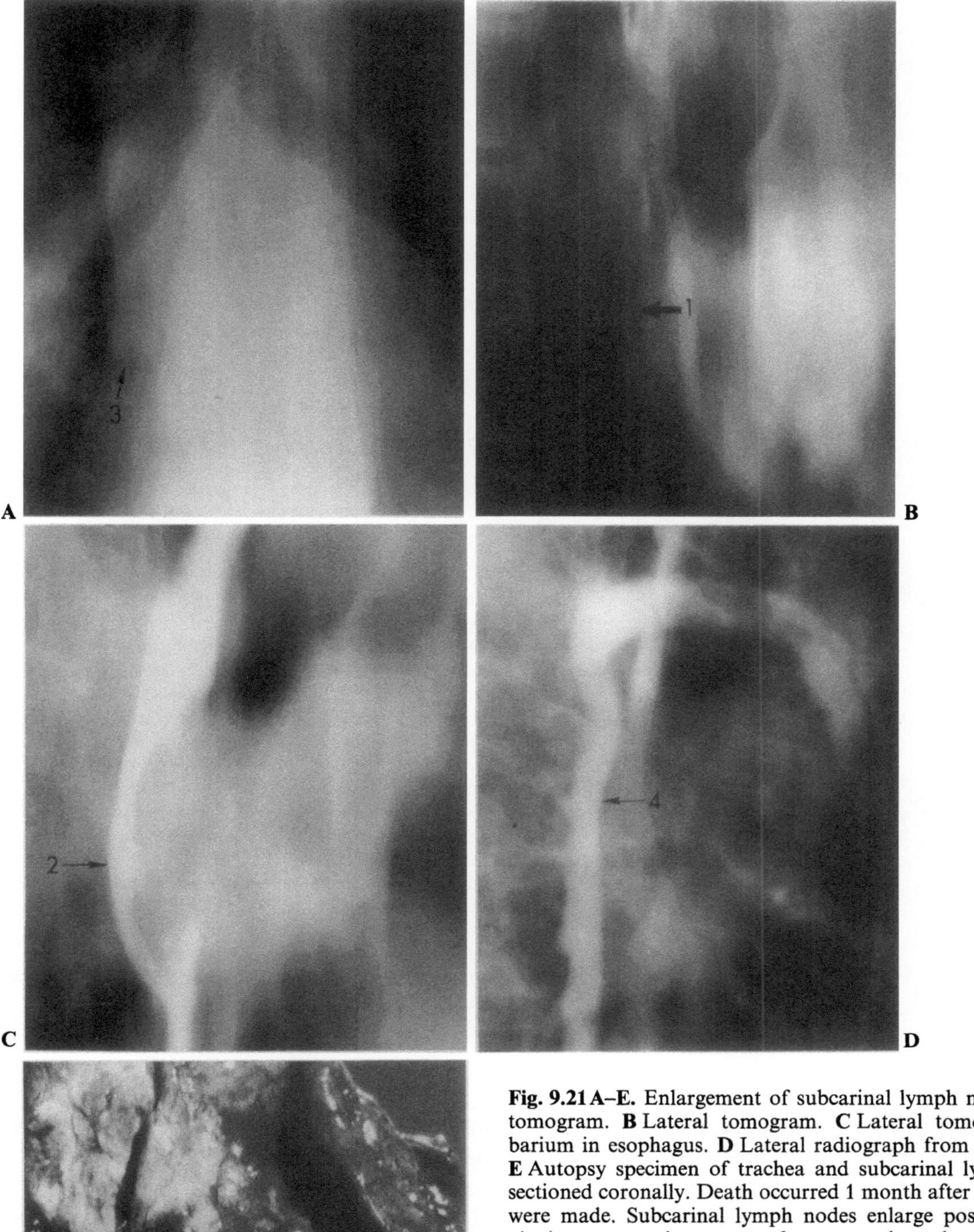

Fig. 9.21 A–E. Enlargement of subcarinal lymph nodes. **A** AP tomogram. **B** Lateral tomogram. **C** Lateral tomogram with barium in esophagus. **D** Lateral radiograph from azygogram. **E** Autopsy specimen of trachea and subcarinal lymph nodes sectioned coronally. Death occurred 1 month after films (**A–D**) were made. Subcarinal lymph nodes enlarge posteriorly impinging on anterior aspect of azygoesophageal recess (*1*) and displacing esophagus posteriorly (*2*). Nodal mass is commonly outlined on its right side (*3*) by lung in recess. Note that on cross-table lateral azygogram (**D**), nodal mass compressed anterior wall of ascending portion of azygos vein (*4*), whereas on lateral tomograms (**B**) and (**C**), posterior aspect of nodal mass was situated well forward of spine. Nodal mass therefore dropped posteriorly when patient was supine, attesting to mobility of mediastinal structures despite presence of pathology (**A, B,** and **E** From [22])

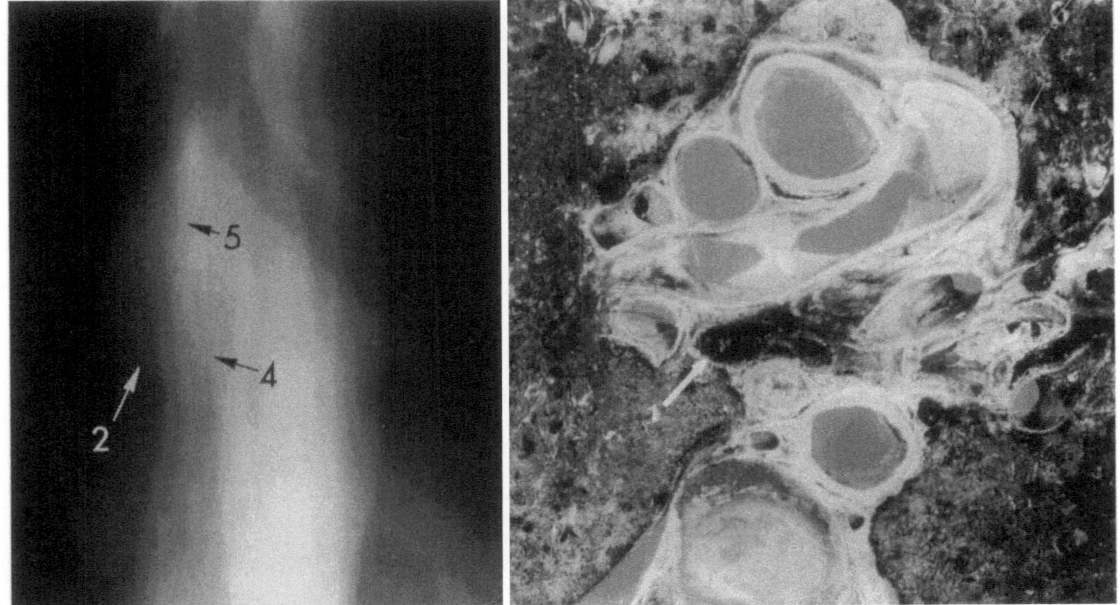

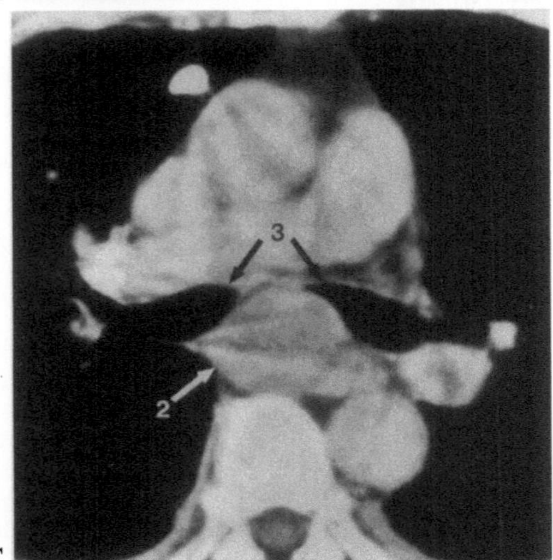

Fig. 9.22 A–C. Enlargement of subcarinal lymph nodes. **A** AP tomogram. **B** Transverse body section. **C** Computed tomogram. Subcarinal lymph nodes can be identified in **B** (*1*). Overpenetrated AP films and AP tomograms will commonly show enlarged subcarinal lymph nodes to be outlined by lung in azygoesophageal recess (*2*). Interface that results is convex to right, always an abnormal configuration for the recess. Lung is extruded to right by presence of subcarinal mass because recess is open only to right side and when it is compromised, this is the only direction available for displacement. Note that line representing medial aspect of azygoesophageal recess can be followed cephalad of inferior border of nodal mass due to presence of minimal lung in recess behind mass (*4*). Since, however, anterior posterior depth of recess has been diminished by compression of nodal mass, line is usually less distinct and tends to become fainter at its cephalad extent (*5*). Computed tomography (**C**) is almost always confirmatory of subcarinal adenopathy (*2*) and is more sensitive than plain films. The subcarinal mass, if large, can displace the carina forward (*3*). (**A** From [22])

showed subcarinal nodes greater than 15 mm in diameter. Only 23% showed abnormality of the contour of the azygoesophageal recess on PA radiographs. Forty percent showed increased density in the region of the recess. Muller et al. [33] also found that the medial wall of the right main stem and intermediate bronchi was visible on PA films in only 27% of patients with subcarinal adenopathy as compared with a visualization rate of 87% in normal patients.

Exclusion of lung from the upper portion of the azygoesophageal recess is often very well demonstrated by computed tomography (Fig. 9.22). A smooth or lobulated mass is seen producing a convex bulge into the azygoesophageal recess. Minimal subcarinal convexity may be a normal finding on computed tomography [37]. Keep in mind that, as previously discussed, this fact does not alter the principle that, on frontal radiographs, any right-sided convexity of the azygoesophageal recess is abnormal. Large subcarinal masses may displace the bronchial tree forward, an occurrence well shown on computed tomograms (Fig. 9.22).

9.3.3.2 Left Atrial Enlargement

Enlargement of the left atrium posteriorly characteristically causes deviation of the barium-filled esophagus, which lies in immediate contact with the atrium (Fig. 9.23). It is apparent, therefore, that enlargement of the atrium posteriorly will cause this chamber to intrude into the azygoesophageal recess from the front. This will cause lung in the azygoesophageal recess to be extruded somewhat to the right side, an effect similar to that produced by enlarged subcarinal nodes.

Changes that result from enlargement of the left atrium differ from those caused by enlarged subcarinal nodes in several significant ways. If enlargement of the left atrium is only to a minimal degree (Fig. 9.24), the lung is excluded from the recess by the atrium at a level of T-6, T-7, or T-8. The normal arcuate configuration of the cephalad portion of the recess on frontal radiographs is usually preserved since a slightly enlarged atrium does not impinge upon the recess at this higher level. As the atrium enlarges farther superiorly, it may extend to the level of the carina, sometimes widening it (Fig. 9.25). In such instances the cephalad portion of the recess is obliterated. The enlarged left atrium usually produces a smooth, gently rounded contact with left lung; a lobulated contour strongly suggests subcarinal adenopathy. When the left atrium enlarges to the degree of becoming truly subcarinal in location, one can usually follow the margin of the obliterated recess inferiorly to the point of entry of the pulmonary veins, thus establishing the "mass" as left atrium. In these patients, lung extending into the almost totally obliterated recess forms a line that extends laterally as it progresses caudally (Figs. 9.24, 9.25). This is in contradistinction to the appearance of subcarinal lymph node enlargement; the interface of lung in the recess with enlarged nodes characteristically produces a lobulated line that extends medially as it progresses caudally (Figs. 9.21, 9.22).

The point of entry, or confluence, of the right pulmonary veins can interrupt the configuration of the azygoesophageal recess even if the atrium is not enlarged (Fig. 9.26) [4]. This is particular-

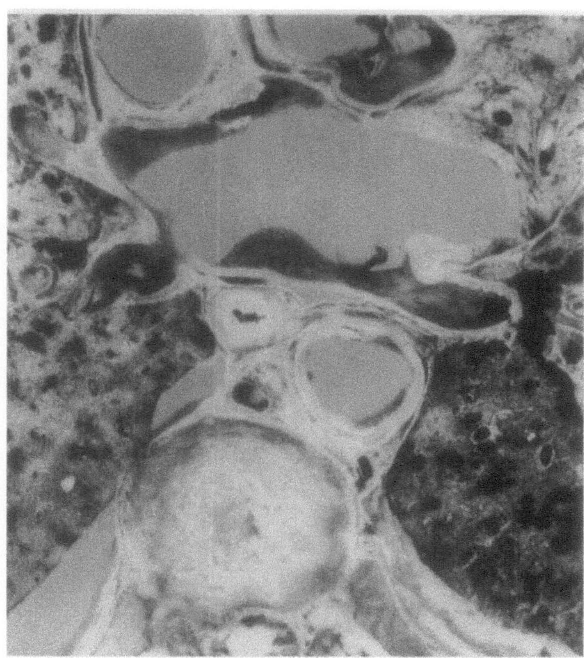

Fig. 9.23. Anatomic relationships of left atrium (transverse body section). Enlargement of left atrium can cause chamber to bulge into right lung or left lung. Left atrium also can enlarge posteriorly, resulting in backward displacement of esophagus and exclusion of lung from azygoesophageal recess. (From [22])

ly true when there is considerable loss of volume of the left lung. This finding is somewhat difficult to explain since the confluence is in a coronal plane anterior to the esophagus and hence is in front of the azygoesophageal recess (see chapter 10). The following thesis is offered as a possible explanation. The point of entry of the left pulmonary veins into the left atrium may sometimes lie in the identical sagittal plane with the lung-mediastinal interface in the azygoesophageal recess. If this anatomic circumstance obtains, both profiles will be superimposed on a frontal radiograph and the line representing contact of lung in the recess with the mediastinum may appear to be lost.

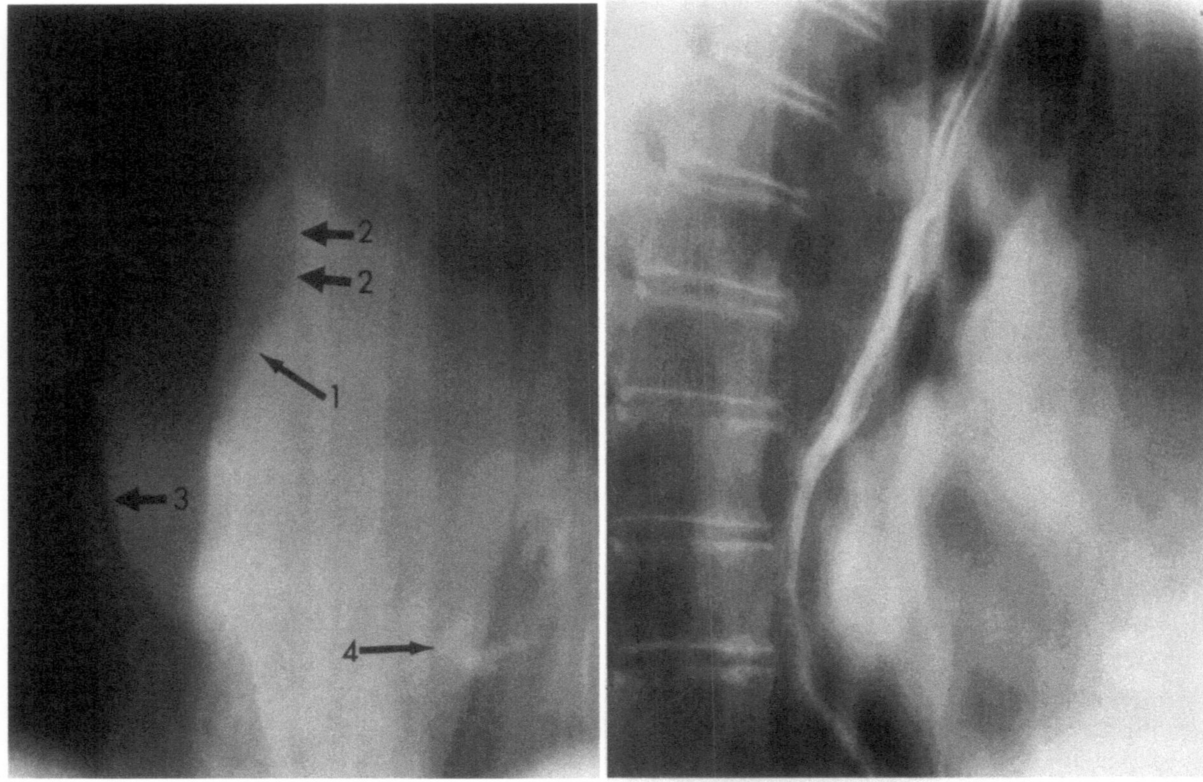

Fig. 9.24 A, B. Enlargement of left atrium. A AP tomogram. B Lateral tomogram with barium in esophagus. Enlargement of left atrium will displace crista pulmonis from azygoesophageal recess at a lower level (*1*) than does enlargement of subcarinal nodes. If left atrial enlargement is not extreme, lung can be seen in relatively normal position in azygoesophageal recess immediately below carina (*2*). Confluence of right pulmonary veins is well demonstrated (*3*), as is calcification in mitral valve (*4*). (A From [22])

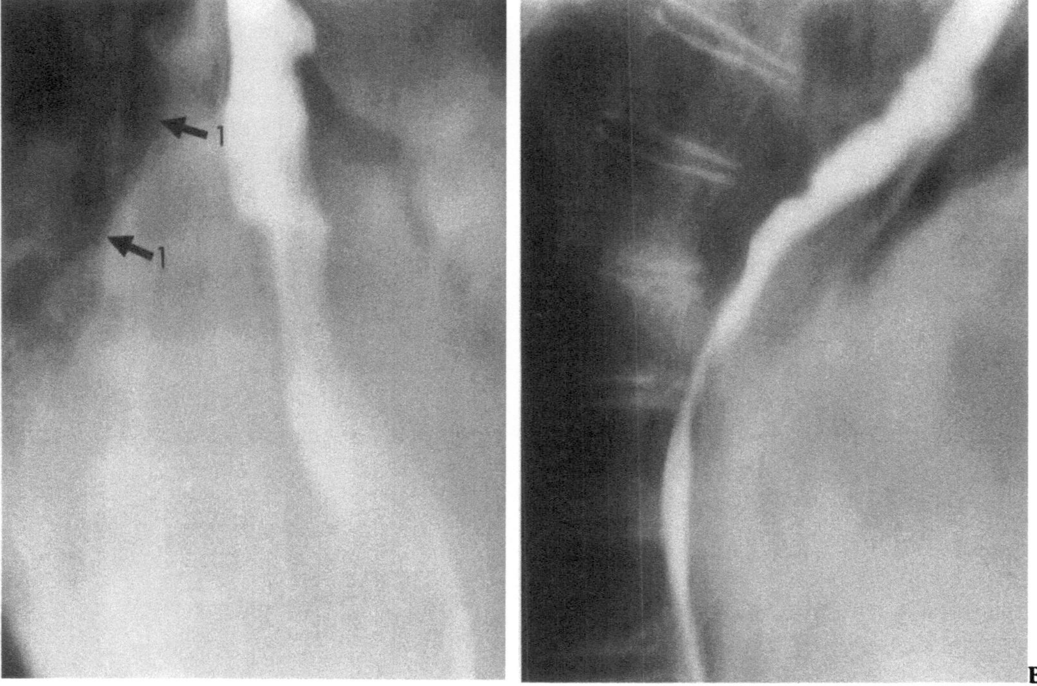

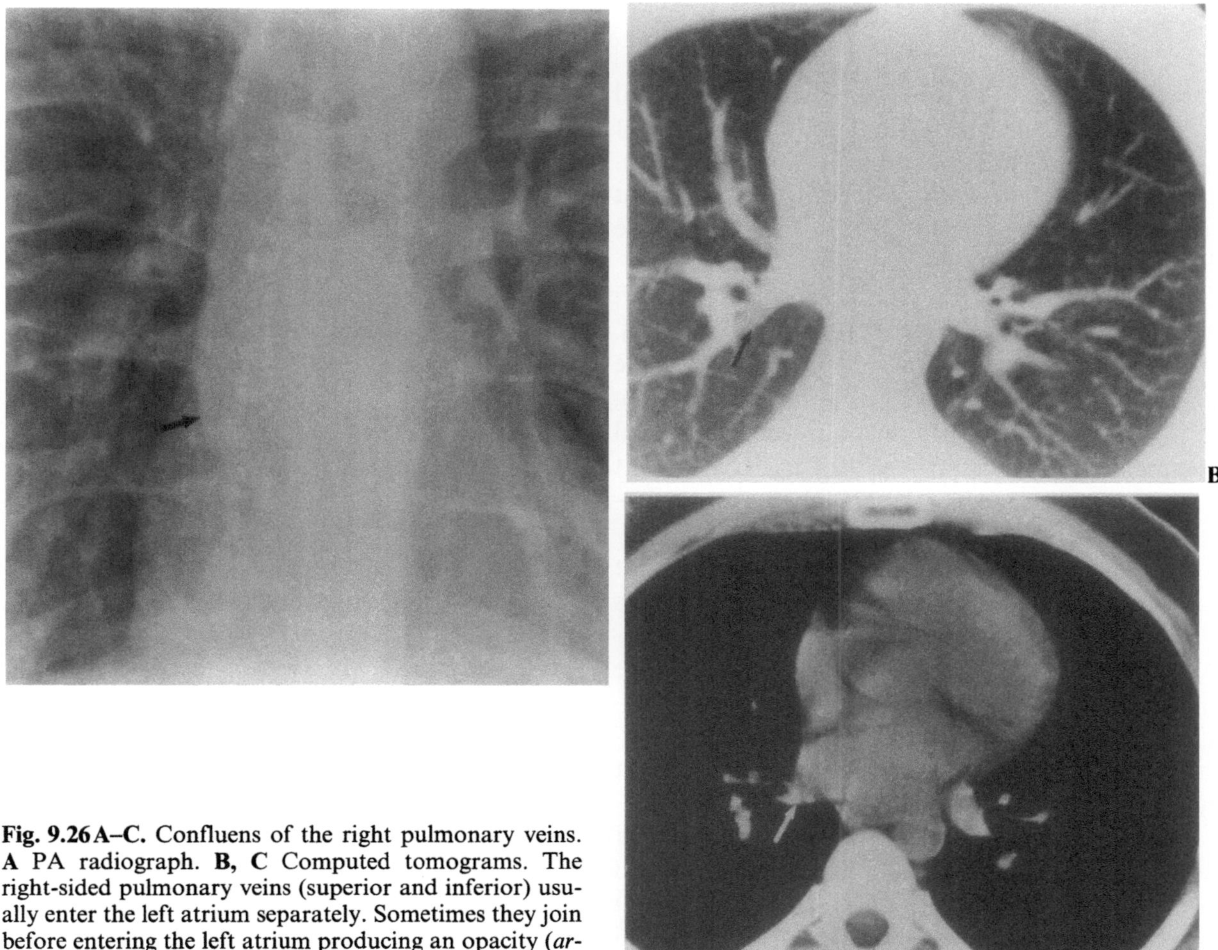

Fig. 9.26 A–C. Confluens of the right pulmonary veins. **A** PA radiograph. **B, C** Computed tomograms. The right-sided pulmonary veins (superior and inferior) usually enter the left atrium separately. Sometimes they join before entering the left atrium producing an opacity (*arrow*) seen through the right atrium

◁ **Fig. 9.25 A, B.** Enlargement of left atrium. **A** AP tomogram. **B** Lateral tomogram. Marked enlargement of left atrium, as shown in this case, causes chamber to rise superiorly and posteriorly between major bronchi to widen carinal angle. Lung is thus excluded from cephalad portion of azygoesophageal recess. Under these circumstances, configuration of interface between lung and enlarged atrium is different from configuration produced by subcarinal adenopathy. When left atrium is enlarged, interface deviates laterally as it extends toward diaphragm (*1*). Due to the fact that vector forces against lung are at higher level with subcarinal adenopathy, this condition produces interface with lung that deflects medially as it extends toward the diaphragm (see Figs. 20, 21, and 22). (**A** From [22])

9.3.3.3 Bronchogenic Cyst

Bronchogenic cysts may be either parenchymal or mediastinal; mediastinal bronchogenic cyst most often occurs in a subcarinal location somewhat more frequently extending to the right side, hence its inclusion in this chapter on the infra-azygos area.

The respiratory tract and the esophagus both arise from the embryonic foregut [39, 43, 44]. Bronchogenic cysts are a type of cyst of the foregut and are the result of abnormal budding of the tracheal primordium or abnormal branching of the tracheobronchial tree [44]. It has been theorized that parenchymal bronchogenic cyst is the result of a rather late embryologic event and mediastinal bronchogenic cyst to an earlier aberration [44]. Enterogenous cysts are thought to represent an even earlier embryologic fault [44]. Thoracic cysts of congenital type frequently have bronchial and enterogenous elements, making separation into distinct categories difficult. Nevertheless, a study of 86 foregut cysts reported by Reed and Sobonya [43] classified 77 as respiratory and nine as enteric. Of the respiratory cysts, 66 were mediastinal and only 11 intrapulmonary. This distribution is at variance with the earlier series of Rogers and Osmer [44] who found only 14 of 46 bronchogenic cysts to be present in the mediastinum.

Most mediastinal bronchogenic cysts are grouped about the carina [42], typically in a subcarinal location. Of the 30 mediastinal bronchogenic cysts that they considered to be carina based, Reed and Sobonya [43] found that 15 extended posteriorly, 13 inferiorly, and only two anteriorly. Rogers and Osmer [44] reported two of 46 mediastinal bronchogenic cysts located in the right paratracheal area [44]; among 66 bronchogenic cysts of the mediastinum, Reed and Sobonya found 11 in a paratracheal position [43].

The subcarinal location of most bronchogenic cysts with inferior and posterior extension causes them to intrude into the azygoesophageal recess from in front in a manner analogous to enlarged subcarinal lymph nodes (Fig. 9.27) [28]. In contrast to the often lobulated character of the interface made by enlarged nodes with

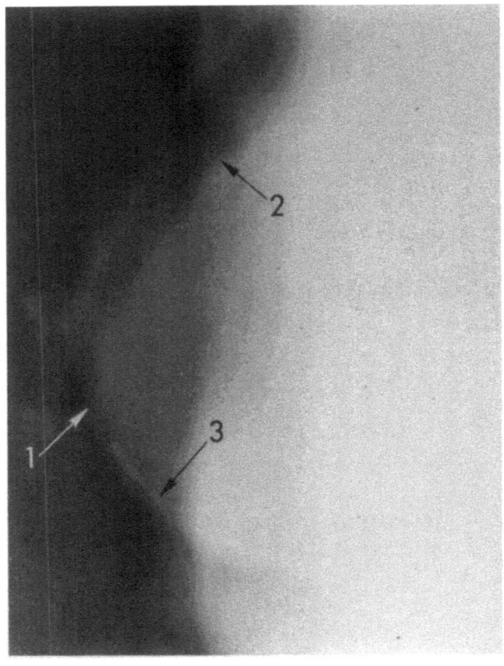

Fig. 9.27. Bronchogenic cyst (AP tomogram). Mediastinal bronchogenic cysts are found near carina, typically in subcarinal location. They extend posteriorly and inferiorly as they enlarge and cause lung to be displaced from azygoesophageal recess (*1*). They produce smooth, round, or oval imprint on lung. They may impinge against bronchi (*2*). Exceptionally, they may calcify (*3*)

the right lower lobe, bronchogenic cysts produce a smooth spherical or oval impression on adjacent lung (Fig. 9.27). Of the 14 cases reported by Reed and Sobonya [43], 12 were oval and two spherical. Bronchogenic cysts commonly displace the esophagus posteriorly, and because of their common extension to the right side, the esophagus is more often deviated to the left than it is to the right.

Bronchogenic cysts are fluid filled. The fluid may be clear and serous or turbid and mucoid. Although bronchial communication in intrapulmonary bronchogenic cyst is the rule, such communication in mediastinal bronchogenic cyst is rare. A review of the literature has shown that only four mediastinal bronchogenic cysts have been reported in which an air-fluid level was demonstrated [44]. All were subcarinal in location. Calcification in bronchogenic cysts is uncommon (Fig. 9.27). Ziter et al. [52] have reported two mediastinal bronchogenic cysts with calcification in their walls, and at least three examples of milk of calcium in mediastinal bronchogenic cysts have been reported [3, 11]. A similar example of milk of calcium in an intrapulmonary bronchogenic cyst has also been recorded [12].

Mediastinal bronchogenic cysts are usually asymptomatic, and most are discovered at routine examination. If a round or oval subcarinal mass is found to contain fluid of water density at computed tomography, a presumptive diagnosis of bronchogenic cyst is secure. It should be emphasized that not all bronchogenic cysts will show Hounsfield numbers consistent with water density; higher numbers are often encountered due to the presence of proteinaceous fluid, mucus, or blood within the cyst [30, 32, 34]. Intrapulmonary bronchogenic cysts bleed and commonly become secondarily infected. In infants, their bulk may compress lung and shift the mediastinum [18]; they should be removed [17].

9.3.3.4 Esophageal Masses, Paraesophageal Lymph Node Enlargement, and Other Masses Lying Posteriorly in the Mediastinum

Masses that arise in the esophagus will also distort the azygoesophageal recess. The changes produced are of course dependent on the location of the esophageal lesion and on its size. In general the alterations are similar to those caused by subcarinal lymph-adenopathy or left atrial enlargement; such findings should be anticipated because the esophagus courses behind the subcarinal nodes and left atrium, in front of the azygoesophageal recess. If the mass lies at the level of the carina, distortion of the smooth arcuate sweep of the upper portion of the recess may be seen (Fig. 9.28).

The paraesophageal lymph nodes drain lymph from the midportion of the esophagus. They are most commonly found from the level of the inferior pulmonary vein to the diaphragm, lying in loose areolar tissue that surrounds the esophagus. They are located adjacent to the para-aortic nodes, and their efferents pass to the subcarinal nodes [31]. McCort [31]

found a high incidence of paraesophageal nodes when carcinoma involved the lower half of the esophagus. He infrequently found them to be involved by metastases from carcinoma of the bronchus. On the other hand Nohl [35, 36] states that paraesophageal nodes are "often" involved by metastases from lower lobe carcinoma. Filly et al. [15] found that posterior mediastinal nodes were involved in 10% of patients with non-Hodgkin's lymphoma and in 5% of patients with Hodgkin's disease. Involvement of posterior mediastinal nodes as the only evidence of thoracic disease was encountered in non-Hodgkin's lymphoma but not in Hodgkin's disease [15].

Paraesophageal nodes commonly produce smooth or lobulated masses indenting the lower half of the azygoesophageal recess and frequently deviate the esophagus (Figs. 9.29, 9.30). It is easy to appreciate that almost always the impressions on the recess caused by paraesophageal nodes cannot be distinguished from deviations produced by the contiguous primary tumor. McCort [31] states that paraesophageal nodes do not impinge against the left lung because of the intervening position of the descending aorta. Enlarged nodes lying to the left of the lower portion of the esophagus are therefore difficult and sometimes impossible to identify on plain radiographs. Exceptionally, when they are quite large, they can be detected (Fig. 9.30B).

Saks et al. [46] have recently reported deviation of the contours of the azygoesophageal recess following injection therapy for esophageal varices. Other masses situated in a position contiguous to the recess will also alter its appearance on radiographs. The changes they produce will be dependent upon their size and location. Such masses may impinge upon the esophagus causing impressions which must be distinguished from those made by normal structures. Such impressions have been reviewed throughout this book, especially in chapters 6, 7, and 8 and have also been summarized in the recent article by Chasen et al. [6].

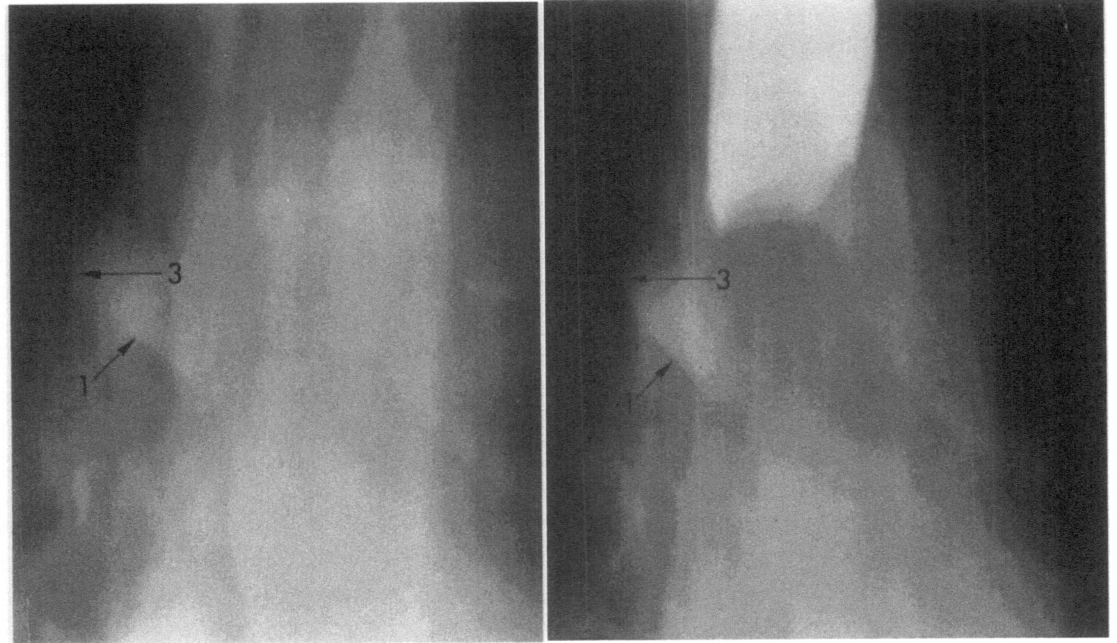

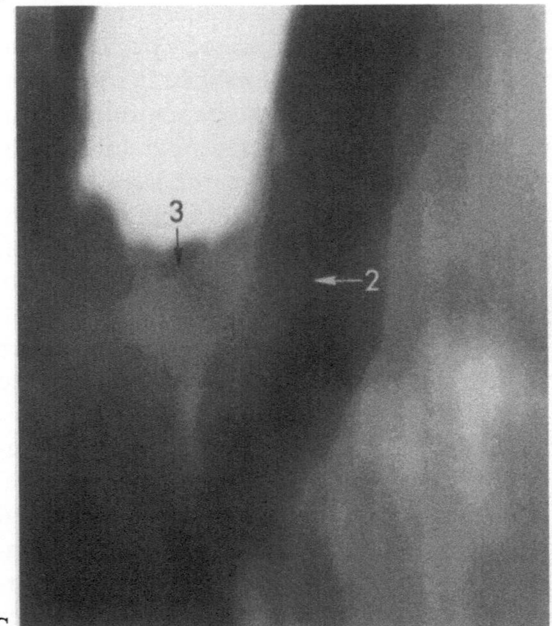

Fig. 9.28 A–C. Esophageal carcinoma. Distortion of azygoesophageal recess. **A** AP tomogram. **B** AP tomogram with barium in esophagus. **C** Lateral tomogram with barium in esophagus. Carcinoma involving middle or lower third of esophagus can distort azygoesophageal recess. In this patient with carcinoma of middle third of esophagus, lesion lies immediately in front of cephalad portion of azygoesophageal recess and intrudes into recess from in front. Lung is displaced to right. Configuration of upper part of recess has an angulated contour with minimal convexity directed to the right (*1*) instead of being a smooth arc with convexity to left. Anterior margin of mass can also be identified (*2*). Note that azygos arch is carried laterally into right lung and is visible on frontal and lateral radiographs (*3*). (**A** and **B** From [22])

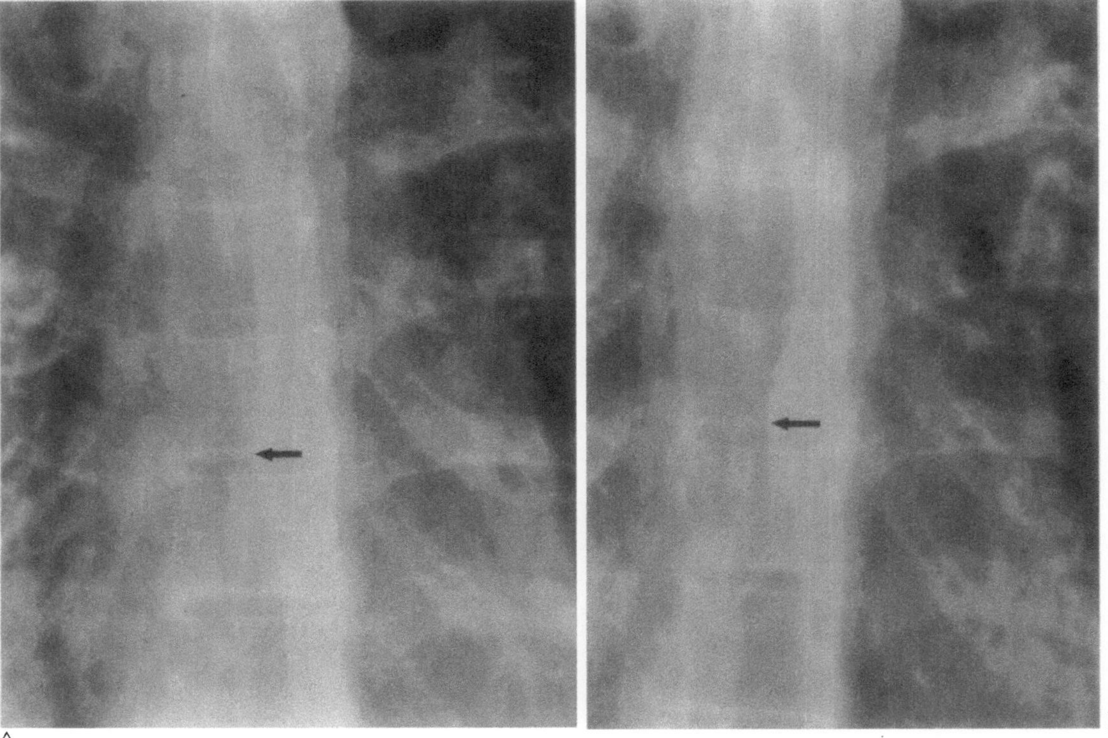

A

B

Fig. 9.29 A, B. Distortion of the azygoesophageal recess. Paraesophageal lymph node enlargement. PA radiographs. These films made 4 months apart on a patient with carcinoma of the cervix show distortion of the midportion of the azygoesophageal recess by enlarged paraesophageal lymph nodes (*arrow*). Nodes are numerous about the lower esophagus. Note that nodes do not contact left lung, apparently due to the position of the descending aorta (see text)

Fig. 9.30 A, B. Distortion of the azygoesophageal recess. Paraesophageal lymph node enlargement. **A** PA radiograph. **B** Computed tomogram. Paraesophageal lymph node enlargement is readily identified at computed tomography. Nodes contact right lung in the azygoesophageal recess (*single arrow*). Enlarged paraesophageal nodes less commonly abut against left lung, being separated from left lower lobe by aorta. If they are considerably increased in size, they may be visible in preaortic position (*double arrows*)

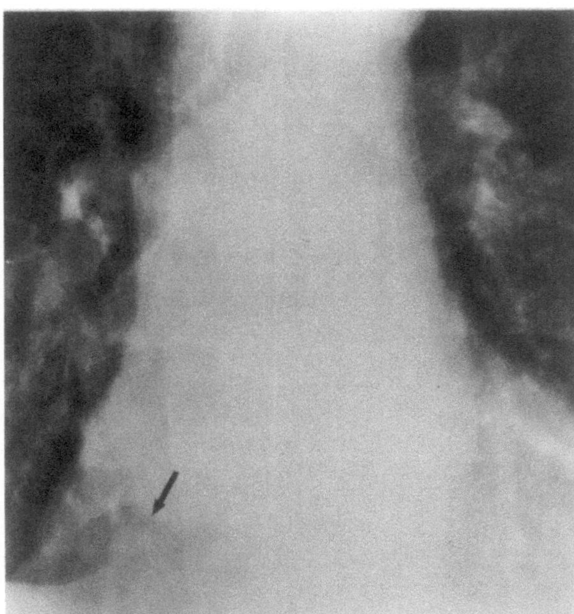

A

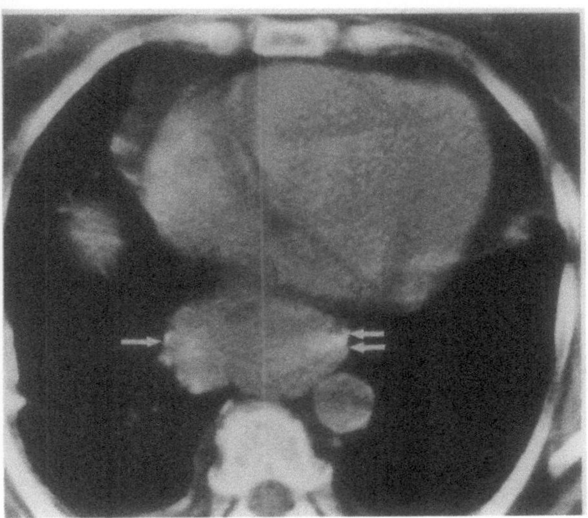

B

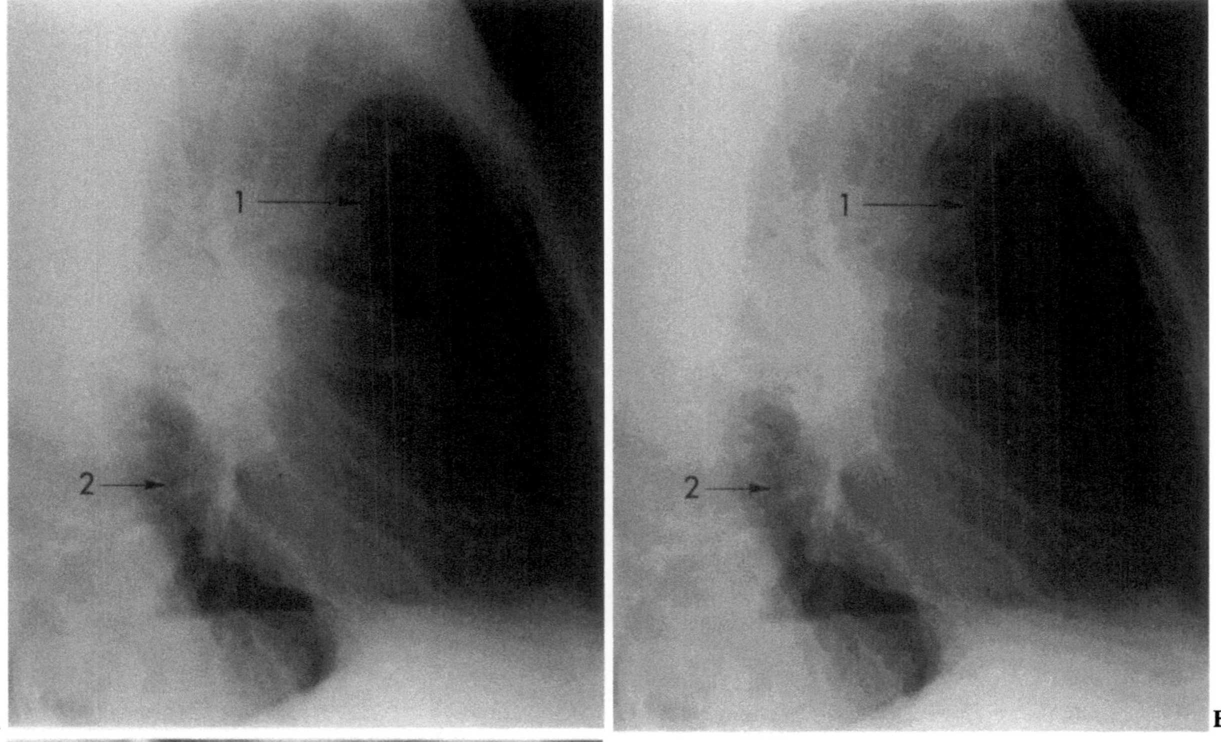

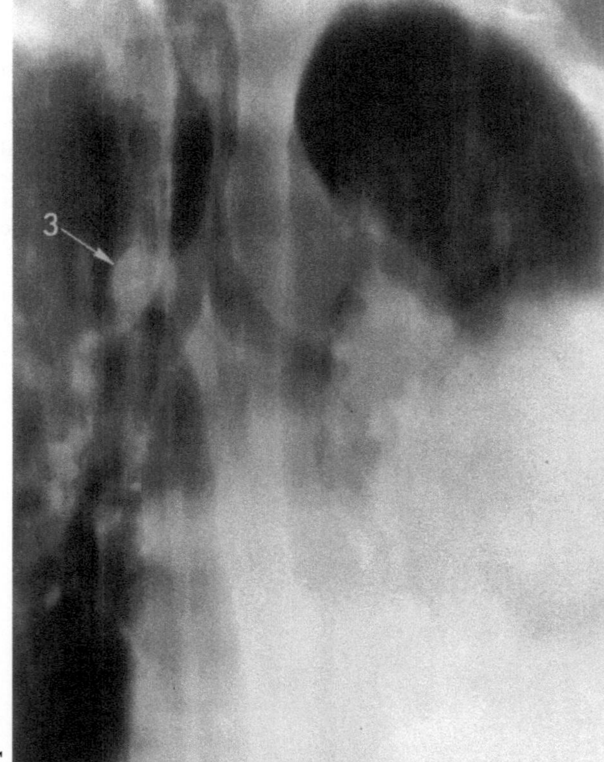

Fig. 9.31 A–C. Posterior "herniation" of lung. A and B PA and lateral radiographs. C AP tomogram. When all of left lung or portion of it has been removed surgically or is atelectatic, right lung may herniate into left hemithorax. Herniation is often anterior (1) (see chapter 5), but may be posterior. A prespinal line is present (2), indicative of right lung in front of spine. Posterior herniation occurs behind esophagus above and below azygos arch. Best demonstrations of azygos arch are seen on radiographs of patients with posterior herniation of lung (3)

9.3.3.5 Posterior "Herniation" of Lung

Left pneumonectomy and extensive degrees of collapse of the left lung characteristically produce rotation and posterior displacement of the heart into the left hemithorax. The anterior portion of the right lung then crosses the anterior mediastinum in compensation. Occasionally, however, so-called posterior herniation of the lung into the left hemithorax also occurs [26, 29]. Posterior herniation of the right lung occurs through the supra-azygos recess above the azygos arch and through the azygoesophageal recess below it. Under such circumstances, the extremely deep intrusions of lung over and under the azygos arch produce some of the best demonstrations of the roentgen anatomy of the azygos arch and its pleural reflections (Fig. 9.31).

A marked protrusion of the right lung into the left thorax behind the esophagus is common in cases of total collapse of the left lung. Occasionally masses involving the posteromedial portion of the left lung may be outlined by virtue of their contact with the herniated right lung. The posterior aspect of a left hilar mass may abut against herniated right lung posterior to the inferior pulmonary ligament. The radiologic significance of the latter structure will be discussed in greater detail in the section on the hila.

It is curious that although right-to-left posterior herniation is an almost constant occurrence in cases of left pneumonectomy or total left lung collapse, left-to-right herniation in right pneumonectomy or total right lung collapse is rare. The position of the descending aorta is most often used to explain this peculiar circumstance. Lodin [26] has noted that there is a potential for left-to-right hernia anterior to the aorta and behind the esophagus but also feels that left-to-right herniation is rare.

Air in the pleural space may fill the recesses above and below the azygos arch. As would be expected, this happens most often in cases of tension pneumothorax. Frequently, a tube in the right pleural space will be seen with its tip overlying the thoracic spine and sometimes extending to the left of the spine on frontal radio-

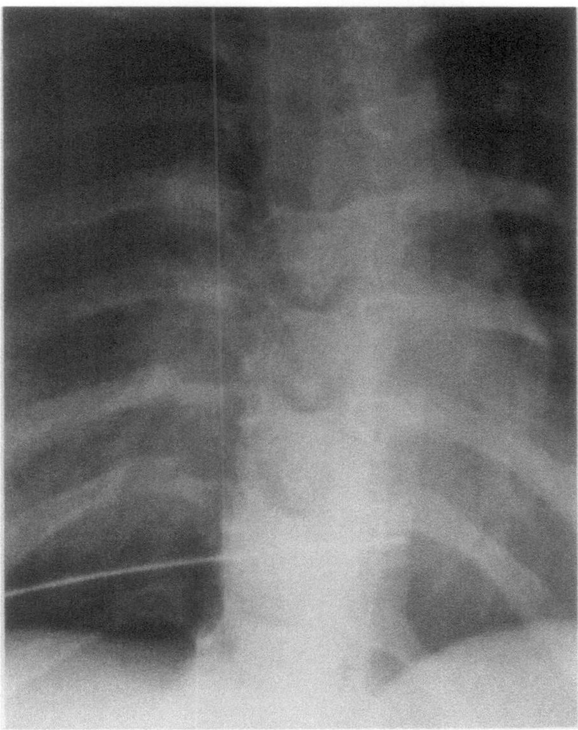

Fig. 9.32. Chest tube in azygoesophageal recess (AP radiograph). It is a common experience to see chest tubes extending from right hemithorax well across midline to left side. Although such tubes may exceptionally extend anterior to heart, they almost universally cross from right to left through azygoesophageal recess

graphs. Tubes in this position are most often posterior crossing the azygoesophageal recess from right to left (Fig. 9.32). The presence of a tube in the left hemithorax crossing to the right has not been encountered.

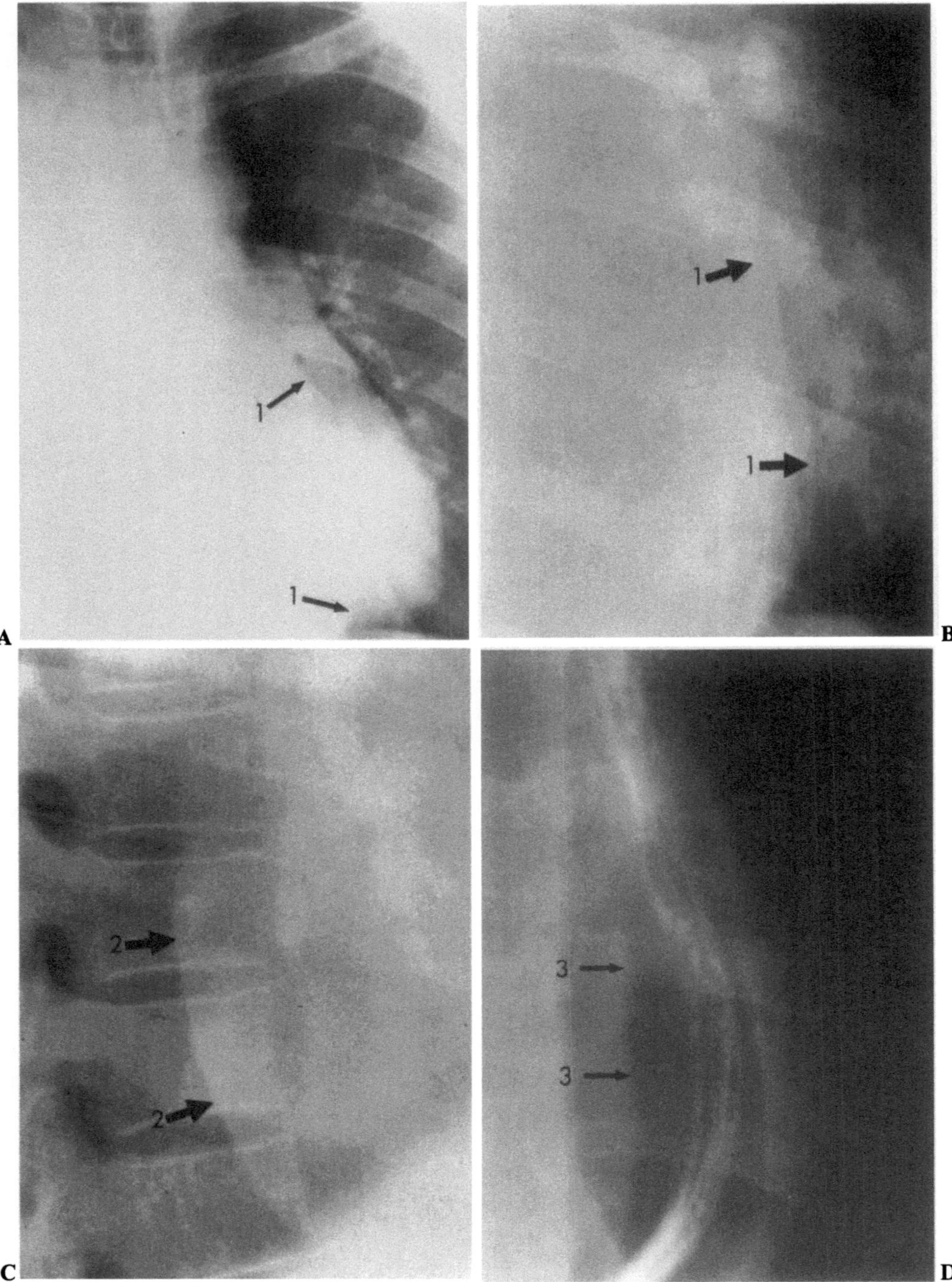

Fig. 9.33 A–D

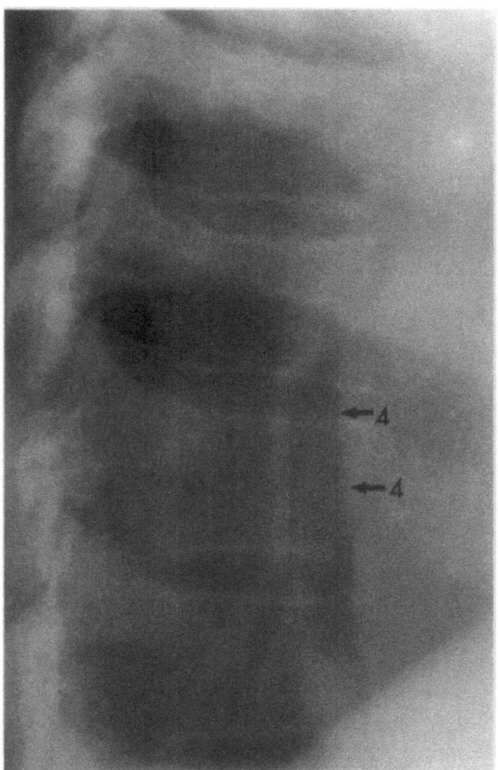

Fig. 9.33E

Fig. 9.33A–E. Massive right pleural effusion. Presentation as left retrocardiac mass. **A** PA radiograph. **B** and **C** PA and lateral radiographs of left lower thorax. **D** and **E** Right lateral decubitus and prone lateral radiographs of left lower thorax following installation of gas into right pleural space. This patient with massive right pleural effusion showed left retrocardiac mass (*1*). Posterior aspect of mass appeared to overlie spine (*2*). Following right-sided thoracentesis, small quantity of air was instilled into right pleural space, and patient placed in decubitus position with right side down. Gas could be seen to rise into retrocardiac shadow, proving it to be the azygoesophageal recess distended with fluid and extending far to left side (*3*). Subsequently patient was placed prone and cross-table lateral film was obtained (**E**) again showing air-fluid level in posterior aspect of azygoesophageal recess (*4*). (**B–E** From [22])

9.3.3.6 Posterior "Herniation" of Massive Pleural Effusion

With truly massive pleural effusions, the right or left pleural space distended by fluid may herniate across the midline. When effusion is right sided the herniated azygoesophageal recess extends to the left behind the esophagus and in front of the spine to contact the left lung. In our experience, this occurrence is uncommon, and left-to-right herniation is even more rare. Nevertheless, Sukumaran and Berger [49] reported 50 patients with massive effusions resulting in 16 herniations. In ten patients, herniation was right to left; in six individuals it was left to right. In all cases herniation was infra-azygos and infra-aortic. Massive right pleural effusion may result in the appearance of a left retrocardiac density [40]. The shadow produced is the outline of the fluid-filled azygoesophageal recess extending far to the left (Figs. 9.33, 9.34). The fluid-filled recess crossing the mediastinum behind the esophagus and in front of the descending aorta becomes truly sac-like and may drape itself around the descending aorta, obliterating the outline of the lateral edge of the aorta on frontal films. This is particularly true of radiographs made in the recumbent position. Although a left-sided presentation of a right-sided pleural effusion is an unusual occurrence, this possibility should always be considered when a retrocardiac mass is encountered in association with a massive right pleural effusion. It should not be confused with a mediastinal or pulmonary mass. Reduction in the size of the shadow following thoracentesis will confirm the diagnosis; a small quantity of air instilled following thoracentesis can be positioned into the recess, confirming beyond question the nature of the shadow (Fig. 9.33). Right-sided presentation of a massive left-sided pleural effusion is not as common (Fig. 9.35), again presumably due to the position of the descending aorta. The radiologic findings in massive pleural effusion are thus analogous to the changes encountered in posterior herniation of lung.

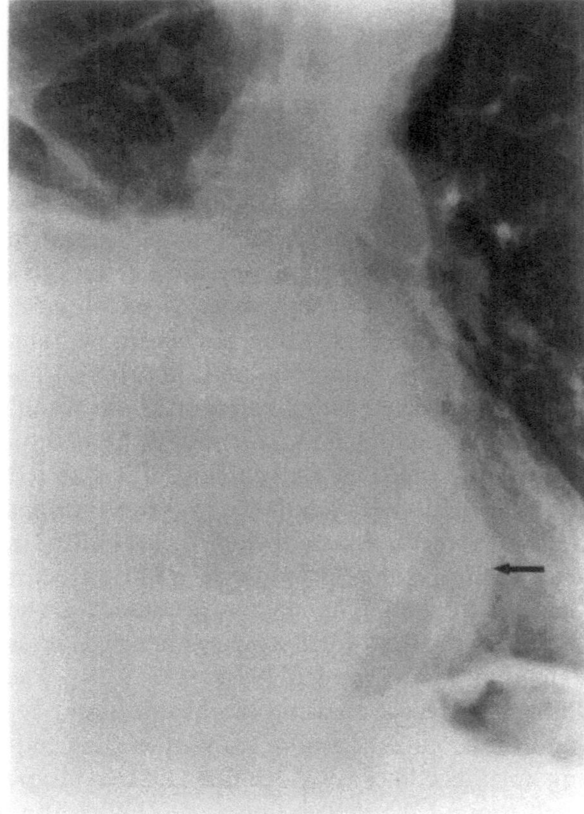

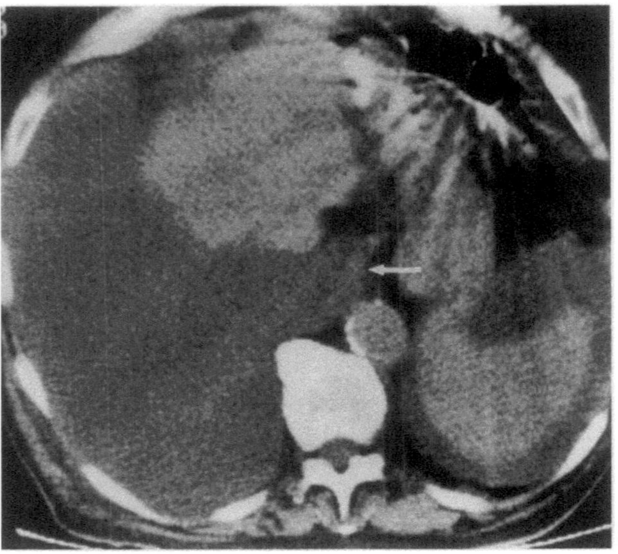

Fig. 9.34A, B. Right pleural effusion. Presentation as a left retrocardiac mass. **A** PA radiograph. **B** Computed tomogram. Distension of the azygoesophageal recess to the left side to produce a retrocardiac mass (*arrow*) can be demonstrated by computed tomography. Extension of the recess to the left is more evident on the erect PA radiograph than on the supine computed tomogram due to the effect of gravity

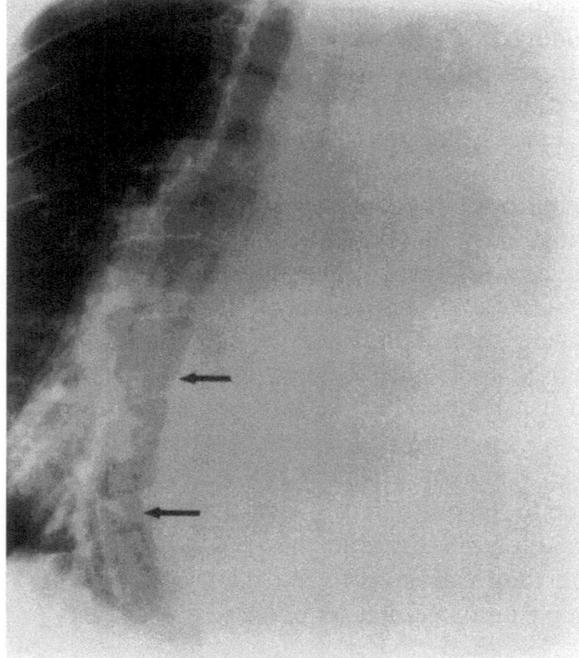

Fig. 9.35. Left pleural effusion. Presentation as a right retrocardiac mass. PA radiograph. Bulging of the left pleural sac to the right across the azygoesophageal recess (*arrows*) as the result of a large left-sided effusion is less common than left-sided presentation of right effusion. Of 16 herniations reported by Sukumaran and Berger [49], ten were right to left and six were left to right

9.3.3.7 Visualization of Pulmonary and Pleural Masses by Virtue of Their Contact with Contralateral Lung Across the Azygoesophageal Recess

The fact that the right and left lungs are able to contact one another across the posterior junction lines above and below the azygos and aortic arches does on infrequent occasions allow a pulmonary or pleural mass on one side to be partially outlined by air in the contralateral lung. An example of a mass in the left lower lobe silhouetted by right lung is shown in Fig. 9.42, and an example of a diffuse mesothelioma over the crista pulmonis of the right lower lobe in contact with left lung is demonstrated in Fig. 9.36.

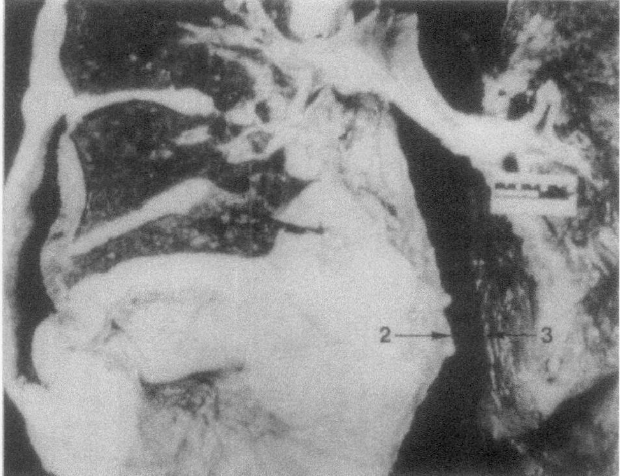

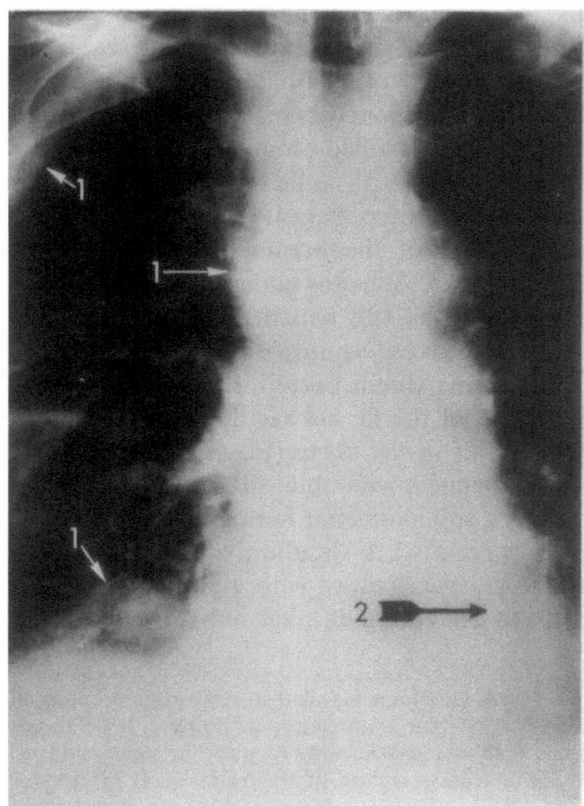

Fig. 9.36A, B. Visualization of pleural masses due to their contact with contralateral lung across azygoesophageal recess. A PA radiograph. B Coronal section through plane of trachea made at autopsy. In this patient with diffuse mesothelioma, multiple pleural masses were identified in right side of thorax. A retrocardiac mass was also present (2). Coronal body section at autopsy shows this density was mesothelioma covering surface of crista pulmonis (2) visualized by virtue of its contact with air in left lower lobe (3). (Courtesy A. Templeton, Kansas City, MO)

9.3.3.8 Hiatus Hernia

Hernias through the esophageal hiatus intrude into the inferior portion of the mediastinum behind the heart and in front of the spine and thus impress upon and distort the inferior portion of both lungs. Although hernias are more commonly found to extend into the left chest, they may also protrude to the right, displacing the inferior portion of the azygoesophageal recess to the right. Since the esophagus lies anterior to the recess, the intrusion into the recess by a hiatus hernia is usually from the front. At times a hernia may impinge upon both lungs; well-penetrated frontal radiographs and AP

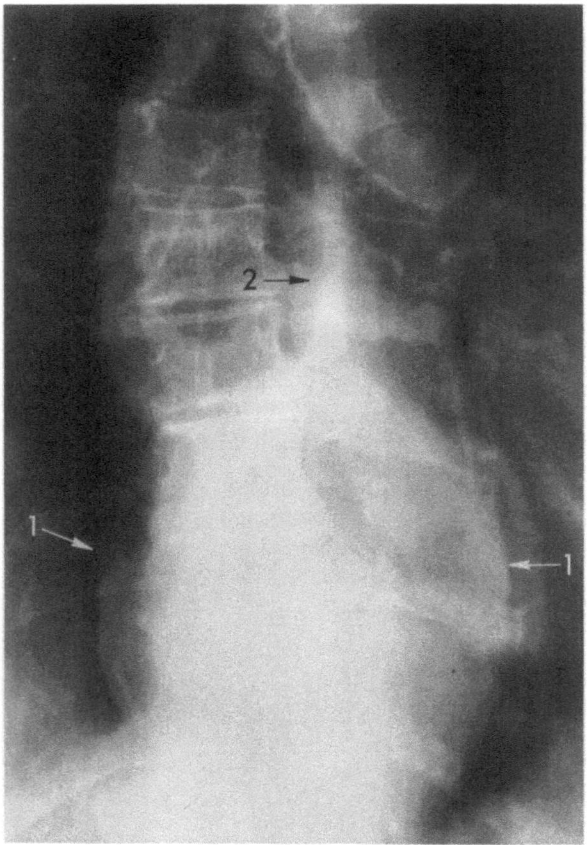

Fig. 9.37. Hiatus hernia distorting azygoesophageal recess (AP radiograph). Esophageal hiatal hernias intrude into inferior portion of mediastinum behind heart and in front of spine and may impress upon medial aspect of left and right lungs (*1*). In this patient with deep medial extension of each lung against mediastinum, pleurae sweep off top of hernia sac and contact one another to produce posterior junction line (*2*)

conventional tomograms may show the hernia insinuating itself between the right and left mediastinal pleurae (Fig. 9.37). In patients with deep medial extension of each lung, the pleurae may be seen to sweep off the top of the hernia sac, contacting one another to produce the posterior junction line (Fig. 9.37). If the hernia is very large, it may extend cephalad to the carina as in Fig. 9.38. When this occurs, the right lung can be excluded totally from the azygoesophageal recess – the displaced posterior lung outlining the hernia on its right side (Fig. 9.38). At times the hernia may compromise the recess anteriorly but not totally obliterate it. The arcuate line of lung in the recess may then be visualized through the air-filled stomach. Note that the line seen in Fig. 9.38 could have been considered to be the pleuroesophageal stripe. However, the interposition of the hernia between the right lung and the esophagus makes this an anatomic impossibility in this patient. The line is merely lung in the recess against the fibro-fatty tissues of the mediastinum posteriorly. Note also that a portion of the hernia sac lies against the left lateral wall of the aorta (Fig. 9.38). If the herniated stomach were fluid filled, the aortic outline on a supine frontal radiograph would have been obliterated, a situation similar to the loss of the aortic shadow with right-sided pleural effusion presenting as a left retrocardiac mass.

Fig. 9.38 A–D. Hiatus hernia distorting azygoesophageal ▷ recess. **A** AP tomogram made post mortem. **B** AP tomogram with nasogastric tube in place in same cadaver. **C** Coronal body section of this cadaver. **D** Transverse body section of same cadaver made at lower end of **C**. This postmortem examination shows hiatus hernia excluding lung from anterior aspect of azygoesophageal recess from diaphragm to carina (*1*). Line representing contact of right lung with mediastinal soft tissues behind hernia is also shown (*2*). Note that this line, which simulates pleural esophageal stripe, could not represent this structure, since nasogastric tube shows course of esophagus to lie far to right of this line. Coronal body section (**C**) clearly demonstrates interposition of hernia (*3*) between esophagus (*4*) and right lung (*5*). In this patient, there is no way in which right lung could have contacted esophagus to produce line simulating pleural esophageal stripe in **A** and **B**. Transverse body section made immediately above diaphragm shows contact of right lung with mediastinum behind hernia (*6*). Hernia sac lies against left lateral wall of descending aorta. (**B–D** From [22])

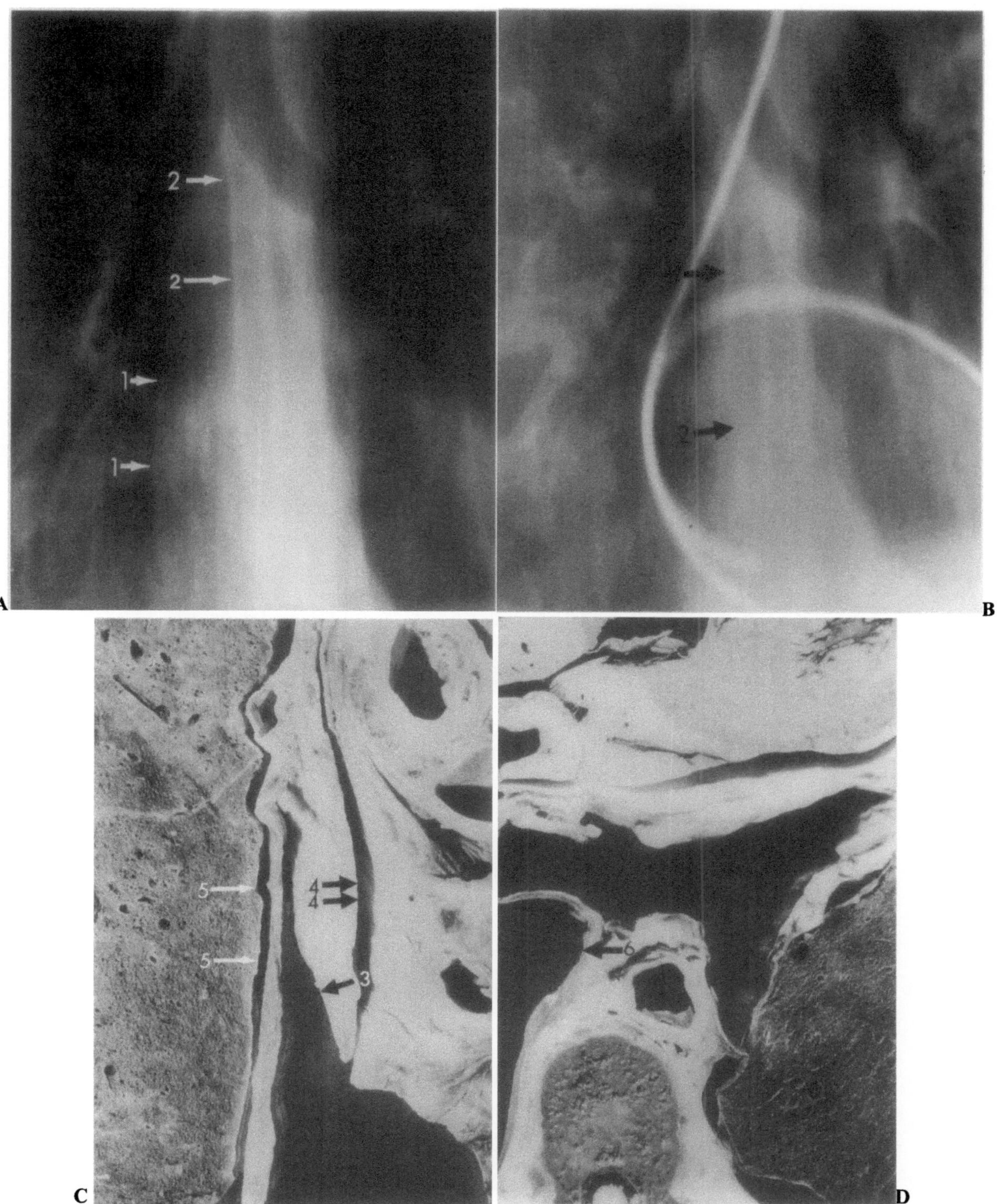

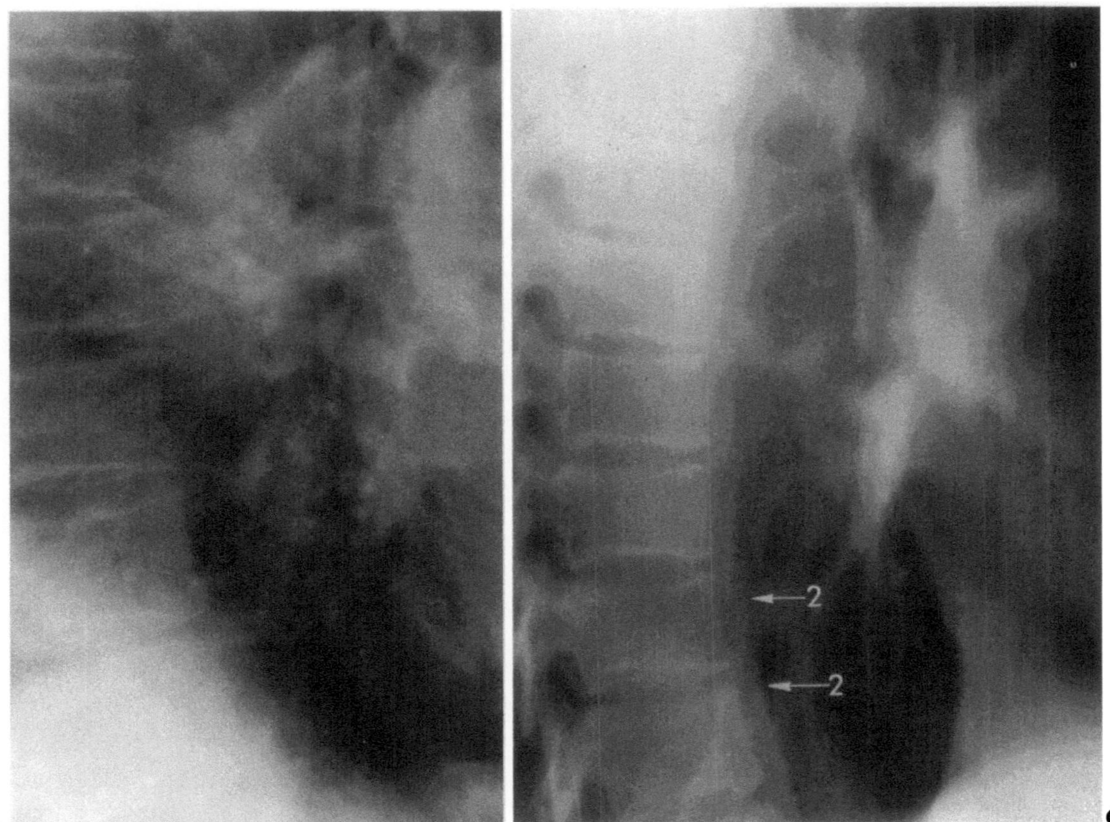

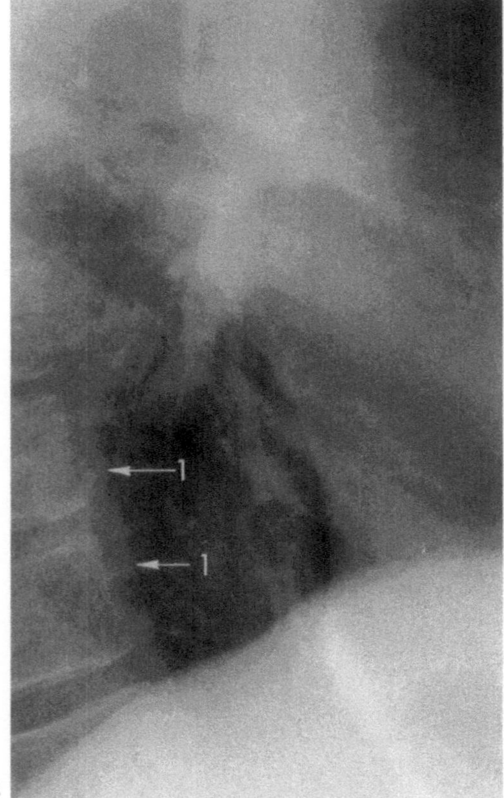

Fig. 9.39 A–C. Prespinal line. A and B Lateral radiographs. C Lateral tomogram. Normally no stripe of soft tissue density is seen in front of spine on lateral radiograph (A). If, however, there is a considerable volume of lung in prespinal location, as when azygoesophageal recess is deep, soft tissue stripe may be seen outlined between anterior margins of vertebral bodies and posterior aspect of lung in azygoesophageal recess. This line has been called "prespinal line" and may be used in radiographic interpretation in manner analogous to use of paraspinal line in diagnosis. In this patient with left lower lobe atelectasis in A, prespinal line developed following total collapse of left lung and herniation of right lung to left through azygoesophageal recess (1). Normal prespinal line was clearly shown by tomography (2)

9.3.4 The Prespinal Line

It has been stated many times previously that lung in the azygoesophageal recess and sometimes in the supra-azygos recess may extend well to the left in front of the spine. Lung in the azygoesophageal recess adopts this position in about three-fourths of older patients. In the series of normal patients studied by Lunn and Lien [27], lung extended to the midline or to the left of it in 17 of 22 patients over 50 years of age. Lung permits visualization of the soft tissues anterior to the spine on well-penetrated lateral radiographs and lateral tomograms (Figs. 9.39, 9.40, 9.41). It is ideally demonstrated at computed tomography. This stripe has been called the "prespinal line" [20, 22]. Al-

though no standards have been determined, this soft tissue plane outlined between the anterior surfaces of the vertebral bodies and lung in the recesses is probably no more than 2 or 3 mm thick in normal subjects. The incidence of its visualization on lateral radiographic examinations has not been established. At the T-4 or T-5 level the prespinal line is interrupted as lung in the supra-azygos and azygoesophageal recesses swings forward over the posterior turn of the azygos arch.

The prespinal line can be utilized in radiographic interpretation in exactly the same way that the paraspinal line is used to analyze films. Figure 9.40 demonstrates bilateral paraspinal masses in a patient with multiple myeloma. Involvement of the body of T-4 is also evident. A lateral tomogram made on this patient shows marked thickening of the prespinal line, which can be seen in contact with the posterior turn of the azygos arch (Fig. 9.40).

In the case illustrated in Fig. 9.42, it was not possible to determine with certainty from the radiographs whether the large lesion in the left lower thorax medially arose in the lung or in the mediastinum. Lateral tomograms showed that the prespinal line was deviated forward at

Fig. 9.40 A, B. Abnormality of prespinal line. **A** AP tomogram. **B** Lateral tomogram. In this patient with proven multiple myeloma, involvement of vertebral body (*1*) was accompanied by paravertebral masses (*2*) and by marked diffuse thickening of prespinal line (*3*). No standards for normal range of thickness or prespinal line are available. Note that anterior edge of prespinal line has been carried forward to contact posterior turn of azygos arch (*4*). (**B** From [22])

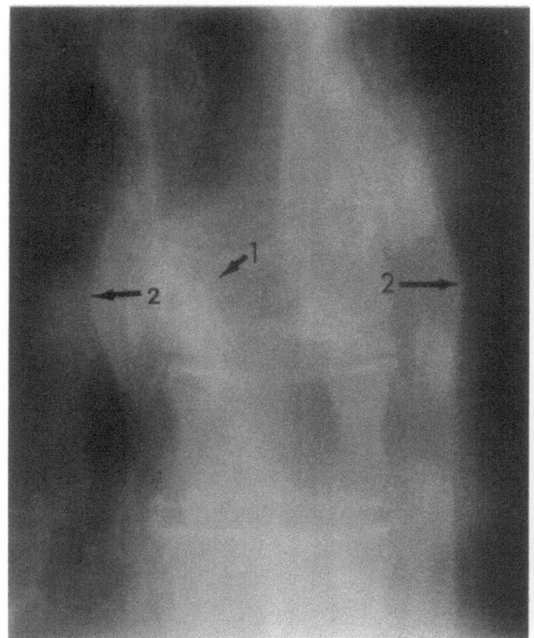

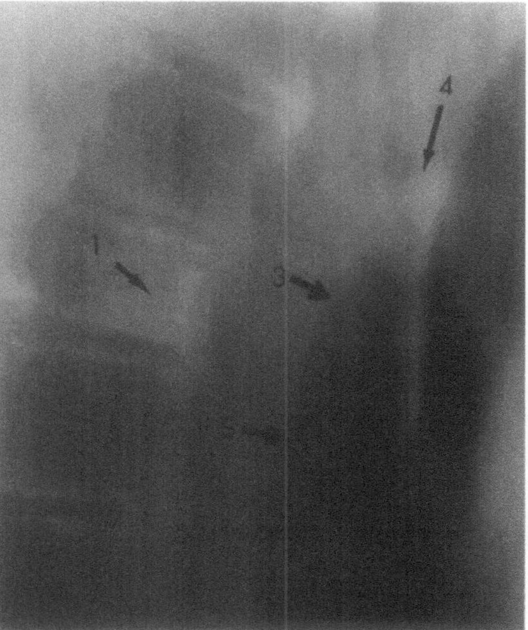

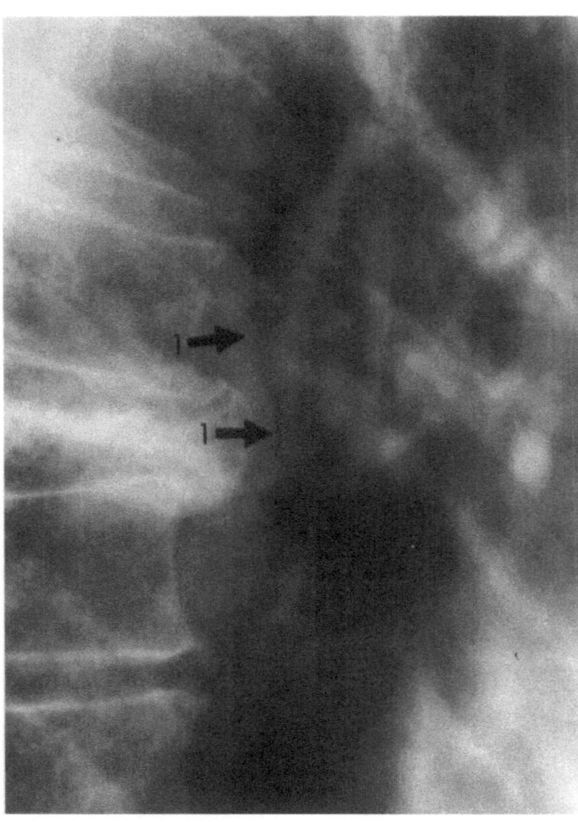

Fig. 9.41. Abnormality of prespinal line (lateral radiograph). Forward deviation of prespinal line in this patient with metastatic carcinoma to spine is clearly shown (*1*). (From [22])

Fig. 9.42 A, B. Abnormality of prespinal line. **A** AP tomogram. **B** Lateral tomogram. AP tomogram shows large mass in left inferior thorax medially. It could not be determined with certainty whether this mass was of mediastinal, pleural, or parenchymal origin. Lateral tomogram (**B**), showing distinct anterior deviation of lower aspect of prespinal line (*1*), proved unequivocally that whatever the process was, an element of extrapleural disease was present. At surgery, large bronchogenic carcinoma was found involving left lower lobe. Upon incision of parietal pleura, large prespinal nodes involved by metastatic tumor were encountered

▽

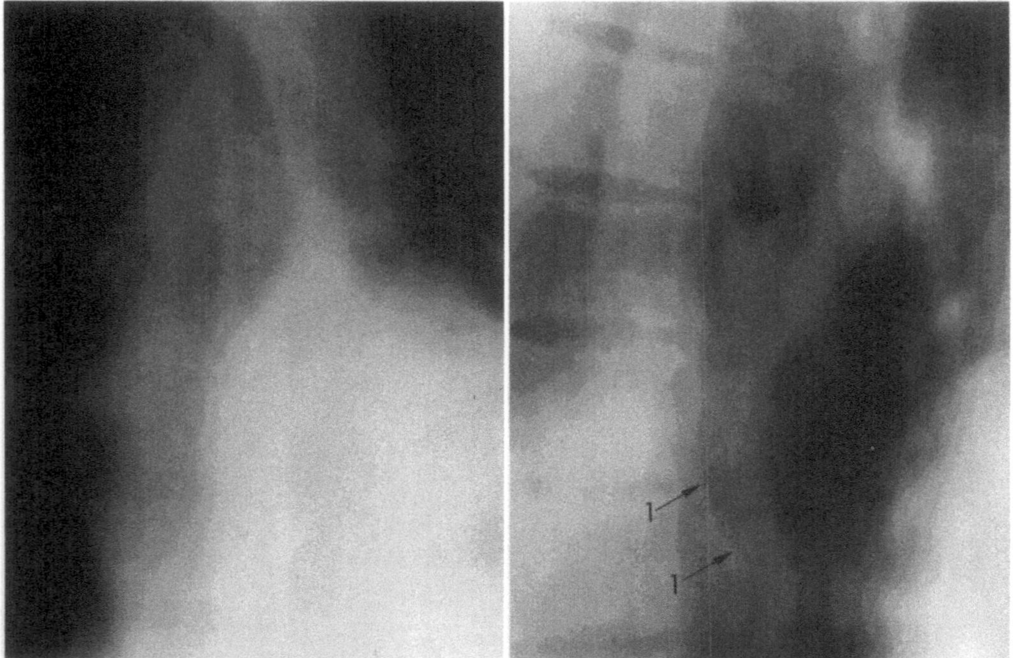

A   B

the T-8 to T-9 level. The point of this anterior displacement coincides with the upper margin of the impression made by the mass on the azygoesophageal recess on the AP tomograms. On the basis of this deviation in the prespinal line, it was concluded that whether the large mass was pulmonary or mediastinal, there must be extrapleural disease anterior to the spine. At surgery a large left lower lobe carcinoma was encountered. Prespinal lymph nodes at the T-8 to T-9 level were found to be considerably increased in size secondary to metastatic involvement. The prespinal line is deviated by osteophytes as well as by infectious processes, hematomas, and a wide variety of less commonly encountered pathologic processes.

9.4 The Paraspinal Area

The right lung posterior to the azygoesophageal recess usually makes some contact with the soft tissues anterior to the spine but invariably meets the soft tissues lateral to the spine. The radiographic counterpart of this contact is the paraspinal line. On the right the paraspinal line is not seen in many patients, presumably because the lung-soft tissue interface is in an oblique rather than a sagittal plane and hence does not present itself in profile to a frontal X-ray beam. The right paraspinal line is identifiable more often in left anterior oblique and right posterior oblique projections. A more complete discussion of the concept of the paraspinal line and its application to radiologic diagnosis is included in chapter 7.

References

1. Bachman AL, Teixidor HS (1975) The posterior tracheal band: a reflector of local superior mediastinal abnormality. Br J Radiol 48:352–359
2. Beck E, Beattie EJ Jr (1958) The lymph nodes in the mediastinum. J Int Coll Surgeons 29:247–251
3. Bergstrom JF, Yost RV, Ford KT, List RM (1973) Unusual roentgen manifestations of bronchogenic cysts. Radiology 107:49–54
4. Berne AS, Gerle RD, Mitchell GE (1969) The mediastinum – normal roentgen anatomy and radiologic techniques. Semin Roentgenol 4:3–21
5. Cahan WG, Watson WL, Pool JL (1951) Radical pneumonectomy. J Thorac Surg 22:449–473
6. Chasen MH, Rugh KS, Shelton DK (1984) Mediastinal impressions on the dilated esophagus. RCNA 22:591–605
7. Cimmino CV (1956) The esophageal-pleural stripe on chest teleroentgenograms. Radiology 67:754–756
8. Cimmino CV (1961) Further notes on the esophageal-pleural stripe. Radiology 77:974–978
9. Cimmino CV (1981) The esophageal-pleural stripe: an update. Radiology 140:609–613
10. Cimmino CV, Snead LO (1965) The posterior mediastinal line on chest roentgenograms. Radiology 84:516–518
11. Cornell SH (1965) Calcium in the fluid of mediastinal bronchogenic cyst – a new roentgenographic finding. Radiology 85:825–827
12. Cubillo E, Rockoff SD (1971) Milk of calcium fluid in an intrapulmonary bronchogenic cyst. Chest 60:608–610
13. Doppman J (1967) Effect of Valsalva maneuver on the inferior vena cava in man. Invest Radiol 2:332–338
14. Doppman JL, Rubinson RM, Rockoff SD, Vasko JS, Shapiro R, Morrow AG (1966) Mechanism of obstruction of the infra hepatic portion of the inferior vena cava in the presence of increased intraabdominal pressure. Invest Radiol 1:37–53
15. Filly R, Blank N, Castellino RA (1976) Radiographic distribution of intrathoracic disease in previously untreated patients with Hodgkin's disease and non-Hodgkin's lymphoma. Radiology 120:277–281
16. Gladnikoff H (1948) A radiographic study of the mediastinum in health and pulmonary carcinoma. Acta Radiol [Suppl] 73:1–87
17. Grafe WR, Goldsmith EI, Redo SF (1966) Bronchogenic cysts of the mediastinum in children. J Pediatr Surg 1:384–393
18. Gwinn JL, Lee FA (1975) Radiological case of the month. Contributed by Pottenger LK, Kirks DR: Parenchymal bronchogenic cyst. Am J Dis Child 129:953–954
19. Heitzman ER (1975) Roentgen anatomic correlations in the mediastinum. In: Margulis AR, Gooding CA (eds) Diagnostic radiology. University of California Press, Berkeley
20. Heitzman ER (1984) The lung. Radiologic-pathologic correlations. Mosby, St. Louis

21. Heitzman ER, Scrivani JV, Martino J, Moro J (1971) The azygos vein and its pleural reflections. I Normal roentgen anatomy. Radiology 101:249–258

22. Heitzman ER, Scrivani JV, Martino J, Moro J (1971) The azygous vein and its pleural reflections. II Applications in the radiological diagnosis of mediastinal abnormality. Radiology 101:259–266

23. Heller RM, Dorst JP, James AE Jr, Rowe RD (1971) A useful sign in the recognition of azygous continuation of the inferior vena cava. Radiology 101:519–522

24. Knutsson F (1955) Mediastinal pleurae. Acta Radiol 43:265–275

25. Lachman E (1942) Comparison of the posterior boundaries of the lungs and pleura as demonstrated on the cadaver and on the roentgenogram of the living. Anat Rec 83:521–542

26. Lodin H (1957) Mediastinal herniation and displacement – studied by transversal tomography. Acta Radiol 48:337–350

27. Lund G, Lien HH (1982) Computed tomography of the azygoesophageal recess. Acta Radiol [Diagn] 23:225–230

28. Lund G, Lien HH (1983) Abnormalities of the azygo-esophageal recess at computed tomography. Acta Radiol [Diagn] 24:3–10

29. Maier HC (1938) Mediastinal hernia in the absence of pneumothorax. Am J Roentgenol 39:687–697

30. Marvasti MA, Mitchell GE, Burke WA, Meyer JA (1981) Misleading density of mediastinal cysts on computed tomography. Ann Thorac Surg 31:167–170

31. McCort JJ (1952) Radiographic identification of lymph node metastases from esophageal carcinoma. Radiology 59:694–711

32. Mendelson DS, Rose JS, Efremidis SC, Kirschner PA, Cohen BA (1983) Bronchogenic cysts with high CT numbers. AJR 140:463–465

33. Muller NL, Webb NR, Gamsu G (1985) Subcarinal lymph node enlargement: radiographic findings and CT correlation. AJR 145:15–19

34. Nakata H, Nakayama C, Kimota T, Nakayama T, Tsukamoto Y, Nobe T, Suzuki H (1982) Computed tomography of mediastinal bronchogenic cysts. J Comput Assist Tomogr 6:733–738

35. Nohl HC (1956) An investigation into the lymphatic and vascular spread of carcinoma of the bronchus. Thorax 11:172–185

36. Nohl HC (1962) The spread of carcinoma of the bronchus. Year Book Medical Publishers, Chicago

37. Onitsuka H, Kuhns LR (1980) Dextroconvexity of the mediastinum in the azygo-esophageal recess: normal CT variant in young adults. Radiology 135:126

38. Ormond RS, Jaconette JR, Templeton AW (1963) The pleural esophageal reflection: an aid in the evaluation of esophageal disease. Radiology 80:738–742

39. Panicek DM, Heitzman ER, Randall PA, Groskin SA, Chew FS, Lane EJ, Markarian B (1987) The continuum of developmental pulmonary anomalies. Radiographics 7:747–772

40. Pantoja E, Kattan KR, Thomas HA (1984) Some uncommon lower mediastinal densities. A pictorial essay. RCNA 22:633–646

41. Proto AV, Speckman JM (1979) The left lateral radiograph of the chest. Med Radiogr Photogr 55:30–74

42. Reed JC, Reeder MM (1974) Middle mediastinal lesion. Topics in radiology gamut. JAMA 230:891–892

43. Reed JC, Sobonya RE (1974) Foregut cysts in the thorax. Am J Roentgenol Radium Ther Nucl Med 120:851–860

44. Rogers LF, Osmer JC (1964) Bronchogenic cyst – a review of 46 cases. Am J Roentgenol Radium Ther Nucl Med 91:273–281

45. Rubinson RM, Vosko JS, Doppman JL, Morrow AG (1967) Inferior vena caval obstruction resulting from increased intra abdominal pressure – experimental hemodynamic and angiographic observations. Arch Surg 94:766–770

46. Saks BJ, Kilby AE, Dietrich PA, Coffin LH, Krawitt EL (1983) Pleural and mediastinal changes following endoscopic injection therapy of esophageal varices. Radiology 149:639–642

47. Schnur MJ, Winkler B, Austin JHM (1981) Thickening of the posterior wall of the bronchus intermedius – a sign on lateral chest radiographs of congestive heart failure, lymph node enlargement and neoplastic infiltration. Radiology 139:551–559

48. Snider GL, Gildenhorn HD, Rubenstein LH (1956) Dextroposition of the descending thoracic aorta. Radiology 67:333–338

49. Sukumaran M, Berger HW (1979) Mediastinal herniation of pleural sac in massive pleural effusion. Chest 75:382–383

50. Tisi GM, Friedman PJ, Peters RM, Pearson G, Carr D, Lee RE, Selawry O (1983) Clinical staging of primary lung cancer. Am Rev Resp Dis 127:659–664

51. Tonkin JL, Keats JE, Capp MP (1977) Radiographic isolation of the inferior vena cava. AJR 129:657–659

52. Ziter FMH, Brammit DH, Halloman KR, Conte PJ (1969) Calcified mediastinal bronchogenic cysts. Radiology 93:1025–1026

10 The Pulmonary Hilum

Each lung is connected to the mediastinum by a bronchovascular pedicle enclosed in a connective tissue envelope. Although there has been some discussion in the literature [20, 39] over the most appropriate term for this pedicle, standard medical dictionaries prefer "hilus" as being semantically proper. In everyday parlance, "hilum" is much more commonly used; this designation will be maintained in the following discussion.

10.1 General Anatomic Considerations

10.1.1 Vessels and Bronchi

The main or undivided pulmonary artery passes upward and posteriorly from its point of origin to divide into the right and left pulmonary arteries behind the ascending aorta (Fig. 10.1). The main pulmonary artery lies entirely within the pericardium, as do the proximal portions of the right and left pulmonary arteries [9]. From its point of origin the right pulmonary artery courses posteriorly and laterally in a gentle arc in front of the right main and intermediate bronchus and behind the superior vena cava (Fig. 10.2). It exits the pericardium just after giving rise to the truncus anterior, the artery

to the right upper lobe. The left pulmonary artery has a shorter intrapericardial course than the right (Fig. 10.3). Following its exit from the pericardium, it swings cephalad over the left main and upper lobe bronchi which, since they lie below the vessel, are designated as being "hyparterial" [5] (Figs. 10.1, 10.5). The right upper lobe bronchus lies above the right pulmonary artery and, hence, is "eparterial" [5] (Figs. 10.1, 10.4).

In general, the arterial supply to the lobes of the lungs follows the pattern of bronchial branching [9]. The right pulmonary artery bifurcates into two branches, an upper trunk, termed the "truncus anterior" by Boyden [5], and a lower or interlobar trunk [39]. The truncus anterior branch, given this name because it passes anterior to the right upper lobe bronchus (Fig. 10.4), is distributed to the right upper lobe, whereas the lower trunk supplies the middle and

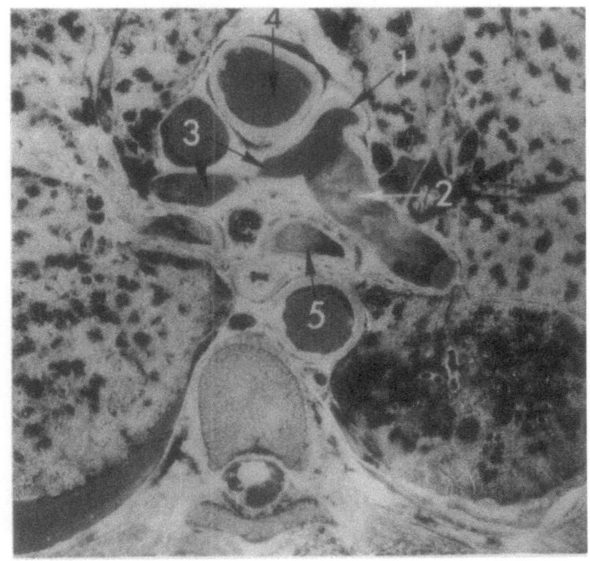

Fig. 10.1. Division of main pulmonary artery. Undivided pulmonary artery (*1*) passes upward and posteriorly from its point of origin to divide into the left pulmonary artery (*2*) and right pulmonary artery (*3*) behind ascending aorta (*4*). Note that left pulmonary artery passes above left main bronchus (*5*) and left upper lobe bronchus. These structures are therefore designated as being "hyparterial." Right upper lobe bronchus coursing behind right pulmonary artery lies predominantly above artery and is therefore designated as "eparterial"

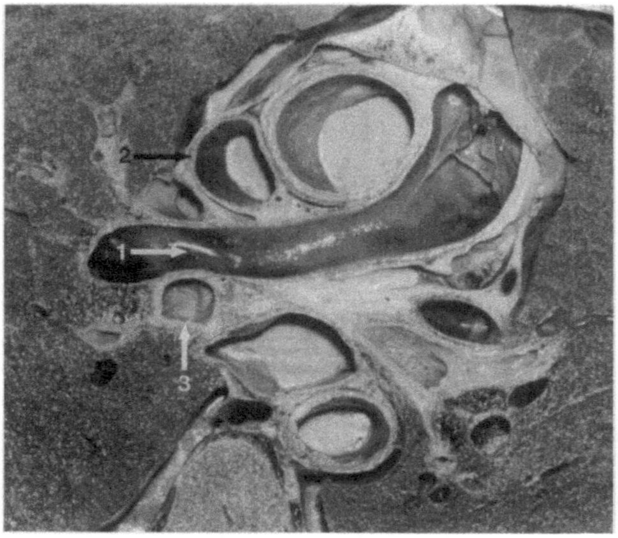

Fig. 10.2A–C. Course of right pulmonary artery. **A** Transverse body section. **B** Roentgenogram of same body section. **C** Computed tomogram made at same level on the same cadaver before sectioning. From its point of origin, right pulmonary artery (*1*) courses posteriorly and laterally, passing behind superior vena cava (*2*) and anterior and inferior to right main bronchus (*3*) to enter lung

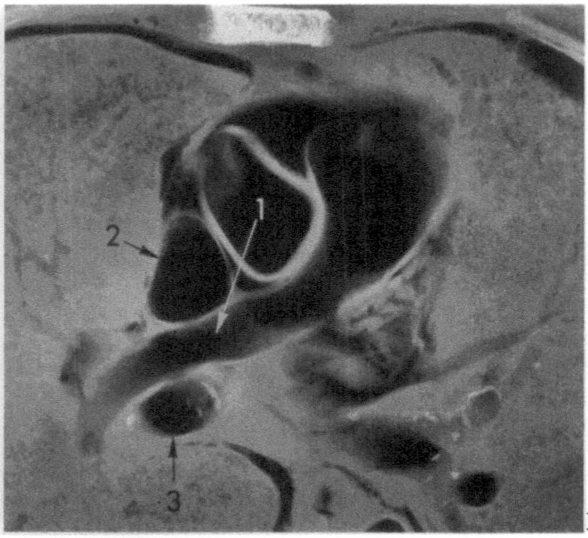

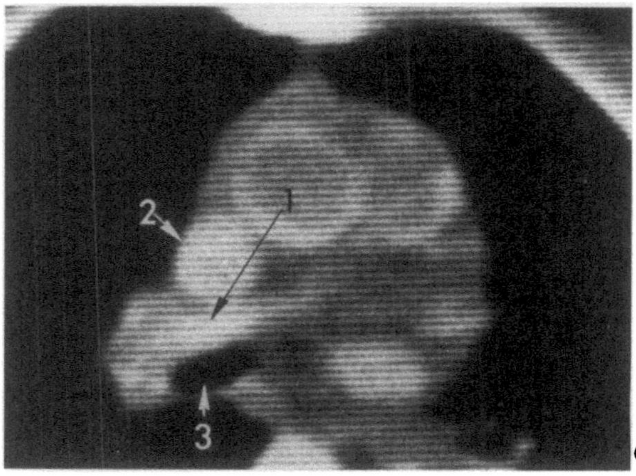

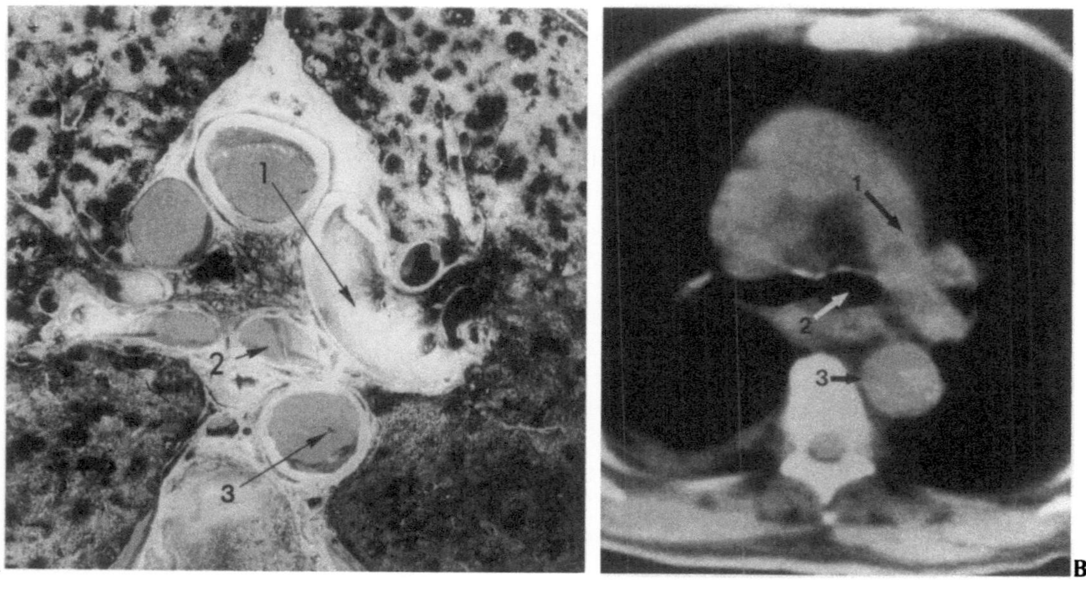

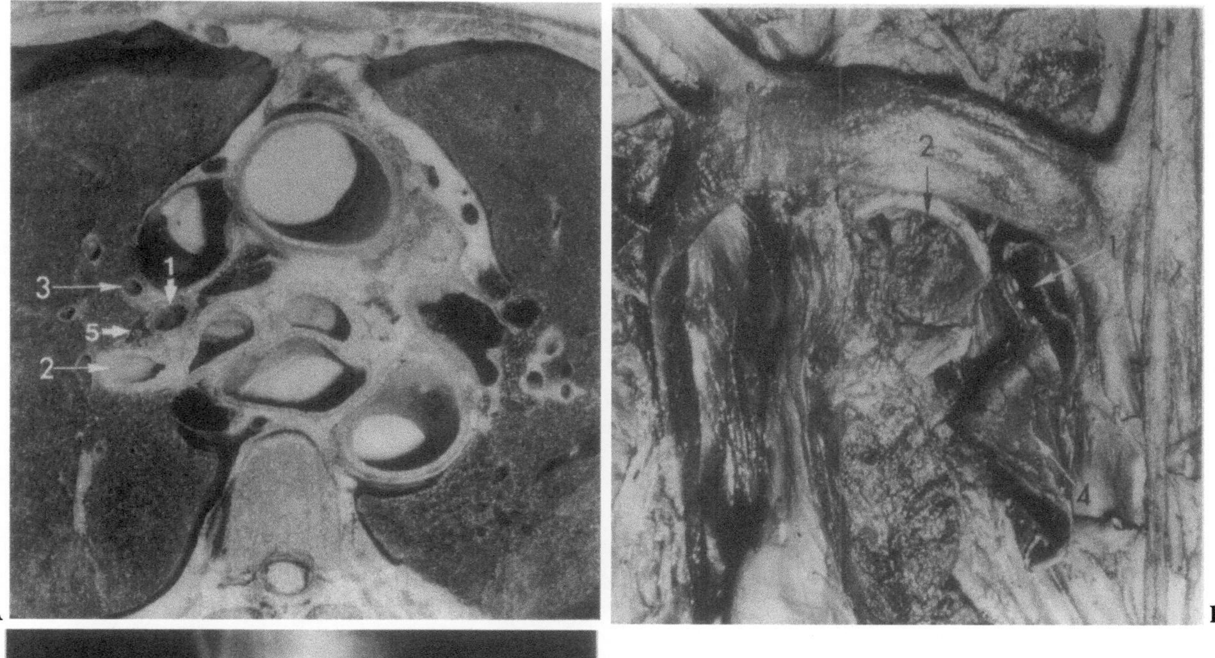

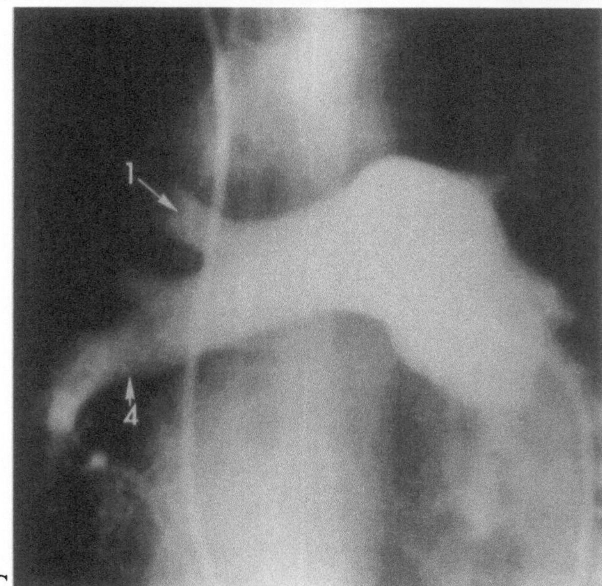

Fig. 10.4A–C. Relationship of vessels and bronchi in right hilum. A Transverse body section. B Right side of mediastinum with mediastinal pleura removed. C AP radiograph from pulmonary arteriogram. Just before its exit from pericardium, right pulmonary artery gives off branch called "truncus anterior" (*1*), which is distributed to right upper lobe. This artery is so designated because it lies anterior to right upper lobe bronchus [*2*]. The bronchus also lies slightly higher than the artery and thus is referred to as being "eparterial." The truncus anterior, along with right superior pulmonary vein (*3*), forms upper portion of right hilar shadow. Note that vein lies anterolateral to artery. Arterial branch to right lower lobe (*4*) forms lower portion of right hilar shadow and is situated immediately above inferior pulmonary veins. Note the lymph node (*5*) lateral to the "truncus anterior"

◁ **Fig. 10.3A, B.** Course of left pulmonary artery. **A** Transverse body section. **B** Computed tomogram. Left pulmonary artery (*1*) has shorter intrapericardial course than the right. Major portion of vessel lies anterior and superior to left main bronchus (*2*) and left upper lobe bronchus. Vessel continues posterior to left main bronchus as arterial branch to left lower lobe. At this point it is in intimate association with descending aorta (*3*)

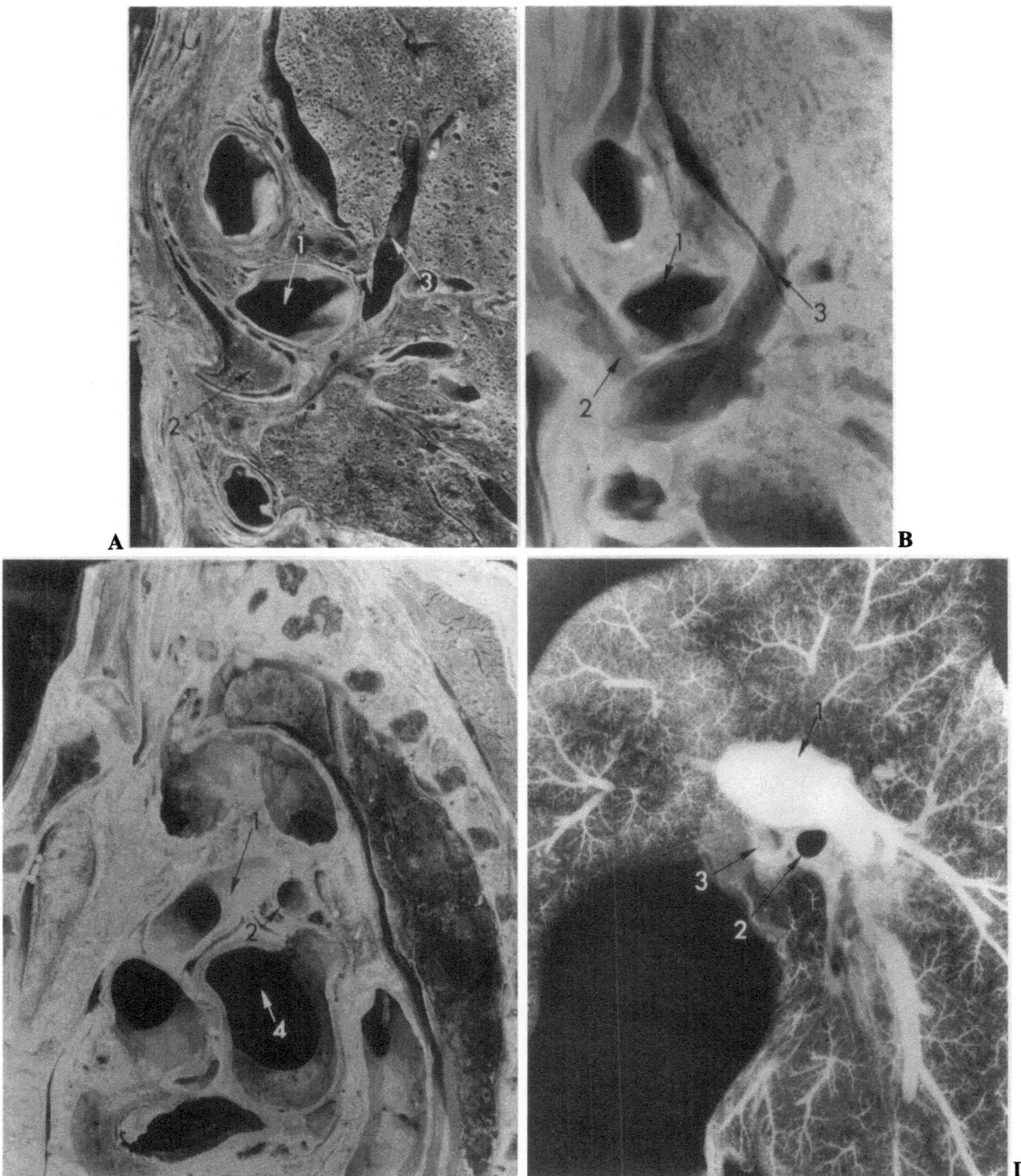

Fig. 10.5A–D. Relationship of vessels and bronchi in left hilum. **A** Coronal body section. **B** Roentgenogram of same coronal body section. **C** Sagittal body section through left hilum. **D** Radiograph of sagittal section of left lung through hilum following barium arteriography. Left pulmonary artery (*1*) courses superiorly and posteriorly from its point of origin passing above left upper lobe bronchus (*2*) which is therefore referred to as being "hyparterial." Where vessel turns to descend as artery to left lower lobe, it is intimately associated with descending aorta. Left superior pulmonary vein (*3*) passes anterior to left upper lobe bronchus (see also Fig. 10.23). Left upper lobe bronchus in turn lies immediately above left atrium (*4*). Bronchus is therefore ringed by vascular structures. Inferior pulmonary veins join atrium below level of hilum and thus do not contribute to formation of hilar shadow

the lower lobes. The branching of the left pulmonary artery grossly resembles that of the right side, although there is more variation in the arterial distribution to the left upper lobe than there is to the right upper lobe.

The pulmonary veins are quite variable in their size and course [78]. Nevertheless, it is convenient to consider that the superior pulmonary veins are formed by the union of anterior (apical-anterior) and posterior venous tributaries. The radiographic anatomy of these segmental vessels is best appreciated on computed tomograms and will be reviewed in section 10.2.4. The right superior pulmonary vein courses downward from a position that is usually lateral to the upper lobe artery and passes in front of the right pulmonary artery to enter the left atrium immediately below the pulmonary artery. The left superior pulmonary vein passes downward lateral to the left pulmonary artery and then in front of the left upper lobe bronchus, although at times a venous branch from the upper lobe may lie posterior and inferior to the bronchus. The left upper lobe bronchus is thus ringed by vascular structures – the artery above and behind, the superior vein in front and the left atrium and inferior vein below.

The inferior pulmonary veins cross the lower lungs almost horizontally and enter the left atrium separately or in common with the upper lobe veins. The lower lobe veins are too low in position to contribute to the density of the hilar shadows. The point of entry of the pulmonary veins into the left atrium is often termed the "venous confluens." It is frequently identifiable on the right (see Fig. 9.26) and sometimes on the left (see Fig. 7.24) and should not be mistaken for a mediastinal mass. Recent comprehensive reviews of the correlated radiographic anatomy of the pulmonary veins have been provided by Genereux [28] and by Godwin and Chen [33]. The bronchi are relatively thin walled and of course are air filled; therefore they contribute little to the production of the hilar shadow. The hila are thus radiographic representations of the pulmonary arteries and the superior pulmonary veins.

In summary, then, the major structures of each hilum are similarly arranged from front to back on the two sides. The superior pulmonary veins are in front, the arteries in the middle and the bronchi behind (Figs. 10.4, 10.5). On the left the arterial branch to the left lower lobe descends behind the bronchus (Fig. 10.5D).

10.1.2 Hilar Lymph Nodes

Several classifications of the lymph nodes of the thorax have been developed and are reviewed by Nagaishi [53]. There has been considerable controversy in the literature over which lymph nodes should be designated as hilar. Nodes clustered about the major bronchi, particularly at their points of bifurcation, have generally been considered to belong in the hilar group. Some authors would include nodes more peripheral in lung in this group while others feel that only the nodes about the main bronchi should be considered hilar in location. In the past, such differences were of little practical significance, but in more recent years, the clinical staging of lung cancer by the TNM staging system [1] has led to the need for a more precise and standardized system for identifying hilar and mediastinal lymph node stations. Relatively recently, the American Thoracic Society, recognizing that "commonly accepted, specific anatomic definitions of each nodal stations are lacking" formed a committee on lung cancer and charged it with the responsibility of developing a map of regional pulmonary lymph nodes that would be acceptable to all physicians who care for the patient with lung cancer. It was requested that the terminology should avoid the use of the words "mediastinal" and "hilar" because they lack clinical-anatomic specificity [77]. Following this mandate the committee developed a classification which was adopted by the American Thoracic Society in November of 1981. In this scheme nodes formerly designated as "hilar" are referred to as "right tracheobronchial nodes" and "left peribronchial nodes." "Right tracheobronchial nodes" are defined as nodes to the right of the midline of the trachea from the level of the cephalic border of the azygos vein to the origin of the right upper lobe bronchus. "Left peribronchial nodes" are defined as being to the left of the midline of the trachea between the carina and the left upper lobe bronchus, medial to the ligamentum arteriosum. Nodes designated as "intrapulmonary" or "pulmonary ligament nodes" in this new classification might have previously been considered to be hilar by some observers. This new classification along with the significance of the reporting of hilar and mediastinal lymph node size and location in patients with bronchogenic carcinoma is considered in detail in chapter 3.

Nodes in right tracheobronchial and left peribronchial areas and intrapulmonary nodes may be anterior, posterior, medial, or lateral to the bronchi, predominantly situated at their angles of bifurcation. The nodes tend to ring some bronchi, and their enlargement may cause bronchial compression leading to atelectasis. Particularly vulnerable to this type of impingement are the bronchi to the right middle lobe, the left upper lobe, and the anterior segment of the right upper lobe.

The efferents of the hilar lymph nodes drain into the paratracheal lymph node chain of the homolateral side. The major bronchi and the hilar lymph nodes are supplied by the bronchial arteries and are drained by the bronchial veins. Normally, the hilar nodes are of small size and contribute little to overall hilar density.

10.1.3 The Inferior Pulmonary Ligament

All of the structures of the hilum are enclosed in a connective tissue sheath that is prolonged inferiorly, where it is known as the inferior pulmonary ligament (Figs. 10.6, 10.7). To understand the anatomy of this area, visualize the structures of the hilum as a clothesline running between the mediastinum and the lung. Consider that a sheet is thrown over this clothesline and extends downward in front of and behind it. Below the inferior pulmonary veins the pleural layers (analogous to the sheet) are apposed and are referred to as the "inferior pulmonary ligament" (Figs. 10.6, 10.7).

Inferiorly, it may extend to the diaphragm or not quite to the diaphragm (Fig. 10.7). Rost

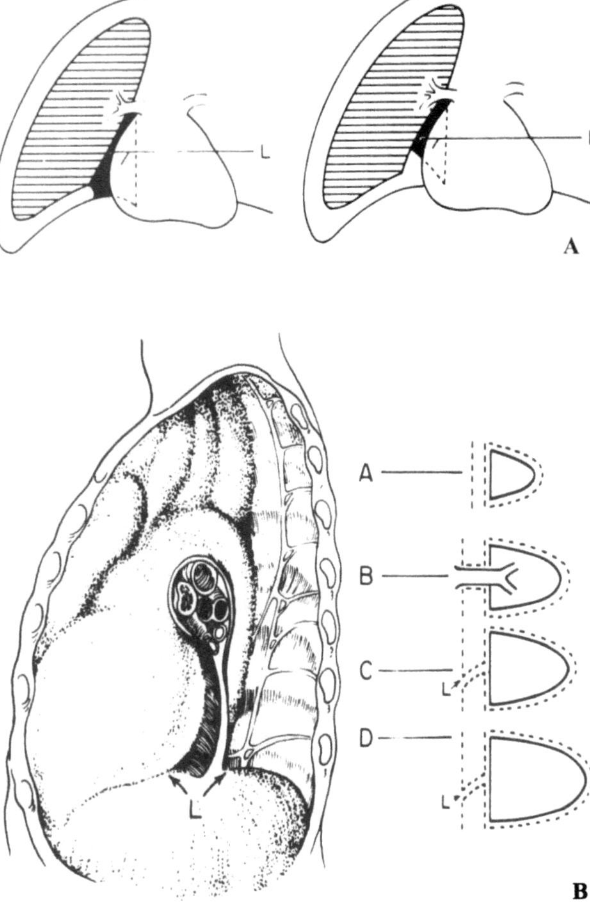

Fig. 10.6A, B. Anatomy of inferior pulmonary ligament. Structures of each lung root are enclosed in sheath of parietal pleura that is continuous with mediastinum medially and with visceral pleura over lower lobe laterally. This sheath extends inferiorly to diaphragm, sometimes ending just short of it. Ligament encloses within its leaves structures of hilum, inferior pulmonary veins, and lymph nodes, which are designated as "nodes of inferior pulmonary ligament." Note that dimension of inferior pulmonary ligament from side to side is greater inferiorly than it is superiorly. This configuration is thought to account for triangular configuration of paramediastinal collections of pleural fluid. (From [66])

and Proto have emphasized that it courses posteriorly as it descends [73]. Its dimension from side to side is less at the hilum than it is below creating a triangular configuration (Figs. 10.6, 10.7). Medially, the ligament becomes continuous with the parietal pleura of the mediastinum anterior to a coronal plane through the esophagus, whereas laterally it

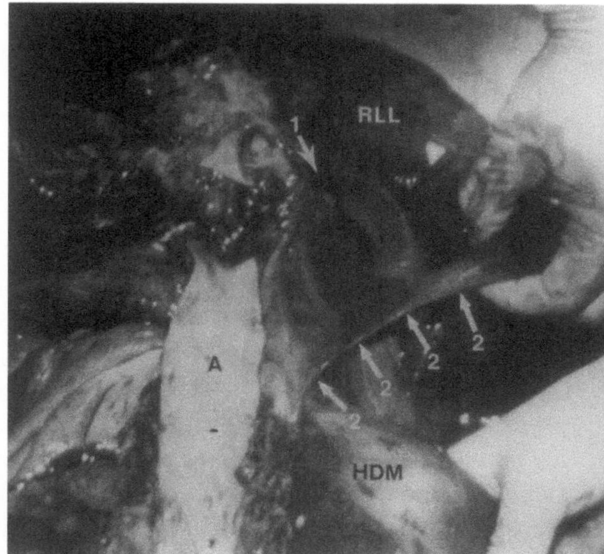

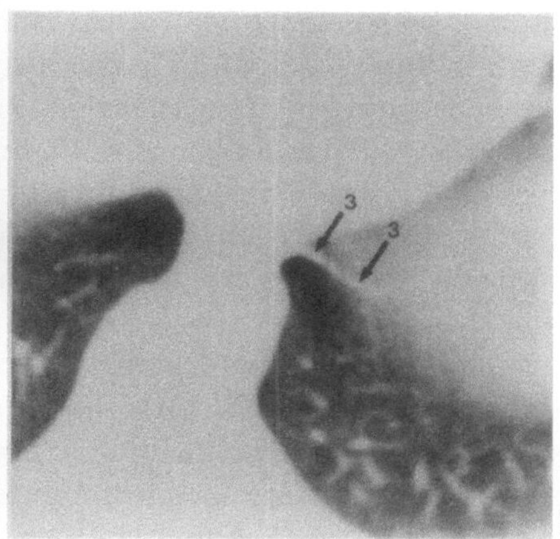

Fig. 10.7A, B. The inferior pulmonary ligament. **A** Right ligament as viewed from behind. **B** Computed tomogram. The inferior pulmonary ligament medially becomes continuous with the parietal pleura of the mediastinum anterior to a coronal plane through the esophagus. Laterally, it merges with the visceral pleura of each lower lobe (*RLL*). Note again that the side-to-side dimension of the lobe is less superiorly (*1*) than it is inferiorly (*2*). In this patient the ligament does not extend to the hemidiaphragm (*HDM*) and has a free falciform lower edge (*2*). The ligament is commonly identified at computed tomography (*3*) more often on the left side than on the right (see text). (**A** From [73])

merges with the visceral pleura over the lower lobes. The inferior pulmonary ligament lymph nodes lie within the leaves of the ligament below the inferior pulmonary veins. They number one to five on each side and receive lymphatic flow from the basal segments of each lower lobe [53]. Radiographic aspects of the inferior pulmonary ligament have been authoritatively reviewed by Rabinowitz and Wolf [67] and Rabinowitz et al. [68]. The inferior pulmonary ligament is rarely identified on PA, lateral, or oblique radiographs in normal subjects. Similarly it is uncommon to identify it in pathological states, although exceptionally it can be identified in cases of pneumothorax.

The inferior pulmonary ligament is commonly seen at computed tomography [12, 34, 52, 73] (Fig. 10.7). On computed tomograms it

was identified on the left in 38% and on the right in 12% of patients in the series reported by Cooper et al. [12]. It was identified on the left in 67% and on the right in 37% of patients studied by Rost and Proto [73]. It was seen by them only at the diaphragm or slightly above it. They could offer no explanation for the greater frequency of its demonstration on the left side, but Cooper et al. [12] has theorized that the fact that the right ligament is shorter than the left and the projection of the dome of the liver into the right hemithorax makes detection of the right ligament more difficult. Since the ligament runs between the lung and the mediastinum, structures which are normally apposed, it is in a sense surprising that the ligament is seen at all. It is thought that lung in front of and behind the ligament outlines it [73]. The ligament probably does not "collapse" against the mediastinum because of its attachment to the diaphragm. This fact also probably explains why the ligament is seen most often at the diaphragm or immediately above it.

An understanding of the anatomy of the inferior pulmonary ligament is useful in the analysis of many intrathoracic abnormalities. However, its influence on the appearance of the chest radiograph in disease states is primarily an indirect one. The ligament binds the lower lobe to the mediastinum and significantly affects the pattern of lower lobe atelectasis. The collapsed lobe swings posteriorly and medially like a door on a hinge to lie against the mediastinum and the paraspinal soft tissues. Even when the degree of collapse is severe, the anteromedial margin of the lower lobe is displaced posteriorly to only a limited degree because it is fixed in place by the inferior pulmonary ligament. It has been theorized that atypical, mass-like forms of left lower lobe collapse may result when the ligament fails to extend all the way to the diaphragm [29].

The ligament lies in a coronal plane with a side-to-side dimension less at its upper margin than at its lower end; that is, the lower lobe is bound more closely to the mediastinum at the hilum than it is at the diaphragm. It has been conjectured that this anatomic arrangement is responsible for the triangular configuration of paramediastinal fluid collections seen on frontal radiographs [67, 68].

Theoretically, when the inferior pulmonary ligament reaches all the way to the diaphragm, it should compartmentalize the medial side of the inferior pleural space. This fact might also influence the appearance of paramediastinal pleural fluid. In fact, no convincing example of such fluid compartmentalization exists in our material, presumably because movement of pleural fluid with change in body position soon causes it to be distributed on both sides of the ligament.

Rabinowitz and Wolf [67] state that lymph node masses and fluid collections, the latter having extended from the mediastinum, may be present between the leaves of the pulmonary ligament. There is no doubt that this is the case in surgical and autopsy material. However, it is difficult to do more than suggest this possibility on the basis of radiographic examinations.

Ravin et al. [69] have reported three cases of post-traumatic pneumatocoel occurring in the inferior pulmonary ligament. Volberg et al. [79] have discussed air collections in the inferior pulmonary ligament in neonates with respiratory distress. Recently, however, Godwin et al. [35] and Friedman [22] have presented rather strong evidence to suggest that such collections are usually, if not always, loculated pneumothorax or loculated pneumomediastinum unrelated to the pulmonary ligament. For a review of this subject in greater detail, refer to chapter 3.

10.2 Radiologic Correlations with Anatomy and Pathology

The hilum can and often must be studied in a variety of projections – frontal, lateral, oblique, and axial or transverse. Frontal examination is achieved by means of PA and AP radiographs and by conventional tomography in the AP plane. Lateral examination may be by means of lateral radiographs, conventional tomography in the lateral plane, and by magnetic resonance imaging. Oblique examination is achieved through use of oblique plain films, angled conventional tomography and magnetic resonance imaging. Axial or transverse imaging is achieved through the use of computed tomography and magnetic resonance.

Conventional radiographs made in PA or AP projection are standard studies for investigation of the hilum in frontal projections. Occasionally conventional tomograms made AP or PA are of value; in the opinion of this author, conventional AP or PA tomograms are the preferred examination for detailed evaluation of the trachea and main bronchi. The ability to study the major airway in profile rather than in cross section as in computed tomography or magnetic resonance is sometimes a distinct advantage. For all other indications, most observers now prefer computed tomography and/or magnetic resonance imaging over conventional tomography for detailed investigation of the hilum [31, 48, 51, 61]. It is generally felt that examination in the axial projection is superior to evaluate hilar anatomy and pathology, but in addition much better delineation of the mediastinum can be achieved by such techniques than can be obtained by conventional tomography.

From the earlier discussion of hilar anatomy it should be inferred that the radiographic shadow known as the "hilum" is primarily a representation of the pulmonary artery. Lavender [45] and Lavender and Doppman [46] have pointed out that the upper portion of the hilar shadow is a reflection of the upper lobe pulmonary veins as well as the upper lobe arteries. The lower portion of the hilum represents the lower pulmonary artery trunk only; the inferior pulmonary veins are too low to contribute to the hilar shadow. As mentioned previously, the bronchi and normal lymph nodes also add little to the production of hilar density.

The left hilum is higher than the right in 97% of normal individuals; in 3% the hila are at the same level [20]. In Felson's series the right hilum was never normally higher than the left [20]. The higher position of the left hilum is explained by the anatomic position of the two pulmonary arteries. The left pulmonary artery, arching upward over the left main and upper lobe bronchi, rises to a higher level than does the right pulmonary artery.

10.2.1 Frontal Projection

Evaluation of the questionably abnormal hilum on frontal radiographs is a common and often challenging task. A pathologic process involving the hilum may present itself as a hilum which is too large, too small, or too dense (Figs. 10.8, 10.9). Abnormalities of size may result from a variety of pathologic states. Rigler et al. [71] pointed out that enlargement of the hilum is one of the most commonly overlooked signs of bronchogenic carcinoma (Figs. 10.8, 10.9); enlargement is often subtle. Thickening of central bronchial walls or narrowing of them should always be looked for with great care and, when present, support the probability that an otherwise equivocal hilum is abnormal (Figs. 10.8, 10.9 B). Such observations on plain films are unfortunately infrequent [83]. The distinction of hilar mass from a prominent pulmonary artery has always been a particularly common and vexing problem. At the present time this dilemma is usually easily resolved by computed tomography (Fig. 10.12). Many other congenital and acquired conditions will cause an increase in hilar size; these processes and their differential diagnosis have been discussed thoroughly by Felson [20] and by Reeder and Felson [70] and will not be considered further here. Reeder and

Felson [70] have also provided a gamut list for the abnormally small hilum. It is perhaps worthy of emphasis that one of the most common causes for a small hilum, and one which is often overlooked, is lobar atelectasis (Fig. 10.9 C). When a lobe is collapsed, the artery to that lobe cannot be seen because it is surrounded by airless lung. Only the pulmonary artery or arteries supplying the noncollapsed lung are visualized, and the hilum thus appears small. This is particularly evident in cases of lower lobe collapse. Since atelectasis is one of the most frequent radiographic manifestations of lung cancer, a small hilum should raise suspicion of bronchogenic carcinoma just as a large hilum does.

Discussions of the large and small hilum naturally raise the issue of the standards by which the size of the hilar shadow should be judged. An attempt to provide such a standard of measurement has been made by Rigler et al. [71]. Suffice it to say that variation in size of the hilum is great and that assessment by measurement is not useful. The most worthwhile approach to assessing whether or not a hilum is enlarged is to compare its size with that of the opposite hilum (Figs. 10.8, 10.9). The density of the two hilar shadows should also be compared and frequently provides a useful clue to hilar pathology (Figs. 10.8, 10.9). Assessment of density is, however, highly subjective and should be approached in a conservative manner [49].

A form of hilar measurement that has some degree of reliability and reproducibility is a determination of the diameter of the descending trunk of the right pulmonary artery [6]. This vessel, when measured at its widest point on frontal radiographs, should not exceed 16 mm in men or 15 mm in women. If measurements are greater than these maximum figures, the inferior portion of the hilum can be said to be enlarged and pulmonary arterial hypertension, either due to increased flow or increased resistance, should be considered likely [6]. Unfortunately in many cases of hilar enlargement the descending trunk of the right pulmonary artery is difficult or impossible to measure.

The intrapericardial portion of the right pulmonary artery is easy to measure in all subjects.

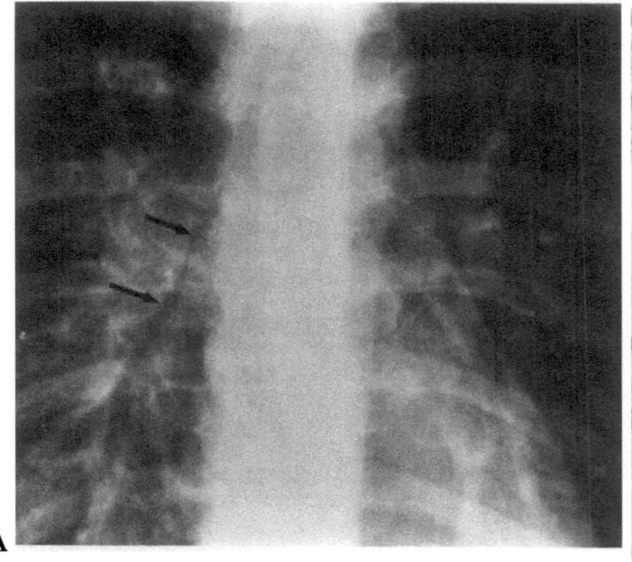

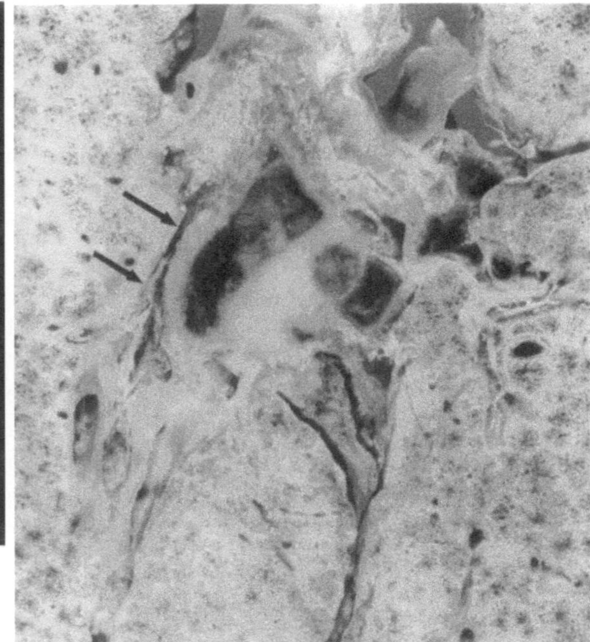

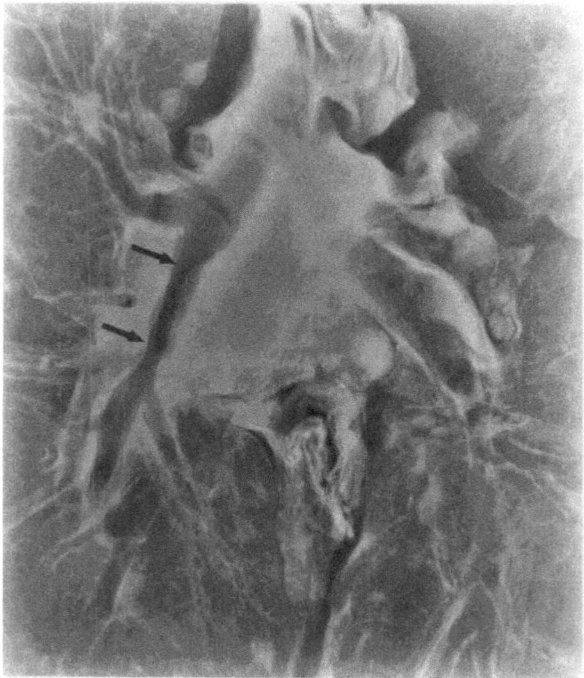

Fig. 10.8A–C. The abnormal hilum. **A** PA radiograph. **B** Coronal section through the carina of this patient at postmortem examination. **C** Radiograph of the slice shown in **B**. In this patient with bronchogenic carcinoma, the right hilum is large and dense (compare it to the left hilum). The intermediate bronchus is narrowed (*arrows*). Primary lung cancers originating in the hilum develop from cells of the bronchial mucosa and may grow intralumenally or extend through the bronchial wall. In this patient, both types of extension of the tumor occurred. Since it is difficult to detect slight changes in hilar size or density, hilar masses usually are diagnosed late in their course, are often not resectable, and have a poor prognosis

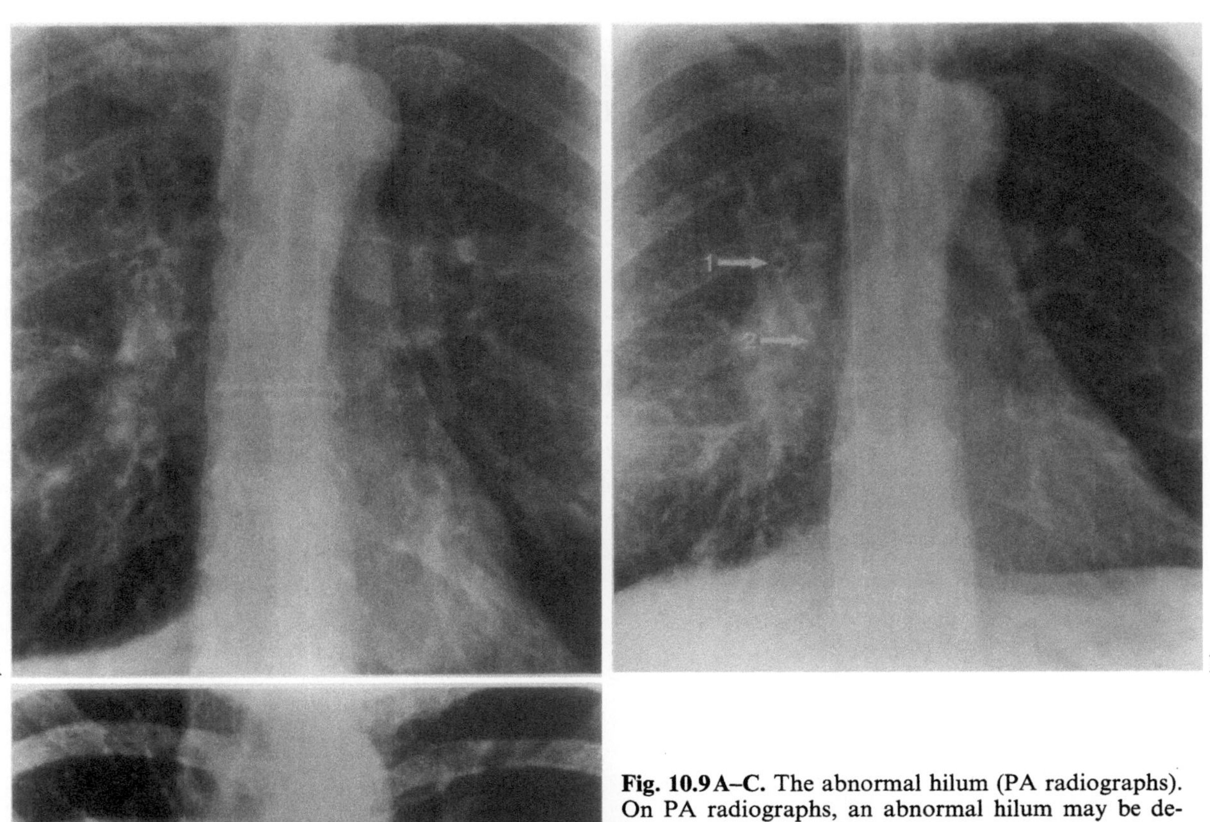

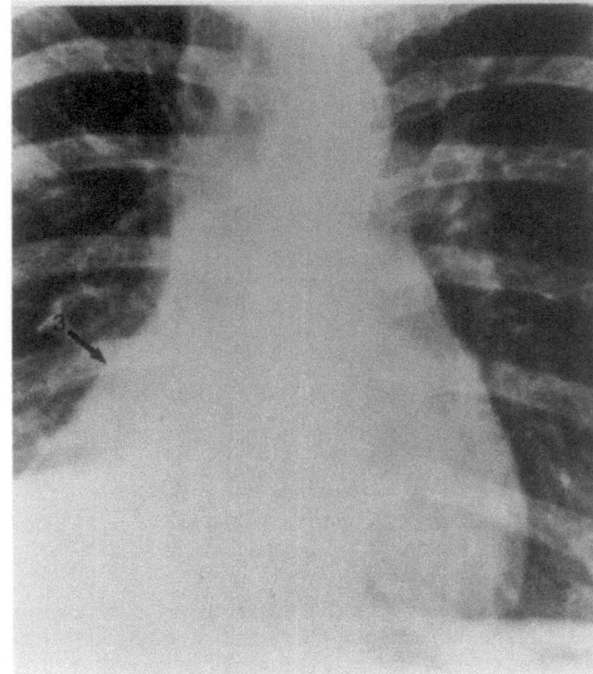

Fig. 10.9 A–C. The abnormal hilum (PA radiographs). On PA radiographs, an abnormal hilum may be detected because it is too large, too small, or too dense. Hilar measurements are not worthwhile; comparison with the opposite hilum is mandatory. Abnormal hila xusually result from bronchogenic carcinoma or from adenopathy. **A** and **B** are radiographs made on the same patient a few months apart. In **A** subtle enlargement of the right hilum proved to be due to bronchogenic carcinoma. **B** Shows a clearly enlarged hilum. Note that it is also much more dense than the left hilum. The peribronchial cuff (*1*) and the medial displacement of the intermediate bronchus (*2*) are findings confirming abnormality. In **C** the right hilum is small since only the right upper lobe artery is visible. The lower lobe artery cannot be seen in the collapsed right lower lobe (*3*). The collapse was secondary to bronchogenic carcinoma. Since collapse is so often caused by carcinoma and because collapse usually results in an ipsilateral small hilum, a small hilum should raise the strong suspicion of underlying neoplasm just as a large or dense hilum does

If it is enlarged, it is reasonable to assume that a large hilum seen on conventional radiographs is a reflection of an enlarged extrapericardial right pulmonary artery [59].

10.2.1.1 Enlargement of Hilar Lymph Nodes

Increase in size of the hilar lymph nodes is common and is produced by a wide variety of inflammatory and neoplastic conditions. When these nodes, at the points of bifurcation of the lobar and segmental bronchi, are enlarged, they are sometimes almost circumferentially surrounded by aerated lung, giving a "potato-like" configuration said to be quite characteristic of sarcoidosis and silicosis. A less classic but more frequently encountered appearance is one of mild or moderate hilar lobulation. Such a configuration of the hilum suggests that enlarged nodes are present; this feature is frequently easier to identify on lateral films than it is on frontal radiographs (Fig. 10.10). Commonly adenopathy produces a relatively nonspecific hilar prominence on frontal radiographs; at times, this appearance too is more easily confirmed as being due to enlarged lymph nodes on lateral radiographs. Chang and Zinn [7] have

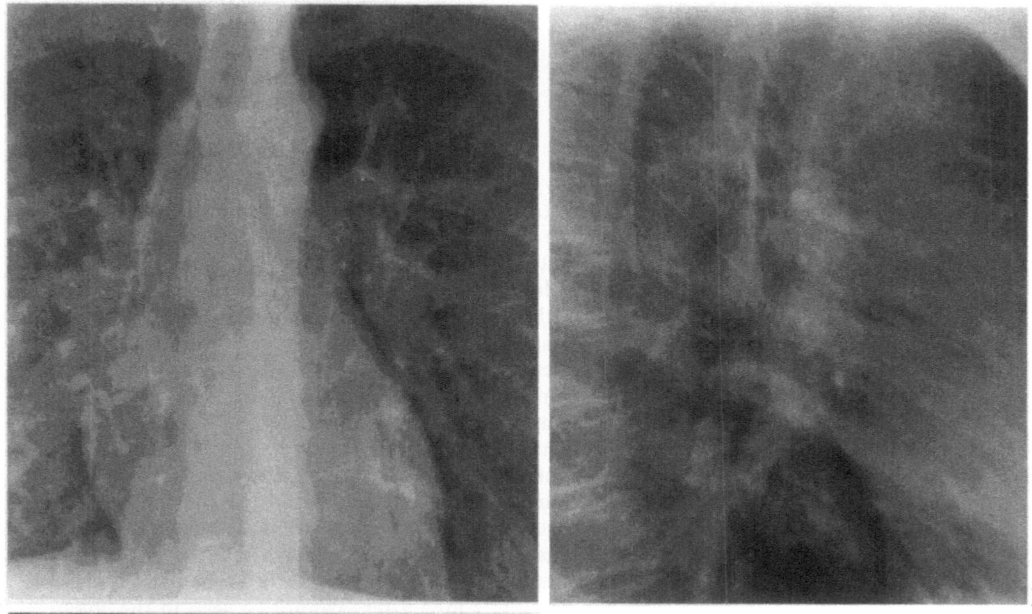

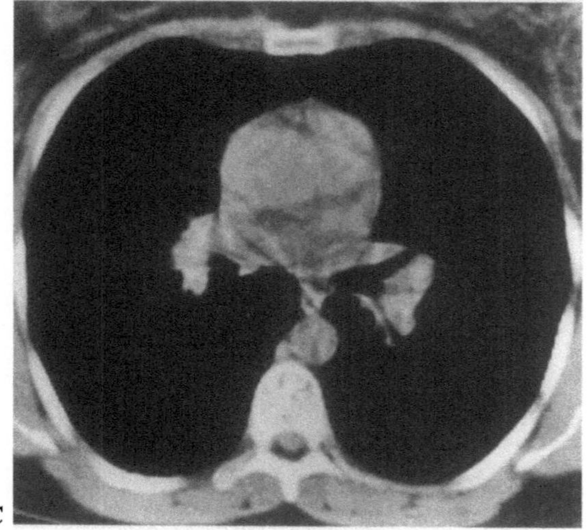

Fig. 10.10 A–C. Hilar adenopathy. A PA radiograph. B Lateral radiograph. C Computed tomogram. When extreme enlargement of hilar nodes occurs, they frequently present a "potato-like" appearance on radiographs. Less extreme degrees of enlargement show lobulated configurations (A and B). If anterior or posterior hilar nodes are predominantly involved, as in this patient, enlargement is often best seen on lateral view. If nodes in lateral aspect of hilum are involved, changes are best identified on PA view. Computed tomography often clearly demonstrates hilar adenopathy (C). Minimal degrees of enlargement may be difficult to detect and contrast enhancement may be necessary to determine whether the shadows in question are entirely vascular or not. The disease was sarcoidosis

pointed out that anteriorly and posteriorly situated hilar nodes are often hidden on frontal radiographs by the pulmonary arteries superimposed upon them. However, they feel that enlargement of the nodes in the lateral portion of the hilum is more easily appreciated on frontal radiographs.

In the absence of the lobulated appearance characteristic of adenopathy, it may be very difficult to determine whether hilar nodes are enlarged or not. If more central, mediastinal nodes can be shown to be increased in size, the statistical likelihood that a prominent hilar shadow is due to adenopathy is increased. The distinction between enlarged nodes and a prominent pulmonary artery on PA radiographs can be a challenging exercise. Computed tomography readily resolves the problem (Fig. 10.10 C). Computed tomography is the most useful adjunct to plain films to diagnose hilar adenopathy, but even with this study, determination of minimal nodal enlargement is difficult.

10.2.1.2 The Hilum Convergence Sign

A simple but practical aid in determining whether the prominent hilum is due to an enlarged pulmonary artery is to follow the peripheral arteries centrally to their origin. The structure from which they emanate is thereby identified as the pulmonary artery. This observation has been called the "hilum convergence" or "bifurcation sign" by Felson [18, 19, 20]. In applying this sign it should be recalled that some anterior and posterior branches of the pulmonary artery may project slightly medial to the most lateral margin of the vessel from which they arise.

10.2.1.3 The Hilum Overlay Sign

Felson has described another sign related to the hilum that is of value in distinguishing mediastinal masses, particularly anterior mediastinal masses, from a prominent cardiac silhouette. This observation is called the "hilum overlay sign" [18, 20]. Felson's studies found that the first branching of each main pulmonary artery

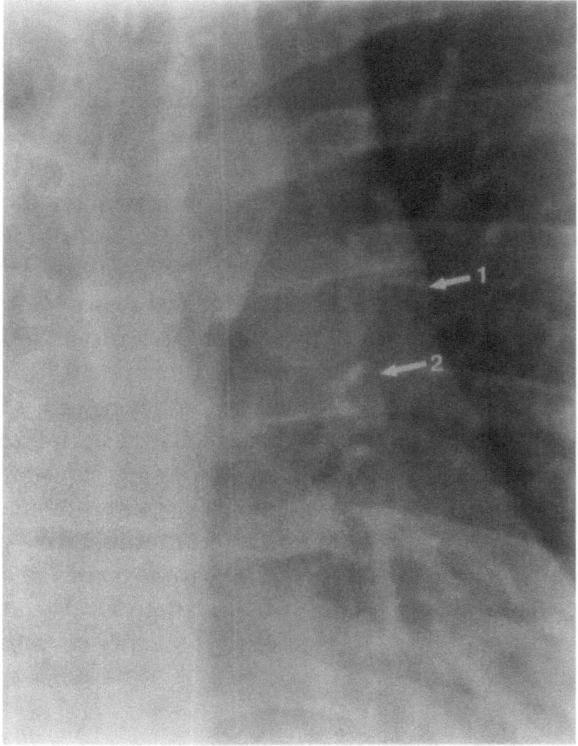

Fig. 10.11. The hilum overlay sign. PA radiograph. Felson [20] found that the first branching of either main pulmonary artery is lateral to the cardiac shadow or just within its outer aspect in 98% of normal individuals. In this patient there was prominence of the left side of the mediastinum (*1*). The fact that the first branching of the left pulmonary artery (*2*) lies well medial to the shadow in question strongly suggests that the abnormality is the result of a mediastinal mass. This observation is useful in distinguishing mediastinal masses from enlarged cardiac silhouette and is called "hilum overlay sign." In this case, the abnormal mediastinal contour extended cephalad lateral to the aortic knob further supporting the diagnosis of a mediastinal mass lesion. The process was Hodgkin's disease

is observed lateral to the cardiac shadow or just within its outer aspect in over 98% of individuals and lies less than 1 cm within the border in the remainder [20]. Therefore, in the analysis of radiographs showing a questionably abnormal mediastinum, the finding of the first bifurcation of the right or left pulmonary artery more than 1 cm medial to the edge of the shadow in question strongly suggests the density to be a mediastinal mass, not a prominent cardiac silhouette (Fig. 10.11).

10.2.1.4 The Posteriorly Directed Right Pulmonary Artery

Occasionally, the right pulmonary artery, in the lower portion of the right hilum, will appear to be round, rather than tubular, on frontal radiographs. A mass in the inferior hilum then becomes a major differential consideration, for how could the normal interlobar artery present an arcuate interface with lung superiorly and inferiorly in frontal projection? An explanation is readily offered by reference to Fig. 10.12. In some individuals, the right pulmonary artery in the major fissure passes directly posterior for a part of its course and is viewed "end-on" by the frontal X-ray beam. This orientation may be hard to appreciate on lateral radiographs or oblique views and computed tomography may be necessary to confirm this anatomic variant with certainty. In this author's experience the

Fig. 10.12A, B. The posteriorly directed right pulmonary artery. **A** PA radiograph. **B** Computed tomogram. Occasionally, the right pulmonary artery in the lower portion of the right hilum will appear as a round rather than tubular shadow on frontal radiographs (*1*). It may simulate a hilar mass. In this projection, a tubular structure can present convex superior and inferior margins only if the vessel is being imaged on end. In some individuals the interlobar portion of the right pulmonary artery adopts a horizontal, posterior course (*2*) before turning inferiorly. This variant has not been seen on the left side

left interlobar pulmonary artery has not been seen to adopt a similar orientation.

10.2.1.5 The Hilar Angle. The Vascular Converging Points of the Right Hilum

At the point where the right superior pulmonary vein crosses the descending portion of the pulmonary artery their lateral margins form an obtuse angle, sometimes referred to as the "hilar angle" [14, 45, 46]. The angle is not present on the left. In patients with pulmonary venous hypertension the superior pulmonary veins may dilate, making the angle more acute. If pulmonary arterial hypertension is superimposed on venous hypertension, the lower lobe artery may increase in size as well, making the hilar angle still more acute. The lateral edge of the superior pulmonary vein is normally quite straight; with pulmonary venous hypertension it may bow laterally, producing an abnormal upper hilar configuration with convexity directed laterally. Due to variability in the configuration and vertical course of the superior pulmonary vein, this sign is only of limited usefulness in the diagnosis of venous hypertension. The angle may be lost as the result of hilar mass or lymphadenopathy.

Don and Hammond [13] have recently discussed a radiographic appearance of the right hilum in frontal projection which can be considered as being analogous to the hilar angle. They

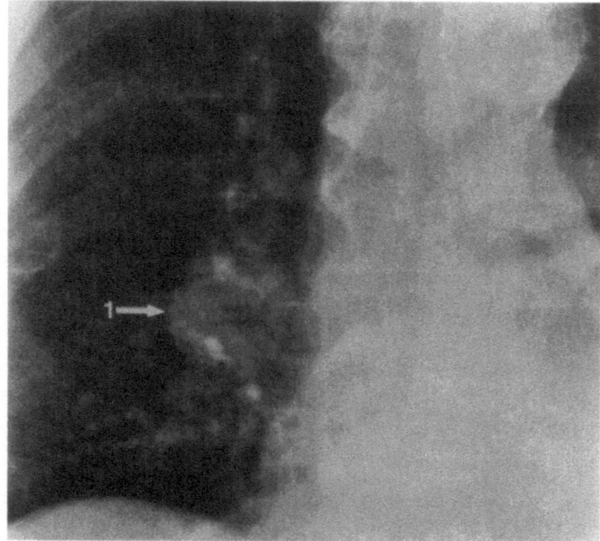

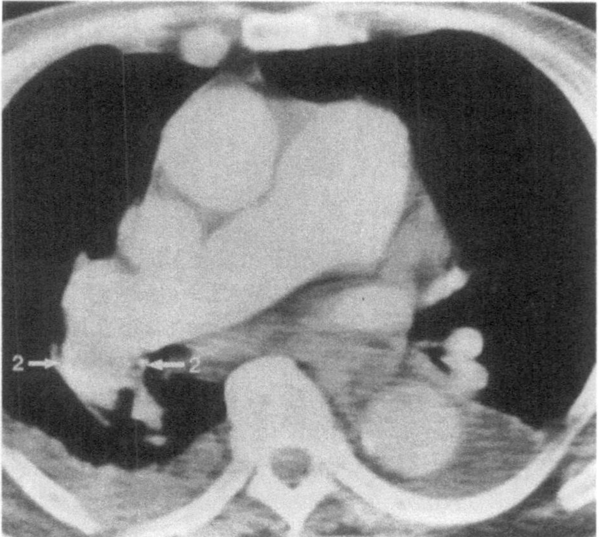

point out that there are two vascular converging points in the right hilum. The upper point represents the trifurcation of the truncus anterior in the right upper lobe while the lower point is the crossing of the superior pulmonary vein and the descending pulmonary artery – the hilar angle. Similar converging points are not present on the left side. Absence of the two converging points on the right supports the diagnosis of lobar collapse or resection.

10.2.1.6 The Hilar Height Ratio

It has been previously stated that the normal left pulmonary artery lies higher, or more cephalad, than the right; hence, the left hilum is normally higher than the right. Homer has stated this point somewhat differently: the left hilum is in the upper half of the hemithorax, the right hilum is in the lower half. As an extension of this anatomic point, Homer developed the concept of the hilar-height ratio [41]. He draws a line parallel to the thoracic spine from the highest point of the pulmonary apex to the diaphragm. A second line through the midpoint of the hilum intersects the first line at right angles. The ratio of the distances from the apex to the hilum and the hilum to the diaphragm are then obtained. Alterations in the normal ratios are encountered in a variety of conditions, most notably atelectasis [42]. Although most radiologists do not make a numerical determination of the hilar-height ratio, the practical importance of taking careful note of hilar position is emphasized by Homer's observations.

10.2.2 Lateral Projection

The plain lateral chest radiograph is extremely useful to study the normal and the abnormal hilum. The efficacy of the routine use of lateral chest radiographs has been addressed by Sagel et al. [74]. Excellent reviews of the anatomy of the hila as seen in the lateral projection have been produced by Austin [2], Proto and Speckman [63, 64], and by Vix and Klatte [78]. Their observations have been used freely in the development of this discussion.

The right pulmonary artery usually gives rise to its superior trunk, the truncus anterior, within the pericardium (see Fig. 10.4). The extrapericardial course of the inferior trunk usually is horizontal for only a matter of millimeters. As a result, an end-on demonstration of the normal right pulmonary artery is uncommon. When seen, the vessel is located anterior to the intermediate bronchus and above the lower portion of the right superior pulmonary vein (Fig. 10.13).

The left pulmonary artery has a short intrapericardial course. Its longer extrapericardial portion is surrounded by lung in the left lung root and, as a result, is very commonly visualized as it passes above the left main and left upper lobe bronchi. Lung inserting itself into the aortic-pulmonic window usually outlines clearly the superior aspect of the left pulmonary artery, particularly when the window is deep as when the pulmonary artery or aortic arch is ectatic or when the lungs are hyperinflated (see Figs. 7.6 and 7.7). In fact, failure to visualize the left pulmonary artery clearly on lateral radiographs should raise the suspicion of a left hilar mass (see Fig. 7.8).

Vix and Klatte [78] emphasized the influence of film projection on the visualization of arterial anatomy on lateral chest films. When a lateral film is made with slight rotation so that the right side of the chest is projected somewhat anterior to the left side, the arc of the left pulmonary artery is widened (Fig. 10.16), and the shadow of the right superior pulmonary vein becomes more prominent. On films made in this slight obliquity, the vein may be mistaken as a mass. When a lateral film is made with the right side of the patient rotated posteriorly, the hila are superimposed, and the arc of the left pulmonary artery is foreshortened. Films made with this deviation from a true lateral projection are the least desirable for the study of hilar detail (Fig. 10.16).

On lateral radiographs the lower end of the right superior pulmonary vein is seen just below the right pulmonary artery (Fig. 10.13). Just prior to entering the left atrium it lies immediately anterior to the right middle lobe bronchus (Fig. 10.19). The lower portion of the left supe-

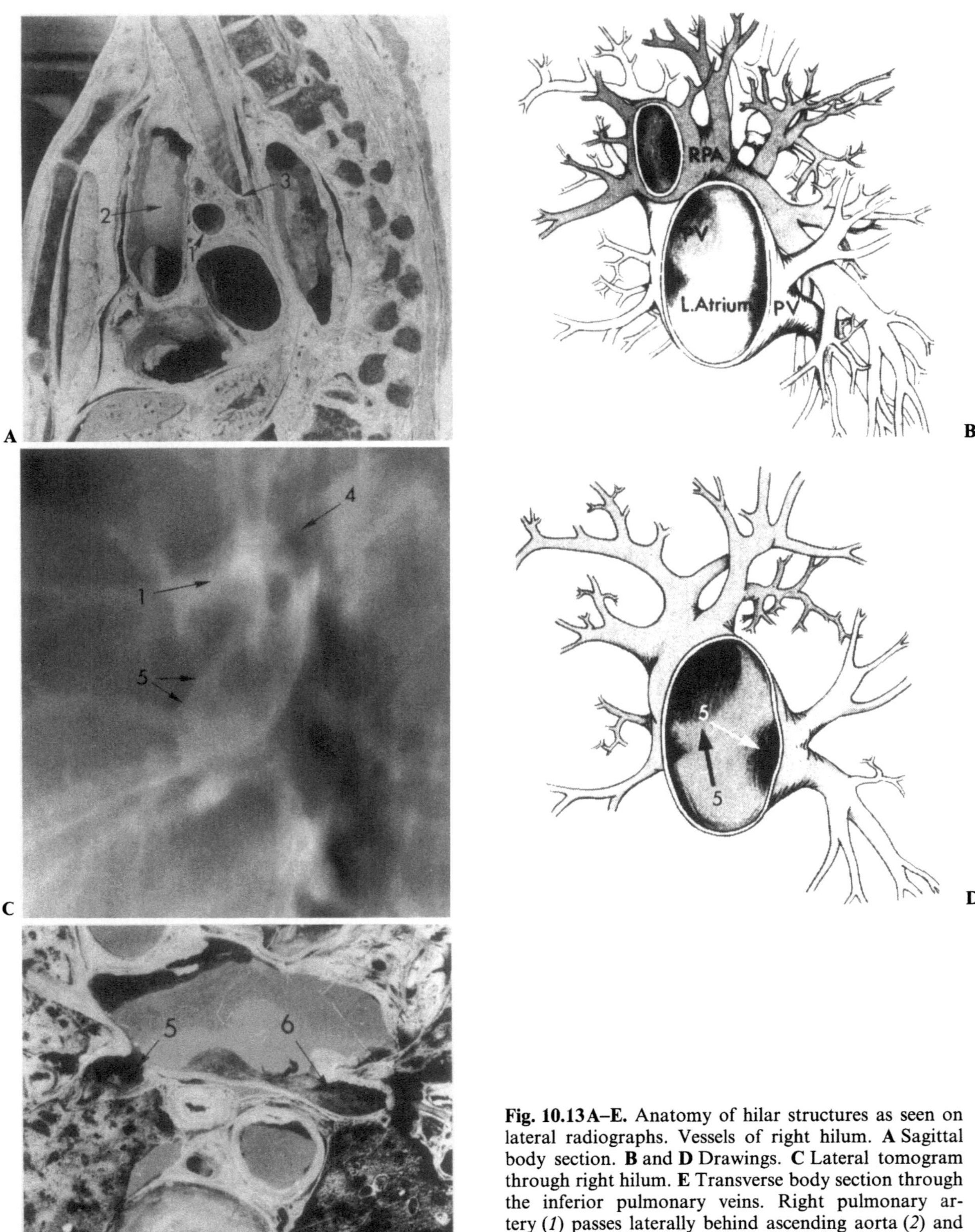

Fig. 10.13A–E. Anatomy of hilar structures as seen on lateral radiographs. Vessels of right hilum. **A** Sagittal body section. **B** and **D** Drawings. **C** Lateral tomogram through right hilum. **E** Transverse body section through the inferior pulmonary veins. Right pulmonary artery (*1*) passes laterally behind ascending aorta (*2*) and superior vena cava, in front of and slightly below carina (*3*). It courses into lung in front of and somewhat below right upper lobe bronchus (*4*) (see also Fig. 10.1). Confluence of right pulmonary veins (*5*) lies below artery and in coronal plane slightly anterior to confluence of left pulmonary veins (*6*). (**B** and **D** From [78])

rior pulmonary vein lies mainly anterior to the left upper lobe bronchus, although a branch of this vein may course from behind the bronchus and below it to join other superior pulmonary vein branches (Fig. 10.14). Both right and left inferior pulmonary veins are situated below and behind the superior pulmonary veins. The right inferior pulmonary veins enter the left atrium anterior to the left veins (Fig. 10.13). End-on visualization of the veins sometimes simulates a mass in the mediastinum or in the lung requiring oblique films or computed tomograms for differentiation.

The carina, usually lying at the level of the sixth thoracic vertebra, is rarely identified on lateral radiographs [63, 64]. The right upper lobe bronchus originates about 2.5 cm from the carina; the left, about 5 cm from it [44]. Both bronchi pass horizontally from their origin for a short distance and therefore can be seen end-on on most lateral chest radiographs (Fig. 10.15). Each bronchus is located in the plane of the trachea; a line drawn down the tracheal air column usually transects them both. Sometimes, the left upper lobe bronchus lies slightly posterior to this plane. The right upper lobe bronchus is higher than the left. In Lane and Whalen's [44] series, the distance between the two bronchi on the lateral radiograph varied from 1.0 to 3.7 cm and was the least in hyposthenic individuals and the greatest in hypersthenic persons. The left upper lobe bronchus is surrounded by vascular structures with the pulmonary artery above and behind, the superior pulmonary vein in front, and the left atrium and sometimes a branch of the superior pulmonary vein below and anterior (Figs. 10.5 and 10.14). Since it is so encompassed by vascular structures, the left upper lobe bronchus is usually easy to see on lateral radiographs. The right upper lobe bronchus is less easy to identify since it is surrounded primarily by lung. Only along its anteriosuperior margin, where it is in contact with the truncus anterior, is it marginated by a vessel [63, 64]. Proto and Speckman [63, 64] identified the left upper lobe bronchus on end in 77% of lateral films and the right upper lobe bronchus on end in only 15%.

Both of the figures are lower than those reported by Lane and Whalen [44].

Bachman et al. [3] commented on the demonstration of bronchial anatomy in true lateral radiographs and in radiographs made slightly off true lateral projection (Fig. 10.16). They identified the left upper lobe bronchus in 78% of true lateral projections. If the patient was turned into a position with the right hemithorax 10° anterior to the left, the left upper lobe bronchus was seen in 88% of patients whereas films made with the right chest 10° posterior to the left showed it in only 43%. The more frequent demonstration of the left upper lobe bronchus on lateral films made with the right chest slightly forward is due to the slightly posterior course of this bronchus. The right upper lobe bronchus was identified in 35% of true lateral projections, in 33% of examinations in which the patient was rotated into a position with the right chest 10° forward, and in 22% of radiographs in which the patient was rotated so that the right chest was 10° posterior to the left side. For a complete review of the effects of mild obliquity on the appearance of the hila on lateral radiographs, the reader is referred to the comprehensive article by Bachman et al. [3].

The demonstration of an abnormal position of the upper lobe bronchi, anterior or posterior to the plane of the trachea, can be an important diagnostic finding on lateral chest radiographs. Lane and Whalen [44] found posterior displacement of the left upper lobe bronchus (and the left main bronchus as well) in 92 of 100 patients with proven left atrial enlargement. In some patients, such displacement was the only abnormal radiographic finding. The bronchi may be displaced forward with upper lobe atelectasis and backward with lower lobe collapse [88]. Proto and Merhar [62] have emphasized that forward displacement of central bronchi identified on lateral radiographs or computed tomograms helps to distinguish large posterior pleural fluid collections from an expanded, opaque lower lobe. Posterior displacement of the bronchi, especially the left, may be associated with hiatus hernias of large size [88]. (A further discussion of displacement of the left main bronchus is included in chapter 7.)

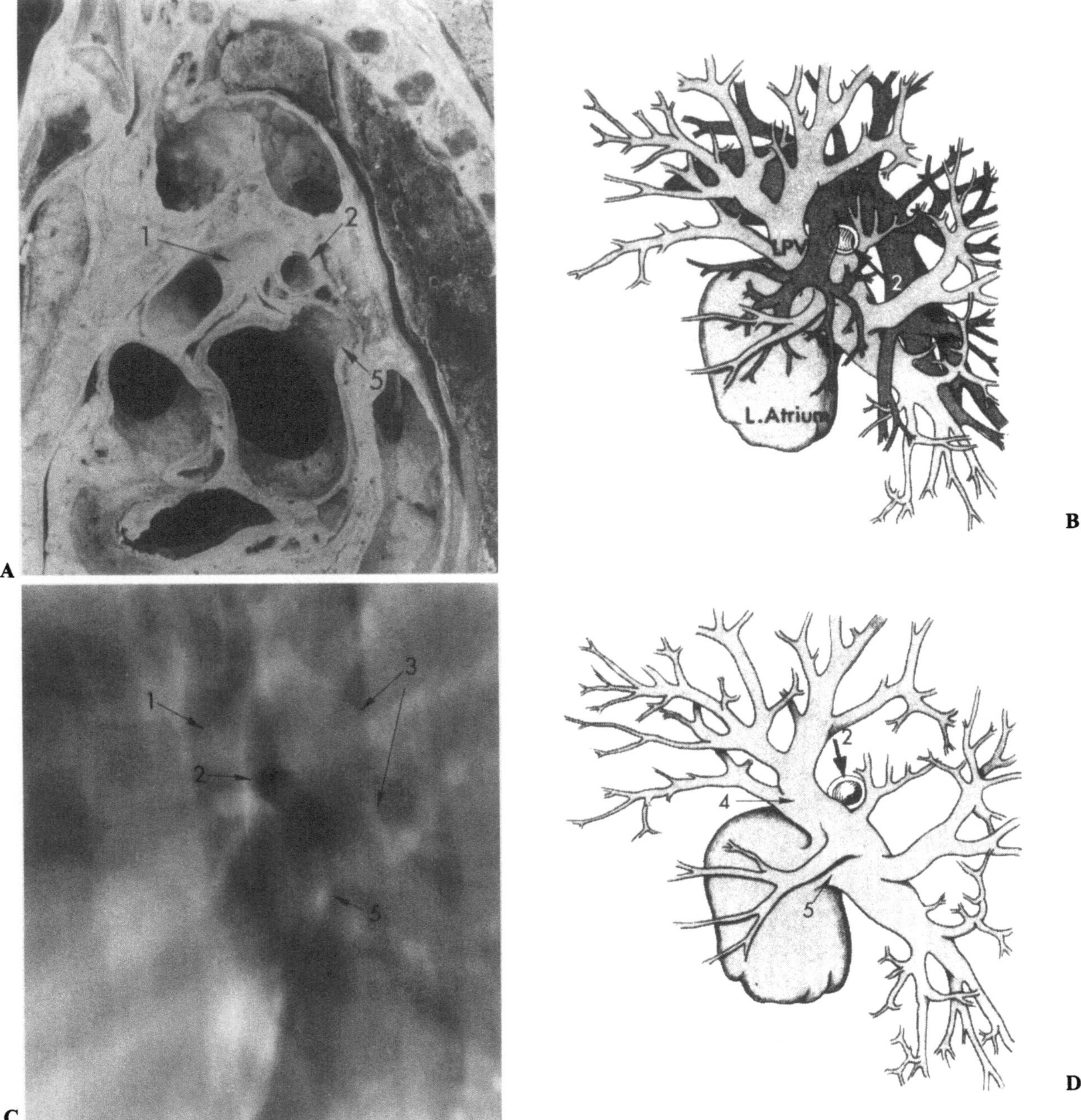

Fig. 10.14A–D. Anatomy of hilar structures as seen on lateral radiographs: vessels of the left hilum. **A** Sagittal body section. **B** and **D** Drawings. **C** Lateral tomogram through left hilum. Left pulmonary artery (*1*) courses superiorly and posteriorly from its point of origin, passing above left upper lobe bronchus (*2*). Descending branch of left pulmonary artery (*3*) passes behind bronchus. Left superior pulmonary vein (*4*) lies in front of bronchus. Confluence of left pulmonary veins (*5*) lies below left upper lobe bronchus in coronal plane slightly posterior to confluence of right pulmonary veins (see Fig. 10.13E). (**B** and **D** From [78])

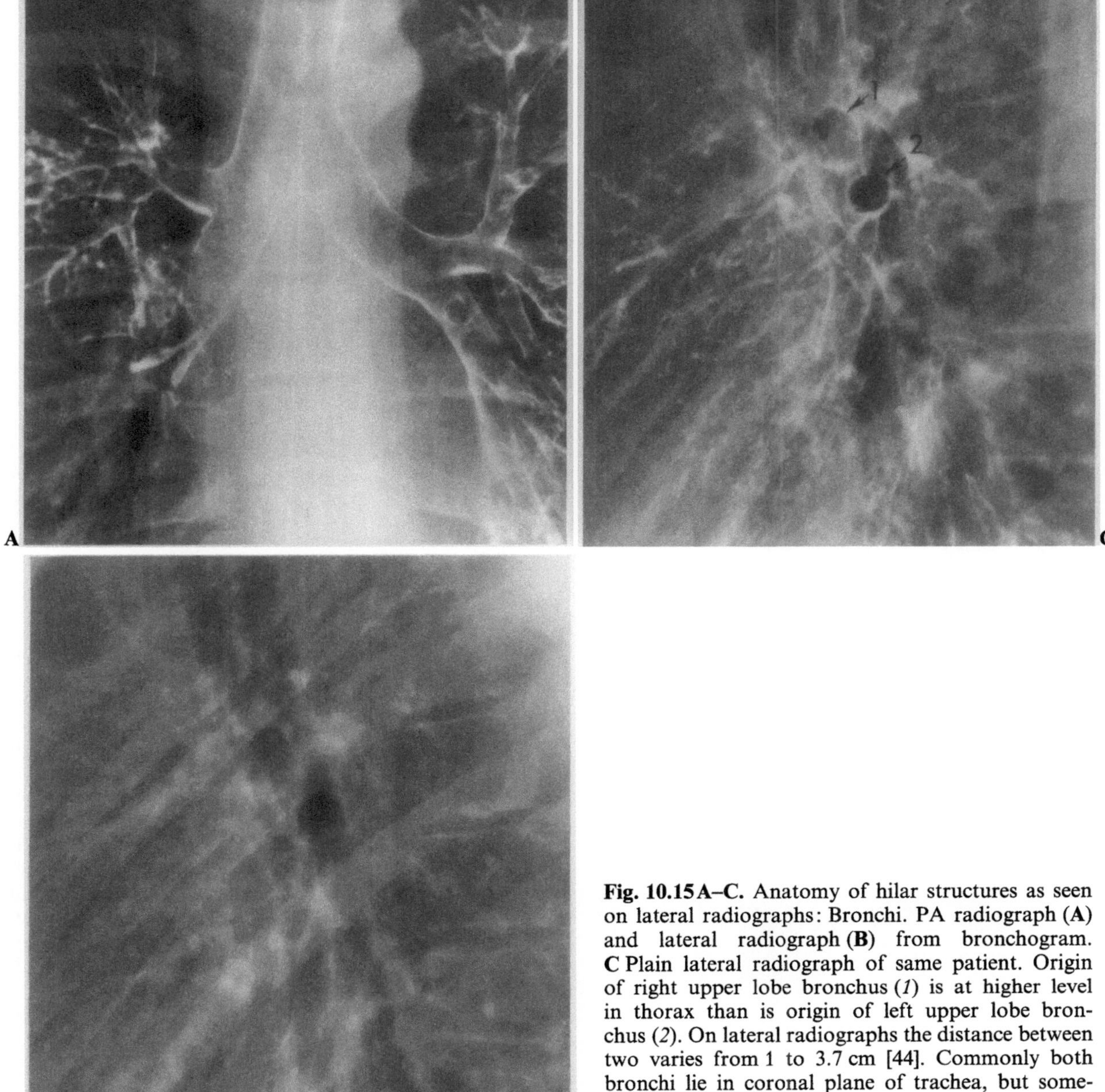

Fig. 10.15A–C. Anatomy of hilar structures as seen on lateral radiographs: Bronchi. PA radiograph (**A**) and lateral radiograph (**B**) from bronchogram. **C** Plain lateral radiograph of same patient. Origin of right upper lobe bronchus (*1*) is at higher level in thorax than is origin of left upper lobe bronchus (*2*). On lateral radiographs the distance between two varies from 1 to 3.7 cm [44]. Commonly both bronchi lie in coronal plane of trachea, but sometimes left upper lobe bronchus lies slightly posterior to this plane

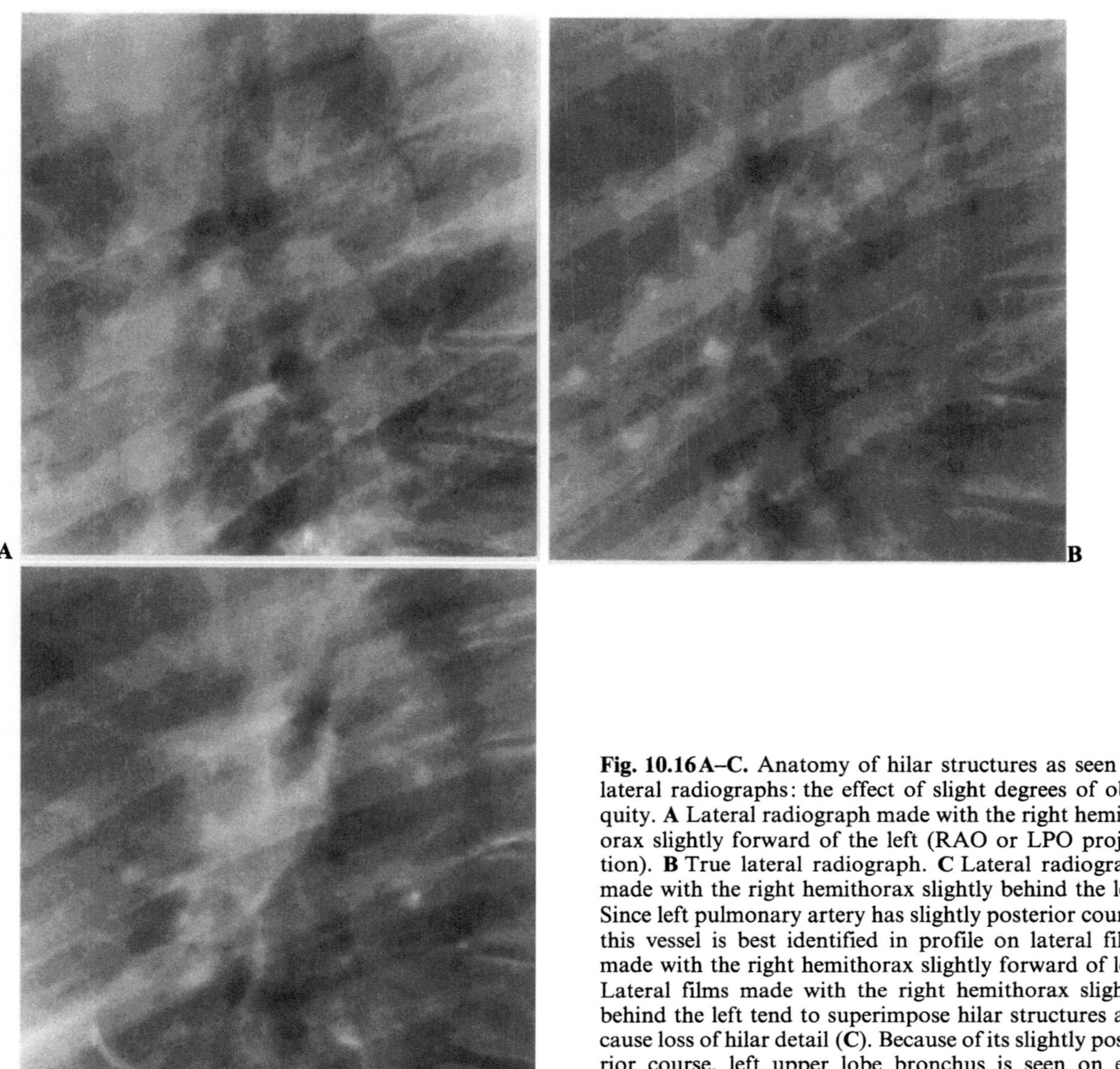

Fig. 10.16A–C. Anatomy of hilar structures as seen on lateral radiographs: the effect of slight degrees of obliquity. **A** Lateral radiograph made with the right hemithorax slightly forward of the left (RAO or LPO projection). **B** True lateral radiograph. **C** Lateral radiograph made with the right hemithorax slightly behind the left. Since left pulmonary artery has slightly posterior course, this vessel is best identified in profile on lateral films made with the right hemithorax slightly forward of left. Lateral films made with the right hemithorax slightly behind the left tend to superimpose hilar structures and cause loss of hilar detail (**C**). Because of its slightly posterior course, left upper lobe bronchus is seen on end somewhat more frequently on lateral films made with the right hemithorax anterior to the left

The posterior walls of the major bronchi can often be identified as they extend from each hilum. Proto and Speckman [63, 64] were able to see the posterior walls of the right main and intermediate bronchus in about 95% of patients.

Schnur et al. [75] identified the posterior wall of the intermediate bronchus well in 50% of patients and less well in another 40%. Visualization of the wall is improved on lateral films made with the right chest slightly forward of the left. Contrast allowing demonstration of the posterior wall of the right main and intermediate bronchus is provided by lung in the azygoesophageal recess. This interface is well shown at computed tomography. The anterior walls of the right main and intermediate bronchi are rarely seen due to their intimate contact with vessels anterior to them (Figs. 10.1–10.4). The posterior wall of the left main bronchus is much less commonly seen and was identified in about 45% of patients by Proto and Speckman [63, 64]. When seen, it was usually at or just below the left upper lobe bronchus where it was contacted by preaortic lung. The walls of the central bronchi are fine structures; abnormality can be suspected if they are more than 3 mm in thickness. Localized thickening or lobulation is more suggestive and raises the possibility of adjacent edema, lymph node enlargement or neoplasm [27, 75].

The right middle lobe bronchus is rarely seen in lateral projection and was identified in only 1.8% of Proto and Speckman's patients [63, 64].

In contrast to the more proximal airway, the posterior walls of the lower portions of the lower lobe bronchi cannot be seen due to the passage of the inferior pulmonary veins behind them. The anterior wall of the left lobe bronchus was seen in about 41% of Proto and Speckman's cases [63, 64]. The wall is said to be comma shaped on lateral radiographs and extends in a curvilinear course from the left upper lobe bronchial orifice (Figs. 10.14C and 10.15B). Its course is more posteriorly directed than is the right lower lobe bronchus (Fig. 10.15B), an anatomic feature thought to account for the greater frequency of aspiration into the left lower lobe than into the right lower lobe in supine patients.

10.2.3 Oblique Projection

It is unfortunate that today oblique radiographs at 30° or 45° are seldom used to evaluate hilar anatomy or pathology since they are simple, inexpensive and have considerable diagnostic value [89].

Favez and Soliman [16], and Favez et al. [17], and others [8, 50] have, however, popularized 55°-angled tomography of the hilum as an improved method of assessing hilar disease. In this technique, the plane of the patient's back is made to form an angle of 55% with the table top and conventional tomographic sections are made through the dependent hilum. The technique is said to be preferable to conventional tomography made in frontal or lateral projections since the bronchi are thrown into better profile and enlarged lymph nodes are better seen at the bronchial bifurcations. Tomograms at 55° are not easy to interpret and require considerable experience and skill [8].

In the era of computed tomography, 55°-angled tomography still has its advocates. However, most observers feel that computed tomography performed with state-of-the-art equipment provides more information about hilar anatomy and pathology [31, 48, 83] (see chapter 3). It is preferred by many experienced radiologists because of the additional information concerning lung and mediastinum which it provides.

10.2.4 Axial Projection

Study of the hilum in the axial or transverse plane may be achieved by computed tomography or by magnetic resonance imaging.

10.2.4.1 Computed Tomography

Computed tomography is, at the present time, the definitive modality for imaging the pulmonary hilum. Optimum demonstration of the hilum at computed tomography requires state-of-the-art equipment and meticulous attention to technique. Glazer et al. [30, 32] have suggested a standard protocol for the performance of computed tomography of the hilum. Initially, a drip infusion of 30% meglumine iothalamate is started and contiguous sections 1 cm in thickness are obtained from the pulmonary apices to the right upper lobe bronchus. Scanning is then stopped and an intravenous bolus injection of 40–50 cc 60% meglumine iothalamate is begun. After one-half of the bolus has been injected, rapid sequence scanning is started again using 1 cm contiguous slices. Usually, six sections extending caudally from the right upper lobe bronchus are adequate to demonstrate the entire hilum. Thin section analysis is sometimes performed using 5 mm thick sections. Images should be observed at both lung and mediastinal settings. Many problems related to the hilum can be evaluated satisfactorily without contrast enhancement, although it is the opinion of authors such as Sone et al. [76] that an ideal study always employs contrast.

Since the anatomy of the two hila is considerably different, radiologic correlations with anatomy will be discussed separately for each side. The studies of Gamsu [23–25], Naidich et al. [54–57], and Webb et al. [81, 82] were heavily relied upon for the development of the ensuing sections. Jardin and Remy [43] have provided a detailed study of the segmental bronchovascular anatomy of the lower lobes with computed tomographic correlations. Review of these papers is strongly recommended.

The Right Hilum

The right pulmonary artery can be identified in all computed tomographic scans as it courses in a gentle arc, with convexity posterior, across the pericardium (see Figs. 10.2, 10.18). It can always be seen to pass between the superior vena cava anteriorly and the right main and intermediate bronchi posteriorly (see Figs. 10.2, 10.18). Just before exiting from the pericardial sac, the right pulmonary artery gives rise to the truncus anterior, the branch to the right upper lobe (see Figs. 10.4, 10.17). The truncus anterior is visible in all computed tomographic scans. Depending upon the angle of ascent of the vessel and the level of computed tomographic section, it can be imaged as a round or oval structure (Fig. 10.17). In non-enhanced scans it can be difficult to distinguish the vessel from a node or a mass (Fig. 10.19 B). Its AP dimension is usually equal to or less than the diameter of the right main bronchus, but in one-third of the cases studied by Webb et al. it was larger than the right main bronchus [81]. A soft tissue aggregate 0.3–1.5 cm in diameter composed of lymph nodes and fat is present lateral to the truncus anterior in normal subjects [76, 84] (see Figs. 10.4, 10.30). Large opacities or lobulated densities in this area are abnormal (see Figs. 10.27 B, 10.30). The right interlobar artery passes downward anterolateral to the upper portion of the bronchus intermedius and lateral to the lower portion of the bronchus intermedius [81] (Fig. 10.18). An exception to this rule occurs when the upper portion of the interlobar artery adopts a posterior course (Fig. 10.12, see section 10.2.1.4). In such instances, the artery will lie lateral to the upper portion of the intermediate bronchus and may simulate a mass. In its descent, the interlobar artery passes between the origins of the right middle lobe and superior segmental bronchi and presents a single rounded prominence against adjacent lung (Fig. 10.18). Lobulation at this level is abnormal [81, 82]. On the appropriate computed tomographic section, the interlobar artery and the superior segmental artery arising from it produce a vascular configuration resembling a comma [81] (Fig. 10.18). The descending branch

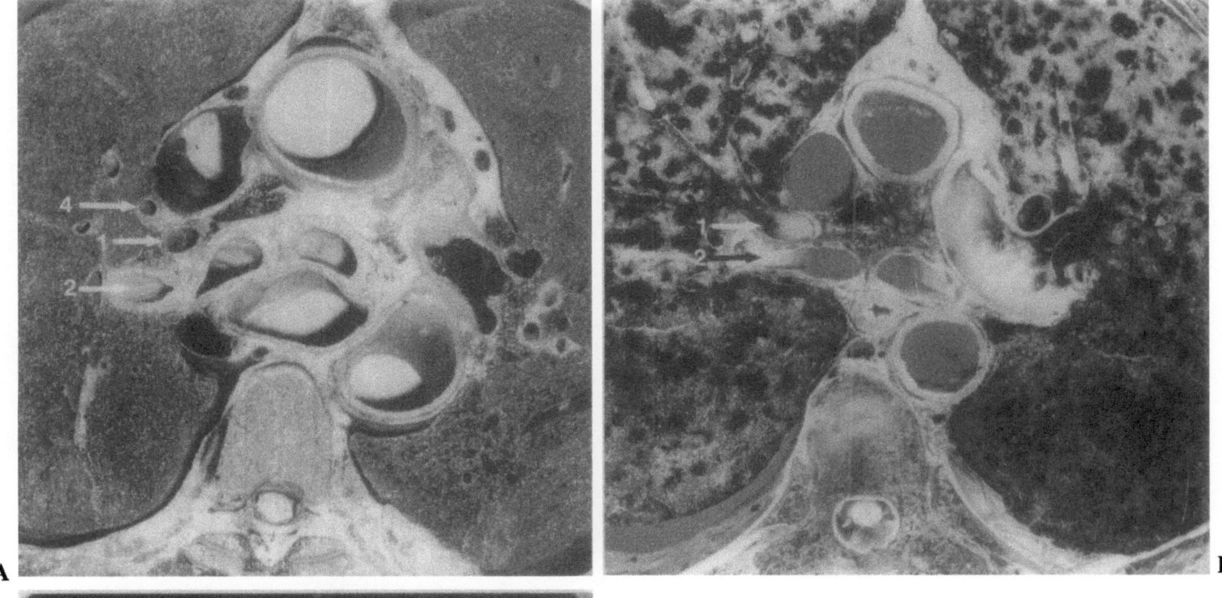

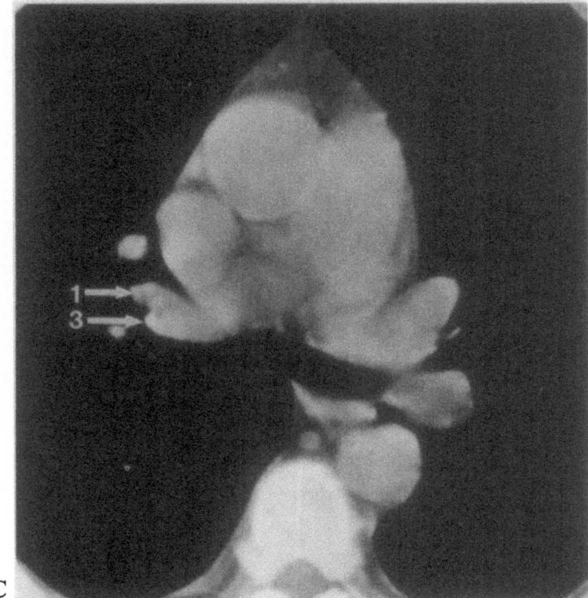

Fig. 10.17 A–C. Arterial anatomy of the right hilum at computed tomography. The truncus anterior. **A** and **B** Transverse body sections. **C** Computed tomogram with contrast enhancement. The arterial branch to the right upper lobe, the truncus anterior (*1*) is so named because it lies immediately anterior to the right upper lobe bronchus (*2*). Depending upon the degree of its ascent from the hilum, its appearance in cross section may be round (**A**) or oval (**B**). Either configuration may simulate a mass on computed tomograms and contrast enhancement may be necessary to prove the vascular nature of the shadow. In **C** the truncus anterior (*1*) is seen as an oval structure of the same density of the parent right pulmonary artery (*3*). Note also the anterior branch of the right superior pulmonary vein (*4*)

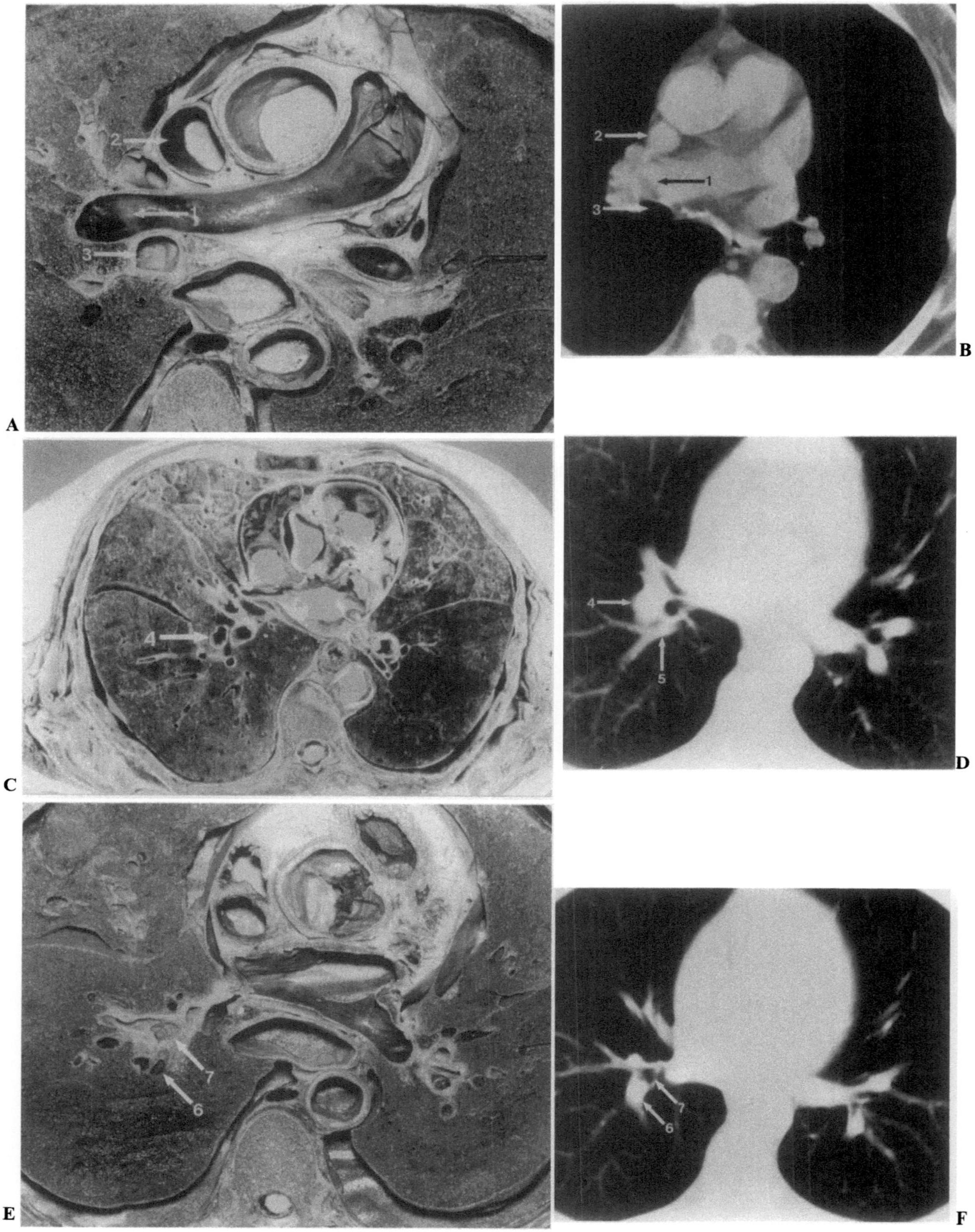

A
B
C
D
E
F

◁ **Fig. 10.18 A–F.** Arterial anatomy of the right hilum at computed tomography. **A, C,** and **E** Transverse body sections. **B, D,** and **F** Computed tomograms. The right pulmonary artery (*1*) courses in a gentle arc, with convexity directed posteriorly, across the mediastinum. On all computed tomograms it can be identified between the superior vena cava (*2*) and intermediate bronchus (*3*). After giving rise to the truncus anterior branch (see Fig. 10.17) it exits the pericardium, turning inferiorly or occasionally posteriorly (see section 10.2.1.4). The right interlobar artery (*4*) passes downward anterolateral to the upper portion of the bronchus intermedius (**A** and **B**) and lateral to the lower portion of the bronchus intermedius (**C** and **D**). In this part of its course, the vessel produces a single rounded mass against lung (**C** and **D**). In **D** the interlobar artery and the superior segmental artery (*5*) combine to produce a shadow resembling a comma [81]. The vessel continues caudad between the middle and superior segmental bronchi. At the origins of the basal segmental arteries, a lobulated shadow may be seen. The basal segmental arteries (*6*) lie lateral and/or posterior to the corresponding bronchi (*7*)

of the right pulmonary artery gives rise to the basal segmental arteries. At the origin of these vessels, the right pulmonary artery can adopt a lobulated configuration [81] (Fig. 10.18).

The venous anatomy of the lungs is quite variable, but a knowledge of the usual configuration of the superior pulmonary veins is necessary to avoid misinterpretation of a normal vein as a node or a mass (see Fig. 10.24). The right superior pulmonary vein is formed as a result of confluence of anterior (apical anterior) and posterior tributaries. The posterior branch always can be identified in the notch formed by the anterior and posterior segmental bronchi to the right upper lobe (Fig. 10.19). As it descends, the anterior vein can be seen lying in front of the truncus anterior and behind the superior vena cava where it can simulate a node or a mass (Figs. 10.17, 10.19). The two veins converge to form the superior pulmonary vein and are joined by the middle lobe vein or veins anterior to the middle lobe bronchus [5] (Fig. 10.19). Anterior to the middle lobe bronchus, the superior pulmonary vein can be mistaken for a node or a mass (Fig. 10.19).

Lung in the azygoesophageal recess always contacts the posterior wall of the right main and upper lobe bronchi and allows assessment of the thickness of the bronchial walls at this point (Fig. 10.21). Wall thickness should not exceed 3 mm and is usually less than 1.5 mm [63, 64]. Irregular thickening is highly suspect (see Fig. 10.27). Masses anterior to the right upper lobe bronchus on computed tomographic scans often distort or obstruct the anterior segmental bronchus and may displace it laterally [25].

The segmental bronchi to the right upper lobe adopt a trifurcate pattern [5]. The apical and anterior segmental bronchi can be identified in all computed tomographic examinations; the posterior segmental bronchus is not seen in all studies due to its obliquely cephalad course [81]. In most subjects, the apical bronchus lies with the main branch of the truncus anterior on its medial side; the posterior division of the superior pulmonary vein lies on its lateral aspect [81] (Fig. 10.20). Thus, a round density lateral to the apical bronchus is to be expected as a normal

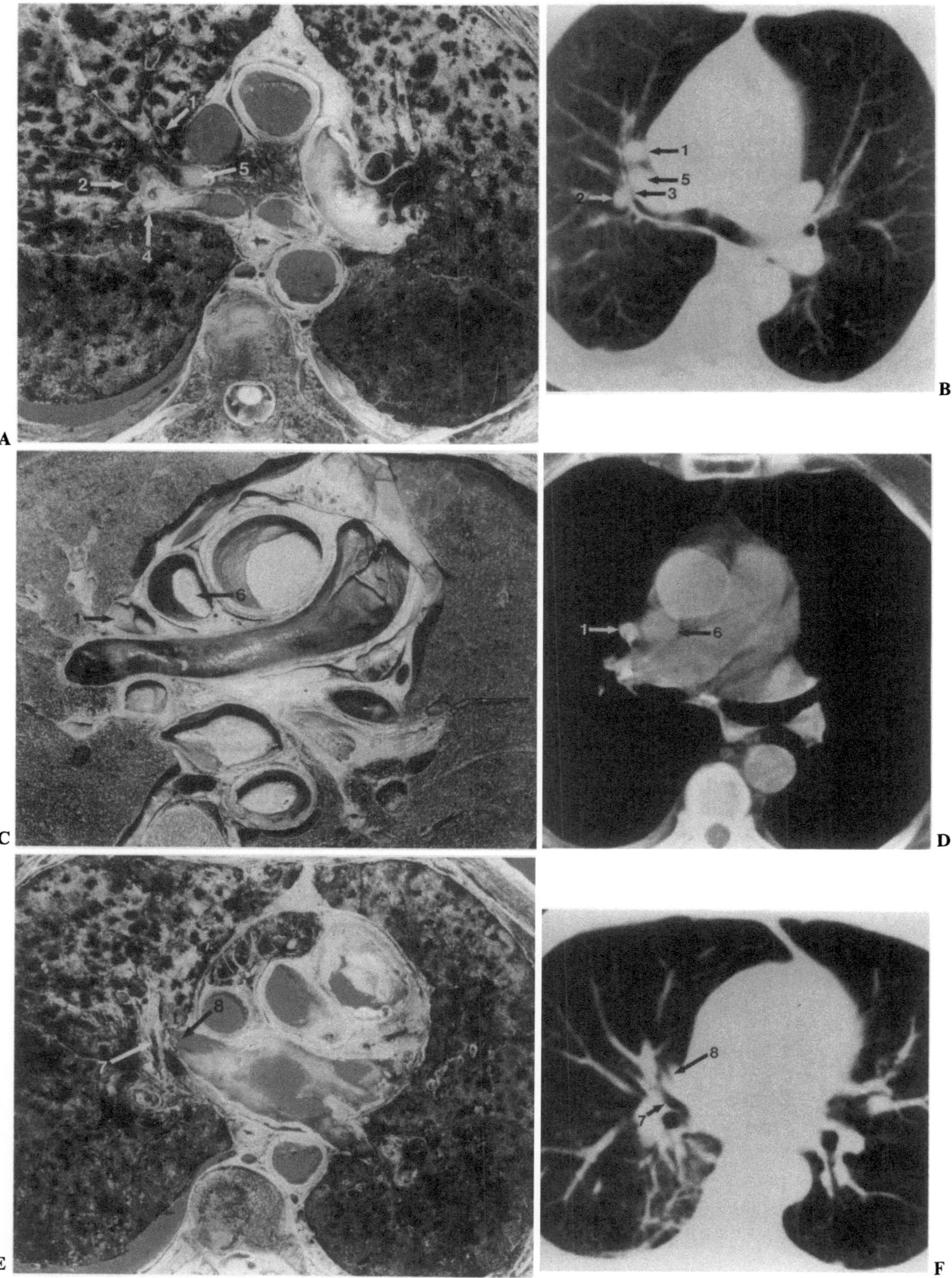

◁ **Fig. 10.19 A–F.** Venous anatomy of the right hilum at computed tomography. **A, C,** and **E** Transverse body sections. **B, D,** and **F** Computed tomograms. The anterior (apical anterior) (*1*) (see also Fig. 10.17 A) and posterior (*2*) veins of the right upper lobe combine to form the right superior pulmonary vein. The posterior branch is easily identified between the anterior (*3*) and posterior (*4*) segmental bronchi. In its descending course the anterior vein lies in front of the truncus anterior (*5*) and lateral or posterolateral to the superior vena cava (*6*). At this point, as in **B**, it may simulate a node or mass. In the computed tomogram shown in **D**, contrast enhancement proved the shadow to be vascular. Anterior to the right middle lobe bronchus (*7*) the superior pulmonary vein is joined by the middle lobe vein or veins where it again can simulate a node or a mass (*8*)

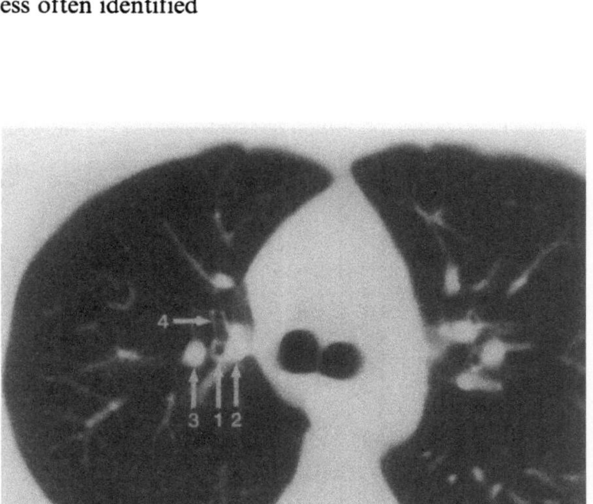

Fig. 10.20. Bronchial anatomy of the right hilum at computed tomography. Apical bronchus of the right upper lobe. The apical bronchus to the right upper lobe can be identified in all computed tomograms. Usually, the bronchus (*1*) lies between the main branch of the truncus anterior (*2*) medially and the posterior tributary of the right superior pulmonary vein laterally (*3*). In this patient, the anterior segmental bronchus (*4*) can also be identified. The posterior segmental bronchus usually runs a course oblique to the plane of section and is less often identified

finding. An ill-defined opacity is abnormal and raises the question of mass.

The intermediate bronchus is seen on two or three contiguous 1 cm thick sections in all patients [85] (Fig. 10.21). It is always contacted on its posterior aspect by lung in the azygoesophageal recess. Its thickness is similar to that of the right main and right upper lobe bronchi [63, 64]. It is commonly engulfed and distorted by right hilar neoplasms [75, 85] (see Fig. 10.27). The right middle lobe bronchus is seen in all patients, although its segmental bronchi are variably demonstrated [81] (Fig. 10.21). The superior segmental bronchus is visible in about 90% of patients [81] (Fig. 10.21). Sometimes its origin is opposite the take-off of the bronchus to the middle lobe but about as often it arises about 1 cm lower [54, 81].

Below the origin of the superior segmental bronchus, the common basal bronchus (the basal stem) [5] can be seen anterior to the lower lobe artery and the inferior pulmonary veins. Since the vessels lie behind the bronchus, density anterior to the bronchus should raise the likelihood of mass. The basal bronchi are often well seen at computed tomography, but it is commonly difficult to identify them precisely by segment (Fig. 10.21). Attempts can be made to identify them by level of origin (B-7 higher than B-8, etc.) and by their distribution. Rotation caused by collapse or pleural effusion can, however, make this a very frustrating exercise.

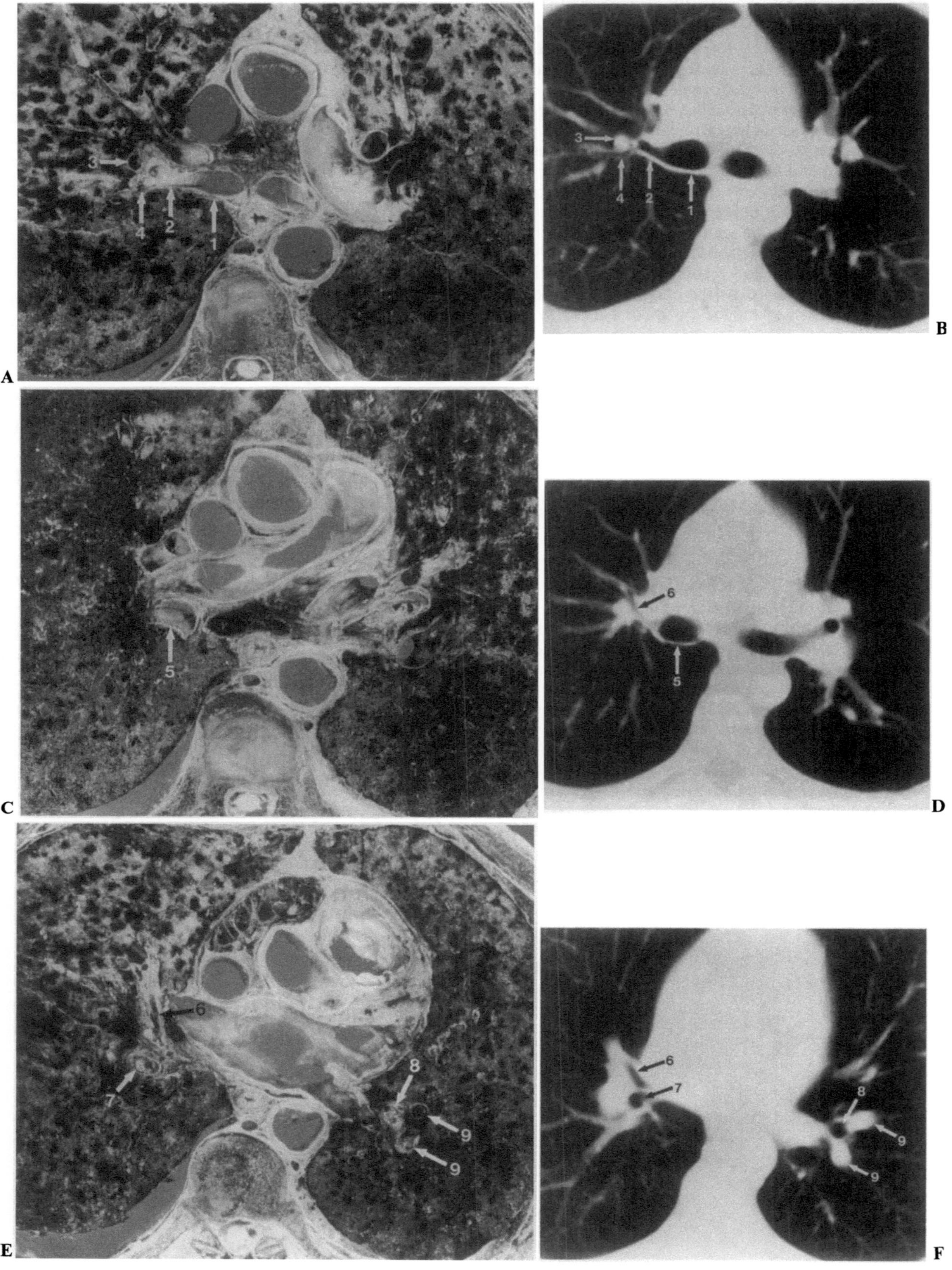

◁ **Fig. 10.21 A–F.** Bronchial anatomy of the right hilum at computed tomography. **A, C,** and **E** Transverse body sections. **B, D,** and **F** Computed tomograms. Lung in the azygoesophageal recess always contacts the posterior wall of the right main (*1*) and right upper lobe bronchi (*2*). Wall thickness should not exceed 3 mm and is usually less than 1.5 mm [63, 64]. Again note the posterior tributary of the right superior pulmonary vein (*3*) immediately anterior to the posterior segmental bronchus (*4*). The posterior wall of the intermediate bronchus (*5*) is also consistently identified and the right middle lobe bronchus (*6*) is always seen. Segmental bronchi to the middle lobe are variably shown. The superior segmental bronchus (*7*) is seen in about 90% of patients [81], arising at the level of the middle lobe bronchus or slightly below. Basal segmental bronchi (*8*) are inconstantly shown; they lie anterior and/or medial to their respective arterial branches (*9*)

The Left Hilum

The left pulmonary artery of course lies higher than the left (Fig. 10.22). On its downward course as the interlobar artery, it gives rise to the left superior segmental artery. The combination of the interlobar portion of the vessel and the superior segmental artery create a "comma-shaped" configuration on computed tomographic scans made through the inferior portion of the hilum [81]. The lower portion of the interlobar artery produces a rounded configuration against adjacent lung (Fig. 10.22). A lobulated configuration may be encountered at the level where the basal arteries take origin (Fig. 10.22).

Like the right superior pulmonary vein, the left superior pulmonary vein is formed by confluence of anterior (apical-anterior) and posterior branches. The posterior branch can often be seen lateral to the apical segmental bronchus [81] (Fig. 10.23). The superior pulmonary vein can be seen on computed tomographic scans as a distinct convexity anterior to the left pulmonary artery at its exit from the pericardium. It was identified by Webb et al. [81] in two-thirds of patients. Since this point is at the back of the lateral aspect of the aortic-pulmonic window, it is possible to confuse the vessel with a window node (Fig. 10.24). More inferior, the left superior pulmonary vein just above its entry into the left atrium can cause another convexity anterior to the lingular bronchus (Fig. 10.23).

The left upper lobe bronchus is lower (hyparterial bronchus) than the right upper lobe bronchus and on computed tomographic scans is usually seen on a section 1 cm below the right upper lobe bronchus. The left main and upper lobe bronchi are usually seen in a continuum on the same level of section (Fig. 10.26). The shadow of the left pulmonary artery, partially volumed, can be seen through the left upper lobe bronchus which usually demonstrates mild concavity of its posterior wall [54] (Fig. 10.26).

On computed tomographic examinations 86% of patients demonstrate lung in contact with the posterior wall of the left main and proximal lower lobe bronchi [80, 81] (Fig. 10.26). This "retrobronchial stripe" was seen by Proto and Speckman [63, 64] in 43% of plain

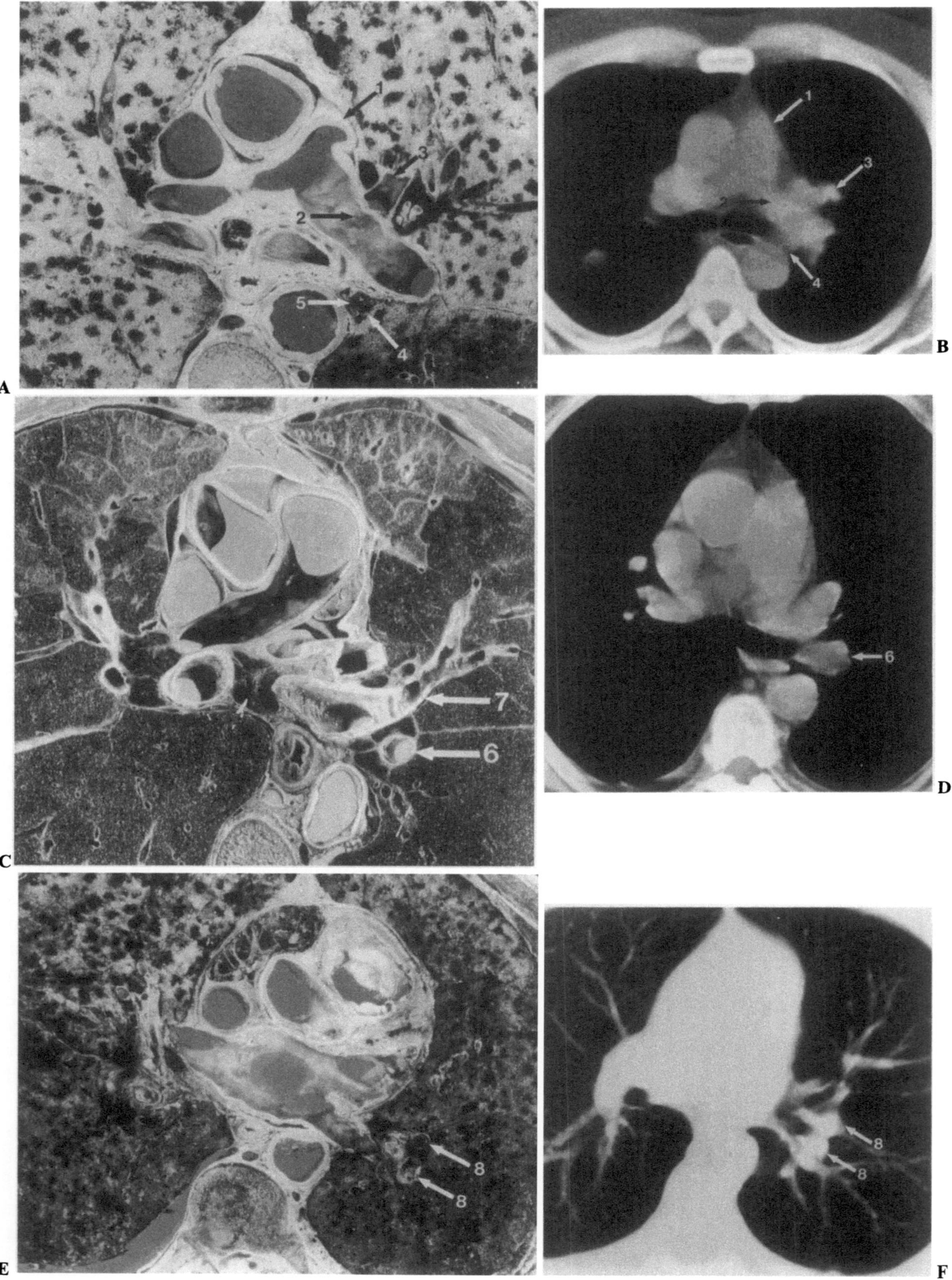

◁ **Fig. 10.22 A–F.** Arterial anatomy of the left hilum at computed tomography. **A, C,** and **E** Transverse body sections. **B, D,** and **F** Computed tomograms. The left pulmonary artery lies higher than the right pulmonary artery and is usually imaged on a section 1 cm higher. It can be identified arising from the main pulmonary artery (*1*) and adopts an arcuate posterior course (*2*) over the left main and upper lobe bronchi. The left superior pulmonary vein (*3*) is constantly identified anterior to the distal portion of the vessel. The posteromedial aspect of left pulmonary artery, proximal to its turn inferiorly, contacts the aorta permitting a beak-like intrusion of lung into the back of the aortic-pulmonic window (*4*). A lymph node (*5*) is commonly found at this point. The interlobar portion of the artery (*6*) descends between the lingular (*7*) and superior segmental bronchi. Its division into the basal arteries can result in a distinct lobulated appearance (*8*) on the appropriate level of section

lateral radiographs of the chest. In Proto and Speckman's series the thickness of this stripe did not exceed 2 mm. Greater thickening suggests mass [80]. The point of contact of bronchial wall with lung is posteromedial to the left pulmonary artery and anterolateral to the descending aorta and is made by lung which is preaortic in position (see chapter 7). Sometimes a "beak" or "tongue" of lung extends into the mediastinum posteromedial to the left pulmonary artery and anterolateral to the descending aorta (Fig. 10.22). A posteriorly directed convexity at this point is abnormal and commonly results from enlargement of a lymph nodes or nodes situated at this spot (see Fig. 7.14).

In 75% of individuals, the left upper lobe bronchus bifurcates into a superior and an inferior or lingular division [5]. In this circumstance the anterior segmental bronchus originates from the apical posterior bronchus [5] (Fig. 10.23). In 25% of persons, the anterior segment arises independently and a trifurcate branching pattern is present.

These anatomic variations are usually established at computed tomographic study. The apical bronchus is always visible, and the posterior branch of the superior pulmonary vein is seen lateral to it in 50% of examinations [54] (Fig. 10.25). As on the right side, a round opacity lateral to the apical bronchus is normal, any other density lateral to the bronchus is suspicious for mass [81]. The anterior segmental bronchus is seen in the majority of patients [81] (Fig. 10.23); the posterior segmental bronchus, like its right-sided counterpart is less often identified due to its obliquely cephalad course [81].

Sometimes, the lingular bronchus may be difficult to distinguish from the anterior segmental bronchus at computed tomographic examinations. A sharp raphe or "secondary carina" between the upper lobe bronchus at the lingular level and the lower lobe bronchus at the level of the superior segmental bronchus is usually the most helpful distinguishing feature [54] (Fig. 10.26). If, at the same level, a bronchus opposite the bronchus in question can be identified as the superior segmental bronchus (Fig. 10.26), the portion of the airway in question is confirmed as lingula. In many patients,

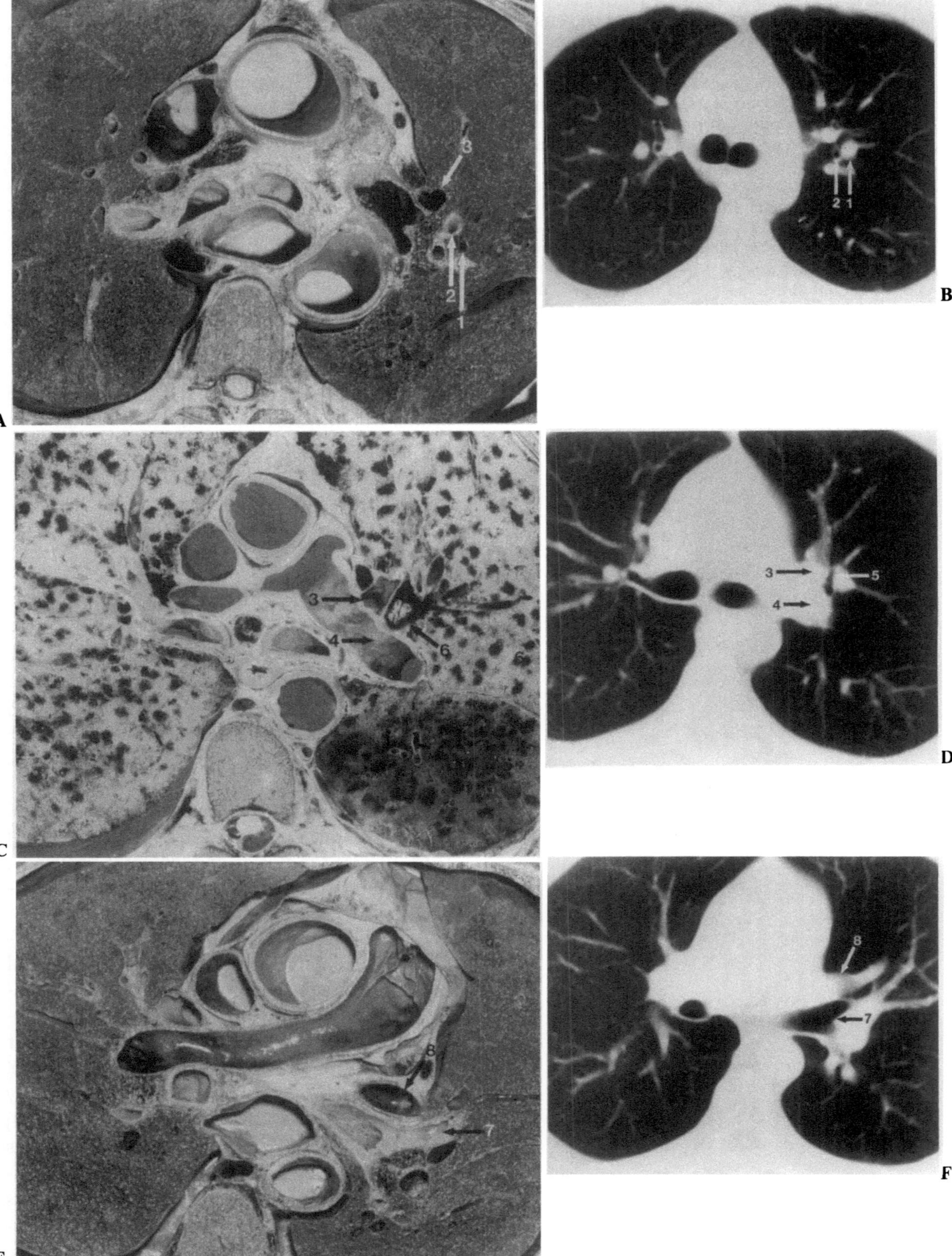

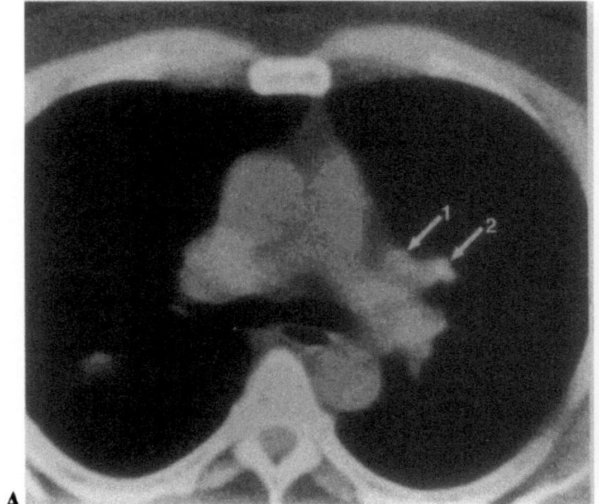

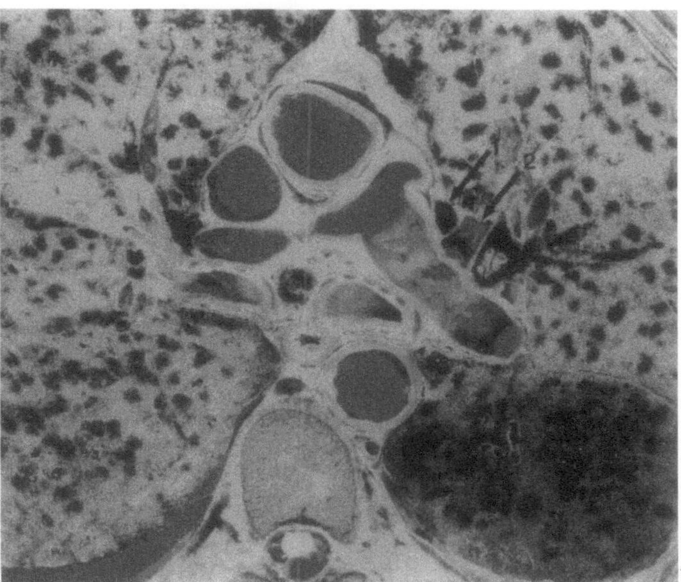

Fig. 10.24 A, B. Involvement of the left hilum by bronchogenic carcinoma. Findings at computed tomography. **A** Computed tomogram. **B** Transverse body section. Analysis of computed tomograms requires thorough knowledge of correlated radiographic anatomy to detect abnormality. In **A** a lymph node (*1*) in the lateral aspect of the aortic-pulmonic window lies adjacent to the left superior pulmonary vein (*2*). Sometimes the vein can be mistaken for a node or mass. Contrast enhancement may be required to determine whether the shadow is vascular. In this patient, several enlarged lateral aortic nodes were also present

◁ **Fig. 10.23 A–F.** Venous anatomy of the left hilum at computed tomography. **A, C,** and **E** Transverse body sections. **B, D,** and **F** Computed tomograms. The left superior pulmonary vein, like its counterpart on the right side, is formed by the union of anterior and posterior tributaries. The posterior division (*1*) is less constant than its right-sided counterpart being seen lateral to the apical bronchus (*2*) in about 50% of individuals [54, 81]. The left superior pulmonary vein (*3*) is consistently seen anterior to the distal portion of the main left pulmonary artery (*4*) and medial to the anterior segmental bronchus (*5*). (Note that this bronchus arises from the apical-posterior segmental bronchus.) A lymph node (*6*) is commonly seen adjacent to the vessel at this level. Not infrequently it is difficult to distinguish the vein from an enlarged lymph node without contrast enhancement. Anterior to the lingular bronchus (*7*) the lower portion of the left superior vein (*8*) just above the left atrium may again simulate a node or a mass

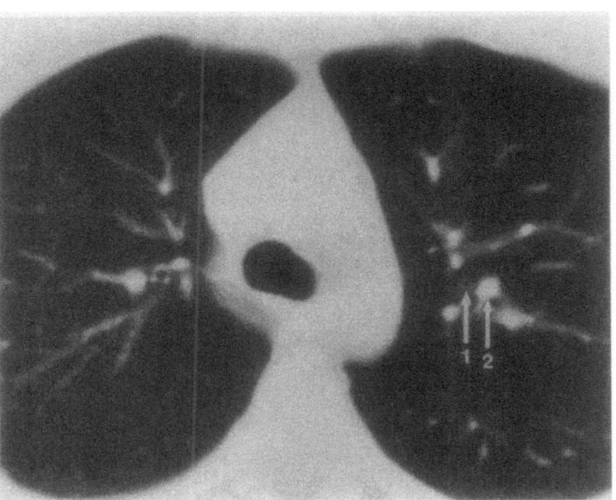

Fig. 10.25. Bronchial anatomy of the left hilum at computed tomography. Apical bronchus of the left upper lobe. The apical bronchus of the left upper lobe (*1*), a branch of the apical posterior bronchus, is seen on all computed tomograms. The posterior division of the left superior pulmonary vein (*2*) is inconstantly seen lateral to it. Usually lung contacts the lateral aspect of the bronchus; ill-defined soft tissue density lateral to it suggests disease [24, 82]

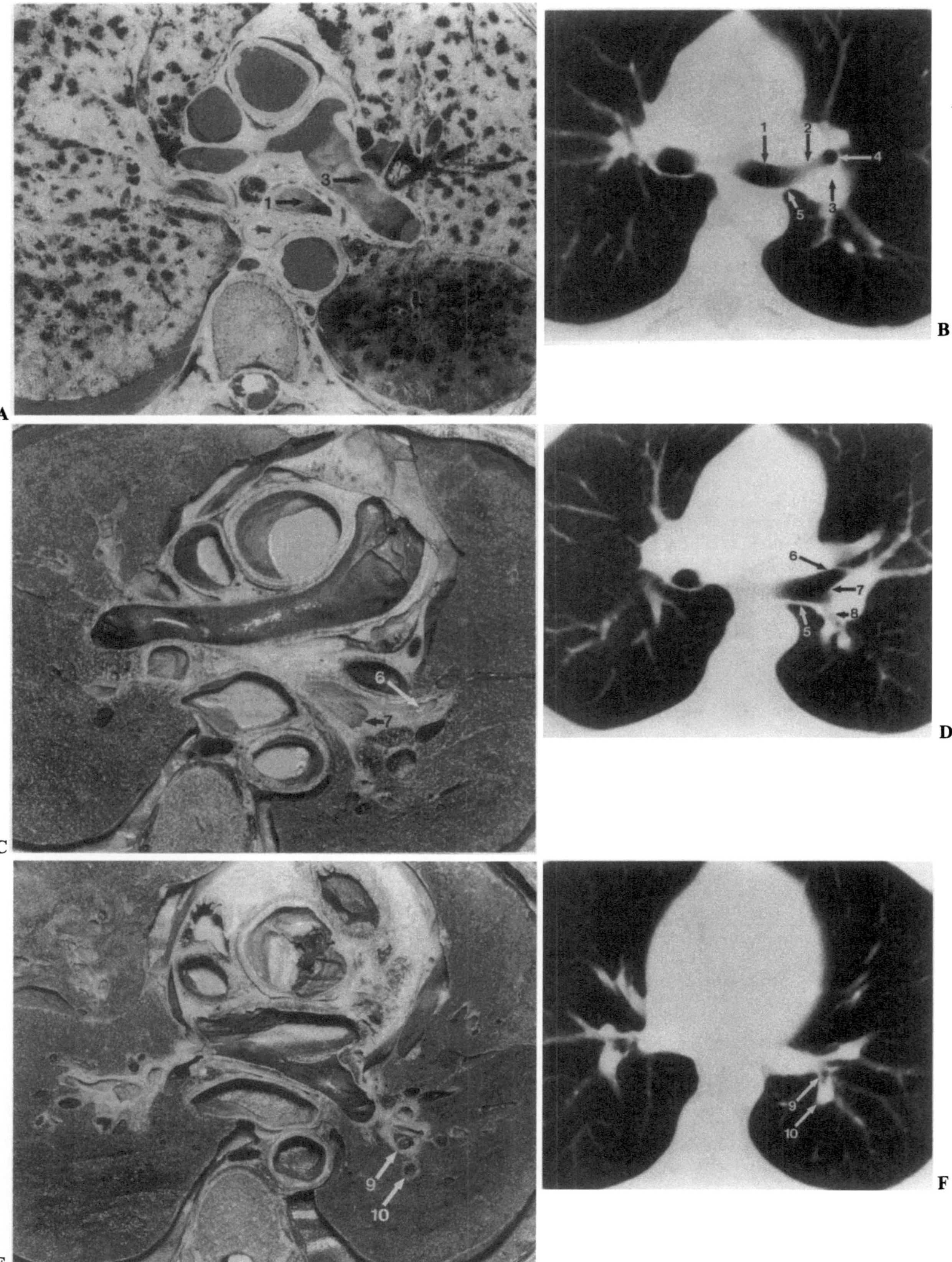

◁ **Fig. 10.26A–F.** Bronchial anatomy of the left hilum at computed tomography. **A, C,** and **E** Transverse body sections. **B, D,** and **F** Computed tomograms. The left main (*1*) and upper lobe (*2*) bronchi can be seen as a continuum in virtually all computed tomograms. Partial volume effect involving the left pulmonary artery (*3*) is also a constant feature. Most examinations show the apical posterior bronchus (*4*) imaged "end-on" at the termination of the left upper lobe bronchus. A large proportion of studies demonstrate lung in contact with the posterior wall of the left main bronchus (*5*) and left lower lobe bronchus. The lingular bronchus (*6*) is usually readily identified by the "secondary carina" or left upper lobe spur (*7*) behind it. The superior segmental bronchus (*8*) usually arises at this level but may originate somewhat lower. As on the right side the basal bronchi (*9*) lie anterior and/or medial to their corresponding arteries (*10*)

however, the superior segmental bronchus arises somewhat lower than the lingular bronchus [81].

The bronchus to the left basal segments, the basal trunk [5], courses anterior to its corresponding artery and the inferior pulmonary veins. Density anterior to the basal trunk suggests disease. Identification of basal bronchi on the left side is subject to the same vagaries that exist on the right.

Computed Tomography in Hilar Carcinoma

From the foregoing discussion it should be clear that the exquisite display of anatomy afforded by computed tomography makes it an excellent tool to study pathological anatomy produced by disease processes, notably bronchogenic carcinoma [15, 37, 38, 40, 65, 66, 83]. Webb et al. [83] have reviewed the findings at computed tomography in 30 patients with microscopically proven bronchogenic carcinoma who had a hilar mass. The principal findings fell into three categories: abnormal hilar contours, thickening of bronchial walls where they contact lung and bronchial narrowing, obstruction or displacement (Figs. 10.27, 10.28). Secondary signs such as atelectasis, mucoid impaction, etc. were seen in some patients.

Assessment of abnormal contours relied on evidence of deviation from the normal computed tomographic anatomy previously described. Nevertheless, judgement was often subjective [83]. On this basis 25 of 30 cases were judged abnormal (Table 10.1).

In the study 80% of patients had abnormal bronchi on computed tomographic scans. Only three of the patients showed bronchial abnor-

Table 10.1. Computed tomography in bronchogenic carcinoma presenting with a hilar mass ($n = 30$). (Adapted from [83])

	Right hilum ($n = 19$)	Left hilum ($n = 11$)
Abnormal hilar contour	16	9
Bronchial wall thickening	11	4
Bronchial narrowing obstruction or displacement	18	8

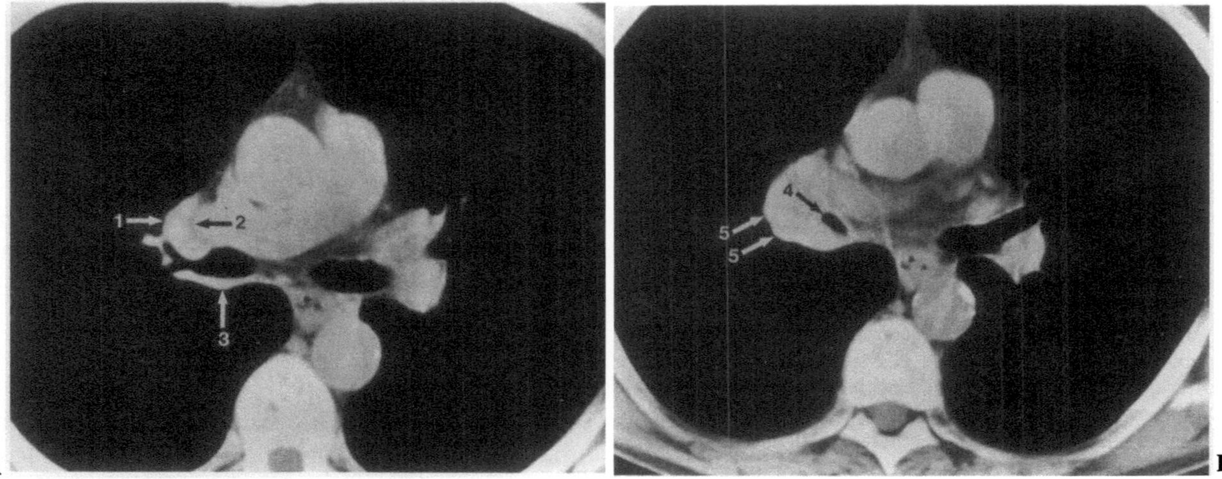

Fig. 10.27 A, B. Involvement of the right hilum by bronchogenic carcinoma. Findings at computed tomography. Computed tomography is an ideal modality to evaluate bronchogenic carcinoma involving the hilum. Principal findings are abnormal hilar contours, thickening of bronchial walls and bronchial narrowing, obstruction, or displacement [83]. In **A** too much soft tissue density (*1*) is seen lateral to the right pulmonary artery (*2*). Also seen is irregular thickening of the posterior wall of the right upper lobe bronchus (*3*). In **B** all detail lateral to the bronchus intermedius (*4*) is lost due to the presence of a lobulated mass (*5*). The intermediate bronchus is narrowed and rotated forward

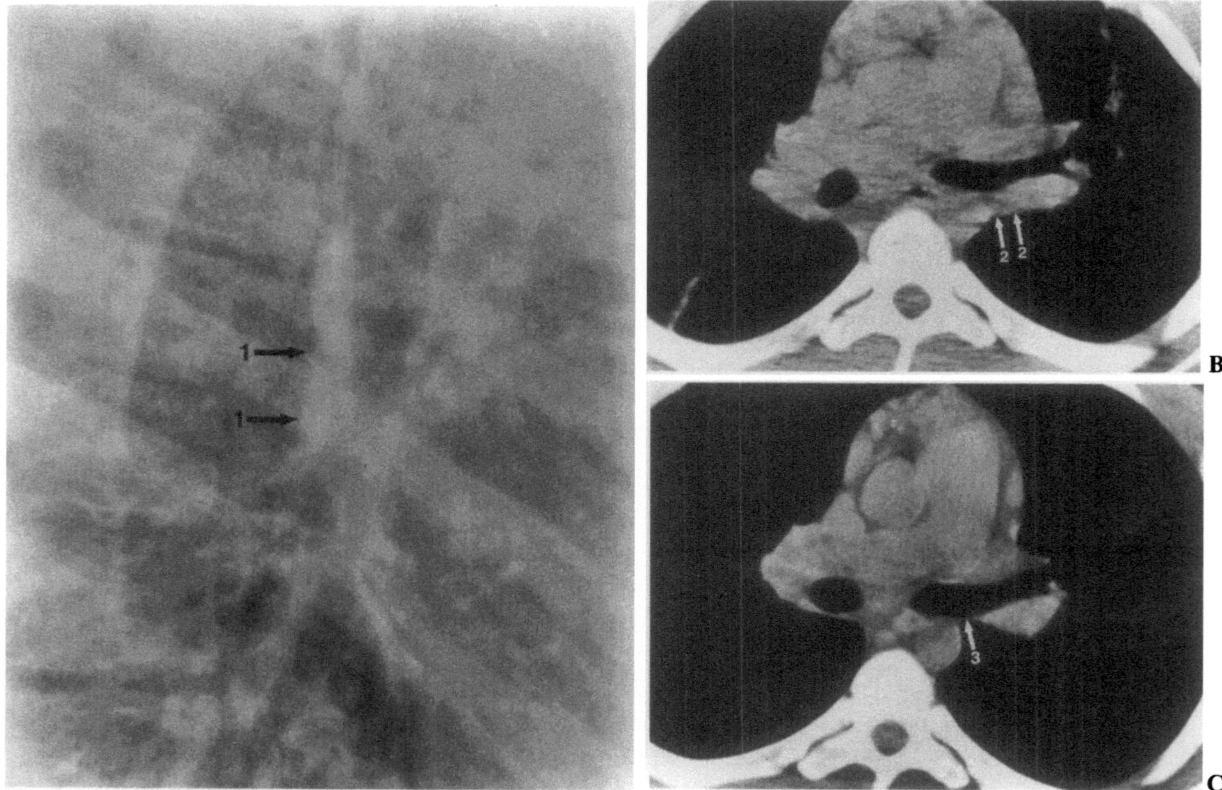

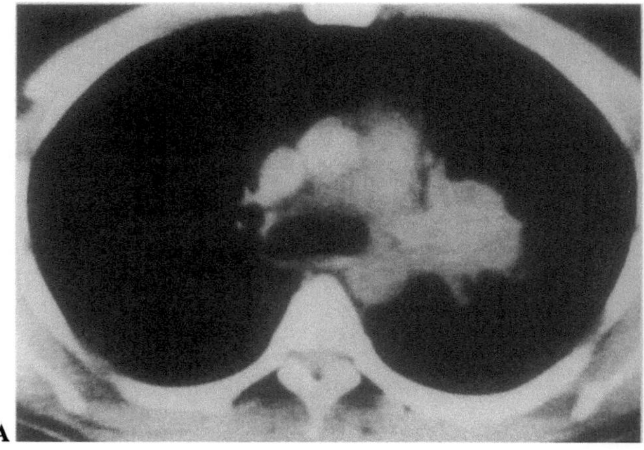

A

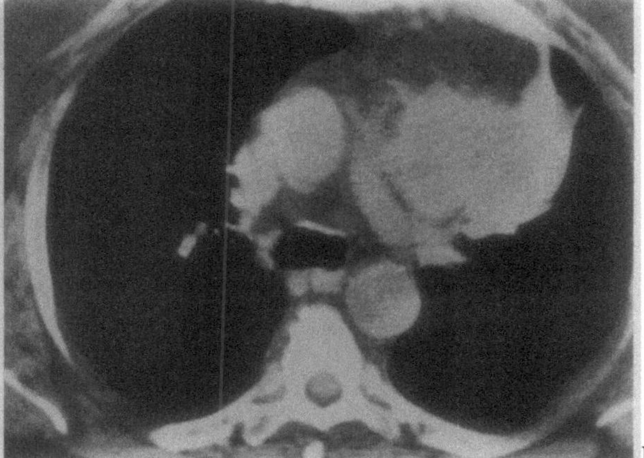

B

mality on plain films. Bronchial wall thickening was identified in 15 patients, and bronchial narrowing, obstruction, or displacement occurred in 26 (Table 10.1). Diagnosis of bronchial narrowing should be approached with caution; bronchi passing obliquely in or out of the plane of section may be incorrectly assessed as abnormal. Mucus or blood in bronchi can be misdiagnosed as tumor. Correlation with bronchoscopic findings are excellent in this series. Computed tomography did, however, show several abnormalities which were beyond the reach of the bronchoscope. Recently, Naidich et al. [58] also demonstrated excellent correlation of computed tomographic findings with findings at fiberoptic bronchoscopy.

A common, and difficult, problem in the evaluation of hilar pathology in proven or suspect bronchogenic carcinoma involves the determination of whether the process has invaded the mediastinum. This judgement has major impli-

◁ **Fig. 10.28 A–C.** Involvement of the left hilum by Hodgkin's disease. Findings at computed tomography. **A** Lateral radiograph. **B** and **C** Computed tomograms. Computed tomography is an excellent modality for judging thickening of bronchial walls, an abnormality often produced by neoplastic disease. In this young man with Hodgkin's disease, thickening of the posterior wall of the left main and lower lobe bronchi (*1*) is strongly suggested on the lateral radiograph and confirmed by computed tomography (*2*). After therapy (**C**), the bronchial wall thickening is no longer apparent. The disease process also involved the right hilum and anterior mediastinal nodes

Fig. 10.29 A, B. Computed tomographic assessment of direct mediastinal invasion by contiguous neoplasm. Direct invasion of contiguous neoplasm into the mediastinum can be difficult to assess at computed tomography. In **A** the left hilar mass did not invade the mediastinum although no fat plane was visible between the mass and the left pulmonary artery. The patient was resectable. Definite determination of mediastinal invasion can be made only if tentacles or wisps of tumor can be seen to interdigitate with mediastinal fat (**B**) or if tumor involves the central bronchi, vessels, or esophagus

cations for tumor staging (see chapter 3). Mere abutment of tumor against the mediastinum is insufficient evidence to conclude that the tumor has invaded the mediastinum; evidence that tumor extension interdigitates with mediastinal fat is required for definitive diagnosis [4] (Fig. 10.29).

Computed Tomography in the Detection of Hilar Adenopathy

Computed tomography has gradually emerged as the primary modality for the diagnosis of hilar lymph node enlargement suspected on plain chest radiography (see Fig. 10.10). In part, computed tomography is preferred because it affords evaluation of all of the lymph node stations in the thorax. A meticulous description of the anatomy of hilar lymphadenopathy has been provided by Sone et al. [76] and the interested reader is directed to this work for a detailed description. Like the diagnosis of bronchogenic carcinoma, lymphadenopathy is diag-

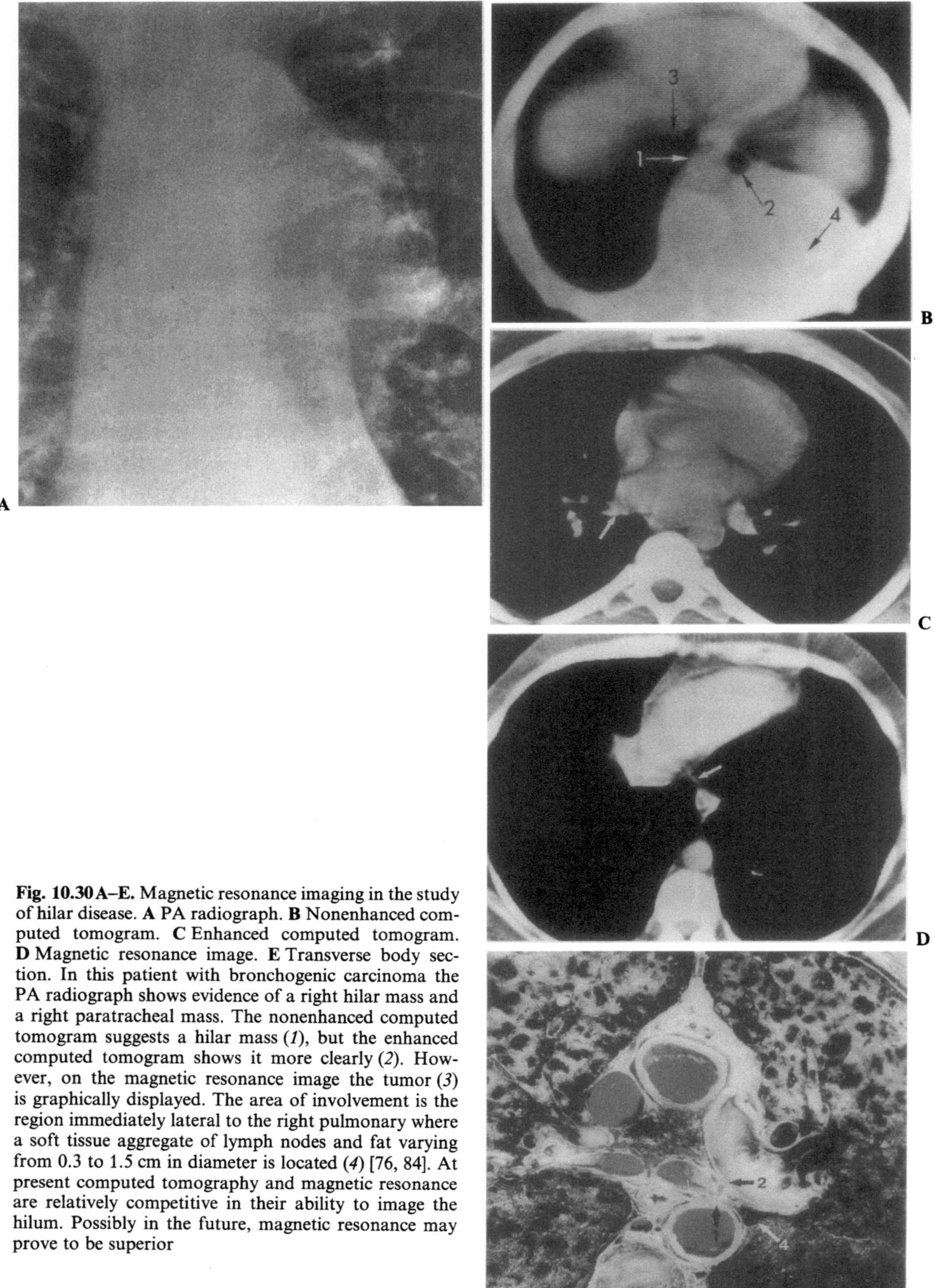

Fig. 10.30 A–E. Magnetic resonance imaging in the study of hilar disease. **A** PA radiograph. **B** Nonenhanced computed tomogram. **C** Enhanced computed tomogram. **D** Magnetic resonance image. **E** Transverse body section. In this patient with bronchogenic carcinoma the PA radiograph shows evidence of a right hilar mass and a right paratracheal mass. The nonenhanced computed tomogram suggests a hilar mass (*1*), but the enhanced computed tomogram shows it more clearly (*2*). However, on the magnetic resonance image the tumor (*3*) is graphically displayed. The area of involvement is the region immediately lateral to the right pulmonary where a soft tissue aggregate of lymph nodes and fat varying from 0.3 to 1.5 cm in diameter is located (*4*) [76, 84]. At present computed tomography and magnetic resonance are relatively competitive in their ability to image the hilum. Possibly in the future, magnetic resonance may prove to be superior

nosed on the basis of deviation from the normal anatomic appearances described previously. Gamsu [23] has studied the diagnosis of hilar adenopathy by computed tomography and found a sensitivity of 0.70, a specificity of 0.84 and a diagnostic accuracy (true positives + true negatives: total patients) of 0.81 in his series by patients.

10.2.4.2 Analysis of the Hilum by Magnetic Resonance Imaging

Imaging of the body by magnetic resonance is in its infancy. The efficacy of magnetic resonance imaging in the evaluation of thoracic disease is incompletely determined [10, 11, 26, 32, 36, 47, 60, 84, 86, 87]. It is certainly true that magnetic resonance imaging allows a ready distinction of hilar mass from vascular structures without the need for contrast enhancement often required in computed tomographic examinations [32, 36, 47]. Preliminary studies comparing computed tomography and magnetic resonance imaging of the hila suggest that in most instances both studies provide essentially the same information. In a few cases, computed tomography proved superior, and in a few others, magnetic resonance imaging was superior (Fig. 10.30). These preliminary studies would suggest that magnetic resonance imaging is as sensitive as computed tomography for the detection of hilar mass or adenopathy [32, 36, 84]. Computed tomography offers better spatial resolution; for example, bronchial anatomy is much better demonstrated by computed tomography than by magnetic resonance imaging because of this important factor. It may be, however, that magnetic resonance imaging will prove to be more sensitive than computed tomography to distinguish neoplasm from other hilar masses. It is generally conceded that T1-weighted images provide the greatest image contrast between hilar tumor and adjacent mediastinal fat, whereas T2-weighted images result in better spatial resolution and the strongest signal from hilar masses [60]. Usually both short and long repetition times are employed. Thus far, exploitation of the capability of magnetic reso-nance to provide imaging in the sagittal or coronal plane without degradation of spatial resolution has not achieved wide popularity [60, 84].

References

1. American Committee for Cancer Staging and End Result Reporting (1973) Clinical staging system for carcinoma of the lung. Chicago
2. Austin JMH (1984) The lateral chest radiograph in the assessment of nonpulmonary health and disease. Radiol Clin North Am 22:687–698
3. Bachman DM, Ellis K, Austin JHM (1978) The effects of minor degrees of obliquity on the lateral chest radiograph. Radiol Clin North Am 16:465–485
4. Baron RL, Levitt RG, Sagel SS, White MJ, Roper CL, Marburger JP (1982) Computed tomography in the preoperative evaluation of bronchogenic carcinoma. Radiology 145:727–732
5. Boyden EA (1955) Segmental anatomy of the lung. McGraw-Hill, New York
6. Chang CH (1962) The normal roentgenographic measurement of the pulmonary artery in 1085 cases. Am J Roentgenol Radium Ther Nucl Med 87:929–935
7. Chang CH, Zinn TW (1976) Roentgen recognition of enlarged hilar lymph nodes. Radiology 120:291–296
8. Chasen MH, Yrizarry JM (1983) Tomography of the pulmonary hili: anatomical reassessment of the conventional 55 degree posterior oblique view. Radiology 149:365–369
9. Clemente CD (1985) Gray's anatomy, 30th Am edn. Lea and Febiger, Philadelphia
10. Cohen AM (1984) Magnetic resonance imaging of the thorax. Rad Clin North Am 22:829–846
11. Cohen AM, Creviston S, LiPuma JP, Bryan PJ, Haaga JR, Alfidi RJ (1983) NMR evaluation of hilar and mediastinal lymphadenopathy. Radiology 148:739–742
12. Cooper C, Moss AA, Buy J-N, Stark DD (1983) CT appearance of the normal inferior pulmonary ligament. AJR 141:237–240
13. Don C, Hammond DI (1985) Vascular converging points of the right pulmonary hilus and their diagnostic significance. Radiology 155:295–298
14. Doppman JL, Lavender JP (1963) The hilum and the large left ventricle. Radiology 80:931–936
15. Faling LJ, Pugatch RD, Jung-Legg Y, Daly BDT, Hong WK, Robbins AH, Snider GL (1981) Computed tomographic scanning of the mediastinum in the staging of bronchogenic carcinoma. Am Rev Respir Dis 124:690–695
16. Favez G, Soliman O (1966) Radiological examination of the lung and mediastinum with the aid of posterior oblique tomography at an angle of 55 degrees. (Karger, Basel), Hafner, New York

17. Favez G, Willa C, Heinzer F (1974) Posterior oblique tomography at an angle of 55 degrees in chest roentgenology. Am J Roentgenol 120:907–915

18. Felson B (1968) More chest roentgen signs and how to teach them. Radiology 90:429–441

19. Felson B (1969) The mediastinum. Semin Roentgenol 4:41–58

20. Felson B (1973) Chest roentgenology. Saunders, Philadelphia

21. Friedman PJ (1981) Practical radiology of the hila and mediastinum. Postgrad Radiol 1:269–304

22. Friedman PJ (1985) Adult pulmonary ligament pneumatocoel; a loculated pneumothorax. Radiology 155:575–576

23. Gamsu G (1983) Computed tomography of the pulmonary hila. In: Moss AA, Gamsu G, Genant HK (eds) Computed tomography of the body. Saunders, Philadelphia, pp 271–319

24. Gamsu G (1986) Computed tomography of normal pulmonary hila. Contemp Diag Radiol 9(5):1–6

25. Gamsu G (1986) Computed tomography of abnormal pulmonary hila. Contemp Diag Radiol 9(6):1–6

26. Gamsu G, Webb WR, Sheldon P, Kaufman L, Crooks LE, Birnberg FA, Goodman P, Hinchcliffe W, Hedgecock M (1983) Nuclear magnetic resonance imaging of the thorax. Radiology 147:473–480

27. Genereux G (1977) Unusual intrathoracic manifestations of bronchogenic carcinoma. In: Margulis AR, Gooding CA (eds) Diagnostic radiology. University of California, San Francisco, pp 553–584

28. Genereux GP (1983) Conventional tomographic hilar anatomy emphasizing the pulmonary veins. AJR 141:1241–1257

29. Glay J, Palayew M (1981) Unusual pattern of left lower lobe atelectasis. Radiology 141:331–333

30. Glazer GM, Francis IR, Gebarski K, Samuels BI, Sorensen KW (1983) Dynamic incremental computed tomography in evaluation of the pulmonary hila. J Comput Assist Tomogr 7:59–64

31. Glazer GM, Francis IR, Shirazi KK, Bookstein FL, Gross BH, Orringer MB (1983) Evaluation of the pulmonary hilum: comparison of conventional radiography, 55 degree posterior oblique tomography, and dynamic computed tomography. J Comput Assist Tomogr 7:983–989

32. Glazer GM, Gross BH, Aisen AM, Quint LE, Francis IR, Orringer MB (1985) Imaging of the pulmonary hilum: a prospective comparative study in patients with lung cancer. AJR 145:245–248

33. Godwin JD, Chen JTT (1986) Thoracic venous anatomy. AJR 147:674–684

34. Godwin JD, Vock P, Osborne DR (1983) CT of the pulmonary ligament. AJR 141:231–236

35. Godwin JD, Merten DF, Baker ME (1985) Paramediastinal pneumatocoel: alternative explanation to gas in the pulmonary ligament. AJR 145:525–530

36. Heelan RT, Martini N, Westcott JL, Bains MS, Watson RC, Caravelli JF, Berkmen YM, Henschke CI, McCormack PM, McCaughan BC, Zaman MD (1985) Carcinomatous involvement of hilum and mediastinum: computed tomographic and magnetic resonance evaluation. Radiology 156:111–116

37. Heitzman ER (1978) Radiologic diagnosis of mediastinal lymph node enlargement. J Can Assoc Radiol 29:151–157

38. Heitzman ER (1981) Computed tomography of the thorax: current perspectives. AJR 136:2–12

39. Herrnheiser G (1962) An anatomico-roentgenological analysis of the normal hilar shadow. Am J Roentgenol Radium Ther Nucl Med 48:595–612

40. Hirleman MT, Yiu-Chiu US, Chiu LC, Schapiro RL (1980) The resectability of primary lung carcinoma: a diagnostic staging review. CT 4:146–163

41. Homer MJ (1978) The hilar height ratio. Radiology 129:11–16

42. Homer MJ (1979) The abnormal hilar height ratio. AJR 133:723–726

43. Jardin M, Remy J (1986) Segmental bronchovascular anatomy of the lower lobes: CT analysis. AJR 147:457–468

44. Lane EJ Jr, Whalen JP (1969) A new sign of left atrial enlargement: posterior displacement of the left bronchial tree. Radiology 93:279–284

45. Lavender JP (1964) Letter to the editor. Br J Radiol 37:243

46. Lavender JP, Doppman J (1962) The hilum in pulmonary venous hypertension. Br J Radiol 35:303–313

47. Levitt RG, Glazer HS, Roper CL, Lee JKT, Murphy WA (1985) Magnetic resonance imaging of mediastinal and hilar masses: comparison with CT. AJR 145:9–14

48. Lewis JW Jr, Madrazo BL, Gross SG, Eyler WR, Magilligan DJ Jr, Kvale PA, Rosen RA (1982) The value of radiographic and computed tomography in the staging of lung carcinoma. Ann Thorac Surg 34:553–558

49. Lodwick GS, Keats TE, Dorst JP (1958) An evaluation of the significance of transverse hilar measurements in the diagnosis of primary lung cancer. Radiology 71:370–374

50. McLeod RA, Brown LR, Miller WE, DeRemee RA (1976) Evaluation of the pulmonary hila by tomography. Radiol Clin North Am 14:51–84

51. McLoud TC, Wittenberg J, Ferrucci FT Jr (1979) Computed tomography of the thorax and standard radiographic evaluation of the chest: a comparative study. J Comput Assist Tomogr 3:170–180

52. Mintzer RA, Hendrix RW, Johnson CS, Neiman HL, Cugell DW (1979) The radiologic significance of the left pulmonary ligament: experience with 26 patients. Chest 76:401–405

53. Nagaishi C (1972) Functional anatomy and histology of the lung. University Park Press, Baltimore

54. Naidich DP, Terry PB, Stitik FP, Siegelman SS (1980) Computed tomography of the bronchi. I Normal anatomy. J Comput Assist Tomogr 4:746–753

55. Naidich DP, Stitik FP, Khouri NF, Terry PB, Siegelman SS (1980) Computed tomography of the bronchi. II Pathology. J Comput Assist Tomogr 4:754–762

56. Naidich DP, Khouri NF, Scott WW Jr, Wang K-P, Siegelman SS (1981) Computed tomography of the pulmonary hila. I Normal anatomy. J Comput Assist Tomogr 5:459–467

57. Naidich DP, Khouri NF, Stitik FP, McCauley DI, Siegelman SS (1981) Computed tomography of the pulmonary hila. J Comput Assist Tomogr 5:468–475

58. Naidich DP, Lee J-J, Garay SM, McCauley DI, Aranda CP, Boyd AD (1987) Comparison of CT and fiberoptic bronchoscopy in the evaluation of bronchial disease. AJR 148:1–7

59. O'Callaghan JP, Heitzman ER, Somogyi JW, Spirt BA (1982) CT evaluation of pulmonary artery size. J Comput Assist Tomogr 6:101–104

60. O'Donovan PB, Ross JS, Sivak ED, O'Donnell JK, Meaney TF (1984) Magnetic resonance imaging of the thorax: the advantage of coronal and sagittal planes. AJR 143:1183–1188

61. Osborne DR, Korobkin M, Ravin CE, Putman CE, Wolfe WG, Sealy WC, Young WG, Breiman R, Heaston D, Ram P, Halber M (1982) Comparison of plain radiography, conventional tomography and computed tomography in detecting intrathoracic lymph node metastases from lung carcinoma. Radiology 142:157–161

62. Proto AV, Merhar GL (1984) Central bronchial displacement with large posterior pleural collections. Findings on the lateral chest radiograph and CT scans. J Can Assoc Radiol 35:128–132

63. Proto AV, Speckman JM (1979) The left lateral radiograph of the chest. Part I. Med Radiogr Photogr 55:30–74

64. Proto AV, Speckman J (1980) The left lateral radiograph of the chest. Part II. Med Radiogr Photogr 56:38–64

65. Pugatch RD, Faling LJ (1981) Computed tomography of the thorax: a status report. Chest 80:618–626

66. Quint LE, Glazer GM, Orringer MB, Francis IR, Bookstein FL (1986) Mediastinal lymph node detection and sizing at CT and autopsy. AJR 147:469–472

67. Rabinowitz JG, Wolf BS (1966) Roentgen significance of the pulmonary ligament. Radiology 87:1013–1020

68. Rabinowitz JG, Cohen BA, Mendelson DS (1984) The pulmonary ligament. RCNA 22:659–672

69. Ravin CE, Smith GW, Lester PD, McLoud TC, Putman CE (1976) Post-traumatic pneumatocele in the inferior pulmonary ligament. Radiology 121:39–41

70. Reeder MM, Felson B (1975) Gamuts in radiology. Audiovisual Radiology of Cincinnati, Cincinnati

71. Rigler LG, O'Laughlin BJ, Tucker RC (1952) Significance of unilateral enlargement of the hilus shadow in the early diagnosis of carcinoma of the lung with observations on a method of mensuration. Radiology 59:683–693

72. Ross JS, O'Donovan PB, Novoa R, Mehta A, Buonocore E, MacIntyre WJ, Golish JA, Ahmad M (1984) Magnetic resonance of the chest: initial experience with imaging and in vivo T1 and T2 calculations. Radiology 152:95–101

73. Rost RC Jr, Proto AV (1983) Inferior pulmonary ligament: computed tomographic appearance. Radiology 148:479–483

74. Sagel SS, Evens RGT, Forrest JV, Bramson RT (1974) Efficacy of routine screening and lateral chest radiographs in a hospital-based population. NEJM 291:1001–1004

75. Schnur MJ, Winkler B, Austin JHM (1981) Thickening of the posterior wall of the bronchus intermedius. A sign on lateral chest radiographs of congestive heart failure, lymph node enlargement, and neoplastic infiltration. Radiology 139:551–559

76. Sone S, Higashihara T, Morimoto S, Ikezoe J, Arisawa J, Monden Y, Nahakara K (1983) CT anatomy of hilar lymphadenopathy. AJR 140:887–892

77. Tisi GM, Friedman PJ, Peters RM, Pearson G, Carr D, Lee RE, Selawry O (1983) Clinical staging of primary lung cancer. Am Rev Resp Dis 127:659–664

78. Vix VA, Klatte EC (1970) The lateral chest radiograph in the diagnosis of hilar and mediastinal masses. Radiology 96:307–316

79. Volberg FM, Everett CJ, Brill PW (1979) Radiologic features of inferior pulmonary ligament air collections in neonates with respiratory distress. Radiology 130:357–360

80. Webb WR, Gamsu G (1983) Computed tomography of the left retrobronchial stripe. JCAT 7:65–69

81. Webb WR, Glazer GM, Gamsu G (1981) Computed tomography of the normal pulmonary hilum. J Comput Assist Tomogr 5:476–484

82. Webb WR, Gamsu G, Glazer GM (1981) Computed tomography of the abnormal pulmonary hilum. J Comput Assist Tomogr 5:485–490

83. Webb WR, Gamsu G, Speckman JM (1983) Computed tomography of the pulmonary hilum in patients with bronchogenic carcinoma. J Comput Assist Tomogr 7:219–225

84. Webb WR, Gamsu G, Stark DD, Moore EH (1984) Magnetic resonance imaging of the normal and abnormal pulmonary hila. Radiology 152:89–94

85. Webb WR, Hirji M, Gamsu G (1984) The posterior wall of the bronchus intermedius: radiographic-CT correlation. AJR 142:907–911

86. Webb WR, Jensen BG, Gamsu G, Sollitto R, Moore EH (1984) Coronal magnetic resonance imaging of the chest: normal and abnormal. Radiology 153:729–735

87. Webb WR, Jensen BG, Sollitto R, de Geer G, McCowin M, Gamsu G, Moore E (1985) Bronchogenic carcinoma: staging with MR compared with staging with CT and surgery. Radiology 156:117–124

88. Whalen JP, Lane EJ Jr (1969) Bronchial rearrangements in pulmonary collapse as seen on the lateral radiograph. Radiology 93:285–288

89. Young JWR, Anderson BL, Reinig JW (1984) Oblique chest film: value in routine and selective use. AJR 142:69–72

Subject Index

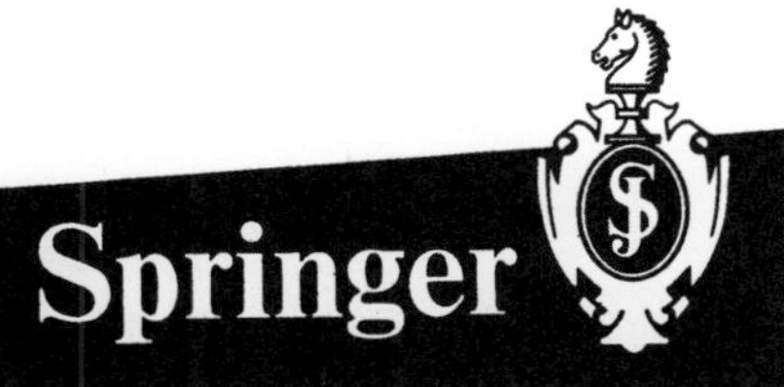
Springer

A. L. Baert, A. Wackenheim, L. Jeanmart

Abdominal Computer Tomography

With collaboration of G. Marchal, G. Wilms

1980. 315 figures in 585 separate illustrations. XI, 185 pages. (Atlas of Pathological Computer Tomography, Volume 2). ISBN 3-540-10093-8

D. Beyer, U. Mödder

Diagnostic Imaging of the Acute Abdomen

A Clinico-Radiologic Approach

1988. 250 figures containing 680 separate figures. Approx. 450 pages. ISBN 3-540-17520-2

H. Bismuth, D. Castaing

Operative Ultrasound of the Liver and Biliary Ducts

1987. 69 figures. VI, 91 pages. ISBN 3-540-17091-X

G. Antes, F. Eggemann

Small Bowel Radiology

Introduction and Atlas

1988. 276 figures. VI, 207 pages. ISBN 3-540-15263-6

Springer-Verlag
Berlin Heidelberg New York
London Paris Tokyo

P. G. Herman (Ed.)

Iatrogenic Thoracic Complications

1983. 256 figures. XIX, 243 pages. (Radiology of Iatrogenic Disorders). ISBN 3-540-90729-7

UICC International Union Against Cancer

B. Hoogstraten, B. J. Addis, H. H. Hansen, N. Martini, S. G. Spiro (Eds.)

Lung Tumors

Lung, Mediastinum, Pleura, and Chest Wall

1988. 100 figures, 33 tables. XX, 272 pages. (Current Treatment of Cancer). ISBN 3-540-16920-2

M. A. Meyers (Ed.)

Computed Tomography of the Gastrointestinal Tract

Including the Peritoneal Cavity and Mesentery

1986. 250 figures in 466 parts, 17 tables. XIV, 279 pages. ISBN 3-540-96232-8

S. Seeber (Ed.)

Small Cell Lung Cancer

1985. 44 figures, 47 tables. VII, 166 pages. (Recent Results in Cancer Research, Volume 97). ISBN 3-540-13798-X

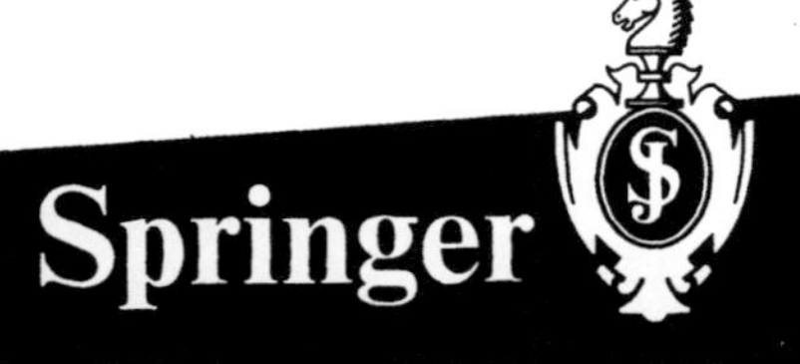

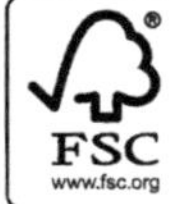

MIX
Papier aus verantwortungsvollen Quellen
Paper from responsible sources
FSC® C105338

If you have any concerns about our products,
you can contact us on
ProductSafety@springernature.com

In case Publisher is established outside the EU,
the EU authorized representative is:
**Springer Nature Customer Service Center GmbH
Europaplatz 3, 69115 Heidelberg, Germany**

Printed by Libri Plureos GmbH
in Hamburg, Germany